Protective Gloves for Occupational Use

This revised text discusses key aspects for protective gloves, including glove materials, the manufacture of gloves, how to perform testing of gloves, and glove performance.

The book provides guidance on how to select gloves to prevent skin contamination from chemical and microbial exposure in the occupational environment and presents hard-to-find information in one easy-to-use resource. It covers important concepts, including prevention of contact dermatitis, clinical testing of occupation-related glove sensitivity, and infection control and preventative measures for pandemics.

The book

- Provides update state-of-the-art information, practices, standards, and guidelines.
- Covers information on protective glove material technology, protective effects, and adverse medical effects.
- Explores ways to select gloves to prevent skin contamination from chemical and microbial exposure in the occupational environment.
- Discusses concepts, including glove materials, the manufacture of gloves, how to perform testing of gloves, and glove performance according to standardized technical methods in vivo.

The text will be useful for professionals in the fields of occupational medicine, occupational health, occupational and industrial hygiene, health care, and public health. It will also help graduate students in the fields of chemistry, chemical engineering, mechanical engineering, biology, pharmacy, and environmental health. This book offers a wealth of information on protective glove material technology, protective effects, and adverse medical effects. It gives detailed discussion of parameters, including the selection and use of gloves for industrial chemicals, acrylates, and pesticides, and gloves as protection against microbial contamination. It will be a valuable resource for professionals and graduate students in the fields of occupational and industrial hygiene, healthcare, public health, chemistry, chemical engineering, mechanical engineering, biology, pharmacy, occupational, and environmental health.

Protective Gloves for Occupational Use

Third Edition

Edited by

Robert N. Phalen and Howard I. Maibach

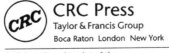

CRC Press
Taylor & Francis Group
Boca Raton London New York

CRC Press is an imprint of the
Taylor & Francis Group, an **informa** business

Third edition published 2023
by CRC Press
6000 Broken Sound Parkway NW, Suite 300, Boca Raton, FL 33487-2742

and by CRC Press
4 Park Square, Milton Park, Abingdon, Oxon, OX14 4RN

CRC Press is an imprint of Taylor & Francis Group, LLC

© 2023 selection and editorial matter, Robert N. Phalen and Howard I. Maibach, individual chapters, the contributors

First edition published by CRC Press 1994
Second edition published by CRC Press 2019

Library of Congress Cataloging-in-Publication Data

Names: Phalen, Robert N., editor. | Maibach, Howard I., editor.
Title: Protective gloves for occupational use / edited by Robert N. Phalen and Howard Maibach.
Description: Third edition. | Boca Raton : CRC Press, 2023. | Revised edition of: Protective gloves for occupational use / edited by Anders Boman ... [et al.]. 2nd ed. c2005. | Includes bibliographical references and index.
Identifiers: LCCN 2022020986 (print) | LCCN 2022020987 (ebook) | ISBN 9780367649005 (hardback) | ISBN 9780367649050 (paperback) | ISBN 9781003126874 (ebook)
Subjects: LCSH: Contact dermatitis--Prevention. | Protective clothing. | Dermatotoxicology. | Industrial hygiene. | Occupational diseases.
Classification: LCC RL244 .P76 2023 (print) | LCC RL244 (ebook) | DDC 616.5/1--dc23/eng/20220629
LC record available at https://lccn.loc.gov/2022020986
LC ebook record available at https://lccn.loc.gov/2022020987

ISBN: 9780367649005 (hbk)
ISBN: 9780367649050 (pbk)
ISBN: 9781003126874 (ebk)

DOI: 10.1201/9781003126874

Typeset in Times
by Deanta Global Publishing Services, Chennai, India

Contents

SECTION I   Introduction to Prevention and Protective Gloves

SECTION II   Regulations and Standards

SECTION III   Glove Sensitivity and Effects on Skin

SECTION IV *Protection against Chemical and Microbial Agents*

SECTION V   Special Topics

Preface

Twenty-eight years after the first edition of *Protective Gloves for Occupational Use*, the topic is still an important and widely discussed area of personal protective equipment. The second edition provided considerable updates on the research and development, providing state-of-the-art information on glove materials, the manufacture of gloves, how to perform testing of gloves, and glove performance according to standardized technical methods. This third edition provides critical updates on the changes in glove manufacturing, the evolving chemistry of rubber contact allergens in gloves, as well as changes in regulations and standardized tests used to evaluate glove performance and aid in their selection. Updates on glove sensitivity and effects on the skin are also provided.

Dermatitis that results from exposure to chemicals, wet work, and even protective gloves themselves remains as common as ever before. Exposure to chemicals occurs in occupational, domestic, and leisure situations. Protective gloves help prevent new cases of dermatitis and enable patients with already established dermatitis to continue to work and enjoy a high-quality life. Information on this subject provides a solid basis for the correct choice of glove materials and offers essential details that help produce guidelines for the occupational use of protective gloves.

This book focuses on protection from chemical and biological agents and adverse reactions caused by protective gloves. Since the second edition was published, rubber chemical additives from both natural and synthetic rubber gloves can be quite complex and rubber accelerator contact allergy remains a problem. The COVID-19 pandemic has also created unique issues concerning glove availability, use, extended use, and disinfection in healthcare.

This third edition draws from and builds on the material of the second edition, with the addition of eight new chapters. Chapter 1 provides an overview of contact dermatitis. Chapters 2 and 22 summarize basic guidelines for when and how to choose protective gloves for occupational use. Chapters 3 and 10 through 12 provide comprehensive information about glove materials, permeation testing, penetration testing, and durability. Chapters 6 through 9 document the current US, European, Japanese, and Australian standards for gloves. Chapters 13 through 19 describe the adverse effects of protective gloves. Chapters 20 and 21 describe dermal exposures to chemicals through gloves and fabrics (e.g., textiles). Chapters 22 through 26 detail selection instructions that will make it easier for workers in specific areas to choose protective gloves for chemical and biological agents. Chapter 23 provides an extensive review of the associated dermatological problems and selection of gloves for work with acrylates. Chapter 27 provides an important update on alcoholic gels and glove use, especially as it pertains to the COVID-19 pandemic. Chapters 28 and 29 provide a further review of the effectiveness of masks for source control, which has become an additional consideration during the COVID-19 pandemic. Chapter 30 provides new information on the extended use and disinfection of N95 respirators and exam gloves during the COVID-19 pandemic.

   This book is a valuable resource for dermatologists involved in clinical research and product development, occupational health physicians and nurses, industrial (occupational) hygienists, chemical safety engineers, and other health and safety professionals who work in areas where skin exposure may occur.

Robert N. Phalen, Ph.D., CIH, FAIHA

Howard I. Maibach, M.D.

Editors

Robert N. Phalen, Ph.D., CIH, FAIHA, is a professor and program chair of Occupational Safety and Health at the University of Houston Clear Lake, Texas, USA. Dr. Phalen is an industrial hygienist with expertise in protective clothing and dermal exposure assessment. He earned his doctoral degree from the University of California Los Angeles in Environmental Health Science with a specialization in industrial hygiene. He is a Certified Industrial Hygienist and a Fellow of the American Industrial Hygiene Association. His primary publications are on chemical permeation and the durability of protective clothing.

Howard I. Maibach, M.D., is a professor of Dermatology at the University of California San Francisco, USA, with expertise in treating contact dermatitis and occupational dermatitis. His specialties include allergic skin disorders and skin conditions caused by exposure to toxic substances. Dr. Maibach earned his medical degree from Tulane University School of Medicine, New Orleans, Louisiana, USA. He has over 2500 publications and has served on the editorial boards of more than 30 scientific journals. He is a member of 19 professional societies, including the American Academy of Dermatology, the San Francisco Dermatological Society, and the International Commission on Occupational Health. Dr. Maibach has been a long-term contributor to experimental research on contact dermatitis, contact urticaria, and other skin conditions.

Contributors

Ayse S. Filiz Acipayam, M.D.
Bakirköy Dr. Sadi Konuk Training and
    Research Hospital
Istanbul, Turkey

Rasmus Overgaard Bach, M.D.
Odense University Hospital Denmark
Odense, Denmark

Ola Bergendorff, Ph.D.
Lund University
Skåne University Hospital
Malmö, Sweden

Jordan L. Bormann, M.D.
University of Utah Health
Salt Lake City, Utah, U.S.A.

Magnus Bruze, M.D., Ph.D.
University of Southern Denmark
Odense, Denmark

Marija Bubaš, M.D., Ph.D.
Croatian Institute of Public Health
Zagreb, Croatia

Taylor Bullock, M.D.
The Cleveland Clinic Foundation
Cleveland, Ohio, U.S.A.

Diana M. Ceballos, Ph.D., M.S., CIH
Boston University
School of Public Health
Boston, Massachusetts, U.S.A.

John W. Cherrie, Ph.D.
Institute of Occupational Medicine
    (IOM)And Institute of Biological
    Chemistry, Biophysics and
    Bioengineering
at Heriot-Watt University
Edinburgh, Scotland

Marie-Noëlle Crépy, M.D.
Paris Descartes University
Paris, France

Steve H. Dou
University of California, Berkeley
Berkeley, California, U.S.A.

Karen S. Galea, Ph.D.
Institute of Occupational
    Medicine (IOM)
Edinburgh, Scotland

**Ana Maria Giménez-Arnau,
M.D., Ph.D.**
Hospital del Mar
Universitat Autònoma de Barcelona
Barcelona, Spain

Yuji Haishima, Ph.D.
National Institute of Health Sciences
Kawasaki-Shi, Kanagawa, Japan

Youssef K. Hamidi, Ph.D.
University of Houston Clear Lake
Houston, Texas, U.S.A.

Nils Hamnerius, M.D., Ph.D.
Lund University
Skåne University Hospital
Malmö, Sweden

**Norman W. Henry III, M.S., CIH,
FAIHA**
Safety, Health, and Environmental
    Consulting
Safety and Health by Protection
    (SHBP)
Elkton, Maryland, U.S.A.

Pierre Hoerner, Ph.D.
Advanced Barrier Solutions SARL
Senlis, France

Jean-Marie Lachapelle, M.D., Ph.D.
Catholic University of Louvain
Brussels, Belgium

Sarah Levitt
California State University,
    Long Beach
Long Beach, California, U.S.A.

**Suzana Ljubojević Hadzavdic,
M.D., Ph.D.**
University Hospital Center Zagreb
University of Zagreb School of
    Medicine
Zagreb, Croatia

Howard I. Maibach, M.D.
University of California San Fransisco
San Francisco, California, U.S.A.

Kayoko Matsunaga, M.D., Ph.D.
Fujita Health University Bantane
    Hospital
Fujita Health University School of
    Medicine
Nagoya, Aichi, Japan

Danielle L. McGeachie, M.D.
Townsville University Hospital
Townsville, Queensland, Australia

Halie N. Mechels
University of South Dakota
Sioux Falls, South Dakota, U.S.A.

Kristian Fredløv Mose, M.D., Ph.D.
Odense University Hospital Denmark
Odense, Denmark

Ryusuke Nakaoka, Ph.D.
National Institute of Health Sciences
Kawasaki-Shi, Kanagawa, Japan

Jesper B. Nielsen, M.Sc., Ph.D.
University of Southern Denmark
Odense, Denmark

Rosemary L. Nixon, M.D.
Occupational Dermatology Research
    and Education Centre
Skin Health Institute
Melbourne, Australia

**Taku Ohhara, M.S. (Pharmaceutical
Sciences)**
Medical Device Evaluation Division
Pharmaceutical Safety and
    Environmental Health Bureau
Ministry of Health, Labour and Welfare
Chiyoda-ku, Tokyo, Japan

Christopher L. Packham
EnviroDerm Services
Longhope, U.K.

**Robert N. Phalen, Ph.D., CIH,
FAIHA**
University of Houston Clear Lake
Houston, Texas, U.S.A.

Andaç Salman, M.D.
Acıbadem Mehmet Ali Aydınlar
    University School of Medicine
Department of Dermatology
and
Marmara University School of Medicine
Department of Dermatology
Istanbul, Turkey

Paul D. Siegel, Ph.D.
Health Effects Laboratory Division
National Institute for Occupational
    Safety and Health
Morgantown, West Virginia, U.S.A.

Apra Sood, M.D., F.A.A.D.
University of California Davis Health
Sacramento VA Medical Center
Mather, California, U.S.A.

Cecilia Svedman, M.D., Ph.D.
Lund University
Skåne University Hospital
Malmö, Sweden

Akimasa Takeuchi, Ph.D.
Medical Device Evaluation Division
Pharmaceutical Safety and
    Environmental Health Bureau
Ministry of Health, Labour and Welfare
Chiyoda-ku, Tokyo, Japan

Helen E. Taylor, Ph.D.
EnviroDerm Services
Longhope, U.K.

James S. Taylor, M.D.
The Cleveland Clinic Foundation
Cleveland, Ohio, U.S.A.

Thaibinh Tran
University of California San Fransisco
San Francisco, California, U.S.A.

**Wenhai Xu, Ph.D., MBA, CIH, CSP,
CHMM**
Tenneco
Southfield, Michigan, U.S.A.

Terminology and Abbreviations

1 TERMINOLOGY

A **protective glove** is an item of personal protective equipment that protects the hand or any part of the hand from hazards. It may also cover part of the forearm. Some of the terms used in technical permeation testing and the dermatological field need some clarification.

Degradation can be defined as the loss of integrity of the glove membrane due to chemical interaction with the penetrating or exposing chemical.

Penetration of a chemical is a process that can be defined as the flow of a chemical through closures, porous materials, seams, pinholes, or other imperfections in a protective clothing material and on a nonmolecular level. It should be pointed out that in experimental dermatology the term penetration is used with a somewhat different meaning.

Percutaneous absorption is defined as the penetration of substances from the outside into the skin and thereafter through the skin and into the blood and lymph vessels. The three routes of penetration are (1) via the sweat ducts; (2) via the hair follicles and associated sebaceous glands (also called transappandageal transport), which can be considered equivalent to the definition of penetration used in connection to material testing; and (3) across the continuous stratum corneum (also called transepidermal transport), which corresponds to the definition for permeation defined below.

Permeation in technical testing means the process by which a chemical migrates through the protective glove material on a molecular level. It involves (1) sorption of molecules of the chemical into the contacted surface of the material, (2) diffusion of the sorbed material within the material, and (3) desorption of the molecules from the opposite surface of the material. Two common measures of chemical permeation include the breakthrough time and steady-state permeation rate.

The **chemical resistance** of protective materials, typically in terms of chemical permeation, can also be tested in vivo using experimental animals and in clinical studies.

Dermatitis is a general term for inflammatory diseases in the skin.

Eczema is an inflammatory disease in the skin engaging the epidermis. It entails one or several of the following morphological changes: erythema, edema, papules, and vesicles. Commonly it also may be scaly, encrusted, oozing, and lichenified (e.g., hyperpigmentation and thickening of the skin).

Contact urticaria is a histamine-mediated, quickly appearing wheal and flare in the skin that follows contact with a histamine-releasing substance. This is either a chemical substance or a protein giving an IgE-mediated reaction.

Contact dermatitis (contact eczema) is dermatitis or eczema that follows the skin contact with a chemical substance or product. It usually needs a long time of exposure to appear. It is caused by contact with either skin-irritating chemicals, i.e., irritant contact dermatitis, or allergens, i.e., allergic contact dermatitis, or both in combination.

A **patch test** is a clinical diagnostic test performed for the diagnosis of allergic dermatitis. It typically involves the use of patches with suspected agents, which are placed on the skin for some time (e.g., 48 hours). Testing is usually done on the back.

A **skin prick test** is a clinical diagnostic test performed for the diagnosis of an immediate skin reaction. It typically involves a skin puncture or scratch that just penetrates the skin surface. Testing is usually done on the arms or upper back.

2 ABBREVIATIONS

Some commonly used abbreviations are listed below. Most abbreviations for chemical names used in the text are explained when first mentioned there and not given in this list.

ACD	Allergic contact dermatitis
ACGIH	American Conference of Government Industrial Hygienists
AIDS	Acquired immune deficiency syndrome
ANSI	American National Standards Institute (US)
AQL	Acceptable quality level
ASTM	American Society for Testing and Materials (now ASTM International)
BT, BTT	Breakthrough time (or breakthrough detection time)
CDC	Centers for Disease Control and Prevention (US)
CE	Conformité Européenne (European health & safety product label)
CEN	European Committee for Standardization (Comité Européen de Normalisation)
CPC	Chemical protective clothing
CR	Chloroprene rubber (Neoprene® or chloroprene)
CU	Contact urticaria
EN	European standard (Norme Européen)
FDA	Food and Drug Administration (US)
HAV	Hepatitis A virus
HBV	Hepatitis B virus
HCV	Hepatitis C virus
HIV	Human immunodeficiency virus
HSV	Herpes simplex virus
ICD	Irritant contact dermatitis
ICDRG	International Contact Dermatitis Research Group
ICU	Immunologic contact urticaria
IS0	International Organization for Standardization
IVDK	Information Network of Departments of Dermatology
NBR	Nitrile butadiene rubber (or nitrile rubber)
NBT	Normalized breakthrough time
NFPA	National Fire Protection Association (US)
NICU	Nonimmunologic contact urticaria

NIOSH	National Institute for Occupational Safety and Health (US)
NRL	Natural rubber latex (or natural rubber)
OA	Occupational asthma
OSHA	Occupational Safety and Health Administration (US)
PCR	Polymerase chain reaction
PE	Polyethylene, polyethene
PEL	Permissible exposure limit
PPE	Personal protective equipment
PR	Permeation rate
PU	Polyurethane
PVC	Polyvinyl chloride (or vinyl)
RAST	Radioallergosorbent test
SBT	Standardized breakthrough time
SSPR	Steady-state permeation rate
TDDS	Transdermal drug delivery systems
TEWL	Transepidermal water loss
TLV	Threshold limit value
TPE	Thermoplastic elastomer

Section I

Introduction to Prevention
and Protective Gloves

1 Prevention of Contact Dermatitis

S. H. Dou and H. I. Maibach

CONTENTS

1.1 INTRODUCTION

A distinction is usually made between *primary prevention*, i.e., inhibition of the infection and onset of contact dermatitis, and *secondary prevention*, i.e., early diagnosis and inhibition of relapses. In tertiary prevention, also known as rehabilitation, a chronically diseased patient is treated and reintegrated into the working environment. The value of disease prevention is evident to individuals, society, and the medical community. For human, social, and economic reasons, it would be of great benefit if people exposed to harmful chemicals and products could be protected from developing contact dermatitis. Therefore, it is important to focus on methods in primary prevention.

Multiple prophylactic means are available, as summarized in Table 1.1, which can be used as a checklist; the means are grouped under the following subheadings: Chemicals, Individual Screening, Avoidance of Contact, Skin Care Program, and, finally, Miscellaneous Means.

These aspects of prevention have been reviewed.[1-5] When facing the current or imminent skin problems of a single patient, all of these prophylactic means should be considered. However, the responsibility for primary prevention rests mainly with manufacturers and producers of chemicals and products, government agencies, consumer organizations, occupational health physicians and nurses, occupational (industrial) hygienists, and safety engineers. This is because primary prevention is much broader and requires less personalized care compared to secondary prevention. However, all forms of treatment must be tailored to the severity of dermatitis when applicable.

For secondary prevention, a greater responsibility is placed on physicians treating the cases (dermatologists, occupational health physicians, and others) and on nurses occupational (industrial) hygienists, and safety engineers.

DOI: 10.1201/9781003126874-2

TABLE 1.1

Prophylaxis of Contact Dermatitis

Chemicals

- Identification of the allergen in the patient
- Occurrence, the concentration of the allergen in the environment
- Allergen removal or replacement
- Modification or inactivation of the allergen
- Knowledge of how to read ingredient labels, i.e., safety data sheets (SDS)
- Medication administration to the patient against the allergen
- Friction should be minimized
- Soaps usage should be limited
- Predictive testing: skin irritating potential
- Predictive testing: sensitizing potential

Individual Screening: Individuals identified at preemployment examination and periodic health screening

- Those with increased susceptibility or predisposition, i.e., atopics
- Patients with a history of contact dermatitis
- Patients with stasis eczema and/or venous leg ulcers

Avoidance of Contact: Avoidance of direct contact with causative products and materials

- Protective gloves
- Aprons, sleeves, boots, glasses, face masks, hair net, ear protection, etc.
- Protective (barrier) creams for a specific patient
- Dishwasher, washing machine, long-handled brushes
- Automation, closed systems
- Efficient ventilation

Skin care program

- Soaps, detergents, cleansing agents with low irritancy potential
- Hot water, shower, sauna, maintaining hygiene
- Soft towels
- Emollient and moisturizing creams

Miscellaneous Means

- Legislation
- Labeling of products and chemicals; safety sheets
- Information to patients, consumers, workers, supervisors
- Awareness in medical and civilian sectors
- Training of workers in special industrial processes
- Good housekeeping
- Modifying work processes
- Minimizing wet/humid work conditions
- Research on prevention and dissemination of results obtained
- Interference with mechanisms of inflammation
- Finding of new biomarkers

1.2   PROTECTIVE GLOVES AND OTHER METHODS OF PREVENTION

The use of protective gloves is one of several possibilities to avoid developing contact dermatitis or a relapse; however, they are only one of many proactive measures. All items listed in Table 1.1 should be considered, and, according to our experience, optimal results are achieved when several of the recommended prophylactic means are combined in a wise and fruitful way.

To rely on just one of these recommendations—sometimes to reduce costs—is less effective. Just as the conditions leading to contact dermatitis are often multifaceted, preventative measures should also be so. However, it is up to the persons involved in preventive dermatology to demonstrate that the suggested methods and measures are efficacious and cost-effective.

Current protective gloves are not perfect. As documented in the following chapters, most are permeable to various chemicals and do not always provide the promised protection. Side effects, such as irritancy and contact allergy, occur and are sometimes reasons for discontinuance of their use by patients and exposed workers.

Gloves that will give more efficient protection and fewer side effects are then highly desirable. We are optimistic that devoted people from industry, universities, and research institutes will meet this challenge and provide us with the desired products.

REFERENCES

1. Rycroft, R.J.G. 1998. Occupational dermatoses, in *Rook's Textbook of Dermatology*, Vol. 1, 8th ed., Burns, D.A., Breathnach, S.M., Cox N., Griffiths C.E.M., Eds. Oxford: Black-Well Scientific Publications, chap. 21, page 821.
2. Lachapelle, J-M. 2001. Principles of prevention and protection in contact dermatitis (with special reference to occupational dermatology), in *Textbook of Contact Dermatitis*, Rycroft, R.J.G., Menné, T., Frosch, P.J., and Lepoittevin, J-P., Eds. Berlin: Springer-Verlag, 979.
3. Agner, T. and Held, E. 2002. Skin protection programmes. *Contact Dermatitis* 46:253.
4. John, S.M., Johansen, J.D., Rustemeyer, Th., Elsner, P., and Maibach, H.I. 2020. *Kanerva's Occupational Dermatology*, 3rd ed. Heidelberg: Springer-Verlag.
5. Lachapelle, J-M. and Maibach, H.I. 2020. *Patch and Prick Testing*, 4th ed., Heidelberg: Springer-Verlag.

2 Occupational Hygiene Assessments for the Use of Protective Gloves

W. Xu

CONTENTS

2.1 INTRODUCTION

Historically, skin disorders and diseases along with hearing loss are the most prevalent occupational illnesses in the United States.[1,2] Employers are required to assign protective clothing or equipment, wherever needed, to prevent work-related diseases and injuries affecting the skin and other organs. Employers must assess the hazards and the risks associated with performing the work to determine the need. Such occupational hygiene assessment, also called hazard assessment or risk assessment, should incorporate the nature and extent of the hazards involved, the potential severity of adverse effects of exposure to the worker, the likelihood of exposure to hazardous materials or agents, and solutions other than personal protective equipment (PPE).

2.2 REQUIREMENTS FOR ASSESSMENT

Some countries have a legal requirement for a "hazard assessment" before the selection and use of gloves and personal protective equipment. For example, the

DOI: 10.1201/9781003126874-3

US Occupational Safety and Health Administration (OSHA) in its several standards (personal protection equipment, hazard communication, lead, sanitation, and hand protection) requires the employer to assess the workplace to determine whether hazards are present or likely to be present and, if so, to select the appropriate personal protective equipment for the specific hazards involved. It also requires that the selection decision be communicated to the affected employee, that the equipment fits properly, and that training of employees in the use and limitations of the equipment is provided. The occupational hygiene process incorporates these required elements of the assessment.

2.3   THE OCCUPATIONAL HYGIENE PROCESS

Occupational hygiene (also known as industrial hygiene) is the art and science of anticipating, recognizing, evaluating, and controlling health and safety hazards from biological, chemical, and physical agents and other stressors in the workplace and community.[3]

Anticipation of health and safety hazards is based on a review of plans for a process, on proposed changes in materials, or on job descriptions alone. It requires the most sophisticated level of occupational hygiene knowledge and skill to anticipate potential problem areas before the problems occur.

The next aspect of the occupational hygiene process—recognition of a problem from an existing operation—though somewhat less difficult, still relies on both experience and knowledge. Ideally, the health and safety hazards are recognized before any adverse events. In reality, this step of the occupational hygiene process is often triggered by employee complaints or reports of near-miss, injury, or illness.

Evaluation of the problem follows the recognition phase. The ultimate goal of the evaluation phase, together with the previous steps, is to assess the risk from exposure. Occupational hygiene evaluations can be either qualitative or quantitative, or both. For materials that present a skin hazard or that are absorbed through the skin and present a systemic hazard, the evaluation will often be completed on a qualitative basis, as there are few standard measures for quantifying dermal hazards in the workplace. While some specific OSHA standards (e.g., lead, cadmium) contain housekeeping provisions that address the issue of surface contamination, there are currently no surface contamination criteria or quantifications for skin absorption included in OSHA standards.[4] ACGIH has established only two surface TLVs related to Skin and DSEN notations for methyltetrahydrophthalic anhydride isomers and o-phthalaldehyde.[5]

The subsequent consideration is controls available to eliminate or limit the risk to a point considered acceptable. One control method common to many applications is the use of personal protective equipment, especially gloves, for the protection of the hands. For most jobs, the hands that are most likely to suffer the consequences of contact with a hazardous chemical or physical agent. Organizations such as the National Institute for Occupational Safety and Health (NIOSH) have recognized skin diseases and disorders as a major occupational health problem. Therefore, gloves play a significant role in protecting workers from chemical and physical hazards.

Overall, the occupational hygiene process is to assess and control the risks to the workers based on general occupational hygiene knowledge and specific knowledge about the tasks performed. It should also be reevaluated after the controls are implemented for continuous improvement opportunities.

2.4   OVERVIEW OF RISK ASSESSMENT

The occupational hygiene process is integrated into and essential for risk assessment and management. Risk can be defined as the likelihood of an undesirable effect. In our application, this is often an adverse health effect. Risk assessment is the systematic process of determining the probability and magnitude of the undesired effect, either quantitatively or qualitatively. Risk assessment is frequently described as a four-phase process: hazard identification, hazard characterization, exposure assessment, and risk characterization.[6]

Risk characterization is based on both the hazard characterization and the exposure. For example, the greatest hazard of working in a refinery is the danger of fire and explosion. Major fire is an extremely rare event (very low frequency), but the severity is so great that most companies are willing to go to great lengths and expenses to protect against it. This has included the mandated use of fire-resistant clothing by all workers as well as other measures. Another example of severe health effects is dimethyl mercury. Several drops over a hand wearing a disposable latex glove had been fatal.[7] On the other hand, gasoline is universally recognized as a hazardous compound. It is extremely flammable and toxic. It contains a wide range of organic constituents, some of which probably exhibit skin permeability, toxicity, and carcinogenicity (e.g., benzene). Most would not argue these points, yet few of us use gloves when putting gasoline into our cars even though they are provided at most gasoline pumps. Even the gas station attendants in the few remaining nonself-service stations rarely use gloves. There are probably several reasons why gloves are not worn, including the matter of convenience. Nevertheless, a key aspect is that we consider the secondary contact (i.e., contact from the dispensing nozzle, not the actual fluid) and frequency of exposure to represent a trivial risk. This personal risk assessment is also greatly aided by the fact that gasoline is a familiar product with which almost everyone has had some experience. Nevertheless, we generally apply more stringent risk characterization at work.

2.5   HAZARD CHARACTERIZATION

Occupational hazards to the skin and other organs from dermal exposure can be physical hazards or health hazards. Examples of physical hazards are the following:

- Tears, cuts, and punctures to the skin or glove
- Abrasion of the skin or glove
- Thermal injury
- Flammability of the protective equipment
- Radiation

Adverse health effects from dermal exposure can be skin disorders localized to the contacted skin. Other organs away from the contact skin can also be damaged as the chemicals can be absorbed through the skin and transferred to other parts of the body. Such effects are systemic effects. Additionally, dermal contact can also sensitize the exposed person, and a small amount of the same substance exposed to later may trigger a severe allergic reaction.[8]

Safety Data Sheets (SDSs), which are required under hazard communication standard, can be a great resource for identifying adverse health effects. Appendix A of the OSHA hazard communication standard highlighted the dermal acute toxicity, sensitization, and irritation/corrosivity reporting under the framework of the Globally Harmonized System of Classification and Labelling of Chemicals (GHS).[9] Examples of other great resources include International Chemical Safety Cards (ICSCs), Hazardous Substances Data Bank (HSDB) now within PubChem, and NIOSH Pocket Guide to Chemical Hazards.

2.6 SKIN NOTATIONS

Dermal exposure is often overlooked as an important route of exposure contributing to the systemic health effects.[8] Various regulatory agencies and occupational hygiene organizations have attempted to address dermal exposure with a "skin" notation along with the airborne occupational exposure limits (OELs) they set.

The American Conference of Governmental Industrial Hygienists (ACGIH) assigns a Skin notation to chemicals for which air sampling alone is insufficient to quantify exposure accurately and measures to prevent significant cutaneous absorption may be required.[5] In general, these chemicals have significant potential for absorption via the hands and forearms during the workday. Highly toxic materials having a relatively low dermal LD50 (i.e., 1 g/kg of body weight or less) would be given a Skin notation. Examples of these chemicals include carbon disulfide, carbon tetrachloride, and the common solvent methyl alcohol. ACGIH also includes a notation for dermal sensitization (DSEN). Methyl acrylate is an example of a chemical that has both a Skin and DSEN notation.[5] ACGIH does not assign a Skin notation if a chemical only causes irritation or corrosive effects after dermal exposure.[5]

The OSHA "skin" notation serves as a warning that skin contact with the substance can cause irritation and/or that cutaneous absorption should be prevented to avoid exceeding the permissible exposure limit (PEL).[4]

NIOSH, in its current Pocket Guide, merely states that the "skin" designation indicates the potential for dermal absorption; skin exposure should be prevented through the use of good work practices, gloves, coveralls, goggles, and other appropriate equipment.[10] NIOSH also published and revised A Strategy for Assigning New NIOSH Skin Notations and Skin Notation Profiles for their chemicals with skin notation.[11]

Although these "skin" notations are not the same, the organizations emphasize that the dermal route should be considered in control measures for such designated chemicals. It should also be noted that the absence of a "skin" notation does not mean that the chemical is not absorbed through the skin.[6]

2.7 EXPOSURE ASSESSMENT

The following discussion is for chemical exposure, and a similar dose approach applies to exposure to physical agents. There can be a wide variation in duration and frequency of contact:

- Continuous direct contact
- Intermittent direct contact
- The potential for direct contact

The physical state of chemicals (solids, liquid, or vapor) also affects the exposure (affinity with and uptake by the exposed skin). Additional factors include relative humidity, sun exposure, presence of other chemicals in the mixture, hand washing, glove use, and change schedule.[8]

In addition to the exposure duration and frequency, the surface area exposed and the concentration of the chemical are required to calculate the overall exposure. A wipe sampling method can be used to quantify the concentration of certain chemicals on the skin. The results may directly inform risk determination for localized health outcomes.

However, for systemic health effects, it is more difficult to define the uptake rate through the skin and subsequent pharmacokinetics. As a result, dermal exposure is often ignored or underestimated for its contributions to the systemic health effects.[8]

Dermal exposures can be monitored with the analytical/sampling approach or be estimated with the modeling approach. The analytical approach can be the direct measurement of the skin with patches, wipes, or video imaging. It can also be indirect to investigate the processes before dermal exposure occurs (migration and transfer approaches) or measure the concentrations of the substance in body fluids or tissues after absorption (biomonitoring). Currently, there is no guide to selecting an analytical method in a specific circumstance, and more research is needed in this area.[12]

In the absence of measured values, dermal exposure modeling is a valuable alternative. Various models are summarized in WHO's Environmental Health Criteria 242 Dermal Exposure.[12] American Industrial Hygiene Association (AIHA) published IHSkinPerm, a practical Excel application for estimating dose from dermal exposure.[13]

2.8 RISK CHARACTERIZATION

Risk characterization can be qualitative or quantitative. A classical approach is to estimate both the effects of contact (severity) and the exposure level/probability for the hazards present. A risk matrix can be developed using this approach by estimating the relative risk represented by the intersection of probability and severity, as shown in Table 2.1. The risk levels shown in the table are estimates of relative risk that can be determined by a group or a single person. For example, the combination of the "probable" contact of a chemical with a "serious health effect" results in a very high-level risk. In this case, the protective equipment choice is critical to the safety of the worker. For gloves, this might be the case when handling dimethyl mercury or a dangerous virus.

TABLE 2.1

An Example of a Simple Relative Risk Matrix Based on Severity and Exposure Probability

Exposure or Probability	No Effect	Minor Effect	Temporary Health Effect	Serious Health Effect	Death
Certain	Very low	Medium	High	Very high	Very high
Very probable	Very low	Medium	High	Very high	Very high
Probable	Very low	Medium	Medium	Very high	Very high
Possible	Very low	Low	Medium	High	High
Unlikely	Very low	Very low	Low	Medium	Medium

We can use a numeric scoring scheme ranging from 1 to 5, where number 1 would represent the lowest risk and number 5 the greatest risk. Exposure probability can also be rated from 1 to 5, with 5 representing dermal exposure level by itself equivalent to airborne exposure levels over airborne OELs, in terms of absorbed dose. As discussed earlier, the exposure level is often not measured. AIHA has proposed a framework to semi-quantitatively estimate the exposure level by examining contact area, chemical loading/concentration, contact frequency, chemical retention time, and chemical penetration potential.[8]

With glove selection guidance provided later in this book and elsewhere,[14] appropriate gloves can be chosen for a specific hazard and exposure scenario. For example, a low-risk application might permit the use of a glove that could or does allow permeation, whereas a high-risk application would require the use of a glove that offers complete permeation resistance for the length of the operation. In some cases when the risks are very high, the assignment of protective equipment may not be acceptable, as a failure in gloves would result in serious consequences to the user. In the example of the battery charging operation as discussed in Section 2.11, this might represent a moderate (e.g., level three) level of risk because the hazard is acute and the acid is somewhat diluted. This means that a failure of the protective device (i.e., glove) would not likely result in a serious permanent injury. Hence, we would probably consider the use of protective gloves for this work task acceptable. By using this "acceptable risk concept," we can assign gloves that might exhibit permeation at low levels for certain tasks. An example is the application of isopropyl alcohol for cleaning in a hospital, as the major effect of failure would be mild dermatitis from defatting of the skin.

2.9   CONSIDERATION OF CONTROL MEASURES

Before assigning workers protective gloves or other personal protective equipment in high-risk jobs, other control measures should be considered. These include the following:

- Elimination or substitution of a hazard with a less hazardous alternative
- Changes in work practices, such as the use of tools

- Engineering controls or other process changes
- Robotics and other forms of automation

A key factor in the occupational hygiene and risk assessment process is the evaluation of actual work practices. There may be effective alternatives to the actual hand manipulation of an item or work task that are much less expensive and also less difficult to implement than engineering controls. Gloves and other forms of personal protective equipment should be assigned after we have evaluated the risk to the user in case of a failure. They should be used as an additional layer of protection instead of the single critical layer. For those jobs where the risk of serious injury remains after assigning the protective clothing, we will have to incorporate other options.

2.10　REASSESSMENT

After initial control measures are proposed or implemented, the dermal exposure may or may not be reduced to acceptable levels. There can also be changes in operations that increase dermal exposure potential significantly. Therefore, the tasks should be reviewed under the new work configuration periodically to determine if the risks are removed or lowered to an acceptable level. Reassessment is intended to drive continuous improvement in reducing the risks to workers. Again, gloves and PPE are important tools, and they should be used as the last resort or additional layer in the hierarchy of control.

Glove choice should be periodically evaluated. There can be a glove more protective against exposure. It also should be checked if glove choice introduces an added safety hazard (e.g., around rotating machinery) or reduces the dexterity required. One example is in the processing of specialty paints and inks on small roller mills. The glove choice should balance the need to protect skin and avoid additional risks of gloves being caught and pulling the hand into the mill. One possible solution is to wear loose-fitting outer gloves, which can be easily pulled off if caught, with chemically resistant and tight-fitting inner gloves. Another example is from surgeons who need gloves protecting against cuts, punctures, and blood-borne pathogens. However, such gloves may not permit enough dexterity for sensitive and complex tasks. In this case, there may be a balance between personal risk to the doctor and risk to the patient.

2.11　INDUSTRIAL BATTERY CHARGING: AN EXAMPLE

An effective approach to evaluate the risks associated with work is to divide the work being performed or planned into the separate steps required to complete the work task. This process is essentially the same as that used in job safety analysis or the more traditional time study analysis. An industrial battery changing and charging operation for forklift trucks can be used to illustrate this approach. For our example, we concentrate on the charging of batteries removed from the operating vehicle (some sites charge in place and do not remove batteries). The work steps are as follows:

1. Put on protective clothing consisting of a Neoprene apron, Neoprene gloves, and a face shield (estimated average duration of 2 min).
2. Use an overhead hoist to transport a battery from the receiving rack to the charging area (estimated average duration of 5 min).
3. Remove a battery cap and obtain a sample to check the specific gravity of the battery acid (estimated average duration of 2 min).
4. Add battery acid (sulfuric) as required using a bulk dispenser hose with a squeeze spigot (2–10 min estimated average duration).
5. Clean tools by rinsing in water (estimated average duration of 2 min).
6. Clean battery top using baking soda, water, and a brush (estimated average duration of 4 min).
7. Place battery on charge by connecting terminals (estimated average duration of 2 min).
8. Wash and neutralize protective clothing before doffing.
9. Remove protective clothing for proper storage.

Following the description of distinct tasks within the overall job, a listing of chemical, physical, biological, radiological, or other hazards needs to be developed for each step in the task. In our situation described above, the principal hazards are chemical and physical. The temperature of the chemical compound or material and the concentration are important factors. Additionally, the type of contact and the duration or frequency of contact are also important.

Using our example, the following exposure assessment analysis and control measures are developed:

1. Put on protective clothing consisting of a Neoprene apron, Neoprene gloves, and a face shield (requires inspection of protective equipment; face shield may limit visibility).
2. Use an overhead hoist to transport a battery from the receiving rack to the charging area (potential for exposure to battery acid by splash contact or by physical contact with the battery housing; requires the protective gloves to have a moderate level of abrasion resistance).
3. Remove a battery cap and obtain a sample to check the specific gravity (potential for direct liquid contact with battery acid; this requires gloves that do not have a slippery surface when wet and that permit enough dexterity to remove the battery cap and handle the instrument).
4. Add battery acid (sulfuric) as required using a bulk dispenser hose with a squeeze spigot (potential for direct liquid contact with the glove by acid and potential for splash).
5. Clean tools by rinsing in water (requires gloves that will permit water washing and resistance to residual acid).
6. Clean battery top using baking soda and water and a brush (requires gloves that have a good puncture and tear resistance).

7. Place battery on charge by connecting terminals (requires gloves that have a moderate level of cut resistance; electrical resistance is also beneficial).
8. Wash and neutralize protective clothing before doffing (requires decontamination-water washing to remove any sulfuric acid that may have contaminated the gloves or other items of clothing).
9. Remove protective clothing for proper storage (requires gloves to be capable of being water-washed, air-dried, and stored without any degradation).

2.12   WORKER TRAINING

Worker information and training are very important parts of the risk-reduction process. Users should be provided with the following information:

- Nature and extent of the hazards
- Signs and symptoms of overexposure
- Use and limitations of the protective equipment assigned
- Proper fitting, wearing, and doffing of the equipment assigned
- Decontamination procedures, if required
- Inspection, maintenance, and storage procedures
- First aid and emergency procedures

The occupational hygiene evaluation of the job should provide the information necessary to inform the worker of the nature and extent of the hazards and the level of risk the worker will face. This should include the specific nature of the hazard (e.g., corrosive, flammable, toxic) and the extent of the hazard.[9] Other important information includes the signs and symptoms of overexposure so that the worker knows if the protective equipment has failed. The proper use and limitations of the protective equipment are important to provide the worker with the limits to the range of protection provided. The proper fitting of the equipment, how it should be worn, and how to take it off are also important. For example, the correct sizing of gloves, how to put them on properly, how to wear them, and how they should be removed (especially if potentially contaminated) are all part of the information and training that should be given to users. How or when to decontaminate protective equipment is important in those situations where the equipment is likely to become contaminated and before reuse of the equipment. Inspection of the gloves prior to use by the employer will greatly decrease the potential for accidents. Before each use, the worker should also inspect the gloves for imperfections, discolorations, etc. If the gloves are clean, they should be inflated by blowing into them or by quickly folding them at the opening (leaving some air in the glove) and immersing them in water. Bubbles are an indication of pinholes or other discontinuities. Previously contaminated gloves should not be used before they are decontaminated. Finally, it is important to ensure that the worker knows what to do in the event of an emergency.

Knowledge of the hazard and how to use protective equipment properly not only reduces risk but also provides the health and safety professional with a worker capable of contributing feedback on the effectiveness of the protective equipment.

REFERENCES

1. U.S. BLS. 2021. *Industry Injury and Illness Data.* Washington, DC: Bureau of Labor Statistics, U.S. (BLS). Available at: https://www.bls.gov/iif/oshsum.htm (accessed Jan. 31, 2021).

2. NIOSH. 2021. *National Occupational Research Agenda: Disease & Injury.* Washington, DC: National Institute for Occupational Safety and Health (NIOSH). Available at: https://www.cdc.gov/niosh/docs/96-115/diseas.html (accessed Jan. 31, 2021).

3. Milz, S.S. 2011. Principles of evaluating worker exposure, Chapter 7, in *The Occupational Environment: Its Evaluation, Control, and Management*, 3rd ed., Anna, D.H., Ed. Fairfax, VA: American Industrial Hygiene Association, pp. 146–163.

4. OSHA. 2021. *OSHA Standards Do Not Include Surface Contamination Criteria or Quantifications for Skin Absorption.* Washington, DC: Occupational Safety and Health Administration. Available at: https://www.osha.gov/laws-regs/standardinterpretations/1985-06-21 (accessed Jan. 30, 2021).

5. ACGIH. 2020. *2020 TLVs AND BEIs.* Cincinnati, OH: American Conference of Governmental Industrial Hygienists (ACGIH) Publications.

6. Bratt, G., Nelson, D.I. and Maier, A. 2011. Occupational and environmental health risk assessment/risk management, Chapter 8, in *The Occupational Environment: Its Evaluation, Control, and Management*, 3rd ed., Anna, D.H., Ed. Fairfax, VA: American Industrial Hygiene Association, pp. 164–226.

7. Nierenberg, D.W., Nordgren, R.E., Chang, M.B., Siegler, R.W., Blayney, M.B., Hochberg, F., Toribara, T.Y., Cernichiari, E. and Clarkson, T. 1998. Delayed cerebellar disease and death after accidental exposure to dimethylmercury. *N Engl J Med* 338(23):1672–1676. DOI: 10.1056/NEJM199806043382305.

8. Sahmel, J. and Boeniger, M. 2015. Dermal exposure assessment, Chapter 13, in *A Strategy for Assessing and Managing Occupational Exposures*, 4th ed., Jahn, S.D., Bullock, W.H. and Ignacio, J.S., Eds. Fairfax, VA: American Industrial Hygiene Association, pp. 171–195.

9. OSHA. 2021. *Appendix A to 1910.1200: Health Hazard Criteria.* Washington, DC: Occupational Safety and Health Administration. Available at: https://www.osha.gov/dsg/hazcom/hazcom-appendix-a.html (accessed Jan. 30, 2021).

10. NIOSH. 2021. *Pocket Guide to Chemical Hazards, Introduction.* Washington, DC: National Institute for Occupational Safety and Health (NIOSH). Available at: https://www.cdc.gov/niosh/npg/pgintrod.html (accessed Jan. 30, 2021).

11. NIOSH. 2021. *Skin Notation Profiles.* Washington, DC: National Institute for Occupational Safety and Health (NIOSH). Available at: https://www.cdc.gov/niosh/topics/skin/skin-notation_profiles.html (accessed Jan. 30, 2021).

12. WHO. 2014. *Dermal Exposure (Environmental Health Criteria 242).* Geneva: International Program on Chemical Safety and Inter-Organization Programme for the Sound Management of Chemicals, World Health Organization.

13. AIHA. 2021. *IH Apps & Tools.* Fairfax, VA: American Industrial Hygiene Association. Available at: https://www.aiha.org/public-resources/consumer-resources/topics-of-interest/ih-apps-tools (accessed Jan. 31, 2021).

14. Forsberg, K. and Mansdorf, S.Z. 2007. *Quick Selection Guide to Chemical Protective Clothing*, 5th ed. Hoboken, NJ: Wiley-Interscience.

3 Gloves
Types, Materials, and Manufacturing

Marie-Noëlle Crépy and Pierre Hoerner

CONTENTS

DOI: 10.1201/9781003126874-4

3.1   GLOVE TYPES

Gloves are protective equipment intended for various purposes, such as prevention of transfer of microorganisms or harmful agents or protection of the hands against mechanical, thermal, radiation, or electrical risks. Gloves can also be used to protect delicate or clean products from human contamination or damage. Examples of this are clean and sterile gloves used to protect microelectronic components or pharmaceutical products during manufacture.

Protective gloves can be classified into various types according to their usage and market segments. The following three main categories are generally considered: medical gloves, industrial gloves, and household gloves.

3.1.1   MEDICAL GLOVES

Medical gloves are disposable gloves that are used to protect the wearer and/or the patient from the spread of infection or illness during medical procedures and examinations. They are one part of an infection-control strategy and are classified as Medical Devices.[1]

Medical gloves can be subcategorized into two main categories, examination gloves, and surgical gloves, with an additional specialized category termed procedure gloves.

1. *Examination gloves* are disposable devices intended for medical purposes that are worn on the examiner's hands or fingers to prevent contamination between patient and examiner. Examination gloves are thin (50–150 µm, depending on materials), ambidextrous, and, as a standard, conditioned in boxes of 100 pieces. For most applications, examination gloves are worn only for a few minutes. Current examination gloves are made either from natural rubber (NR) or from synthetic rubber, mostly nitrile butadiene rubber (NBR) and, marginally, polychloroprene rubber (CR). Thanks to an attractive price, thermoplastic material, namely polyvinyl chloride (PVC), is still widely used despite its lower barrier performance. Some examination gloves, such as those made of nitrile rubber, can also claim some level of chemical resistance against most chemotherapy agents. NBR has become the material of choice for examination gloves.

2. *Surgical gloves* are more sophisticated than examination gloves. They are to be worn on the hands of operating room personnel to protect a surgical wound from contamination. Surgical gloves are packed in pairs, with

differentiated right and left hands in a sterile pouch and should meet stringent performance criteria, such as leak resistance, mechanical resistance, and biocompatibility. Surgical gloves should be easy to don and provide an outstanding feel and fit and comfort to the user, as well as allow a good grip for instrument prehension. Surgical gloves are thicker than examination gloves (180–250 µm for conventional surgical gloves) and are used for a longer period, sometimes up to a few hours (it is recommended to change the glove every 90 minutes or less in case a perforation is noticed).[2] Current surgical gloves are made either from natural rubber or synthetic rubber, mostly synthetic polyisoprene (IR) and CR. Conversion to powder-free gloves, and now to synthetics, is in progress to mitigate type I allergies to natural rubber.[3] So far, NBR rubber didn't find any great traction for usage as a surgical glove, as the material remains too stiff and is sensitive to water hydration when used for prolonged times. Surgical gloves made from thermoplastic materials, namely Styrenic Block Copolymers (SBC) or polyurethanes (TPU), are also being developed as accelerator-free alternatives to conventional synthetic rubbers,[4] but as of now the market of these products remains marginal. Finally, innovative integrated antimicrobial surgical gloves have been designed to offer some added protection against microbial contamination in case of glove breach. The antimicrobial chemical could be incorporated inside the glove, in the form of drop-like compartments,[5] or the form of a coating at the glove inner surface.[6]

3. *Procedure gloves* are a niche market segment for examination-like gloves being used for medical procedures where sterility is needed outside of the operating room.

3.1.2   INDUSTRIAL GLOVES

Industrial gloves are mostly heavier and nondisposable (reusable). They are designed to provide specific levels of protection against chemical, mechanical, biohazards, thermal, electrical, or radiation risks and are classified as Protective Personal Equipment.

Industrial gloves are made with a wide variety of materials and thicknesses. Various rubber types, such as NR, CR, and NBR, but also Butyl Rubber (IIR), Ethylene-Propylene Diene Monomer (EPDM), Fluoroelastomers (FKM or FPM), Chlorosulfonated Polyethylene (CSM), and Silicone Rubbers (VMQ), are used for the manufacture of industrial gloves. In addition, various other materials which are not conventionally classified as "rubbers," such as thermoplastics (PVC, TPU, SBC), polyolefins (polyethylene (PE)), polyvinyl alcohol (PVA), polyamides (PA), or leather, can also be used. Each of these materials is selected for its specific features and performance levels, as described in detail in Section 2.

Most of the reusable gloves are laminated with an inner fabric liner made of cotton or synthetic fibers that provide easy donning and comfort and could also improve the cut-resistance performance. Some gloves can also have at their inner surface a flock coating of fibers that create a silky and comfortable touch and provide some additional level of comfort during usage. This flock is composed of finely cut natural or synthetic fibers deposited over the glove substrate with the help of an adhesive, typically an acrylic polymer.

The nondisposable glove market also includes very specialized gloves, such as long-sleeve gloves for dry-box application, gloves for electrical insulation, and gloves filled with radiopaque particles to reduce the exposure to harmful ionizing radiation on the operator's hands.

Multilayered materials have been developed for specific applications that require a set of properties that could not be reached by a single material. This is especially the case for chemical resistance, but also for mechanical resistant gloves where materials with good abrasion performance, such as TPU, can be used at the outer glove surface. Examples of multilayered materials currently in the market include NBR-CR and NBR-CR-NBR,[7] IIR-FKM,[8] and CSM-TPU.[9]

The disposable industrial gloves market includes gloves intended to be used for life science applications (pharmaceutical), food industry, semiconductor industry, and electronic industry. These gloves are mainly made from NBR or CR and on a first approach are comparable to conventional examination gloves. However, these gloves undergo additional washing processes, and in most cases they are processed in a clean room to reduce the particle count to levels as low as <650 ($\leq 0.5\mu m$) per cm^2.[10] For special applications, these gloves could also be sold sterile.

3.1.3 HOUSEHOLD GLOVES

Household or domestic gloves are usually reusable, quite often with a flock coating comprising fibers to minimize discomfort due to hand sweating. They are usually made from natural rubber latex (NRL), CR, NBR, or PVC. Disposable gloves for domestic applications are made from NRL, NBR, and PVC, with features similar to those of examination gloves.

3.2 MATERIALS

As already described, protective gloves can be made from a large variety of materials, which will be individually described in this chapter. The formulation of these materials, as well as their transformation process to make a glove, will be discussed in Section 3.

3.2.1 POLYMERS WIDELY USED FOR GLOVES (MASS MARKET)

3.2.1.1 Natural Rubber

NR is a natural product that is well known since ancient times. It is harvested from rubber trees (mostly *Hevea brasiliensis*). When an incision is made on the bark of the tree, a liquid sap naturally flows to heal this incision. The sap is composed of colloidal particles of polyisoprene of high stereospecificity (99% of cis-1,4-polyisoprene) dispersed in water. The generic name of colloidal polymeric particles dispersed in

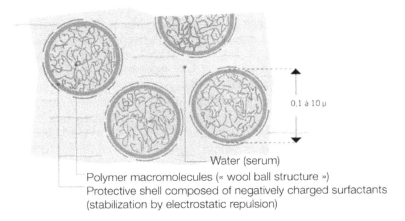

0.1 à 10 µ

Water (serum)
Polymer macromolecules (« wool ball structure »)
Protective shell composed of negatively charged surfactants
(stabilization by electrostatic repulsion)

FIGURE 3.1   Schematic representation of natural rubber particles.

water is "latex"; hence, the rubber tree sap is called "natural rubber latex." The latex particle size ranges from 0.1 µm to 10 µm, as shown in Figure 3.1.

NRL is composed of 27–40% of polyisoprene, 52–70% of water, and 1.5–3% of proteins, which mainly serve for the stabilization of the latex particles.[11]

After collection, the NRL must be preserved and concentrated. Usually, ammonia is used as a preservative, and it must be added at the earliest possible moment. High-ammonia (HA) latex contains about 0.7% ammonia; low-ammonia (LA) latex contains about 0.2% ammonia and additional preservatives. Both are suitable for the manufacture of gloves. The latex suspension is then concentrated to a rubber content of about 60% by centrifugation, creaming, or evaporation before the dipping process. Centrifugation removes the nonrubber chemicals.

NRL was used by the Mayan civilization in thin films as a waterproofing agent, and it was introduced to Europe by Christophe Colomb. In 1845, Goodyear invented the rubber vulcanization process, which transforms the natural rubber gum into an elastic material, displaying remarkable performances such as elasticity and tear resistance.

Unfortunately, NR contains various sensitizing proteins that have been the cause of an epidemic of immediate type I IgE-mediated allergic reactions with different clinical pictures, varying from localized contact urticaria to life-threatening anaphylactic reactions in caregivers and patients.[3] For these reasons, it is gradually being replaced by synthetic materials that are free of any sensitizing proteins.

More than 2,000 species of plants can produce natural rubber, but nowadays it is mainly produced from *H. brasiliensis*. Guayule (*Parthenium argentatum*) is a woody plant growing in the deserts of the US Southwest and Mexico that produces a cleaner natural rubber latex with fewer proteins and thus are less likely to trigger allergies. However, extracting latex from guayule involves cutting the plant, mixing the branches to release the latex entrapped in the cells in the plant, and then extracting/separating the latex from the other residues. This process is far more challenging, lengthy, and expansive than collecting the latex simply by harvesting the bark of the Hevea tree. Despite the complexity, there has been some massive research over the past 30 years on a way to find alternative sourcing to tropical latex.[12]

3.2.1.2 Nitrile Butadiene Rubber and Carboxylated Nitrile Butadiene Rubber (XNBR)

NBR is a copolymer of acrylonitrile and butadiene. XNBR is an improved nitrile rubber with the addition of a carboxylic acid group introduced into the polymer chain through the inclusion of methacrylic acid in the formulation. The acid group's main function is to form ionic crosslinks, for example, with Zinc. The added carboxyl group gives XNBR rubber its high strength; however, this ionic crosslinking also leads to some moisture sensitivity. NBR and XNBR are available in latex form (dispersion in water) at an affordable cost, and XNBR is widely used in the glove industry, especially for thin examination gloves. To prevent complexity and confusion for nonchemists, the name NBR will be used irrespectively if the product is NBR or XNBR.

In addition to examination gloves, NBR is also widely used for household and unsupported industrial gloves. NBR exhibits considerable resistance to oils, fuels, and certain solvents, and it has a very good tensile strength.

3.2.1.3 Polychloroprene Rubber

Polychloroprene rubber was the first commercial synthetic rubber, invented by E. I. DuPont de Nemours & Company in 1930 and sold under the brand name "Neoprene™."

CR is also available in latex form. It is more expensive than NRL and NBR, almost twice the price, but offers an interesting balance of properties, such as good chemical and physical properties, together with good ozone-resistant properties. Therefore, CR is used in all types of gloves, such as thin surgical gloves, household gloves, supported and unsupported industrial gloves, and in combination with NBR or IR gloves.

3.2.1.4 Polyisoprene Rubber

Synthetic polyisoprene can be produced chemically, starting from the isoprene monomer, through various polymerization processes (Ziegler Nata, Anionic). Synthetic polyisoprene is a clone of natural rubber. However, synthetic polyisoprenes would never reach the same level of stereospecificity as natural rubber (99% of cis-1,4-polyisoprene); therefore, some properties of the synthetic copy would not be as good as the natural source (crystalline properties), especially in terms of tear resistance, but IR remains perfectly suitable for application in gloves.

In early 2000, colloidal dispersions (latex) of synthetic polyisoprene have been made available in the market.[13] Despite its higher price (more than two times that of CR), IR latex has gained strong market traction, especially in the surgical glove segment, as the gloves are significantly softer than CR and combine the barrier and comfort properties of natural rubber latex gloves without inducing type I latex allergy.

3.2.1.5 Polyvinyl Chloride

PCV is an economical (cheaper than NBR) and versatile thermoplastic polymer that can be as rigid as industrial pipes or, when formulated with significant amounts of plasticizers, can be as pliable as plastic wrap or as thin and flexible as blood bags or gloves. Phthalates, which used to be the most suitable plasticizers, have been replaced with less toxic substituents such as adipates or vegetal oils. As incineration of PVC generates hydrochloric acid, the use of PVC disposable gloves represents some environmental concerns. PVC is still used for "low price" examination gloves and for some industrial gloves where they provide good protection against many acids, caustics, alkalis, and alcohols. Chemical-resistant PVC gloves offer generally good abrasion resistance but are susceptible to cuts.

3.2.2 Polymers Used for Niche Market Segments

The following materials are currently not used for manufacturing gloves intended for mass market applications but are mostly used for manufacturing industrial gloves where special properties are required. These materials are essentially available as dry rubber, not as water dispersion (latex).

3.2.2.1 Butyl Rubber

IIR is a copolymer of isobutene (97–99.5%), and isoprene (0.5–3%) and is selected for manufacturing gloves, thanks to its low gas permeability and excellent resistance to polar solvents and corrosive chemicals. This material has good flexibility but slightly lower tensile strength than other conventional materials such as NRL, CR, or NBR. It displays poor resistance to petroleum oil and gasoline. Gloves made of IIR for industrial use are available. IIR is the material of choice for CBRN (chemical, biological, radiological, and nuclear defense) protection suits.

3.2.2.2 Chlorosulfonated Polyethylene

Chlorosulfonated polyethylene was initially developed by DuPont, under the trademark Hypalon®, but DuPont closed his US manufacturing plant and stopped this business in 2009. The material is now available through other suppliers under its chemical name CSM.

CSM offers very high resistance to ozone and other oxidizing chemicals, as well as acids and alkalis. It also withstands abrasion. It is often used in gloveboxes and sometimes in connection with other polymers such as TPU.[9]

3.2.2.3 Ethylene–Propylene Diene Monomer

EPDM is a synthetic rubber made from ethylene, propylene, and a diene comonomer with excellent chemical resistance to polar solvents and corrosive chemicals. Just as CSM, EPDM is a rubber with a saturated backbone, and for this reason it has much better resistance to heat, light, and ozone than unsaturated rubbers such as NR, CR, and IR. This makes it suitable to be utilized in harsh environments or for gloves that are regularly sterilized by steam.

3.2.2.4   Fluorocarbon Elastomer

Fluorocarbon elastomers (FKM) are advanced materials obtained by copolymerization of various fluoro-monomers such as vinylidene fluoride and hexafluoropropylene. This elastomer family was discovered by DuPont in 1958 and is sold under the trade name Viton™. Nowadays, a few other suppliers offer similar products under different brands. The main interest of FKM is their unique resistance against a wide variety of chemicals, especially most chlorinated and aromatic solvents, and with extreme heat and oil resistance. However, these products remain significantly more expensive compared to any other elastomers.

3.2.2.5   Styrenic-Block-Copolymers

SBC covers a wide range of block copolymers composed of styrene and butadiene, or styrene and isoprene, with a certain architecture and chain lengths. The SBC family essentially comprises SBS (Styrene–Butadiene–Styrene) and SIS (Styrene–Isoprene–Styrene), as well as their hydrogenated versions, SEBS (Styrene–Ethylene/Butylene–Styrene, obtained after hydrogenation of SBS) and SEPS (Styrene–Ethylene/Propylene–Styrene, obtained after hydrogenation of SIS).

Of all other rubbers discussed above, these materials have the unique advantage of self-organizing in the form of elastic films, thanks to the physical bonding of the polystyrene end blocks, without the need for any additional chemicals, such as cross-linkers, sulfur, or accelerators (Figure 3.2).

Therefore, it is possible to create gloves that offer a better biocompatibility profile, with less or even no extractable chemical.[4] Gloves are soft and flexible with high tensile strength. The drawback of the material is that the gloves do not resist when exposed to low-polarity organic solvents. This drawback can be mitigated with a light chemical crosslinking, which can be achieved without the use of accelerators.[14]

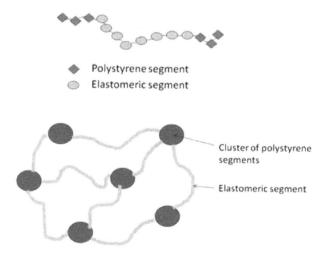

FIGURE 3.2   Self-organization of SBC block copolymers.

SBCs are widely available in dry rubber form. Recently, the first latex dispersion of SIS was introduced in the marketplace.[15] This product was specifically designed for the glove and condom industry.

3.2.2.6 Polyvinyl Alcohol

The polymer of vinyl alcohol is used in industrial gloves for its unique chemical resistance property. PVA is nearly inert to strong solvents, including aromatics, aliphatics, and chlorinated solvents. However, PVA has a limited resistance to water and water-based solutions, which limits its application in the glove industry.

3.2.2.7 Polyethylene

Polyethylene is used to manufacture thin disposable gloves by punching/welding, starting from thin foils of PE. Gloves of different thicknesses and with patterned surfaces are available, as well as gloves with extra-long sleeves (e.g., for veterinarian use). PE gloves offer very good resistance to acids, alkaline, water, and oil and have wide application, such as in food handling, domestic cleaning, hairdressing salons, and nonsterile hospital work. The protective effect is more dependent on the strength of the welded seams than the chemical resistance of the material itself.

3.2.2.8 Polyurethane

Polyurethanes are probably the polymers offering one the highest versatility. They can be designed to fit with the intended usage. TPU normally possesses a very good abrasion resistance and high resistance at the break. However, it is sensitive to degradation by alcohols, which is a major limitation, for example in medical settings. While TPUs can be made having improved alcohol resistance, they tend to produce relatively stiff films, which is problematic for most applications. TPU is mainly processed in solution, particularly in N,N-dimethylformamide (DMF), which is a toxic solvent. TPU latex dispersions developed for the glove and condom dipping industry have recently been introduced in the marketplace.[16]

3.2.2.9 Silicone Rubber (VMQ, LSR)

Silicone rubber is very inert and offers unprecedented insulative properties and thermal stability. Silicone is however not widely used for gloves, except for gloves intended to be exposed to high temperatures.

3.2.3 Materials and Processes Used in Glove Inner and Outer Surfaces

The aspect and performance of glove's inner and outer surfaces are of key importance for their intended purpose. Sometimes, the properties of the glove surface are quite different from those of its core material.

3.2.3.1 Inner Glove Surface

The inner glove surface is aimed to provide easy donning and some comfort during use. Glove donning could be challenging, especially for thin and soft gloves such as medical gloves, which can easily deform when donned. For medical gloves, glove donning was historically achieved using powder. Free particles at the inside layer are extremely efficient in reducing friction, therefore facilitating donning. However, the powder was associated with increased risks of inflammation or sensitization for both wearers and patients, especially when combined with NRL; therefore, many countries, such as the United States, have banned the use of powdered surgical gloves.[17] Nowadays, conventional powder-free medical gloves are designed with either a polymer coating or a surface modification by chlorination:

- **A polymer coating** is a thin coating, usually composed of polyurethane or polyacrylate, located at the inner glove surface. This layer is harder and stiffer than the rubber and generally contains silicone to decrease friction and help with donning.
- **Chlorination** is a chemical modification performed on the surface of the core rubber. Free chlorine, a strong oxidant, is used for its quick reaction with the unsaturation of the rubber material, generating increased surface hardness and roughness. This process is possible only for rubber materials having enough reactive double bonds, such as NRL, IR, NBR, and unsaturated SBC (SBS, SIS), but cannot be used for less reactive rubbers such as CR, EPDM, IIR, CSM, and hydrogenated SBC (SEBS, SEPS). Chlorination can be performed directly during manufacturing (in-line chlorination) and is a cheaper alternative than polymer coating. However, chlorinated gloves are more sensitive to degradation by aging. Also, in-line chlorination involves significant safety and environmental challenges.

Nondisposable gloves are thicker (less prone to deformation during donning) and are shaped to be less fitted to the hand; therefore donning is normally less challenging.

In addition, most nondisposable gloves are laminated with an inner fabric liner made of cotton or synthetic fiber that provides better donnability and comfort. Some gloves can also comprise at their surface a flock coating comprising fibers that create a silky and comfortable touch and provide some additional level of comfort during usage.

3.2.3.2   Outer Glove Surface

The surface of the glove can be smooth or rough in all or parts of the glove. In general, thin gloves have textured fingertips to facilitate instrument prehension.

In addition, the outside glove surface can be modified to decrease the natural tackiness of rubber materials and offer an adequate grip level to the users. Off-line chlorination is very widely used as it offers a permanent modification. Performed in a closed vessel, off-line chlorination is less complicated and risky from both safety and environmental aspects.

For some polymers which cannot be chlorinated, surface modification can be achieved through the specific formulation of the rubber (hardness, the addition of fillers) or by treatment such as applying or spraying a thin layer of a hard polymer at the glove surface.

3.3 MANUFACTURING

Gloves can commonly be manufactured by a dipping process, by punching and welding of plastic film sheets, by an injection molding process, by knitting, or by sewing. Gloves with linings are manufactured by a combination of the sewing and dipping procedure.

Most rubber and thermoplastic gloves are manufactured by the dipping process, which will be exhaustively described in this chapter.

3.3.1 GLOVES MADE BY DIPPING

The dipping process is the method of choice for the manufacturing of thin-walled, extensible articles such as gloves and condoms. The precursor of glove dipping was Ansell, who designed and built the first automatic dipping machine in 1945 and introduced the first disposable surgical gloves in 1964.[18]

Molds or formers made of porcelain, metal, or plastic in the shape of hands of different sizes are mounted on a rack and are slowly dipped into a mixture comprising either a solution or a suspension of the polymeric material. A thin liquid layer is deposited on the mold upon removal from the mixture.

There are two main dipping technologies, depending on the state of the starting polymer that must be transformed: dispersion in water (also called 'latex dipping') or solution in solvent (also called 'solution dipping').

3.3.1.1 Latex Dipping Technology

Latex dipping technology is by far the broadest process currently used for the manufacturing of thin-walled films. As a reminder, latex is the generic name for a stable dispersion of polymer microparticles in water; therefore, the starting point is an aqueous liquid dispersion. Originally, this technology was designed to transform natural rubber latex into protective gloves and is now applied to most synthetic latexes such as NBR, CR, and IR.

In this chapter, a better description of this technology will be provided, considering chemical, physico-chemical, and material properties, with the aim of explaining how it is possible to create a continuous film starting from a heterogeneous biphasic system. This shall provide a better understanding of some common glove-related issues such as leachable chemicals, hydration, or glove microporosity. The authors also recommend the exhaustive book from David M. Hill, *Latex Dipping: Science and Technology*,[19] for those willing to gain further technical details of latex formulation and transformation by dipping.

As mentioned earlier, the starting point for this process is the "latex," i.e., a colloidal suspension of polymer particles in water. The particles have a common submicron size typically ranging from 0.1 to a few μm: NRL has a broad size repartition (typically 0.3–0.8 μm), whereas synthetic latexes such as NBR or CR have narrower size distribution (typical NBR latex size is around 0.1–0.2 μm).

a.   Concept of Latex Destabilization and Stabilization Mechanisms

As a rule, colloidal dispersions are not stable:

- Due to gravity, polymer microparticles would either move upward ("cream") or sediment over time, depending on the density of the polymer compared to water. Most rubber particles are slightly less dense than water (NRL = 0.92; IR = 0.93) and will cream, whereas some are denser (CR = 1.1) and will sediment. Creaming and sedimentation can be addressed by properly stirring the latex to generate some motions and flow to compensate for gravity.
- There are other destabilization mechanisms that are independent of gravity: as the individual microparticles are always in movement (Brownian movement), collisions between particles occur very frequently. If the particle surface is not properly protected, the particles would "stick" together to form larger agglomerates (like a bunch of grapes) in a process called flocculation. It is also possible for the particles to "coalesce," but this mechanism is more adequate for emulsions rather than for latexes. For latexes, flocculation creates a major issue in the dipping technology, as the starting latex shouldn't contain any agglomerates that would impair the film-forming mechanism.

The four common destabilization mechanisms of latexes are represented in Figure 3.3.

To prevent flocculation, the external surface of the microparticle should be modified with some specific chemicals.[20] Latex stabilization can be performed through either electrostatic or steric mechanism, as shown in Figure 3.4.

Electrostatic stabilization consists of covering the particle surfaces with charged molecules. When the particles are getting closer, the same type of charges triggers a repulsion force that prevents particles from sticking together.

Particle stabilization can also be achieved by adding some long polymeric chain at the surface of the particle, which would act as a "long hair" to provide some protection.

Conventional rubber latexes used in the glove industry are mostly electrostatically stabilized. The latex, therefore, comprises some "nonrubber chemicals" introduced to provide enough stability to the latex particles. Additional stabilizers are incorporated to provide better stability before compounding the latex with other chemicals.

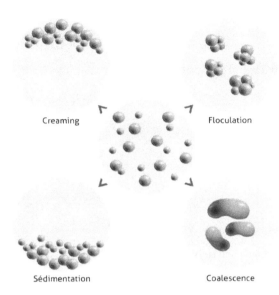

Creaming

Floculation

Sédimentation

Coalescence

FIGURE 3.3   Four common destabilization mechanisms of latexes.

Natural rubber latex is a special case; the stability is provided in this rubber, thanks to a sophisticated mechanism involving a phospholipidic membrane and proteins acting as a membrane surrounding the rubber particle, as shown in Figure 3.5.

b.   Latex Formulation

Elastomers must be formulated with chemical additives to reach the glove's desired properties such as mechanical resistance, barrier integrity, color, and aging protection. In the latex dipping process, these various chemicals should be incorporated directly into the water dispersion. As most of these chemicals are not water-soluble, they should be introduced as dispersions. Such dispersions need to be prepared and stabilized properly.

A conventional latex is generally formulated as below.

Stabilization of the Latex

The commercial latexes need to be sur-stabilized before the addition of the other chemicals; as such, chemicals modify the latex ionic strength, thus impairing the latex stability. Generally, the latex pH is increased to 10–11 by the addition of KOH, and it is also common to add other surfactants (ionic/ nonionic) to further improve its stability. Proteins such as casein were used but are almost no longer used today. Some synthetic latexes such as CR and IR are compounded with rosin resins (also known under the

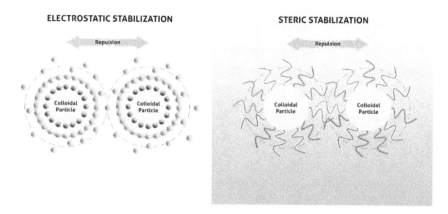

FIGURE 3.4   Electrostatic and steric stabilization mechanisms.

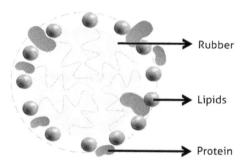

FIGURE 3.5   Schematic representation of a microparticle of natural rubber latex.

name of colophonium) that efficiently serve the purpose of particle stabilization and film formation.

Crosslinking Package

Once the latex is properly stabilized, "crosslinking" agents are generally added. Crosslinking is a chemical reaction that links polymeric chains
together to create a tridimensional network that provides material elasticity
and required (mechanical, chemical) performances.

For rubbers, crosslinking is generally achieved, thanks to sulfur bonds
in a crosslinking process called "vulcanization."

Vulcanizing agents are mostly composed of sulfur and zinc oxide, and a
cocktail of accelerators (in general a blend of two to four chemicals) can be
added.

Vulcanization additives, in water dispersion form, are gently added to
the stabilized latex. The formulated latex then needs to be stored for several

hours, under gentle stirring, until the chemical additives, which have good compatibility with the rubber microparticles, penetrate inside the latex particles. This stage is called "maturation" and could last from 8 hours to 20 hours, depending on the latex type and storage conditions. For rubber latexes with a high chemical reactivity, such as NRL and IR, the migration of the chemicals inside the particles brings some crosslinking among the polymeric chains, even without the application of heat.

As a result, the surface of the particles could become harder, which to a certain extent could impair the film-forming properties as exposed below. For such latexes, there is a window time frame of optimal usage after formulation.

Although vulcanization is, by far, the most common crosslinking route in the glove industry, the use of organic peroxides in replacement for conventional sulfur/accelerator systems is also possible. This alternative route offers some advantages toward conventional vulcanization (accelerator-free) but remains very marginally used for gloves. One reason is that peroxides are sensitive to oxygen, making the glove curing process difficult to reliably control using conventional dipping equipment.

Finally, some thermoplastic elastomers, such as SBC or TPU, do not need any crosslinking package as the molecules are already bonded through physical or ionic interactions.

Colors and Antioxidants

All glove formulations contain antioxidants that enable resistance against attack by oxygen and ozone while gloves are stored, as well as pigments and colorants enabling glove opacification while providing the desired color.

Typical latex formulations and ingredients are provided in Table 3.1.

c. *Film-Forming Mechanism*

Film formation is a critical stage from which the individual rubber particles, together with the additives, are transformed into a film.

Latex film-forming mechanisms have been exhaustively studied.[21] Film-formation occurs in several steps; during this process individual particles group together and then stick and progressively deform due to pressure, as shown in Figure 3.6. As particles remain "soft," they can stick together and deform quite easily.

Resins and colloidal stabilizers, which are added to most synthetic latexes, are aimed to favor the coalescence of the particles. However, straight latex dipping is almost not used in practice. Usually, the formers are first dipped in a solution of an electrolyte, such as calcium nitrate, to pick up a thin layer of salt which is dried before dipping in the latex, as shown in Figure 3.7. This process is called coagulation dipping.

When immersed in the latex, the salt hydrates and the ions destabilize the latex microparticles situated in the vicinity of the former by neutralizing their electrostatic stabilization mechanism. The build-up of the film is extremely rapid and occurs when the former is inside the latex tank. Therefore, after formal removal, the former is covered by a wet-gel film that doesn't flow. This provides an even thickness repartition on the former.

TABLE 3.1

The Main Chemicals Used in Rubber Glove Formulation

Vulcanization Mix

- Sulfur
- ZnO
- Stearic acid (not common for latexes)
- Accelerators (mostly thiazoles, carbamates, thiurams, thiourea, guanidines, xanthates)
  - Thiazoles: typically, MBT, ZMBT. Rarely used on their own, synergistic to carbamates. Less widely used now due to safety concerns about MBT[32]
  - Carbamates: are probably the most commonly used accelerators for glove applications with ZDBC and ZDEC being the most popular. Carbamates are considered fast accelerators
  - Thiurams: they are closely related to carbamates in terms of chemical structures but are rarely used in glove formulation due to allergy concerns
  - Thiourea: typically used in combination with DPG in CR glove formulation
  - Guanidines: principally DPG, widely used in CR and IR glove formulation
  - Xanthates: is a nitrosamine-free safer accelerator that can be used in combination with carbamates

Plasticizers

Seldom used for rubbers processed in latex form

Waxes and several types of plasticizers, such as mineral oils, naphthenic oils, ester-type plasticizers can be used for rubbers or thermoplastics processed in solution

Pigments and Dyes

Mostly mineral pigments are selected among a broad range based on the specific color and opacity required. Grades should be approved for skin contact

Fillers

Seldom used for surgical and industrial gloves. Fillers, especially calcium carbonate (CaCO3), are widely used in NRL examination gloves for cost reduction purposes

Carbon black and finely dispersed silica are used for most rubbers processed in solution

Antioxidants

The most common ones are sterically hindered phenols, sometimes used in combination with a secondary antioxidant

---

Heat-sensitive dipping is another widely used process to manufacture thin-walled articles. In this case, the latex is modified with a heat sensitizing agent, for example, poly vinyl methyl ether (PVME), to allow the latex to gel above a certain temperature. The former are heated to 50–80°C and then dipped in the same way as for straight dipping. The thickness after a single heat-sensitive dip can be up to 4 mm and is dependent on the characteristics of the mix, the temperature and heat capacity of the former, and the dwell time in the latex mix. This process is used for thick-walled products such as electricians' gloves.

d. Other Processing Stages

The wet gel is then immersed in several tanks filled with hot water to leach out the various water-soluble chemicals (e.g., surfactants), which initially act as

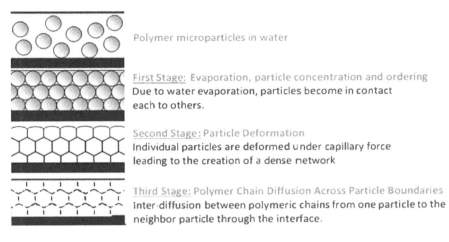

FIGURE 3.6   Latex film-forming common mechanism.

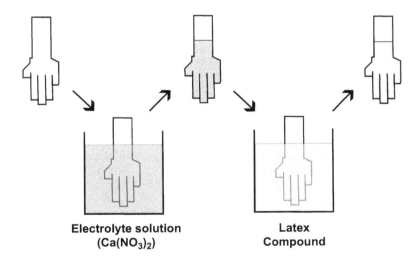

FIGURE 3.7   Coagulant dipping.

particle stabilizers and which have been expelled from the particles during film-forming. These nonrubber chemicals can have a detrimental impact on the film's properties and glove behavior. For these reasons, leaching is an important stage that would directly affect the quality of the glove and its amounts of residual chemicals.

For polymer-coated gloves, after leaching, the mold is dipped in the polymer coating tank. In most cases, the polymer coating is used in the form of a water dispersion (polyacrylates, polyurethanes), but the polymer can also be used in the form of a solution in alcohol or other organic solvents.

While still on its mold, the glove is then dried to remove water and further cured at temperatures ranging from 110°C to 140°C for vulcanization in an oven with hot air. After vulcanization, the gloves are further leached to further remove chemicals and then stripped. During the stripping, the product is usually turned inside out. Before stripping the gloves from the formers, flocking and powdering processes may take place.

For gloves that are not polymer-coated, in-line chlorination is generally performed after vulcanization of the glove. The product is immersed in a dilute aqueous chlorine solution for a short time (a few seconds). The chlorine rapidly reacts with the rubber surface of the product, which results in a lower coefficient of friction. The chlorination also results in a reduced level of extractable latex proteins, both due to the extra leaching achieved by the water and also due to the formation of insoluble forms of some proteins.[22] After chlorination, it is necessary to wash the products to remove excess chlorine, and this is done by using dilute aqueous ammonia solution and then rinsing in water.

After stripping, the molds are washed to remove traces of coagulants before a new cycle. The complete dipping process can be summarized as depicted in Figures 3.8 and 3.9.

To achieve improved physical properties of the gloves, such as tensile strength, tear strength, and swelling, together with excellent solvent resistance, it is sometimes

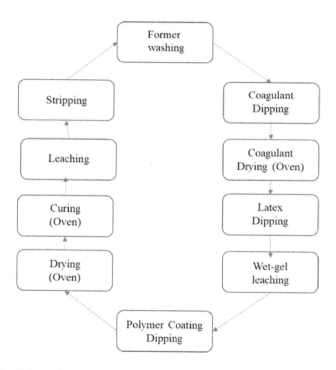

FIGURE 3.8 Schematic representation of a continuous dipping line (polymer coating).

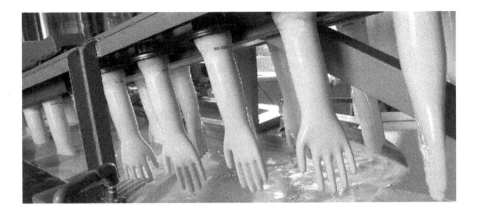

FIGURE 3.9 Automatic glove-dipping process.

interesting to use combinations of different polymers. This can be achieved by using either a blend of polymers or multilayered materials. As polymers are generally not miscible, blends rarely provide the best of each polymer.

Multilayered gloves are more interesting. It is possible to dip gloves with several layers, using different polymers for each layer, for example, NBR–CR–NBR.

e. *Latex Dipping Challenges and Limitations*

As can be seen, producing a "homogeneous" film starting from a latex dispersion, which is heterogeneous, is a complex process: latexes must be properly formulated, macerated, and filtered before usage. Film-forming can be hindered by the presence of any amount of nonrubber chemical additives present at the particle surface or in the serum. Once formed, the film needs to be immersed in water to extract most of these nonrubber chemicals, which can have a detrimental impact on the film properties.

Consequently, the manufacturing of gloves from latex dispersions is water-intensive: the amount of water needed to make one glove can range from 0.3 liter to 1 liter for most common examination gloves, and up to several liters for more demanding applications. After leaching, the water is contaminated by both organic (surfactants, resins) and nonorganic (zinc, salts) chemicals and needs to be processed before discharge.

It should be noted that conventional leaching is not able to remove all the "nonrubber" water-soluble chemicals, especially those that are entrapped in the core of the film. As a consequence, during glove usage, a "hydration" phenomenon could occur, i.e., absorption of small quantities of water in the glove.[23] The mechanism of hydration can be favored by the presence of micro-porosity in the film as well as residual ionic surfactants and electrolytes in the film. Hydration can impact the barrier performance of the film. When special requirements are needed (such as for electrical insulative properties), the gloves must be leached during an extended period to extract higher contents of those chemicals.

3.3.1.2 Solution Dipping Technology

This process can also be described as "solvent-cast or "solution-dipping" technology. The continuous solvent cast process was developed almost a century ago, driven by the needs of the emerging photographic industry.[24] Currently, solution dipping is restricted to the manufacture of gloves made with rubbers that are not commercially available in latex form.

For this production process, the polymer is first "dissolved" (by opposition to "dispersed" as is the case in the latex technology) in one of its good solvents. Dissolved means that the solvent can diffuse into the polymer to provoke chain disentanglement so that each polymer chain can be arranged at a molecular level.

The choice of the solvent depends on the nature of the polymer. The most common polymer and solvent combinations used in the glove industry are represented in Table 3.2.

The dipping principles are different compared with latex dispersions: for example, as there is not any chemical pick-up (coagulation), the film build-up requires several superposed layers.

Interestingly, films obtained from the solution-dipping present the highest level of quality in terms of barrier integrity (less likelihood of microporosity and pinhole) and durability as compared with gloves made starting from a latex. The reason lies in the difference in "scale" at which the polymer chains are arranged: the film formation is controlled at the "molecular" level (nanometer size) and not at the "particle" level (micrometer size) as it is the case for films produced out of dispersions and coagulations. This results in a homogeneous film, as compared with "latex" that presents intrinsic micro-porosity. In addition, films obtained through "molecular" control are cleaner since the starting liquid is not dispersion and therefore does not contain surfactants or processing agents.

Figure 3.10 provides a comparison of the film-forming mechanisms between a latex dispersion (left: micron size scale) and a solution dipping technology (right: nano size scale).

TABLE 3.2
Common Solvents Used in
Solvent-Dipping Technology

Polymer	Recommended Solvents
IIR	Petroleum (aliphatics, aromatics)
EPDM	Petroleum (aliphatics, aromatics)
CSM	Petroleum (aromatics)
SBC	Petroleum (aliphatics, aromatics)
FKM	Ketones
TPU	DMF, DMSO

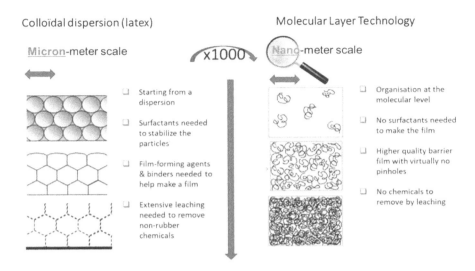

FIGURE 3.10   Film-forming comparison between latex and solution dipping technologies.

The compounding rules and manufacturing process principles are fundamentally different as compared with conventional vulcanized gloves made from latex.

1) Compounding is generally prepared in the factory starting from the various individual chemicals. Conventional additives can directly be incorporated into the solution without the need to use dispersions. Chemicals that are not soluble in the selected solvent need to be finely ground before use.
2) The system works in a close loop: all the solvent evaporated is recovered and used back in the compounding.
3) Only steam or hot inert gas is required to trap and recover the organic solvent.

A typical solution-dipping process is represented in Figure 3.11.

PVC gloves are manufactured in almost the same way. The polymer is solubilized in a significant amount of low volatile plasticizer in a masterbatch called "plasti-sol," which usually contains stabilizers, lubricants, and pigments. The plasticizer plays the role of a solvent. Other organic solvents such as aromatic hydrocarbons or ketones can be added.

a.   Solution Dipping Challenges and Limitations

As most solvents are classified as flammable, solution-dipping factories are significantly more complex to design and operate than latex-dipping, for which water dispersions are used. Also, due to the film pick-up mechanism, the "speed" of the dipping line conveyor chain cannot be as fast as for conventional latex technology, resulting in lower production yields.

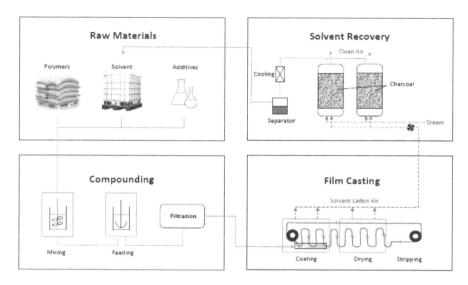

FIGURE 3.11   Solution-dipping process basic schematics.

The areas where flammable gases or vapors could be present shall be designed to properly control vapor concentrations outside explosive limits. A proper risk assessment should be performed to identify and properly assess each risk and put in place control measures. Explosion-proof equipment need to be used in environments where flammable vapors and gazes could be present in sufficient quantities to form explosive mixtures. Overall, the cost of acquisition of such equipment is higher than equipment for usage in a latex factory. Despite these limitations, there are currently several solution-dipping factories in operation, scaled for both niche or high-volume market applications.

Also, the technology suffered from the popular opinion that solvents are not environmentally friendly. This is not true: this belief probably comes by analogy with the paint industry, which progressively shifts from "solvent" to "latex" over the last 30 years. However, what is applicable for a paint (where the solvent is emitted in the open air, contributing to the generation of VOC) is not applicable for a glove where production can be performed in a fully enclosed system, allowing recycling of up to 95% of the overall solvent used in the process. In summary, when designed properly with a solvent recuperation system (SRS), solvent dipping could be a clean and green technology, probably more environment friendly than latex technology, which is a water-intensive process.

Table 3.3 summarizes the main manufacturing process currently used for each of the common elastomers used in the glove industry.

3.3.2   Supported Gloves

Supported gloves are based on natural or synthetic latex-coated fabric liners, which can be made of knitted cotton or woven fabrics of cotton, wool, or synthetic blends. In the manufacturing of this kind of gloves, the fabric-covered former is dipped into

TABLE 3.3

Survey of Natural and Synthetics Polymeric Materials Used for Protective Gloves, and Their Main Manufacturing Process

	International Abbreviation	Main Manufacturing Transformation Process
Natural rubber	NR	Latex (mainly), solution
Nitrile rubber	NBR and XNBR	Latex
Polychloroprene rubber	CR	Latex (mainly), solution
Synthetic polyisoprene	IR	Latex
Polyvinyl chloride	PVC	Solution (plastisol)
Butyl rubber	IIR	Solution[a] or injection molding
Chlorosulfonated polyethylene	CSM	Solution [a]
Ethylene propylene diene monomer	EPDM	Solution
Fluorocarbon elastomer	FKM	Solution
Styrenic block copolymer	SBC (SBS, SIS, SEBS)	Solution [a]
Polyvinyl alcohol	PVA	Solution
Polyethylene	PE	Other
Polyurethanes	TPU	Solution [a]
Silicone rubber	VMQ, LSR	Other

[a] Latex dispersions are commercially available, but now solution dipping remains the main transformation route for these polymers.

the coagulant solution and then into the latex mix, dried, and vulcanized. The rubber layer should penetrate only the outer part of the fabric and not through the complete fabric. There are two alternative methods of dipping fabric-lined gloves. In the first, the viscosity of the latex mix is increased so that fabric penetration is controlled on immersion. After the first straight dipping, the thickness of the polymer layer can be built up by additional dips. Another method without excessive penetration of the fabric is to use hot formers and a heat-sensitive latex mix. The former is fitted with the liner and heated to 60–80°C and then dipped into the latex mix. The heating of the former sets up a temperature gradient across the fabric, which allows the latex to penetrate only the surface before the heat causes the compound to gel. Natural latex or synthetic latex can be used separately or in blends for manufacturing-supported gloves for heavy-duty industrial applications. Partly dipped gloves where only the palms of the gloves are coated can also be made. Some supported gloves are also designed with higher levels of coating penetration. This is typically done to improve certain mechanical properties such as abrasion resistance.

3.3.3 Cut and Sewn Gloves

Gloves manufactured by sewing can be made of knitted fabric (cotton, nylon stretch, Kevlar®, and other synthetic blends, fiberglass, and metal yarn), woven fabric (cotton, synthetic blends), woven and/or knitted fabric impregnated with natural latex or synthetic latex, and leather (chromium or vegetable-tanned) and leather/woven fabric combinations. This kind of working gloves has a wide range of applications. Thin gloves of cotton or nylon stretch can be used as inner gloves to reduce discomfort due to hand sweating and to avoid the risk of rubber contact allergy. They are also commonly used to avoid soiling or light friction. Gloves made from cut-resistant materials are used in situations where sharp materials or tools are handled. Gloves for work in cold areas have extra thick linings or synthetic fur linings, and gloves for work with hot objects are made of fabrics from heat-resistant fibers. Gloves for heat and arc flash are composed of selected para-aramid fiber technology, anti-static yarns, and can also be coated with NBR or NBR/CR foam to provide additional flame resistance. Cut and sewn gloves are not suitable for contact with liquids.

3.3.4   Gloves Made by Punching and Welding

These gloves are made from two plastic polymer films (single-layered or laminates) punched out and welded simultaneously. They are manufactured in different sizes but with a flat shape (2D, not anatomical design in 3D); therefore, the fitness to the hand and the fingers is not comparable with gloves manufactured by the dipping procedure. The welded seams are usually the weak point of the glove, even if some of the polymer materials themselves have good strength and excellent resistance to hazardous chemicals. Laminated gloves containing, among PE, other thin layers made of polymers with a different polarity, such as polyamide or PVA, have been developed to provide gloves offering improved chemical resistance against a wide range of chemicals.[25]

3.3.5   Gloves Made by Molding

The injection molding process allows producing gloves without any solvent or liquid process. This technology commonly used in the dry rubber industry is barely used for gloves: injection molding of a thin-walled article with 3D hand design is a real industrial challenge.

However, this process allows transforming rubber-like IIR[26] and FKM for special application gloves. The injection molding process is not considered a seamless process like the solution-dipping process and does not allow high volume production or thin-walled articles.

3.4   CONCLUDING REMARKS

There are a large variety of rubbers but also thermoplastics or plastic materials that enter the composition of disposable gloves. The choice of the materials is a function of the desired properties of the glove.

Latex and solution dipping are the two main industrial processes used to produce thin-walled articles. Both techniques are complementary and offer advantages and disadvantages. Whereas the latex technology is very widely used, solution-dipping remains more exclusive, restricted today to polymeric materials that cannot be processed in latex (e.g., CSM, IIR, EPDM), or for gloves with high barrier quality requirements.

The *protective effect* of gloves is dependent on several factors:

- Material formulation, manufacturing process, and material thickness.
- Quality control of the product.
- Storage conditions (most gloves are susceptible to UV and oxidation).
- Exposure to chemical mixtures and/or sequential exposures.

The *side effects* on the skin when using protective gloves are well known, and the most common reasons are as follows:

- Occlusive effect causing increased hand sweating
- Several synthetic materials are available to address the type I allergy issues linked to NRL.
- Chemical accelerators remain an issue: while sulfur is "incorporated" within the tridimensional network of the vulcanized polymer, accelerators are not. Therefore, they remain as free components within the glove and as they are poorly soluble in water and are trapped within the film, a large portion remains in the glove even after extensive leaching. During glove storage, accelerators are susceptible to migrating to the surface in what is commonly called "blooming."
- Gloves produced starting from latex also contain some other chemical residues (surfactants, resins) initially used for particle stabilization. For example, exposure to rosin dehydroabietic acid present in CR gloves could be the origin of allergic contact dermatitis.[27]
- Antimicrobials in glove linings.
- Chromium in leather gloves.
- Irritating agents as glove powders (cornstarch or talc).

Latex-free gloves are now widely available. However, surgical gloves made of IR latex can contain high levels of accelerators and other extractable chemicals, which have been found to trigger type IV allergies.[28] Glove manufacturers have designed formulations with less harmful chemical accelerators or even without accelerators. For example, accelerator-free NBR examination gloves have been developed, thanks to ionic crosslinking, for example, with aluminum derivatives.[29] Accelerator-free synthetic surgical gloves have been developed using an innovative UV-curing technology in which the rubber is crosslinked, thanks to other chemical crosslinkers other than a conventional sulfur/accelerator system.[30,31] Finally, accelerator-free surgical gloves made of soft SBC that combine conventional physical crosslinking with some levels of chemical crosslinking are commercially available.[4] Peroxide crosslinking, which can be performed without the use of any chemical accelerators, might also find more interest in the future as a cleaner alternative to conventional vulcanization.

One of the major remaining issues with gloves, especially disposable gloves, is their end-life cycle, and overall, the environmental footprint and sustainability of this industry. Currently, the disposal of used gloves poses a complex and diffuse pollution risk. Considering that billions of disposable gloves are used, pollution involves tens of tons of waste in every single country every year. Only a fraction of those gloves are incinerated. For those, gloves made of NBR generate hydrogen cyanide, whereas PVC releases hydrochloric acid, which has to be captured. Various R&D programs are focused on the development of renewable polymers, biodegradable compositions, as well as reducing the use of energy and water during manufacturing. Gloves made from solvent dipping of block copolymer materials have the potential to be recycled by first cleaning and then re-dissolution in a solvent. This could prove to be a better solution than landfill biodegradation, which will still potentially creates greenhouse gases.

LIST OF ABBREVIATIONS

CR   Polychloroprene Rubber
CSM   Chlorosulfonated Rubber
DPG   Diphenylguanidine
EPDM   Ethylene-Propylene Diene Monomer
FKM, FPM   Fluoroelastomer
IIR   Butyl Rubber
IR   Polyisoprene Rubber
MBT   2, Mercaptobenzothiazole
NR   Natural Rubber
NBL   Natural Rubber Latex
NBR   Nitrile Butadiene Rubber
PA   Polyamide
PE   Polyethylene
PVA   Polyvinyl Alcohol
PVC   Polyvinyl Chloride
SBC   Styrenic Block Copolymers
TPU   Thermoplastic Polyurethane
VMQ   Silicone Rubber
XNBR   Carboxylated Nitrile Butadiene Rubber
ZDBC   Zinc Dibutyldithiocarbamate
ZDEC   Zinc Diethyldithiocarbamate
ZMBT   Zinc Salt of 2, Mercaptobenzothiazole

REFERENCES

1. U.S. FDA. 2008. *Guidance for Industry and FDA Staff.* Medical glove guidance manual. January 22, 2008. Washington, DC: U.S. Food and Drug Administration. Available at: https://www.fda.gov/media/90612/download.
2. Chauvaud, D. 2015. Preventing surgical site infections: Measures other than antibiotics. *Orthopaedics and Traumatology: Surgery & Research* 101:S77–S83.

3. Wrangsjö, K., Boman, A., and Liden, C., Meding, B. 2012. Primary prevention of latex allergy in healthcare–spectrum of strategies including the European glove standardization. *Contact Dermatitis* 66:165–171.

4. Finessis™ Surgical Glove Range. Available at: http://www.finessis.com.

5. Sonntag, P., Hoerner, P., Cheymol, A., Argy, G., Riess, G., and Reiter, G. 2004. Biocide squirting from an elastomeric tri-layer film. *Nature Materials* 3:311–315.

6. Assadian, O., Kramer, A., Ouriel, K., Suchomel, M., McLaws, M.L., Rottman, M., Leaper, D., and Assadian, A. 2014. Suppression of surgeons' bacterial hand flora during surgical procedures with a new antimicrobial glove. *Surgical Infections* 15(N1):43–49.

7. Ansell. *Microflex™ 93–260*. Ansell. Available at: https://www.ansell.com/us/en/products/microflex-93-260.

8. Rex. *ERISTA-BX Butyl Vitric*. Rex. Available at: http://www.rex-gummitechniken.de/en/chemical-protective-gloves/2/erista-bx-butyl-vitric.

9. Piercan. *BAG Y/PUR 7–10*. Piercan. Available at: https://piercan-en.piercan.fr/piercan-gloves/products.

10. IEST. 2013. *IEST-RP-CC005.4 Gloves and Fingercots Used in Cleanroom and Other Controlled Environments*. Schaumburg, IL: Institute of Environmental Sciences and Technology (IEST). Available at: https://www.iest.org/Standards-RPs/Recommended-Practices/IEST-RP-CC005.

11. Jacob, J.L., D'Auzac, J., and Prevôt, J.C. 1993. The composition of natural latex from Hevea brasiliensis. *Clinical Reviews Allergy* 11:325.

12. Cornish, K., Brichta, J.L., Yu, P., Wood, D.F., McGlothlin, M., and Martin, J.A. 2001. Guayule latex provides a solution for the critical demands of the non-allergenic medical products market. *AgroFOOD Industry Hi Tech* 12(6):27–31.

13. Krutzer, B., Ross, M., De Jong, W., Van Dijk, N., and Dik, L. 2013. A comparison of polyisoprene latex to natural rubber latex: Examples in the use of straight-dipped goods. Paper presented at the *Conference on Latex and Synthetic Polymer Dispersions*, Kuala Lumpur, 10–11 September 2013.

14. Treilhes, S., Hoerner, P., and Low, C.G. 2018. *Crosslinked Styrenic Block Copolymers*. Patent WO 2018/224881A1.

15. Kung, A., Krutzer, B., Ling, C.S., Van Dijk, N., and De Jong, W. 2018. Styrene modified synthetic polyisoprene latex for skin friendly latex products. Paper presented at the *9th International Rubber Glove Conference and Exhibition*, Kuala Lumpur, 4–6 September 2018.

16. Suzuki, H., Hui, K.S., and Weiser, M.S. 2018. Water-based polyurethane dispersions for dipping applications. Paper presented at the *9th International Rubber Glove Conference and Exhibition*, Kuala Lumpur, 4–6 September 2018.

17. U.S. FDA. 2016. *Banned Devices; Powdered Surgeon's Gloves, Powdered Patient Examination Gloves and Absorbable Powder for Lubricating a Surgeon's Glove*. Docket No. FDA-2015-N-5017. Washington, DC: U.S. Food and Drug Administration. Available at: https://www.fda.gov/media/102056/download.

18. Ansell – Our History. Available at: www.ansell.com.

19. Hill, D.M. 2019. *Latex Dipping: Science and Technology*, 2nd edition. Berlin: De Gruyter.

20. Keddie, J.L., and Routh, A.F. 2010. An introduction to latex and the principles of colloidal stability, in *Fundamentals of Latex Film Formation*, Keddie, J.L., and Routh, A.F., Eds. Dordrecht: Springer, pp. 1–26.

21. Steward, P.A., Hearn, J., and Wilkinson, M.C. 2000. An overview of polymer latex film formation and properties. *Advances in Colloid and Interface Science* 86:195–267.

22. Subramaniam, A. 1992. Reduction of extractable protein content in latex products, in *Sensitivity to Latex in Medical Devices, Proceedings from International Latex Conference*, Baltimore, MD, November, U.S. Food and Drug Administration, 63.

23. Hentz, R.V., Traina, J.C., Cadossi, R., Zucchini, P., Muglia, M.A., and Giordani, M. 2000. The protective efficacy of surgical latex gloves against the risk of skin contamination: How well are the operators protected? *Journal of Materials Science: Materials in Medicine* 12:825–832.

24. Siemann, U. 2005. Solvent cast technology – A versatile tool for thin film production. *Progress in Colloid and Polymer Science* 130:1–4.

25. Ansell. *Alphatec™ 02–100*. Available at: https://www.ansell.com/us/en/products/alphatec-02-100.

26. Honeywell Safety. *Butoject™ 898*. KCL/Honeywell. Available at: https://www.honeywellsafety.com/SKU.

27. Siegel, P.D., Law, B.F., Fowler Jr, J.F., and Fowler, L.M. 2010. Disproportionated rosin dehydroabietic acid in neoprene surgical gloves. *Dermatitis* 21(3):157–159.

28. Baeck, M., Cawet, B., Tennstedt, B., and Goossens, A. 2012. Allergic contact dermatitis caused by latex (natural rubber) free gloves in healthcare workers. *Contact Dermatitis* 68:54–64.

29. Laskowska, A., Zaborski, M., Boiteux, G., Gain, O., Marzec, A., and Maniukiewicz, W. 2014. Ionic elastomers based on carboxylated nitrile rubber (xnbr) and magnesium aluminum layered double hydroxide. *eXPRESS Polymer Letters* 8(6):374–386.

30. Schaller, R., Holzner, A., Ehrenfeldner, R., Hoechtl, M., Kern, W., Stelzer, F., and Temel, A. 2005. *Method for Producing Crosslinked Elastomer*. Patent US 9279038B2.

31. Crepy, M.N., Lecuen, J., Ratour-Bigot, C., Stocks, J., and Bensefa-Colas, L. 2017. Accelerator-free gloves as alternatives in cases of glove allergy in healthcare workers. *Contact Dermatitis* 78(1):28–32.

32. OEHHA. 2021. *California Prop65: Chemicals (MBT Classified as Cancer-Causing Agent)*. California Office of Environmental Health Hazard Assessment (OEHHA), California Environmental Protection Agency. Available at: http://www.oehha.ca.gov.

4 Extraction and Chemistry of Rubber Allergens

Paul D. Siegel

CONTENTS

Disclaimer: "The findings and conclusions in this report are those of the author and do not necessarily represent the official position of the National Institute for Occupational Safety and Health, Centers for Disease Control and Prevention (NIOSH/CDC). Mention of any company or product does not constitute endorsement by NIOSH/CDC."

4.1 INTRODUCTION

Personal protective gloves are made of natural rubber latex (NRL) or a variety of synthetic rubbers, including styrene-butadiene rubber (SBR), acrylonitrile-butadiene rubber (NBR), butyl rubber (IIR), ethylene propylene diene monomer rubber (EPDM), and polychloroprene rubber (neoprene, CR). NRL can be obtained from several different plants, but the major commercial source is the Pará rubber tree (*Hevea brasiliensis*). These trees are tapped to obtain the latex (isoprene) containing exudate. Notable alternate sources of NRL include the Guayule shrub (*Parthenium argentatum*), goldenrod, and the Russian dandelion (*Taraxacum koksaghyz*), as the latex products produced from these plant extracts have similar properties to that from the Pará rubber tree.[1] *Hevea brasiliensis* proteins, when contacted or inhaled are known to cause allergy and anaphylaxis. Guayule rubber is considered

DOI: 10.1201/9781003126874-5

hypoallergenic as it doesn't contain the same proteins noted in *Hevea brasiliensis* that elicit severe allergic reactions.[2]

Both synthetic and natural latexes, also known as elastomers, are colloidal suspensions of polymeric materials in aqueous systems that require vulcanization to produce rubber gloves. Vulcanization is the process where the rubber molecules are polymerized through cross-linking by sulfur to increase tear and tensile strength, stretch ability, and other desired physical properties. CR vulcanization uses metal oxides such as MgO and ZnO. Sulfur vulcanization of latex is a necessary step in the production of NRL, IIR, NBR, EPDM, and SBR gloves. For sulfur crosslinking to occur, the rubber elastomers must have $C=C$ bonds which require modification of EDPM and IIR to be amenable to sulfur vulcanization. The use of sulfur alone produces very slow vulcanization that requires high temperatures resulting in a product that is prone to oxidative degradation and has poor physical properties. The use of chemical accelerators allows for lower vulcanization temperatures and increases vulcanization efficiency. The type of accelerator(s) used is dependent on the type of rubber and desired product properties. Many of these accelerators are known to cause contact allergies.

The purpose of this chapter is to review analytical chemical and immunochemical methods to assess latex allergenic protein and chemical rubber additive hapten content of rubber gloves. In addition, the chemical mechanisms of vulcanization accelerators that lead to contact sensitization will be discussed.

4.2 LATEX PROTEIN ALLERGENS

Multiple latex proteins are allergenic and cause IgE-mediated Type 1, immediate hypersensitivity reactions. Fifteen allergens that have been identified from *Hevea brasiliensis* NRL are included in the World Health Organization and International Union of Immunological Societies (WHO/IUIS) Allergen Nomenclature database (http://www.allergen.org). Hev b 6 includes both pro- and mature hevein, which are denoted as Hev b 6.01 and 6.02, respectively. The named antigenic latex proteins are listed in Table 4.1. The reactivity profile of IgE from rubber-allergic healthcare workers (HCW) has been reported to be different than that of spina bifida (SB) patients who undergo multiple surgeries and have repeated latex exposures.[3–6] The major allergens recognized by IgE from HCW with glove-related latex allergy are Hev b 5 and Hev b 6.01 or Hev b 6.02, while in SBP, Hev b 1 and Hev b 3 are the major allergens recognized by SB IgE. Others have reported that Hev b 1 is a major allergen in both HCW and SB.[7]

During the powdered latex glove manufacturing process latex proteins can become concentrated onto the powder and become aerosolized, especially when gloves are removed, creating an inhalation hazard. Manufacturers have altered their manufacturing process by adding a chlorination step to provide low-protein content powderless gloves. The chlorination hardens the inner glove surface of the natural or synthetic rubber, making it smooth and allowing for easy donning without the need for powder. It also reduces extractable proteins from the glove surface.[8,9] The public health response to the latex allergy epidemic that arose in the 1980s has been very successful with a drastic reduction in the occurrence of latex protein allergy in the population.[10,11] Analytical immunochemical assays developed to measure latex

TABLE 4.1
Natural Rubber Latex Allergens

Allergen	Protein Name/Description	Molecular Weight (kD)
Hev b 1	Rubber elongation factor	14.6
Hev b 2	Beta-1,3-glucanase	35, 36.5, and 38
Hev b 3	Small rubber particle protein/prenyltransferase	24
Hev b 4	GDSL lipase/esterase family member/ Microhelix	53–55
Hev b 5	Acidic protein	16
Hev b 6.01	Prohevein	20
Hev b 6.02	Mature Hevein protein	4.7
Hev b 7	Patatin homologue	42
Hev b 8	Hevea profilin	15
Hev b 9	Hevea enolase	51
Hev b 10	Manganese superoxide dismutase	26
Hev b 11	Class I Chitinase	30
Hev b 12	Non-specific lipid transfer protein type 1	9
Hev b 13	Esterase	42
Hev b 14	Hevamine	30
Hev b 15	Serine protease inhibitor	7.5

Adapted from World Health Organization and International Union of Immunological Societies (WHO/IUIS) Allergen Nomenclature database (http://www.allergen.org)

allergens from gloves,[12,13] and aerosolizable glove powder[14] played a central role in reducing NRL allergy.

4.2.1 STANDARDIZED TEST FOR ASSESSING RESIDUAL NRL PROTEIN AND ANTIGEN CONTENT

Multiple standardized assays have been developed and subsequently adopted by organizations such as ASTM International. ASTM International adopted assay methods to measure (1) total protein, (2) extractable total antigenic Hev b protein, and (3) specific Hev b proteins. All three methods use the same NRL extraction procedure which allows for multiple analyses on the same extract. Initially, a section of a glove is cut, weighed, and surface area determined. The entire glove is cut into small pieces and suspended in phosphate-buffered saline (PBS) at 5–10 mL/g glove in a polypropylene tube. Extraction is conducted at 25°C for 120 min with either intermittent or constant shaking. Extracts can be filtered or centrifuged to remove insoluble material/particulates.

4.2.1.1 Total Extractable Protein; ASTM D 5712

The ASTM D 5712 titled "Standard Test Method for Analysis of Aqueous Extractable Protein in Latex, Natural Rubber and Elastomeric Products Using the Modified

Lowry Method" was one of the earliest methods standardized during the latex allergy epidemic to assess protein content of exam and surgical NRL gloves.[12] Total aqueous extractable protein by the modified Lowry spectrophotometric assay correlates well, quantitatively, with skin prick test reactivity, but is limited by its high limits of detection (LOD) and quantification, (LOQ).[13] Although ASTM D 5712 contains an acid precipitation step to concentrate the proteins and remove interferences, the LOD and LOQ are 4.7 and 14.1 µg/mL, respectively. This standard method also contains an appendix detailing a high-performance liquid chromatographic (HPLC) method with fluorescence detection for amino acid analysis of proteins for determination of total protein levels in latex gloves or for validation of other protein quantification methods. This HPLC method is based on a study by Schegg et al.[15]

4.2.1.2   Total Antigenic Hev b Protein; ASTM D 6499

The ASTM D 6499 titled "Standard Test Method for Immunological Measurement of Antigenic Protein in Hevea Natural Rubber (HNR) and its Products" employs an inhibition Enzyme-Linked ImmunoSorbent Assay (ELISA) which uses a rabbit polyclonal antiserum that reacts with NRL proteins. The NRL extracts and a reference standard NRL antigen are mixed with the antisera in a serial dilution 96 well plate. The extract/antibody mixture is then transferred to an ELISA plate containing immobilized standard NRL antigen. After an incubation period, the ELISA plate is washed, and a secondary horseradish peroxidase-conjugated anti-rabbit IgG is added. Following incubation and washing, hydrogen peroxide and an o-phenylenediamine substrate are added. After a development period, the enzymatic reaction is stopped, and the absorbance of wells containing the glove extracts and latex protein standards are read at 490 nm. The absorbance reading is inversely related to the protein antigen content of the NRL glove extract. An indirect Hev b antigen ELISA (LEAP assay) that uses the same rabbit anti-Hev b polyclonal antibodies and latex antigen standard as the ASTM method has been reported to correlate well (r = 0.89) with ASTM D 6449.[16]

More recently, a standard method (ASTM D 8238) for extractable guayule natural rubber (GNR) proteins was developed and it is a competitive ELISA that uses rabbit polyclonal anti-GNR IgGs for measurement of GNR protein antigens in GNR gloves. GNR-specific IgG has been reported in workers involved in GNR production; however, no GNR specific-IgE or GNR-related allergic reactions were found.[17]

4.2.1.3   Hev b Allergens; ASTM D 7427

Measures of antigenic latex protein should not be considered equivalent to measures of allergenic protein. The pattern of IgE reactivity toward Hev b proteins varies considerably between latex allergic individuals. Use of IgE from pooled sera taken from latex allergic individuals has been used to measure the allergen content of latex products, but standardization across lots of pooled sera remains a problem. Alternatively, the ASTM D 7427 method uses monoclonal antibodies to quantify 4 Hev b proteins identified as allergens, in two-site, noncompetitive binding immunoenzymetric assays (IEMAs; also known as sandwich ELISAs). The specific Hev b allergens assayed by independent IEMAs are Hev b 1, 3, 5, and 6.02. An Hev b 1, 3,

5, or 6.02 specific monoclonal antibody (mAb) is bound to wells of a 96 well ELISA plate. After blocking nonspecific binding, the glove extracts and respective recombinant Hev b allergen standard are added to the wells and incubated to allow for mAb binding to the allergen. Following an incubation period, the wells are washed, and a second peroxidase bound mAb that recognizes a different epitope on the respective Hev b allergen is added to form the sandwich. Following washing and addition of the peroxidase substrate, 2,2'-azino-di[3-ethylbenzthiazoline sulfonic acid] (ABTS), the color developed is measured spectrophotometrically. The assay optical density is directly proportional to the level of the specific Hev b protein content of the glove extract. The four ASTM D 7427 IEMAs are also available commercially in kit formats (Fitkit®, Icosagen, San Francisco, CA). The sum of the four Hev b allergens is considered an indicator of the glove releasable allergen content. The lowest standards used for quantification are 10 µg/L for the Hev b 1 and 3, and 5 µg/L for Hev b 5 and 6.02.

4.3 RUBBER ACCELERATOR/CHEMICAL CONTACT ALLERGEN ANALYSES

The most common rubber accelerator classes reported causing rubber glove-associated allergic contact dermatitis (ACD) are the thiurams, dialkyldithocarbamates, and benzothiazoles.[18,25] Rubber glove ACD is far more common than the IgE-mediated allergic responses discussed above. More recently, 1,3-Diphenylguanidine (DPG),[19,22] and triphenylguanidine[26] have been reported to be a common cause of synthetic rubber glove-associated ACD. Dialkyl thiourea has been reported to be a major allergen in chloroprene (neoprene) glove ACD.[25,27,28] Table 4.2 lists the rubber accelerators associated with glove contact allergy by chemical analyses and/or patch testing.

Although thiurams are commonly identified by patch testing in cases of rubber glove ACD, residual, extractable thiurams are rarely identified by chemical analyses of rubber gloves. This, in part, may be explained by chemical changes that occur during the rubber vulcanization process. During thiuram-accelerated sulfur vulcanization, tetramethylthiuram disulfide (TMTD) undergoes multiple chemical reactions.[29,30] It will form thiuram polysulfides that react with the rubber polymer forming a side chain (pendant group) on that polymer and this pendant group further reacts with rubber to crosslink polymers. TMTD is also converted to dimethyldithiocarbamic acid (DADCA). DADCA is unstable and decomposes to dimethylamine (DMA) and carbon disulfide. In the presence of ZnO, DADCA reacts further to form zinc dimethydithiocarbamate (ZDMC) and water. In the absence of ZnO, DMA reacts rapidly with and destroys TMTD and pendant groups. Figure 4.1 outlines the various chemical reactions noted above for TMTD-accelerated vulcanization. Bergendorff et al.[31] examined the accelerator chemical content before and after vulcanization of different rubbers. They observed the reduction of TMTD to ZDMC and also the formation of a mixed disulfide in the vulcanized rubber when 2-mercaptobenzothiazole (MBT) and TMTD were together in the process. While these chemical reactions and products have been demonstrated using TMTD, it is reasonable to assume that the same processes hold for other thiuram disulfides.

TABLE 4.2
Rubber Accelerators and Chemical Structures

Rubber Accelerator	Chemical Structure

Thiurams

Tetramethylthiuram
  monosulfide
(TMTM)

Tetramethylthiuram
disulfide
(TMTD)

Tetraethylthiuram
Disulfide
(TETD)

Zinc Dialkyldithiocarbamates
Zinc
Dimethyldithiocarbamate
(ZDMC)

Zinc
Diethyldithiocarbamate
(ZDEC)

(Continued)

TABLE 4.2 (CONTINUED)
Rubber Accelerators and Chemical Structures

Rubber Accelerator	Chemical Structure
Zinc Dibutyldithiocarbamate (ZDBC)	
Zinc Pentamethylenedithio-carbamate (ZPC)	
Benzothiazoles 2-Mercaptobenzothiazole (MBT)	
2-2'-Dithiobisbenzothiazole Disulfide (MBTS)	
Zinc Mercaptobenzothiazole (ZnMBT)	
Dialkylureas	

(Continued)

TABLE 4.2 (CONTINUED)

Rubber Accelerators and Chemical Structures

Rubber Accelerator	Chemical Structure
Diethylthiourea (DETU)	
Dibutylthiourea (DBTU)	
Diphenylthiourea (DPTU)	
Guanidines 1,3-Diphenylguanidine (DPG)	
1,2,3-Triphenylguanidine (TPG)	

Similarly, during thiazole accelerated vulcanization 2-2'-dithiobisbenzothiazole disulfide (MBTS) is reduced to MBT during the formation of the thiazole pendant group on a rubber polymer. Two MBT molecules can react forming additional MBTS molecules. Sulfenamide accelerators will also form MBT and MBTS during the vulcanization process.[29] Thus, due to the multitude of accelerator chemical reactions that occur during the production of rubber products, the residual accelerator(s)

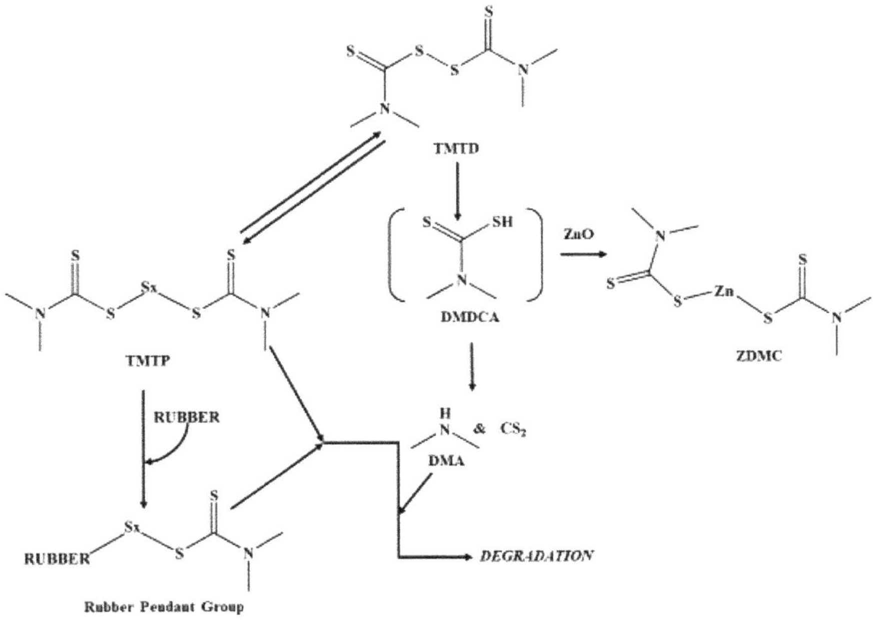

FIGURE 4.1 Pathways demonstrating ZnO requirement for TMTD rubber vulcanization.

found in rubber gloves may be different from that added and declared by the glove manufacturer.

Identification and quantification of rubber glove accelerator levels are technically challenging but may be important in establishing the clinical relevance of a patch test finding, product labeling accuracy, and evaluating trends in glove contact allergy. Chemical analyses include methods of extraction of rubber gloves, spot and screening tests, and quantitative chromatographic analyses.

4.3.1 Glove Accelerator Extraction and Spot Test

Several of the sulfur rubber accelerator spot and screening tests take advantage of zinc dialkyldithiocarbamates (ZDTC) metal reactivity. Two spot tests protocols for accelerator identification are detailed in *The Vanderbilt Latex Handbook*,[32] although a rubber extraction procedure was not described. One spot test uses a cobalt oleate reagent. The cobalt (Co) oleate reagent is made by heating cobalt carbonate in oleic acid to approximately 280°C with dilution in toluene after cooling. Milligram quantities of the accelerator are dissolved in a drop or two of toluene, and a drop of the cobalt oleate reagent is added. Dialkyldithiocarbamates (DTCs) produce a dark yellow-green color, MBT a pale green color, and thioureas a lavender to purple color. The disulfides, thiurams, and MBTS must first be reduced using zinc and dilute hydrochloric acid before the addition of the cobalt oleate reagent to produce a yellow-green or pale green color, respectively. Another method described in *The*

Vanderbilt Latex Handbook uses an aqueous copper solution and concentrated aqueous ammonia to detect DTCs by the formation of a dark brown precipitate.

4.3.2 GLOVE ACCELERATOR QUANTITATIVE ANALYSIS METHODS

Several solvents for the extraction of sulfur accelerators from rubber gloves for chemical analyses have been reported in the literature. These include a 1:1 mixture of acetone:chloroform,[23] acetone,[33] and acetonitrile.[34,24] Hansson et al.[35] recommend the use of methyl butyl ether after determining that acetone can react with mercaptobenzothiazole compounds, causing the formation of new chemical species. It is recommended to use high-grade solvents and metal-free extraction vessels such as polypropylene tubes to avoid transmetalation reactions with ZDTCs.

The ASTM D 7558-09,[36] entitled "Colorimetric/spectrophotometric procedure to quantify extractable chemical ZDTCs, thiurams, and MBT accelerators in NRL and nitrile gloves," describes a simple method adapted from Depree et al.[34,37] to quantify total extractable accelerator levels of three of the most common contact allergen classes in rubber gloves. The assay uses cobalt (Co) to react with ZDTCs and thiurams-producing reaction products that absorb at 320 nm, and producing a shift in the Co-acetonitrile (ACN) solution from blue to green. MBT does not react directly with Co, but is still detected as it has a high molar absorbance at 320 nm. This assay will not identify the specific accelerators; however, it can indicate the accelerator classes present. ZDTCs react rapidly with Co at room temperature, forming stable CoDTCs, while thiurams react very slowly. The glove extract Co reaction mixture is heated to 50°C to drive the reaction of Co with thiurams in this assay. MBT, as stated previously, will absorb at 320 nm in the absence of Co. In addition, CoDTCs, but not MBT, absorb at 370 nm. Zinc dibutyldithiocarbamate (ZDBC) is used as the standard in this assay with a LOD of 15.8 µg/mL.

Several chromatographic methods have been reported in the literature to identify and measure specific allergenic sulfur accelerators from rubber gloves. The extreme metal reactivity of ZDTCs makes it challenging to quantify this class of chemicals as they can react with nickel from stainless steel in the chromatographic instrument's sample path. Kaniwa et al.[38] reported a series of analytical procedures to measure amine, thiuram, "MBT-type" (MBT, MBTS, N-cyclohexyl-2- benzothiazole sulfenamide, morpholinyl-mercaptobenzothiazole), and DTC accelerators from rubber gloves. Glove acetone/chloroform extracts were either evaporated to dryness and reconstituted in dichloromethane for sulfur accelerator analysis or partitioned into 5% HCl for amine analysis by a gas chromatographic (GC) equipped with a nitrogen-phosphorous detector. Thiurams and "MBT-type" accelerators were assayed directly by reversed-phase (RP)-HPLC-UV at 245 and 275 nm. MBT was also assessed by RP-HPLC (UV 275 nm) following methylation. DTCs were reacted with $CoCl_2$ and the resultant CoDTCs were assayed by RT-HPLC (UV 320 nm). Gloves associated with glove ACD were assayed and although thiurams were consistently patch-test positive in the subjects of this study, ZDTCs and amines, but not thiurams, were detected in their gloves. It is common to find multiple ZDTCs in rubber gloves and a drawback to this method is that with multiple ZDTC (differing side chains;

ex. methyl, ethyl, butyl, etc.) containing glove extracts mixed CoDTC species are formed making quantification of the specific ZDTC species difficult.

Single-use medical gloves were surveyed for allergenic rubber accelerators by Knudsen et al.[39] Gloves were extracted with acetone and extracts were evaporated to dryness and reconstituted in chloroform. Extracts were screened qualitatively using high-performance thin-layer chromatography (HPTLC) by developing the plates with dithizone and then with 2,6-Dichloroquinone-4-chlorimide for identification of carbamates, thiurams, and MBT. The accelerator detection limit was approximately 100–200 μg/g of the glove. Extracts were acylated using trifluoroacetic anhydride and analyzed on a GC equipped with a flame ionization detector (GC-FID), and chemical identification was confirmed using a GC-mass spectrometer (GC-MS). The reported limits of detection were between 10 and 20 μg/g of the glove. HPTLC can distinguish between thiurams and their corresponding carbamates, but the GC methods cannot distinguish between these compounds because of the derivatization procedure. Multiple types of accelerators were reported to be present in the gloves, with ZDEC, ZDBC, and zinc MBT (ZMBT) being the most prevalent.

The problem of ZDTC reacting with metal components of a chromatography system can be potentially overcome by using an instrument in which the entire sample flow path, including the injection loop, all tubing, and the analytical column, has been lined with polyether ether ketone (PEEK).[33,40] Using a PEEK-lined HPLC, ZDTCs and MBT were monitored at 280 and 325 nm, respectively. Zinc sulfate was added to the mobile phase to compete with any free residual metals for binding to ZDTCs. Bergendorff et al.[33] reported the presence of ZDEC, zinc pentamethylenedithiocarbamate (ZPD), ZDBC, and MBT from latex and nitrile glove acetone extracts. Several of these gloves contained multiple accelerators. The ZDEC detection limit was reported to be 1 μg/mL. No thiurams were found in any of the 19 gloves analyzed.

Depree et al.[34] used the aforementioned cobalt screening method and an HPLC-UV method modified from their previous study of DTCs in condoms,[37] to survey 38 brands of "off-the-shelf" latex and nitrile exam gloves. This method allows for analyses of ZDTCs on a standard, non-PEEK-lined HPLC system, and aliquots of the same ACN glove extracts can be used for both screening and HPLC-UV analyses. A saturated solution of dimethyldithiocarbamate (ZDMC) in ACN was injected to condition the HPLC sample flow path by binding nickel to prevent loss of other DTCs. ZDMC was added to the sample extracts to help maintain the conditioning. DTCs were quantified by their absorbance at 260 nm and MBT at 320 nm. ZDMC was not added to extracts for MBT analyses. It was determined that ZDMC was not present in the extracts by assaying extracts in which ZDMC was not added to the extract and with ZDEC being used as the HPLC conditioning agent. Only ZDEC, ZDBC, and MBT were found in these gloves. Thiurams were not found in any of the glove extracts. Accelerator content was found to be lower in powder-free vs. powdered gloves. In this study, visible chromatographic peaks ≥ the low standards of 31.3 μg/mL for ZDTCs and 0.24 μg/mL for MBT were quantified. ZDEC and ZDBC detection limits were reported to be 5 and 10 μg/mL, respectively.

1,3-Diphenylguanidine has also been reported to be a common cause of rubber glove-associated ACD.[19,22,41] Pontén et al.[42] reported that DPG, thiuram, and cetylpyridinium chloride (CPC, a cationic quaternary ammonium antimicrobial compound) positive patch tests were prevalent in their rubber glove ACD patients. Glove pieces were extracted in a solvent mixture consisting of 20% ACN, 10% methanol, and 70% 50 mM, pH 5 sodium acetate buffer and analyzed for DPG and CPC using HPLC-UV (254 nm detection) with a cyano column. Limits of detection for DPG and CPC were 0.5 and 10 µg/mL, respectively. Thiurams, ZDTCs, MBT, and MBTS were analyzed by the method of Bergendorff et al.[33] in this study. DPG, CPC, MBT, MBTS, ZDEC, and ZPD were found observed in 3/5, 5/5, 4/5, 2/5, 2/5, and 2/5 of the gloves, respectively.

Neoprene (polychloroisoprene, polychloroprene) is another type of rubber used for making gloves that can cause ACD. A variety of accelerators and additives have been reported to be used in the production of neoprene rubber products, including DTCs and thioureas. Warshaw et al.[28] reported in a retrospective cross-sectional data study that gloves were the most common source of dialkylthioureas in cases of occupational ACD. Ramzy et al.[43] heated chloroprene material in vials at 37°C and extracted the headspace vapor using solid phase microextraction Carboxen-PDMS fibers. The fibers were desorbed in the GC/MS injection port. Diethylthiourea (DETU), dibutylthiourea (DBTU), diphenylthiourea (DPTU), and their respective isothiocyanate breakdown products were assessed. Multiple neoprene products were assayed, but only one single diving sports glove was included in this study. It was concluded that DETU and ethylisocyanate were commonly found in chloroprene materials. In another study, DETU, DBTU, and ethylbutylthiourea were found in an acetone extract of a knee brace used by a thiourea patch-test positive gardener by the previously described HPLC ZDTC method.[40] Even though neoprene surgical and exam gloves are commercially available, residual thioureas in these gloves have not been measured. Siegel et al.[44] extracted four different surgical and exam neoprene gloves using dichloromethane and found dehydroabietic (DHA, colophony) in all four gloves, but not a control polyisoprene surgical glove. Extracts were injected directly into a GC-MS for chemical identification and then quantified by GC-MS following derivatization with N-methyl-N-(trimethylsilyl)trifluoroacetamide and 1% trimethylchlorosilane. DHA is a known prohapten that can cause ACD, but its clinical relevance in neoprene glove ACD has not been established.

4.4   GLOVE ACCELERATOR CHEMICAL MECHANISMS OF ACD

Allergenic rubber accelerators lack sufficient volume and must bind covalently (haptenize) to a protein to cause immune sensitization. Both human and latex proteins may be subject to haptenation, although latex protein haptenation has not been studied. Only a few studies have examined potential rubber glove accelerator chemical reactions that result in protein haptenation, which can lead to dermal sensitization.[45,47] Wang and Tabor studied the reactivity of MBT and related sulfonamides.[48] They reported that MBT can react directly with amino acid carboxyl groups forming thioester bonds, and with amines and the thiol group of cysteine (CYS). Reaction products were identified by the appearance of new spots on TLC plates and spectrophotometric shifts. The actual molecular structures of these reaction products were not elucidated. Based on this study, potential skin penetration, the ability of glutathione (GSH) to reduce MBTS to MBT, and the abundance of GSH in the skin, Hansson et al.[35] suggested that MBT was the main ultimate hapten.

The direct reactivity of MBT with thiol, amine, and carboxyl groups could not be confirmed in subsequent studies by Chipinda et al.[45,47] MBT did not directly react with amino acids or albumin under physiological conditions. MBTS was formed in rubber glove material containing MBT when incubated with either hypochlorous acid, iodine, or hydrogen peroxide; oxidizing agents commonly encountered in the healthcare setting. It was demonstrated that MBTS reacts with the free thiol group of CYS and also can form a mixed disulfide product with CYS34 on bovine serum albumin. Metabolism of MBT or MBTS by isoniazid and dexamethasone-induced rat liver microsomes was not observed. These data support the conclusion that a pre-dominant haptenation mechanism may be through the formation of mixed disulfides with the proteins following oxidization of MBT to MBTS. The central role of the MBT thiol group was confirmed in a chemical structural-allergy activity study conducted using the Guinea Pig Maximization Test (GMPT) in which guinea pigs were sensitized to MBT, and then challenged with MBT, MBTS, and analogs where the -SH group was removed, blocked, or substituted with -OH. MBT sensitized guinea pigs reacted to MBT and MBTS, but not any of the analogs. MBT and MBTS also inhibited both glutathione and thioredoxin reductases that may contribute to the sta-bility of MBT mixed protein disulfides.

Similar to MBT, ZDEC can be oxidized by agents commonly used for disinfec-tion in the healthcare setting to a disulfide (TETD). TETD can form a mixed disul-fide through reaction with free thiol groups on proteins.[46] In addition, ZDEC was demonstrated to directly chelate the active center copper ion of superoxide dismutase (SOD). Transmetalation of ZDEC using cobalt formed the stable CoDEC that was not subject to oxidation to a disulfide and did not chelate SOD copper. ZDEC, TETD, sodium DEC, and another ZEDC oxidation product, tetraethyldicarbamoyl disulfide, but not CoDEC, were positive in the murine local lymph node allergic sensitization assay. Thus, it was demonstrated that ZDEC could act as a prehapten through oxida-tion to disulfides and directly as a hapten through metalloprotein chelation.

4.5   CONCLUSION

Standardized analytical assays are available for measurement of latex protein, anti-gens, and allergens from gloves and their use contributed to the reduction of cases of Type I glove-associated allergic reactions. Chemical analyses to extract, identify, and quantify residual chemical additives from rubber gloves are both complex and instrument intensive and while accelerator-free rubber gloves are available, Type IV rubber glove allergy remains a problem. Contact allergen patch testing of rubber glove allergens suggests that residual thiuram allergy is still prevalent, although chemical analyses of gloves for thiurams are usually negative. This in part can be explained by reduction of thiurams to ZDTCs and formation of other mixed disul-fides during the vulcanization process, cross-reactivity with ZDTCs, and potential for oxidation of ZDTCs back to thiurams during glove use.

REFERENCES

1. van Beilen, J.B., and Poirier, Y. 2007. Guayule and Russian dandelion as alternative sources of natural rubber. *Crit Rev Biotechnol* 27(4):217–31.
2. Siler, D.J., Cornish, K., and Hamilton, R.G. 1996. Absence of cross-reactivity of IgE antibodies from subjects allergic to *Hevea brasiliensis* latex with a new source of natural rubber latex from guayule (*Parthenium argentatum*). *J Allergy Clin Immunol* 98(5 Pt 1):895–902.
3. Peixinho, C.M., Tavares-Ratado, P., Gabriel, M.F., Romeira, A.M., Lozoya-Ibanez, C., Taborda-Barata, L., and Tomaz, C.T. 2012. Different in vivo reactivity profile in health care workers and patients with spina bifida to internal and external latex glove surface-derived allergen extracts. *Br J Dermatol* 166(3):518–24.
4. Raulf-Heimsoth, M., Rihs, H.-P., Rozynek, P., Cremer, R., Gaspar, A., Pires, G., Yeang, H.Y., Arif, S.A., Hamilton, R.G., Sander, I., Lundberg, M., and Brüning, T. 2007. Quantitative analysis of immunoglobulin E reactivity profiles in patients allergic or sensitized to natural rubber latex (*Hevea brasiliensis*). *Clin Exp Allergy* 37(11):1657–67.
5. Yeang, H.Y., Cheong, K.F., Sunderasan, E., Hamzah, S., Chew, N.P., Hamid, S., Hamilton, R.G., and Cardosa, M.J. 1996. The 14.6 kd rubber elongation factor (Hev b 1) and 24 kd (Hev b 3) rubber particle proteins are recognized by IgE from patients with spina bifida and latex allergy. *J Allergy Clin Immunol* 98(3):628–39.
6. Beezhold, D.H., Sussman, G.L., Kostyal, D.A., and Chang, N.S. 1994. Identification of a 46-kD latex protein allergen in health care workers. *Clin Exp Immunol* 98(3):408–13.
7. Chen, Z., Cremer, R., Posch, A., Raulf-Heimsoth, M., Rihs, H.P., and Baur, X. 1997. On the allergenicity of Hev b 1 among health care workers and patients with spina bifida allergic to natural rubber latex. *J Allergy Clin Immunol* 100(5):684–93.
8. Beezhold, D., Pugh, B., Liss, G., and Sussman, G. 1996. Correlation of protein levels with skin prick test reactions in patients allergic to latex. *J Allergy Clin Immunol* 98(6, Part 1):1097–102.
9. Perrella, F.W., and Gaspari, A.A. 2002. Natural rubber latex protein reduction with an emphasis on enzyme treatment. *Methods* 27(1):77–86.
10. Kelly, K.J., and Sussman, G. 2017. Latex allergy: Where are we now and how did we get there? *J Allergy Clin Immunol Pract* 5(5):1212–6.
11. Meade, B.J., Weissman, D.N., and Beezhold, D.H. 2002. Latex allergy: Past and present. *Int Immunopharmacol* 2(2–3):225–38.
12. ASTM International. 1995. *ASTM D5712: Standard Test Method for Analysis of Protein in Natural Rubber and its Products.* West Conshohocken, PA: ASTM International.
13. Beezhold, D., Pugh, B., Liss, G., and Sussman, G. 1996. Correlation of protein levels with skin prick test reactions in patients allergic to latex. *J Allergy Clin Immunol* 98(6 Pt 1):1097–102.
14. Beezhold, D., Horton, K., Hickey, V., Daddona, J., and Kostyal, D. 2003. Glove powder's carrying capacity for latex protein: Analysis using the ASTM ELISA test. *J Long Term Eff Med Implants* 13(1):21–30.
15. Schegg, K.M., Denslow, N.D., Andersen, T.T., Bao, Y., Cohen, S.A., Mahrenholz, A.M., and Mann, K. 1997. Quantitation and identification of proteins by amino acid analysis: ABRF-96AAA collaborative trial. In *Techniques in Protein Chemistry*, Marshak, D.R., Ed. Cambridge, MA: Academic Press, pp. 207–216.
16. Beezhold, D.H., Kostyal, D.A., and Tomazic-Jezic, V.J. 2002. Measurement of latex proteins and assessment of latex protein exposure. *Methods* 27(1):46–51.
17. Hamilton, R.G., and Cornish, K. 2010. Immunogenicity studies of guayule and guayule latex in occupationally exposed workers. *Indust Crops Products* 31(1):197–201.

18. Cao, L.Y., Taylor, J.S., Sood, A., Murray, D., and Siegel, P.D. 2010. Allergic contact dermatitis to synthetic rubber gloves: Changing trends in patch test reactions to accelerators. *Arch Dermatol* 146(9):1001–7.
19. Dejonckheere, G., Herman, A., and Baeck, M. 2019. Allergic contact dermatitis caused by synthetic rubber gloves in healthcare workers: Sensitization to 1,3-diphenylguanidine is common. *Contact Dermatitis* 81(3):167–73.
20. Geier, J., Lessmann, H., Uter, W., and Schnuch, A. 2003. Occupational rubber glove allergy: Results of the Information Network of Departments of Dermatology (IVDK), 1995–2001. *Contact Dermatitis* 48(1):39–44.
21. Goodier, M.C., Ronkainen, S.D., and Hylwa, S.A. 2018. Rubber accelerators in medical examination and surgical gloves. *Dermatitis* 29(2):66–76.
22. Hamnerius, N., Svedman, C., Bergendorff, O., Björk, J., Bruze, M., Engfeldt, M., and Pontén, A. 2018. Hand eczema and occupational contact allergies in healthcare workers with a focus on rubber additives. *Contact Dermatitis* 79(3):149–56.
23. Kaniwa, M.A., Isama, K., Nakamura, A., Kantoh, H., Itoh, M., Ichikawa, M., and Hayakawa, R. 1994. Identification of causative chemicals of allergic contact dermatitis using a combination of patch testing in patients and chemical analysis. Application to cases from industrial rubber products. *Contact Dermatitis* 30(1):20–5.
24. Siegel, P.D., Fowler, Jr., J.F., Storrs, F.J., Sasseville, D., Pratt, M., Bledsoe, T.A., Law, B.F., Beezhold, D., Zug, K., and Fowler, L.M. 2010. Allergen content of patient problem and nonproblem gloves: Relationship to allergen-specific patch-test findings. *Dermatitis* 21(2):77–83.
25. Warshaw, E.M., Raju, S.I., Mathias, C.G., DeKoven, J.G., Belsito, D.V., Maibach, H.I., Taylor, J.S., Sasseville, D., Zug, K.A., Zirwas, M.J., Fowler, Jr., J.F., DeLeo, V.A., Marks, Jr., J.G., Pratt, M.D., and Storrs, F.J. 2013. Concomitant patch test reactions to mercapto mix and mercaptobenzothiazole: Retrospective analysis from the North American Contact Dermatitis Group, 1994–2008. *Dermatitis* 24(6):321–7.
26. Dahlin, J., Bergendorff, O., Vindenes, H.K., Hindsén, M., and Svedman, C. 2014. Triphenylguanidine, a new (old?) rubber accelerator detected in surgical gloves that may cause allergic contact dermatitis. *Contact Dermatitis* 71(4):242–6.
27. Woo, D.K., Militello, G., and James, W.D. 2004. Neoprene. *Dermatitis* 15(4):206–9.
28. Warshaw, E.M., Cook, J.W., Belsito, D.V., DeLeo, V.A., Fowler, Jr., J.F., Maibach, H.I., Marks, Jr., J.G., Mathias, C.G., Pratt, M.D., Rietschel, R.L., Sasseville, D., Storrs, F.J., Taylor, J.S., and Zug, K.A. 2008. Positive patch-test reactions to mixed dialkyl thioureas: Cross-sectional data from the North American Contact Dermatitis Group, 1994 to 2004. *Dermatitis* 19(4):190–201.
29. Nocil Limited. 2014. *Vulcanization & Accelerators*. Arvind Mafatal Group: Technical Notes. Available at: https://www.nocil.com/Downloadfile/DTechnicalNote-Vulcanization-Dec10.pdf (accessed June 30, 2022).
30. Joseph, A.M., George, B., Madhusoodanan, K.N., and Alex R. 2015. Current status of sulphur vulcanization and devulcanization chemistry: Process of vulcanization. *Rubber Science* 28(1):82–121.
31. Bergendorff, O., Persson, C., Lüdtke, A., and Hansson, C. 2007. Chemical changes in rubber allergens during vulcanization. *Contact Dermatitis* 57(3):152–7.
32. Winspear, G.G., Ed. 1987. *The Vanderbilt Latex Handbook*, Third Edition. Norwalk, CT: R. T. Vanderbilt Co.
33. Bergendorff, O., Persson, C., and Hansson, C. 2006. High-performance liquid chromatography analysis of rubber allergens in protective gloves used in health care. *Contact Dermatitis* 55(4):210–5.
34. Depree, G.J., Bledsoe, T.A., and Siegel, P.D. 2005. Survey of sulfur-containing rubber accelerator levels in latex and nitrile exam gloves. *Contact Dermatitis* 53(2):107–13.

35. Hansson, C., Bergendorff, O., Ezzelarab, M., and Sterner, O. 1997. Extraction of mercaptobenzothiazole compounds from rubber products. *Contact Dermatitis* 36(4):195–200.

36. ASTM International. 2014. *ASTM D7558: Standard Test Method for Colorimetric/Spectrophotometric Procedure to Quantify Extractable Chemical Dialkyldithiocarbamate, Thiuram, and Mercaptobenzothiazole Accelerators in Natural Rubber Latex and Nitrile Gloves*. West Conshohocken, PA: ASTM International.

37. Depree, G.J., Bledsoe, T.A., and Siegel, P.D. 2004. Determination of zinc dialkyldithiocarbamates in latex condoms. *J Chromatogr Sci* 42(2):80–4.

38. Kaniwa, M., Isama, K., Nakamura, A., et al. 1994. Identification of causative chemicals of allergic contact dermatitis using a combination of patch testing in patients and chemical analysis. Application to cases from rubber gloves. *Contact Dermatitis* 31(2):65–71.

39. Knudsen, B.B., Hametner, C., Seycek, O., Heese, A., Koch, H.U., and Peters, K.P. 2000. Allergologically relevant rubber accelerators in single-use medical gloves. *Contact Dermatitis* 43(1):9–15.

40. Mathieu, C., Herbreteau, B., Lafosse, M., Morin, P., Renaud, M., Cardinet, C., and Dreux, M. 2000. Liquid chromatography of unstable zinc dithiocarbamates: Application to rubber gloves analysis. *J High Resolut Chrom* 23(9):565–566.

41. Piskin, G., Meijs, M.M., van der Ham, R., and Bos, J.D. 2006. Glove allergy due to 1,3-diphenylguanidine. *Contact Dermatitis* 54(1):61–2.

42. Pontén, A., Hamnerius, N., Bruze, M., Hansson, C., Persson, C., Svedman, C., Thörneby Andersson, K., and Bergendorff, O. 2013. Occupational allergic contact dermatitis caused by sterile non-latex protective gloves: Clinical investigation and chemical analyses. *Contact Dermatitis* 68(2):103–10.

43. Ramzy, A.G., Hagvall, L., Pei, M.N., Samuelsson, K., and Nilsson, U. 2015. Investigation of diethylthiourea and ethyl isothiocyanate as potent skin allergens in chloroprene rubber. *Contact Dermatitis* 72(3):139–46.

44. Siegel, P.D., Law, B.F., Fowler, Jr., J.F., and Fowler, L.M. 2010. Disproportionated rosin dehydroabietic acid in neoprene surgical gloves. *Dermatitis* 21(3):157–9.

45. Chipinda, I., Hettick, J.M., Simoyi, R.H., and Siegel, P.D. 2007. Oxidation of 2-mercaptobenzothiazole in latex gloves and its possible haptenation pathway. *Chem Res Toxicol* 20(8):1084–92.

46. Chipinda, I., Hettick, J.M., Simoyi, R.H., and Siegel, P.D. 2008. Zinc diethyldithiocarbamate allergenicity: Potential haptenation mechanisms. *Contact Dermatitis* 59(2):79–89.

47. Chipinda, I., Zhang, X.D., Simoyi, R.H., and Siegel, P.D. 2008. Mercaptobenzothiazole allergenicity-role of the thiol group. *Cutan Ocul Toxicol* 27(2):103–16.

48. Wang, X.S., and Tabor, M.W. 1988. Studies of the reactivity of morpholine, 2-mercaptobenzothiazole and 2 of their derivatives with selected amino acids. *Contact Dermatitis* 19(1):16–21.

Section II

Regulations and Standards

5 European Standards on Protective Gloves

K.F. Mose, R. Bach, and M-N. Crépy

CONTENTS

5.1 INTRODUCTION

The decision of the European Economic Community (EEC, a precursor to the European Union) to create the Single European Act in 1987 meant that the EEC could facilitate the innovative idea of developing a single European market by the end of 1992. The completion of the single market enabled a free movement of goods between member states and free access to sources of production. However, all the member states have their own laws on product safety, and this can cause technical trade barriers. To eliminate this problem for business and take into account the recommended high level of worker and consumer protection, the European Community ministers agreed on a "New Approach to Technical Harmonization and Standards" in May 1985. This resulted in a Council Directive (Law) in the field of personal protective equipment (PPE) adopted in 1989, containing essential safety requirements. The technical details were left to the European standardization organizations.[1]

Currently, there are three European Standardization Organizations: European Committee for Electrotechnical Standardization (CENELEC), European Telecommunications Standards Institute (ETSI), and European Committee for Standardization (CEN). These organizations are responsible for the continued development and definition of official standards in Europe.[2] In this context, CEN is highlighted because it creates a forum for developing European standards (EN) and technical documents in relation to a plethora of different goods, resources, services, and processes. It is an association composed of the National Standardization Bodies of 27 European countries, the United Kingdom, the Republic of North Macedonia, Serbia, and Turkey, in addition to representatives from the EFTA (European Free Trade Association) countries (Norway, Iceland, and Switzerland). Within the CEN,

DOI: 10.1201/9781003126874-7

preparation of EN is made by Technical Committees (TCs) and their subcommittees, each with its own scope and individual work frame/program. Appointed Working Groups (WGs) composed of a wide field of experts undertake the task of developing drafts for future standards. Of the many active TCs, the Technical Committee CEN/TC 162 "Protective Clothing Including Hand and Arm Protection and Lifejackets" became operational in 1989 and it is currently divided into 13 WGs:

1. General requirements for protective clothing
2. Resistance to heat and fire of protective clothing
3. Protective clothing against chemicals, infective agents, and radioactive contamination
4. Protective clothing against foul weather, wind, and cold
5. Resistance to mechanical impact of protective clothing
6. Lifejackets
7. Visibility clothing and accessories
8. Protective gloves
9. Motorcycle rider protective clothing
10. Buoyant aids for swimming instruction
11. Body protection for sports
12. Diving suits
13. Joint WG between CEN/TC 162 and CEN/TC 161 (Foot and leg protectors) – Test methods for permeation of chemicals through materials for protective footwear, gloves, and clothing.[3]

5.2 DEVELOPMENT OF EUROPEAN STANDARDS

The development of an EN in CEN follows a multistep process:

1. *Proposal development*: A broad range of stakeholders/interested parties (industry, academia, etc.) can make proposals for a new standard. Primarily, proposals are made through CEN members.
2. *Proposal acceptance*: Relevant technical bodies accept the proposal, after which a "standstill" is initiated where all member states immediately cease all national activities within the work frame/program, thus allowing member states to direct all efforts toward a new EN development.
3. *Drafting*: Relevant experts in a technical body make a draft proposal for an EN.
4. *Inquiry*: Upon completion of an EN draft, it is released for public (e.g., public authorities, consumers, and industry) comments and voting. CEN member states collect the comments and submit a national weighted vote, which is finally processed by the CEN technical body. If this enquiry results in an acceptance of the EN, it can then be published by the technical body.
5. *Adoption by weighted formal vote*: In the case of a need for a technical reworking of a draft, the technical body can revise/update, followed by a resubmission and a formal vote (another weighted vote).

6. *EN publication*: After EN approval, it becomes published. Published ENs also work as national standards in the member states, and any national standards that conflict with the new standard must be removed. This, in turn, makes it much easier, e.g., for manufacturers to work and compete in (but also outside) membership countries if they apply the EN.

7. *EN revisions*: ENs need to be reviewed no later than five years after publication.[4,5]

5.3 EUROPEAN DIRECTIVES AND REGULATIONS

5.3.1 PERSONAL PROTECTIVE EQUIPMENT

The work on international standardization in the field of protective clothing was initiated in 1964 by the International Organization for Standardization (ISO)/Technical Committee 94 (ISO/TC 94) "Personal Safety—Protective Clothing and Equipment." Sub-Committee 13 (Protective Clothing) of ISO/TC 94 was formed in 1981 and presently consists of seven working groups.[6,7] In the field of PPE, two complementary directives were adopted in 1989 by the EEC and scheduled to enter into force in 1992; a third directive was adopted in 1993. The Regulation (EU) 2016/425 on PPE (the PPE regulation) was introduced in 2018, and it replaces the former Directive 89/686/EEC.[8] PPE is defined as any device or appliance designed to be worn or held by an individual for protection against one or more safety and health hazards in the execution of the user's activity.[1,9]

The basic outline of the directives is as follows:

1. The council directive on the approximation of the laws of the member states relative to the design of PPE (89/686/EEC).[10] This directive includes PPE for both professional and nonprofessional uses. It defines, in particular, the certification procedures.

2. The council directive concerning the minimum safety and health requirements for the use of PPE by workers at the workplace [(89/656/EEC), third individual directive within the meaning of Article 16(1) of Directive 89/391/EEC]. This directive essentially defines the employer's obligations. It states that PPE shall be used when risks cannot be avoided. The employer must inform his or her workers of the evaluated risks in the workplace, supply appropriate and correctly fitting PPE in compliance with EU standards, and give adequate instruction on the use of PPE. The employer must provide the appropriate equipment free of charge and must ensure that it is in good working order and hygienic condition.[11,12]

3. The council directive concerning the safety of medical devices (93/42/EEC). These devices include gloves for medical use.

4. The PPE transition from council directive 89/686/EEC to the PPE Regulation 2016/425 contains several changes and improvements in terms of the scope, essential health and safety requirements, definitions, economic operators and their obligations, conformity assessment procedures, risk categories, and finally that is functioning more directly as a legal instrument in contrast to the previous directive.[13]

The assessment procedures of PPE relate to control of PPE design and control of PPE production. The target is to give users assurance that the device on the market fulfills the requirements and provides protection and safety at the highest level possible. Application for EC-type examination is to be made by the manufacturer or its authorized representative. The authorized representative is to be established in the European Community. Products meeting the requirements are to carry the CE mark, which implies that they can be marketed anywhere in the European Community countries.[1,9]

According to the risk involved, PPEs are classified into three categories:[10]

- Category I: PPE (previously termed "simple design") intended to protect against minimal risks, which, when the effects are gradual, can be safely identified by the user in good time.
- Category II: All types of PPE that are not included in categories I and III.
- Category III: PPE (previously termed "complex design") intended to protect against mortal danger or against dangers that may seriously and irreversibly harm the health.

Gloves are usually classified as types I or II and rarely as type III.

Directive requirements are dependent on the type of glove:[10]

- **Type I**. Gloves of simple design—for minimal risk application
  - Conform with basic health and safety requirements
  - Technical documentation file
  - Declaration of conformity (requirements as set out in EN420)
  - Affixed CE mark
- **Type II**. Gloves of intermediate design (neither simple nor complex design)—for intermediate risk
  - Conform with harmonized European standard or other verified technical specification
  - Technical documentation file
  - EC-type examination, tested by approved laboratories
  - EC declaration of product conformity
  - Affixed CE mark on conformity, examined and issued by an approved notified body
- **Type III**. Gloves of complex design—for irreversible/mortal risks
  - Conform with harmonized European standard or other verified technical specification
  - Technical documentation file
  - EC-type examination, tested by approved laboratories and surveillance/certification annually by approved notified bodies
  - EC declaration of product conformity
  - Affixed CE mark
  - Manufactured under a formal EC quality assurance system

5.3.2   MEDICAL GLOVES

Medical gloves for single use are gloves intended for use in the medical field to protect patients and users from cross-contamination. They are also designed to protect the user and fall into the definition of personal protective equipment.[12] So they must fulfill the relevant essential requirements of both directives. Up to 2010, single-use gloves in healthcare facilities could only be classified according to either the EU Directive on medical products 93/42/EEC or the EU Directive on PPE for Users 89/656/EEC, despite similar properties.[14] Since 2010, the revised EU Directive 2007/47/EC (2007) allows dual-labeling of products for dual purposes as medical devices and personal protective equipment, as well as the respective dual CE labeling.

The European Union Medical Device Regulation, EU-MDR 2017/745, or MDR replaces the previous European Council Directive 93/42/EEC, or MDD. The MDR is a new set of regulations that governs the production and distribution of medical devices in Europe, including medical gloves and masks, with new requirements in areas such as clinical evaluation, post-market surveillance, and labeling. Compliance with the regulation is mandatory for companies that want to sell medical devices in the European marketplace. While the old MDD was a "directive," the MDR is a "regulation."[15,16]

5.4   STANDARDS RELATED TO PROTECTIVE GLOVES

A comprehensive list of EN Standards for protective and medical gloves of different types and uses are shown in Tables 5.1 and 5.2. The standard (EN 420), "General Requirements for Gloves," defines requirements for most kinds of protective gloves. Key points are the fitness of purpose, innocuousness (the gloves themselves should not cause any harm to the user. Chromium VI—applicable to all leathers; less than 3 mg/kg, pH value is to be greater than 3.5 and less than 9.5), sound construction, storage, sizing, measure of glove-hand dexterity, product information, and labeling.[11,17] Previously only a European standard, it has now been converted into the international standard ISO 21420:2020. The new standard EN ISO 21420 (prepared by Technical Committee ISO/TC 94) provides further alignment with the REACH (Registration, Evaluation, Authorization and Restriction of Chemicals) legislation (Regulation (EC) No 1907/2006) on hazardous substances and adds requirements for:

- Nickel release of all metallic materials in prolonged contact with the skin; less than 0.5 µg/cm² per week),
- for azo colorants. Undetectable release of the carcinogenic amines listed,
- for Dimethylformamide (DMF) in gloves containing polyurethane less than 0.1 % w/w, and
- for Polycyclic aromatic hydrocarbons (PAH's), less than 1 ppm for each of the eight restricted PAH for the rubber/plastic to come in contact with the skin.

TABLE 5.1
List of European Standards (EN) for Protective Gloves Prepared by CEN/TC 162

Document No.	Title
EN 388	Determination of Resistance to Permeation by Chemicals Protective Gloves—Mechanical Test Methods and Specifications
EN 407	Protective Gloves against Thermal Risks
EN ISO 10819	Gloves against the Effect of Vibrations (Work by CEN/TC 231)
EN 659	Protective Gloves for Firefighters
EN 511	Protective Gloves against Cold
EN 420	General Requirements for Gloves
EN 421	Protective Gloves against Ionizing Radiation and Radioactive Contamination
EN 464	Protective Clothing—Protection against Liquid Chemicals—Gas Leak Test
EN 1082-1	Protective clothing—Gloves and arm guards protecting against cuts and stabs by hand knives—Part 1: Chain mail gloves and arm guards
EN 1082-2	Protective clothing—Gloves and arm guards protecting against cuts and stabs by hand knives—Part 2: Gloves and arm guards made of material other than chain mail
EN 1082-3	Protective clothing—Gloves and arm guards protecting against cuts and stabs by hand knives—Part 3: Impact cut test for fabric, leather, and other materials
EN 12477	Protective gloves for welders
EN 13594	Protective gloves for motorcycle riders—Requirements and test methods
EN 14328	Protective clothing—Gloves and armguards protecting against cuts by powered knives—Requirements and test methods
EN 16027	Protective clothing—Gloves with protective effect for association football goalkeepers
EN 16350	Protective gloves—Electrostatic properties
EN 16778	Protective gloves—The determination of Dimethylformamide in gloves
EN ISO 21420	Protective gloves—General requirements and test methods
EN ISO 374-1	Protective gloves against dangerous chemicals and micro-organisms—Part 1: Terminology and performance requirements for chemical risks—Amendment 1
EN ISO 374-2	Protective gloves against dangerous chemicals and micro-organisms—Part 2: Determination of resistance to penetration
EN ISO 374-4	Protective gloves against dangerous chemicals and micro-organisms—Part 4: Determination of resistance to degradation by chemicals
EN ISO 374-5	Protective gloves against dangerous chemicals and micro-organisms—Part 5: Terminology and performance requirements for micro-organisms risks

Note: CEN/TC 162: Protective Clothing, Including Hand and Arm Protection and Lifejackets.

TABLE 5.2
List of European Standards (EN) for Medical Gloves Prepared by CEN/ TC 205

Document No.	Title
EN 455-1	Medical Gloves for Single Use—Part 1: Requirements and testing for freedom from holes
EN 455-2	Medical Gloves for Single Use—Part 2: Requirements and testing for physical properties
EN 455-3	Medical Gloves for Single Use—Part 3: Requirements and testing for biological evaluation
EN 455-4	Medical Gloves for Single Use—Part 4: Requirements and testing for shelf-life determination
EN ISO 21171	Medical gloves—Determination of removable surface powder

Note: CEN/TC 205: Medical Devices.

REFERENCES

1. DTI. 1991. *The Single Market: Personal Protective Equipment*. London, UK: Department of Trade and Industry (DTI) and Central Office of Information.
2. EU. 2021. Key players in European standardisation. An official website of the European Union (EU). [Accessed April 2021]. https://ec.europa.eu/growth/single-market/european-standards/key-players_en.
3. European Committee for Standardization. 2021. Technical bodies: CEN/TC 162 – Protective clothing including hand and arm protection and lifejackets. [Accessed February 2021]. https://standards.cen.eu/dyn/www/f?p=204:29:0::::FSP_ORG_ID,FSP _LANG_ID:6143,25&cs=102A66CBFB980335CEF1DBD3D5340D530#1.
4. European Committee for Standardization. 2021. Standards development. [Accessed April 2021]. https://www.cen.eu/work/ENdev/how/Pages/default.aspx.
5. Karppinen, A. 2015. How are standards developed and structured? Annex A: Detailed description of the standardization process in CEN, in *A World Built on Standards - A Textbook for Higher Education*, Bøgh, S.A., Ed. Nordhavn: Danish Standards Foundation [in English], pp. 53–74.
6. Zimmerli, T. 1992. International standards on protective clothing in ISO and CEN: Cooperation or competition?, in *4th Scand. Symp. Protective Clothing against Chemicals and Other Health Risks, Kittilä, Finland*, Mäkinen, H., Ed. Copenhagen, Denmark: NOKOBETEF IV: 56 [in English].
7. ISO. 2021. *ISO/TC94/SC13 – Protective Clothing*. Geneva: International Organization for Standardization (ISO). [Accessed April 2021]. https://www.iso.org/committee /50626.html.
8. EU. 2021. Personal protective equipment (PPE). An official website of the European Union (EU). [Accessed April 2021]. https://ec.europa.eu/growth/sectors/mechanical -engineering/personal-protective-equipment_en.
9. Mayer, A. 1992. European directives and standards relating to personal protective equipment, in *Performance of Protecting Clothing*, Vol. 4, ASTM STP 1133, McBriarty, J.P. and Henry, N.W., III, Eds. Philadelphia, PA: American Society for Testing and Materials, 990.

10. Anon. 1989. Council Directive of 21 December 1989 on the approximation of the law of the Member States relating to personal protective equipment (89/686/EEC). *Off J Eur Communities* No. L 399/18:30.12.89.

11. Ansell. 2016. *EN Standards Guide: Ansell Summary Guide to EN Standards that Govern EU Certified Hand Protection*, Version 1.0. Belgium: Ansell and Ansell Limited [Accessed December 2021] https://www.ansell.com/us/en/campaigns/enre-sourcecenter/en-standards-guide.

12. Crepy, M.-N., Boman, A., and Zimmermann, F. 2019. Protective gloves, in *Kanerva's Occupational Dermatology*, John, S., Johansen, J., Rustemeyer, T., Elsner, P., and Maibach, H., Eds. Switzerland: Springer Nature, pp. 1663–1684.

13. EU. 2016. *Guidance Document on the PPE Transition from Directive 89/686/EEC to Regulation (EU) 2016/425*. Geneva: European Union (EU). [Accessed April 2021 through an official website of the European Union]. https://ec.europa.eu/docsroom/documents/22106.

14. Kramer, A., and Assadian, O. 2016. Indications and the requirements for single-use medical gloves. *GMS Hyg Infect Control* 11:Doc01.

15. EU. 2017. *Regulation (EU) 2017/745 of the European Parliament and of the Council of 5 April 2017 on Medical Devices, Amending Directive 2001/83/EC, Regulation (EC) 178/2002 and Regulation (EC) No 1223/2009 and Repealing Council Directives 90/385/EEC and 93/42/EEC*. OJ L 117, 55. 2017:1–175. Geneva: European Union (EU).

16. Ansell. 2021. *A Guide to the New European Union Medical Device Regulation (MDR): EU-MDR 2017/745*. Belgium: Ansell and Ansell Limited. [Accessed December 2021] https://www.ansell.com/no/en/medical/eumdr.

17. European Committee for Standardization. 2021. *CEN CENELEC Search Standards*. [Accessed April 2021]. https://standards.cencenelec.eu/dyn/www/f?p=CEN:105::RESET.

6 US Rules, Regulations, and Standards for Protective Gloves for Occupational Use

N.W. Henry and R.N. Phalen

CONTENTS

6.1 INTRODUCTION

Gloves are used to protect one of our most valuable tools—our hands. Our hands can do marvelous things and perform many tasks. These tasks may require the use of gloves for protection against exposure to hazardous physical, chemical, and biological agents during the normal workday. Gloves act as a barrier between our skin and the hazard encountered. Skin is a natural barrier of living tissue sensitive to physical effects, chemical absorption, and biological penetration. Once this natural barrier is broken, our body is susceptible to harm and injury from any one of the three hazards. Gloves provide warmth from cold, insulation from heat, and resistance to sharp objects, chemicals, and biological organisms. They come in various colors, sizes, and shapes and are made of many different types of natural and synthetic materials. Despite the use and nonuse of gloves, hand injuries continue to be one of the most frequently reported occupational injuries. These injuries are preventable if the correct gloves are selected and used for protection against the hazard. The selection of gloves for occupational use is the job of the safety professional. Guides, rules, and regulations for glove use have only recently become available to the safety professional through the efforts of various standard-setting organizations that have developed performance standards for gloves. This chapter discusses some of the current glove standards in the United States.

DOI: 10.1201/9781003126874-8

6.2   RULES, REGULATIONS, AND STANDARDS

Glove standards can be divided into categories depending on the generic type of glove material used, the type of work being done, and the type of hazard encountered. For example, there are standards for gloves made of rubber, for gloves used by electrical workers, and for gloves used against heat and flame. Each standard was generated as a result of a need to evaluate the performance of a material for specific workers against specific hazards. The majority of these standards in the United States have been drafted and written by voluntary consensus of standard-setting organizations such as the American Society for Testing and Materials (ASTM), now ASTM International, and the American National Standard Institute (ANSI). These standard-setting organizations have been the focal point for glove and other protective clothing standards. Various professional organizations representing their constituents have also adopted standards, such as the National Fire Protection Association (NFPA) and the American Dental Association (ADA). Federal standards for the testing of gloves also have been developed to meet military specifications and eliminate unnecessary or undesirable variations in the general sampling and testing procedures. International organizations such as the International Standard Organization (ISO) have also developed standards as well as Europe's EN standard-setting community (see Chapter 5).

Most of the standards that have been adopted have been written to test the performance of gloves under various exposure conditions. The primary parameters evaluated have been physical strength, dexterity, abrasion, and heat and cold resistance. Resistance to swelling, degradation, permeation, and penetration are among the more important chemical parameters evaluated, while biological resistance to liquids and microorganisms also has been evaluated. By measuring key effects in physical and chemical properties, such as tensile strength, thickness changes, and solubility, the performance of materials used to make gloves can be determined. Because much is known about the properties and behavior of natural and synthetic polymers and other materials of construction used for gloves, results of these performance tests conducted under actual use conditions can then be compared to original data on the generic materials to help predict resistance.

There is a broad range of test methods and test conditions. Standard test methods may involve a simple light test in a dark room to look for pinholes or imperfections in gloves, immersion of gloves in a chemical or biological liquid to see if penetration occurs, or more sophisticated permeation tests to determine the breakthrough time and permeation rate. Some tests involve using the whole glove, while others may just require testing a sample or swatch of material. Exposure conditions can range from a splash test to complete liquid contact for varying lengths of time and at different temperatures and pressures. Equipment used for the tests also can vary in degree of complexity, detection sensitivity, level of sophistication, and cost: for example, the inflated-glove water-immersion test for determining pinhole imperfections vs. the use of an tensiometer for measuring tensile strength. Another criterion for these test methods is that they are reproducible and simple enough that most users can do testing for themselves at actual exposure conditions.

For the past 45 years, one technical committee within ASTM, Committee F-23 on Protective Clothing, has been the center of voluntary consensus standards development for items of protective clothing, such as gloves. This committee, charged with the responsibility to develop standard methods of test, terminology, classification, and performance specifications for clothing used to protect against occupational hazards, has generated 44 standards on test methods, specifications, practices, and guides for physical, chemical, biological, and other hazards. These performance standards have set the pace for other standard-setting organizations in the United States and internationally. The committee has sponsored ten international symposia, published standard technical publications (STPs) for each, and compiled a single ASTM Protective Clothing reference on all ASTM protective clothing standards.[1] The tenth international symposium in 2016 focused on risk reduction through research and testing. The purpose of the symposium was to provide a forum for the exchange of ideas on established and emerging protective clothing needs of government and industrial workers, first responders, and civilians. Standards on gloves are included in these presentations and publications. The more recent activity in F-23 was to form a new subcommittee on radiological hazards to promulgate standards for materials used, designed, and constructed to protect against radiation. Agricultural and pharmaceutical specifications for test methods and performance properties for gloves are also being considered. There is very little information about the resistance of gloves to pesticide mixtures and potent chemical therapeutic drugs. Committee F-23 needs more users represented at its meetings to develop more meaningful, useful practical standards and guides for other occupations.

One of the most notable standard methods developed within Committee F-23 was standard test method F 739: *Test Method for Resistance of Protective Clothing Materials to Permeation by Liquids or Gases under Conditions of Continuous Contact*. It was the first standard method developed by F-23 and the one with the most impact on standards for gloves. The key parameters evaluated in this test method are glove breakthrough time and permeation rate. Because gloves and hands can come in direct contact with chemical hazards, it was recognized that they were susceptible to permeation and that some glove materials were more resistant than others. By measuring the chemical breakthrough time and subsequent permeation rate, one could determine chemical hold out (resistance) and protection capacity. This was particularly important for hazardous industrial solvents (benzene) and gases (ammonia). Upon acceptance of this standard, numerous permeation tests were conducted and glove permeation charts and guides were published. Glove users could at least now refer to how long a given glove will protect against exposure. Manufacturers, on the other hand, could work on improving glove performance by developing new products with better resistance. Because of the diversity of chemicals and the need for guidance on test method strategy, a list of a standard battery of test chemicals was developed, F 1001: Guide for the Selection of Chemicals to Evaluate Clothing Materials. Now, most glove manufacturers publish the permeation results of their products using this list as a reference.

While chemical glove permeation standards were the first methods to be developed by Committee F-23 on Protective Clothing, another important area of standards development has been the evolution of medical glove standards.[2] ASTM Committee D-11 on *Rubber* has been the center for this important standard-setting activity since the mid-1970s. Faced with the challenges of determining pinhole leaks in rubber surgeons' and examination gloves, this committee needed to develop better test methods than D 3577: *Specifications for Rubber Surgical Gloves* and D 3578: *Specification for Rubber Examination Gloves* to address healthcare concerns about acquired immune deficiency syndrome (AIDS) and human immunodeficiency virus (HIV). After considerable review, the committee published Standard Method D 5151: *Test Method for Detection of Holes in Medical Gloves* in 1990. This method resulted in an improved, more sensitive test to detect holes in medical gloves. While pinhole leaks were the primary concern in Committee D-11, Committee F-23 focused on penetration test methods for determining leaks with a synthetic blood test and a viral penetration test method using a bacteriophage surrogate to the AIDS and HIV viruses, Phi-X 174. These pass/fail test methods were evaluated in interlaboratory round-robin tests and were Emergency Standards ES 21: *Test Method for Resistance of Protective Clothing Materials to Synthetic Blood* and ES 22: *Test Method for Resistance of Protective Clothing Materials to Penetration by Blood-Borne Pathogens Using Viral Penetration as a Test System.*[3] These two test methods were used to evaluate the performance of clothing and glove materials, but improved methods specifically for whole gloves were being investigated and considered by Committee F-23, as well. Both of these test methods are no longer emergency standards and now have been approved as consensus standards by the Biological Hazards Subcommittee F23.40 of F-23 and redesignated F 1670: *Standard Test Method for Resistance of Materials Used in Protective Clothing to Penetration by Synthetic Blood* and F 1671: *Standard Test Method for Resistance of Materials Used in Protective Clothing to Penetration by Blood-Borne Pathogens Using Phi-X 174 Bacteriophage Penetration as a Test System.* They have been utilized and cited in performance data for several gloves used in the healthcare profession in the United States.

Another test method that was also approved as a consensus standard was F 1819: *Resistance of Materials Used in Protective Clothing to Penetration by Synthetic Blood Using Mechanical Pressure Technique.* This method supplements the previously adopted hydrostatic pressure head techniques and offers the capability of measuring penetration resistance at the greater mechanical pressures that might be encountered in osteoplastic surgery.

A new glove standard was also developed by ANSI and the Industrial Safety Equipment Association (ISEA) in early 2000.[4] This standard, ANSI/ISEA 105-2016, *Standard for Hand Protection Selection Criteria*, provided several different properties for classifying the performance of gloves, including chemical-resistant gloves. The results for a specific glove style are reported according to the level achieved for the respective property. Performance properties are defined in terms of six levels. Gloves not achieving the lowest level are reported as level 0. Properties covered in the standard include:

- Mechanical protection
  - Cut resistance (e.g., ASTM F 1790)
  - Puncture resistance (e.g., ASTM F 1342 and EN 388)

- Hypodermic needle puncture resistance (e.g., ASTM F 2878)
  - Abrasion resistance
- Chemical protection
  - Chemical permeation resistance (e.g., ASTM F 739)
  - Chemical degradation resistance
- Heat and flame protection
  - Ignition resistance (e.g., ASTM F 1358)
  - Heat degradation resistance (e.g., ISO 17493 and ASTM F 2894)
  - Conductive heat resistance (e.g., ASTM F 1060)
- Vibration reduction
- Dexterity

6.3 US STANDARDS ON GLOVES

An updated list of US standards on gloves is shown in Table 6.1. These standard test methods were all developed by various standard-setting organizations such as ASTM, ANSI, NFPA, ISEA, and ADA. They are performance standards used to evaluate gloves used for protection against various hazards in the work environment. These hazards include physical, chemical, and biological agents. The list is not complete, nor is there a description of the actual test method and conditions, since detailed procedures would consume much of this chapter. The list is intended to be a reference for identifying existing standards in the United States. For more specific information on glove performance standards, check organizational websites, such as astm.org, for a complete list of their standards and activities. Governmental regulatory agencies in the United States such as the Occupational Safety and Health Administration (OSHA), Environmental Protection Agency (EPA), Food and Drug Administration (FDA), and the Centers for Disease Control and Prevention (CDC) also have websites with links to a variety of glove information. The National Institute for Occupational Safety and Health (NIOSH) also conducts and supports research on glove materials, methods, and performance.

As new technologies evolve, the need for hand protection and improved glove test methods will continue. Standard-setting organizations in the United States and the rest of the world need to work together in developing these methods, as we now compete in a global market with no boundaries when it comes to protecting our workers. We should wear gloves that the job demands, select gloves that pass performance standards, and remember that many of the accomplishments of man would not be possible without protective gloves.

6.4 RECENT CHANGES, IMPORTANT UPDATES, AND EMERGING ISSUES

It has been over 25 years since the first edition of this book was published, and there have been a lot of changes in rules regulations and improvements in gloves for occupational use. These changes include new types of gloves and updated standards and regulations for use in the workplace environment. One of the most important changes has been the

TABLE 6.1
US Standard Methods for Gloves

Organization	Document No.	Title
ASTM	C 852	Standard Guide for Design Criteria for Plutonium Glove Boxes
ASTM	D 120	Standard Specification for Rubber Insulating Gloves
ASTM	D 3577	Standard Specification for Rubber Surgical Gloves
ASTM	D 3578	Standard Specification for Rubber Examination Gloves
ASTM	D 4108	Test Method for Thermal Protective Performance of Materials for Clothing by Open Flame
ASTM	D 4115	Women's and Girl's Knitted and Woven Dress Glove Fabrics, Performance Specifications
ASTM	D 4679	Standard Specification for Rubber General Purpose, Household or Beautician Gloves
ASTM	D 5151	Standard Test Method for Detection of Holes in Medical Gloves
ASTM	D 5250	Standard Specification for Polyvinyl Chloride Gloves for Medical Application
ASTM	F 496	Standard Specification for the In-Service Care of Insulating Gloves and Mittens
ASTM	F 696	Standard Specification for Leather Protectors for Rubber Insulating Gloves and Mittens
ASTM	F 739	Test Method for Resistance of Protective Clothing Materials to Permeation by Liquids or Gases under Conditions of Continuous Contact
ASTM	F 903	Test Method for Resistance of Protective Clothing Materials to Penetration by Liquids
ASTM	F 955	Test Method for Evaluating Heat Transfer through Materials for Protective Clothing upon Contact with Molten Substances
ASTM	F 1001	Standard Guide for Selection of Chemicals to Evaluate Protective Clothing Materials
ASTM	F 1060	Standard Test Method for Evaluation of Conductive and Compressive Heat Resistance (CCHR)
ASTM	F 1342	Test Method for Protective Clothing Resistance to Puncture
ASTM	F 1383	Test Method for Resistance of Protective Clothing Materials to Permeation by Liquids or Gases under Conditions of Intermittent Contact
ASTM	F 1407	Standard Test Method for Resistance of Chemical Protective Clothing Materials to Liquid Permeation—Permeation Cup Method
ASTM	F 1670	Standard Test Method for Resistance of Materials Used in Protective Clothing to Penetration by Synthetic Blood
ASTM	F 1671	Standard Test Method for Resistance of Materials Used in Protective Clothing to Penetration by Blood-Borne Pathogens Using Phi-X174 Bacteriophage Penetration as a Test System
ASTM	F 1819	Standard Test Method for Resistance of Materials Used in Protective Clothing to Penetration by Synthetic Blood Using a Mechanical Pressure Technique

(Continued)

TABLE 6.1 (CONTINUED)
US Standard Methods for Gloves

Organization	Document No.	Title
ANSI/ADA[a]	No. 76	Non-Sterile Natural Rubber Latex Gloves For Dentistry
ANSI/ISEA[c]	105	American National Standard For Hand Protection Classification
Federal standard	No. 601	Rubber: Sampling and Testing
NFPA[b]	1999	Standard on Protective Clothing and Ensembles for Emergency Medical Operation

[a] ADA—American Dental Association. [b]NFPA—National Fire Protection Association. [c]ISEA—Industrial Safety Equipment Association

acceptance of the Global Harmonization Standard (GHS) passed in 2012. As the name implies, this standard was written to standardize the global use and development of safety standards in the workplace environment. This would include protective gloves used in transportation, distribution, and handling of hazardous materials and agents (chemical, biological, and physical) in research laboratories, industries, medical facilities, and other businesses around the world. In the United States, ASTM International and Committee F23 on Protective Clothing and Equipment continues to be the main leader in developing standards. They have expanded their scope and membership to include members and organizations from other countries complying with the GHS. This committee is composed of users, general interest, producers, and government representatives who participate in the voluntary development of new standards and regulations. Originally, the committee developed performance standards on gloves and suit materials for chemical resistance to hazardous materials, but now has been developing standards for biological and physical hazards (radiation and heat). The need for biological-resistant gloves and suits has been driven by the need for protection in the healthcare industry against HIV, Eboli, and COVID-19 viruses that threaten the world population. Recently, the COVID-19 pandemic resulted in the development of new standards not only for gloves but also for masks.

Since the first edition several of the standards methods, guides, shown in Table 6.1, have been either revised or updated since their original acceptance. These are continually changing; thus it is recommended to check these by accessing them on the ASTM International website (ASTM.org) under technical committee F-23. You will find subcommittees for chemical resistance, biological resistance, and physical resistance with their current standards, guides, specifications, and practices. Table 6.1 also lists other standard-setting organizations such as ANSI (American National Standards Institute) and trade associations in the United States responsible for specific guidance and practices in their profession such as the National Fire Protection Association (NFPA). Internationally, in Europe, the CEN (Community of European Nations) is the main standard-setting organization (see Chapter 5).

In the United States, rules and regulations for occupational use of gloves in the general industry are enforced by OSHA. Specific rules for the construction industry, agricultural, marine, forestry, and mining industries are under their jurisdiction. NIOSH is another organization that is responsible for the research and development and evaluation of protective clothing materials. They have a National Personal Protective Clothing and Research Laboratory (NPPTL) in Pittsburg, Pennsylvania, responsible for testing the safety of gloves and suits in the workplace. Another organization composed of industrial hygienists, the American Industrial Hygiene Association (AIHA) has a technical committee on protective clothing and equipment. This committee is very active in publishing, training, and developing best practices for using and selecting gloves and suits in the workplace. For a complete view of current practices and standards for gloves and test methods, one should read two articles published in the November 2019 issue of the *Journal of Occupational and Environmental Hygiene*.[5,6] The articles compare various standards for testing, identify research gaps, and even discuss the value of whole glove testing and simulated movement. The authors state that the ASTM F739 and the original 1-inch test cell should be the primary permeation test cell for all standards. They also recommend the harmonization among standards, especially in the determination of normalized breakthrough time and steady-state permeation rate. These two parameters are used to compare the performance of the gloves for resistance to hazardous chemicals to continuous liquid contact and/or intermittent (splash) exposures. It is believed that harmonization and further improvement will likely simplify the selection of gloves and chemical protective suits, help expand existing databases, and instill more confidence among users. Ultimately, it will help reduce the number of injuries, illnesses, diseases, and deaths in the workplace environment.

REFERENCES

1. ASTM International. 1992. *ASTM Standards on Protective Clothing, Committee F-23 on Protective Clothing*. Philadelphia, PA: American Society for Testing and Materials.
2. Chatterton, J.R. and Culp, R.D. 1992. The evolution of medical glove standards. *ASTM Standardization News*, August 1992: 26.
3. ASTM. 1993. Atmospheric analysis, occupational health and safety; protective clothing, in *Annual Book of ASTM Standards*, Sec. 11, Vol. 11.03, Philadelphia, PA: American Society for Testing and Materials, pp. 1–858.
4. Henry III, N.W. and Stull, J.O. 2003. Test methods and standards, in *Chemical Protective Clothing*, 2nd ed., Anna, D.H., Ed. Fairfax, VA: AIHA Press, pp. 175–268.
5. Banaee, S, and Hee, SSQ. 2019. Glove permeation of chemicals: The state of the art of current practice, Part 1: Basics and the permeation standards. *J Occup Environ Hyg* 16(12):827–839. DOI: 10.1080/15459624.2019.1678754.
6. Banaee, S, and Hee, SSQ. 2019. Glove permeation of chemicals: The state of the art of current practice-Part 2. Research emphases on high boiling point compounds and simulating the donned glove environment. *J Occup Environ Hyg* 17(4):135–164. DOI: 10.1080/15459624.2020.1721509.

7 Japanese Regulations and Standards for Medical and Dental Grade Gloves

K. Matsunaga T. Ohhara, A. Takeuchi,
R. Nakaoka, and Y. Haishima

CONTENTS

7.1 INTRODUCTION

Japan's population peaked in 2008 and has been declining gradually, reaching 125,570,000 as of January 2021.[1] The proportion of elderly individuals aged 65 years and above in the population is increasing (approximately 28.9% in 2020), making it the world's number-one aging society.[1] The population in need of medical care is increasing year by year, and the medical device market is expanding. The Japanese medical device market is one of the largest in the world, estimated to be $28.1 billion in 2016 and $31.7 billion in 2020.[2] Medical and dental gloves are basic protective equipment that protects medical staff from infection and prevents nosocomial infection.[3] In Japan, measures to prevent infection have become more thorough, and demand for them has increased.[4] COVID-19, which was diagnosed for the first time in Japan in January 2020, soon became a global pandemic, and while the demand for medical and dental gloves increased rapidly on a global scale, a supply shortage

DOI: 10.1201/9781003126874-9

occurred due to the lockdown of the countries concerned. The impact has been enormous, and as of February 2021, the situation is unpredictable. In the second edition, this chapter was written by a US medical doctor and researchers.[5] In this third edition, the chapter is written by a team comprising a Japanese allergy specialist and dermatologist, two medical device examination and management officers from the Ministry of Health, Labour and Welfare (MHLW), and two researchers from the Medical Device Department of the Japanese National Institute of Health Sciences to provide an overview of Japan's current regulations and standards for dental gloves, infection control and glove use, and glove-related allergies, and product selection.

7.2   THE JAPANESE MEDICAL DEVICE REGULATORY SYSTEM

In Japan, the marketing of medical devices is regulated in accordance with the "Act on Securing Quality, Efficacy, and Safety of Pharmaceuticals, Medical Devices (Act No. 145, 1960)" (Pharmaceutical and Medical Device Act).[6] Medical devices are defined in the Pharmaceutical and Medical Device Act as devices and tools intended for use in the diagnosis, treatment, or prevention of diseases or to affect the structure or function of the body and fall under the order for enforcement of the Pharmaceutical and Medical Device Act. Devices and tools include a single program that operates on general-purpose equipment and a product that is a drug or regenerative medical product if used alone but becomes an integrated product when combined with a medical device (i.e., the machinery) and tool part of "combination products."

Medical devices defined in this manner are classified into highly controlled medical devices, controlled medical devices, and general medical devices according to the degree of risk arising from their failure (this will be explained later).

When business operators market medical devices in Japan, they need to follow one of the procedures of pharmaceutical affairs for the acquisition of approval or certification or notification for individual products depending on the class. In addition, before following these pharmaceutical affairs procedures, the license/registration must be obtained separately from the licensing authority for the marketing and manufacturing businesses related to the medical devices. Figure 7.1 shows

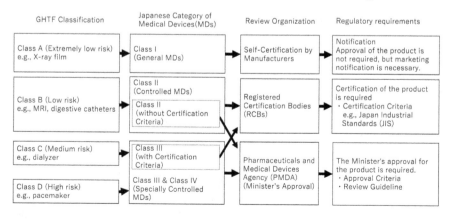

FIGURE 7.1   Medical device approval process.

the relationship between medical device classification and the license/registration required for marketing.

The type of license required for marketing medical devices differs depending on the type of medical device to be marketed. Type 1 medical device marketing business licenses are required for handling highly controlled medical devices; type 2 medical device marketing business licenses are required for handling controlled medical devices; and type 3 medical device marketing business licenses are required for handling general medical devices. Type 1 medical device marketing business operators may also market controlled medical devices and general medical devices, and type 2 medical device marketing business operators may also market general medical devices. Business operators must satisfy all of the following requirements to meet the license requirements for marketing medical devices: (1) the system for manufacturing and quality control shall comply with "The Ministerial Ordinance on Standards for System for Operations of Manufacturing Control and Quality Control for Medical Devices or In-Vitro Diagnostic Agents" (MHLW Ordinance No. 94 in 2014, hereinafter referred to as "QMS System Ordinance"); (2) the post-marketing safety control method shall comply with "The Ministerial Ordinance on Standards for Post-marketing Safety Control for Drugs, Quasi-Drugs, Cosmetics, Medical Devices, and Regenerative Medical Products" (MHLW Ordinance No. 135 in 2004, hereinafter referred to as "GVP Ministerial Ordinance"); (3) business operators must not be applicable for disqualification requirements; and (4) a general marketing manager, domestic quality operation manager, and safety control manager must be assigned.[7,8]

Manufacturers that manufacture medical devices must be registered at the licensing authority for each medical device manufacturing site. Registration must be obtained from the governor of the prefecture where the manufacturing site is located in Japan or from the Minister of Health, Labour, and Welfare in the case where it is located outside Japan. To be registered as a manufacturing site, the applicant needs to meet the requirements and must assign engineers responsible for the on-site control of medical device manufacturing at each manufacturing site. Qualification requirements are also specified for responsible engineers. If a medical device is a biological product, a biological product manufacturing manager who has been approved by the prefectural governor shall be assigned to each domestic manufacturing site handling the biological product for the on-site management of manufacturing. Various matters to be observed are specified for those registered as manufacturers (hereinafter referred to as "manufacturers"). First, the manufacturer of a medical device must adhere to the production management and quality management system (QMS) for medical devices conducted by the marketing authorization holder with approval or certification. Second, the responsible engineer assigned to the manufacturing site must manage and supervise the employees working at the manufacturing site; manage the buildings and equipment, medical devices, and other articles of the manufacturing site; and pay attention to avoid health and hygiene problems. In addition, the manufacturer must respect the opinions of the responsible engineers, which are important for them to fulfill their obligations at these manufacturing sites. The responsible engineer at the manufacturing site also has a duty to prepare and retain the manufacturing and testing records, as well as other management records of the relevant manufacturing site, for a certain period.

The procedures for the acquisition of approval, certification, and notification for individual products differ among manufacturing sites. Approval is an important stage in the licensing process for highly controlled or controlled medical devices. In this system, the Minister of Health, Labour, and Welfare confirms the efficacy and safety of medical devices and ensures that they are appropriate for use. The quality, efficacy, and safety of medical devices are also assured by the review of the Pharmaceuticals and Medical Devices Agency (PMDA) and the approval of the MHLW based on the documents submitted by the applicant. Certification is another stage of the licensing process for highly controlled medical devices and controlled medical devices in which the standards (hereinafter referred to as "certification standards") have been specified by the Minister of Health, Labour, and Welfare (hereinafter referred to as "designated highly controlled medical devices" and "designated controlled medical devices," respectively). The quality, efficacy, and safety of medical devices shall be assured through a review of the conformity with these certification standards confirmed by the third party, the Association of Registered Certification Bodies (ARCB), in a fair and neutral position. Notification is also a stage of the licensing process for general medical devices. Business operators submit a notification to the PMDA on the premise that the quality, efficacy, and safety of the medical devices to be marketed are self-guaranteed.

7.3 REGISTRATION AND APPROVAL

At the research and development stage of a medical device, an evaluation is performed to confirm the basic specifications of a medical device, physical efficacy on living tissue, and various safety levels through benchmark and nonclinical studies using animals. Subsequently, clinical trials and studies were conducted to evaluate the efficacy and safety from the perspective of medical positioning. Subsequently, an application for pharmaceutical approval is filed based on the "Act on Securing Quality, Efficacy, and Safety of Pharmaceuticals, Medical Devices (Act No. 145, 1960)" (Pharmaceuticals and Medical Device Act).[6] Medical devices are manufactured and marketed in our country after obtaining pharmaceutical approval.

For a new medical device to be launched in Japan, various evaluations of quality, efficacy, and safety need to be conducted. In general, the review of medical devices in Japan begins with a clinical background in which the applied product is designed and developed. In other words, it is important to examine the design and development of medical devices for clinical positioning. Based on clinical positioning, the results of nonclinical verification, such as a performance evaluation test or a benchmark test, determine whether the applied product can achieve the intended use and meet the clinical positioning as a medical device. If the results of nonclinical studies are not sufficient to determine whether a medical device can achieve its intended purpose, it is necessary to conduct evaluations through clinical studies or trials.

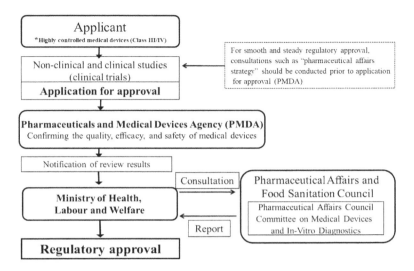

FIGURE 7.2 Flowchart of the regulatory approval process of medical devices.

The process from development to the approval of new medical devices in Japan is shown in Figure 7.2. The business operator who applies for a new medical device shall conduct nonclinical and clinical studies (including clinical trials) to evaluate the quality, efficacy, and safety to guarantee that the intended use of the medical device can be achieved. A consultation, such as a "pharmaceutical affairs strategy consultation," is conducted with the PMDA before filing an application for approval so that the application can be steadily and smoothly prepared. The application for approval will be submitted to the PMDA, which will confirm the quality, efficacy, and safety of the medical device. When the PMDA decides that the applied medical device has been cleared for approval as a result of the approval review, a notification of the review results will be submitted to the MHLW. In the case of new medical devices, the results of the review will be assessed by the Committee on Medical Devices and In-Vitro Diagnostics of the Pharmaceutical Affairs Council of the Pharmaceutical Affairs and Food Sanitation Council, which is the advisory organization of the Minister of Health, Labour, and Welfare. As a result, the Minister of Health, Labour, and Welfare will provide approval based on the report or the results of the consultation.

At the time of approval of all medical devices, including new medical devices, business operators are required to obtain a license from marketing authorization holders according to the type of medical device the business operator applied for. The manufacturing site of the medical device must be registered as a manufacturer.

After obtaining the necessary license and registration, an approval review is conducted for the applied medical device, and approval will be obtained if the product is effective.

Medical devices are not approved in the following cases: if the applied medical device is not considered to have the effectiveness or performance stated in the application in terms of quality, efficacy, and safety; if it is considered to have no value as a medical device because it has a significantly more harmful effect than the effectiveness or performance related to its application; or if its property or quality is considered significantly inappropriate for health and hygiene.

To determine whether or not the product has the effectiveness or performance stated in the application, an evaluation must be conducted to verify the intended use of the applied medical device. In addition, the balance between the effectiveness or performance related to the device's application and adverse effects is assessed by weighing the risks and benefits.

The evaluation indices are specified in Article 41, Paragraph 3 of the Pharmaceuticals and Medical Devices Act. These indices are the standards established by the Minister of Health, Labour, and Welfare based on the opinion of the Pharmaceutical Affairs and Food Sanitation Council to assure the properties, quality, and performance of medical devices. The standards established in the same article are specified in "the standards for medical devices defined by the Minister of Health, Labour, and Welfare in accordance with the provision of Article 41, Paragraph 3 of the Act for Ensuring the Quality, Efficacy, and Safety of Drugs and Medical Devices (MHLW Notification No. 122, dated March 29, 2005)" (hereinafter referred to as the "basic requirement standards").[9]

Currently, these basic requirements consist of 18 provisions. As representative items, requirements related to performance are specified in Article 6, and provisions related to risk management are specified in Articles 2 and 12.

In Article 2 of the basic requirement standards, marketing authorization holders involved in the design and manufacturing of medical devices are required to secure the safety of medical devices based on state-of-the-art technology. In cases where risk is required to be reduced from that perspective, marketing authorization holders shall manage risks such that the residual risks of each hazard are within the acceptable range. In this case, marketing authorization holders should perform the following roles in order and apply them to risk management: identify known or foreseeable hazards; evaluate risks caused by the intended use method and predictable improper use; eliminate risks as much as reasonably practicable through essential safety design and manufacturing, reduce the risks remaining after removal of risks by appropriate protective measures, and indicate remaining risks after removal. Article 6 of the basic requirements stipulates the contents related to the effectiveness of medical devices. All known or foreseeable risks and failures of the medical device should be reduced as much as reasonably practicable under the presumed conditions of use and must be acceptable when compared to the intended effectiveness of the relevant medical device.

If the medical device to be marketed conforms to the certification standards and does not fall under the category of a new medical device, certification shall be obtained through the certification review conducted by the registered certification body. A certification review of the registered certification body is performed by confirming that the following criteria are satisfied: (1) the business operator that filed the application has obtained a medical device marketing business license according to the type of medical device; (2) the manufacturing site that manufactures the medical device has been registered as a manufacturer; (3) the medical device related to the application conforms to the certification standards specified for the medical device; and (4) the method of manufacturing management/quality control of the medical device conforms to the QMS Ministerial Ordinance. The certification standards include the technical standards established by the Notification on Certification Standards (Notification No. 112 issued by the MHLW in 2005) and the standards for primary endpoints that should be evaluated for equivalence to existing products and comply with the Japanese Industrial Standards (JIS).[10] The medical device will not be subject to certification if the shape, structure, principle, method of use, and performance of the medical device are obviously different from those of the existing certified medical device.

7.4 MEDICAL DEVICE CLASSIFICATION

A diverse range of medical devices are subject to regulation in Japan, and their degree of influence on the human body is not fixed. For example, perspectives regarding the method of use, required performance, and degree of risk when a failure occurs are completely different between surgical scalpels and implantable cardiac pacemakers. From this perspective, medical devices are classified and regulated according to the degree of risk worldwide. Japan has a reasonable regulatory system that classifies the characteristics of individual medical devices into three major categories: "highly controlled medical devices," "controlled medical devices," and "general medical devices," as stipulated in the Pharmaceuticals and Medical Devices Act.

"Highly controlled medical devices" refer to those that may have a serious impact on human life and health if an adverse reaction or dysfunction occurs (critical risk) and require appropriate control accordingly. "Controlled medical devices" refer to those that may have an impact on human life and health if an adverse reaction or dysfunction occurs (middle risk) and require appropriate management accordingly. "General medical devices" refer to those that may have a minimal impact on human life and health if an adverse reaction or dysfunction occurs (low risk) and require appropriate control accordingly.

Considering the characteristics of medical devices, "generic names" are used to identify the product group of medical devices with similar risks and performance characteristics (MHLW Notification No. 298, 2004).[11] Generic names are specified for all medical devices, and "highly controlled medical devices," "controlled medical devices," or "general medical devices" are designated for each generic name.

The degree of risk of a medical device is determined for each generic name by classification according to the classification rules. The classification rules are divided into four classes: Class I (A), II (B), III (C), and IV (D), according to the classification rules established by the Global Harmonization Task Force (GHTF). Table 7.1 shows the relationship between the classification of highly controlled, controlled, and general medical devices and the classification of generic name medical devices according to the Pharmaceutical and Medical Device Act.[6]

TABLE 7.1

Classification, Approval, and License of Medical Devices

International Classification	Class I	Class II	Class III	Class IV
Classification of medical devices by risk approval/certification	General medical devices When a failure occurs, the risk to the human body is considered to be extremely low. For example, small items made of copper, and gloves for examination	Controlled medical devices When a failure occurs, the risk to the human body is considered to be relatively low. For example, MRI, CT, electronic sphygmomanometer, and surgical gloves	Highly controlled medical devices When a failure occurs, the risk to the human body is considered to be relatively high. For example, artificial joints, lithotripsy devices, dialyzers, catheters, and contact lenses	Highly controlled medical devices Highly invasive to patients. If a failure occurs, it may directly lead to a life-threatening condition. For example, cardiac pacemaker and stent
Approval, etc. of products	Notification	Third-party certification[a]	Third-party certification[a]	Approval by the minister[b]
Manufacturer	Registration (no category)			
Marketing authorization holder	Type 3 marketing business license	Type 2 marketing business license	Type 1 marketing business license	Type 1 marketing business license
Selling		—	Notification	License
Leasing				
Repairing	License (for each category)			

[a] In the system, the minister's approval is not required for those whose standards have been specified by the Minister of Health, Labour, and Welfare, and compliance with the standards is certified by a private third-party certification organization registered by the Minister of Health, Labour, and Welfare in advance. Note that approval is required for medical devices for which certification standards have not been established.

[b] Among Class 3 highly controlled medical devices, those for which certification standards have been established need to be certified by a third party.

MRI, magnetic resonance imaging; CT, computed tomography

7.5 SPECIFICATIONS OF GLOVES

The JIS are Japanese national standards that document specifications for domestic industrial products and their measurement methods.[11] There are various types of standards, such as those for manufacturing industrial products, including automobiles and electric appliances, information processing, character and program codes, and services. "Standards" are generally considered optional but become mandatory when cited in the laws and regulations. The significance of standardization of tangible and intangible goods, which will be diverse, complicated, and disorderly if left unattended, is to (1) ensure the convenience of economic and social activities such as securing interchangeability; (2) improve the efficiency of production (including mass production through the reduction of product types); (3) ensure fairness (such as safeguarding the interests of consumers and simplifying transactions); (4) promote technological progress (supporting the creation of new knowledge and development and spread of new technologies); (5) secure the safety and health of people; and (6) maintain the environment. Based on these perspectives, "standards" at the national level are established as technical documents and "unified" or "simplified" nationwide. These documents were published as the JIS.

Five JIS related to medical and dental gloves have been published: single-use surgical rubber gloves (JIS T 9107: 2018),[12] single-use dental rubber gloves (JIS T 9113: 2018),[13] single-use dental vinyl gloves (JIS T 9114: 2018),[14] single-use examination rubber gloves (JIS T 9115: 2018),[15] and single-use examination vinyl gloves (JIS T 9116: 2018) (Tables 7.2 and 7.3).[16] The basic document structures of the JIS T 9114: 2018 and JIS T 9116: 2018 are the same. The structures of other JIS are similar, but some parts are slightly different depending on the intended use and materials. Based on normative references, the JIS can be classified into three groups: JIS T 9107: 2018, JIS T 9113: 2018/JIS T 9115: 2018, and JIS T 9114: 2018/JIS T 9116: 2018 (Table 7.4). An outline of the major requirements of each JIS is as follows.

7.5.1 CLASSIFICATION

Single-use surgical, dental, and examination rubber gloves can be classified as either type 1 or 2. Type 1 gloves are mainly made from natural rubber latex, whereas those in type 2 are mainly made from nitrile, polychloroprene, polyisoprene, or styrene-butadiene rubber latex, styrene-butadiene rubber solution, or thermoplastic elastomer solution. Both single-use dental and examination vinyl gloves are composed of vinyl chloride resin.

The shapes of single-use surgical rubber gloves are classified into "shape S," with straight fingers, and "shape C," with curved fingers in the direction of the palm. Single-use dental rubber gloves and single-use dental and examination vinyl gloves are classified into "flat hand type" and "front finger type." The shape of single-use examination rubber gloves was not specified.

The surface finish is, regardless of the glove type, classified as "surface finishing T," in which either part or all of the surface is rough, and "surface finishing P," in which the entire surface is smooth. However, the JIS for single-use dental and examination vinyl gloves does not specify whether they are "T" or "P."

TABLE 7.2

Contents of the Japanese Industrial Standards (JIS) for Medical and Dental Grade Gloves

JIS T 9107: 2018	JIS T 9113: 2018	JIS T 9114: 2018	JIS T 9115: 2018	JIS T 9116: 2018
Single-use sterile surgical rubber gloves—specification	Single-use dental rubber gloves	Single-use dental PVC gloves	Single-use examination rubber gloves	Single-use examination PVC gloves
1. Scope	1. Scope of application	1. Scope of application	1. Scope of application	1. Scope of application
2. Normative references	2. Normative reference	2. Normative reference	2. Normative reference	2. Normative reference
3. Terms and definitions	3. Terms and definitions	3. Terms and definitions	3. Terms and definitions	3. Terms and definitions
4. Classification	4. Classification	4. Classification	4. Classification	4. Classification
4.1 Type	4.1 Types	4.1 Surface finish	4.1 Types	4.1 Surface finish
4.2 Design	4.2 Surface finish	4.2 Shape	4.2 Surface finish	4.2 Shape
4.3 Surface finish	4.3 Shape	5. Materials	5. Materials	5. Materials
5. Materials	5. Materials	5.1 Main materials	5.1 Main materials	5.1 Main materials
5.1 Main materials	5.1 Main materials	5.2 Secondary materials	5.2 Secondary materials	5.2 Secondary materials
5.2 Sub-materials	5.2 Secondary materials	6. Nominal, nominal number, and dimensions	6. Nominal, nominal number, and dimensions	6. Nominal, nominal number, and dimensions
5.3 Biological safety	6. Nominal, nominal number, and dimensions	7. Quality	7. Quality	7. Quality
6. Quality	7. Quality	7.1 Appearance	7.1 Appearance	7.1 Appearance
6.1 Size code and dimensions	7.1 Appearance	7.2 Water tightness (pinhole test)	7.2 Water tightness (pinhole test)	7.2 Water tightness (pinhole test)
6.2 Water tightness (pinhole test)	7.2 Water tightness (pinhole test)	7.3 Performance (tensile test)	7.3 Performance (tensile test)	7.3 Performance (tensile test)
6.3 Properties (tensile properties)	7.3 Performance (tensile test)	7.4 Residual powder	7.4 Water-soluble proteins	7.4 Residual powder

(Continued)

TABLE 7.2 (CONTINUED)

Contents of the Japanese Industrial Standards (JIS) for Medical and Dental Grade Gloves

JIS T 9107: 2018	JIS T 9113: 2018	JIS T 9114: 2018	JIS T 9115: 2018	JIS T 9116: 2018
6.4 Residual powder	7.4 Water-soluble proteins			
	7.5 Residual powder		7.5 Residual powder	
7. Sampling and selection of test pieces	8. Sampling and selection of test pieces	8. Sampling and selection of test pieces	8. Sampling and selection of test pieces	8. Sampling and selection of test pieces
8. Measurement and test methods	9. Measurement and test method	9. Measurement and test method	9. Measurement and test method	9. Measurement and test method
8.1 Measurement of dimensions	9.1 Measurement of dimensions	9.1 Measurement of dimensions	9.1 Measurement of dimensions	9.1 Measurement of dimensions
8.2 Water tightness test (pinhole test)	9.2 Water tightness (pinhole test)	9.2 Water tightness (pinhole test)	9.2 Water tightness (pinhole test)	9.2 Water tightness (pinhole test)
8.3 Properties test (tensile properties)	9.3 Performance (tensile test)	9.3 Performance (tensile test)	9.3 Performance (tensile test)	9.3 Performance (tensile test)
8.4 Residual powder test	9.4 Residual powder	9.4 Residual powder	9.4 Residual powder	9.4 Residual powder
9. Sterilization	10. Sterilization	10. Sterilization	10. Sterilization	10. Sterilization
10. Packaging	11. Packaging	11. Packaging	11. Packaging	11. Packaging
11. Marking	12. Labeling	12. Labeling	12. Labeling	12. Labeling
11.1 Body of gloves	12.1 Glove unit packaging	12.1 Glove unit packaging	12.1 Glove unit packaging	12.1 Glove unit packaging
11.2 Inner package of gloves		12.2 Glove multi-unit packing	12.2 Glove multi-unit packing	12.2 Glove multi-unit packing

(Continued)

TABLE 7.2 (CONTINUED)
Contents of the Japanese Industrial Standards (JIS) for Medical and Dental Grade Gloves

JIS T 9107: 2018	JIS T 9113: 2018	JIS T 9114: 2018	JIS T 9115: 2018	JIS T 9116: 2018
11.3 Unit package of gloves	12.2 Glove multi-unit packing			
11.4 Multi-unit package of gloves				
• Annex A (normative): Water tightness test (pinhole test)	*Annex A (specified): Water tightness test (pinhole test)	*Annex A (specified): Water tightness test (pinhole test)	*Annex A (specified): Water tightness test (pinhole test)	*Annex A (specified): Water tightness test (pinhole test)
• Bibliography	*Reference		*Reference	
• Annex JA (informative): Comparison table between the JIS and corresponding international standards	*Annex JA (reference): the JIS and corresponding international standards	*Annex JA (reference): the JIS and corresponding international standards	*Annex JA (reference): the JIS and corresponding international standards	*Annex JA (reference): the JIS and corresponding international standards
		*Commentary	*Commentary	*Commentary

TABLE 7.3

Scope of the Japanese Industrial Standards (JIS) for Medical and Dental Grade Gloves

JIS No.	JIS Name	Scope
JIS T 9107: 2018	Single-use sterile surgical rubber gloves—specification	Sterilized single-use style surgical rubber gloves used to protect patients and users from cross-infection during medical and dental surgeries
JIS T 9113: 2018	Single-use dental rubber gloves	Sterilized and unsterilized single-use dental rubber gloves used to protect patients and users from cross-infection when used for medical examinations, treatments, and procedures
JIS T 9114: 2018	Single-use dental PVC gloves	Sterilized and unsterilized single-use dental vinyl gloves used to protect patients and users from cross-infection when used for medical examinations, treatments, and procedures
JIS T 9115: 2018	Single-use examination rubber gloves	Sterilized and unsterilized single-use examination rubber gloves used to protect patients and users from cross-infection when used for treatments and procedures
JIS T 9116: 2018	Single-use examination PVC gloves	Sterilized and unsterilized single-use examination vinyl gloves used to protect patients and users from cross-infection when used for treatments and procedures

7.5.2 MATERIALS

The main materials are described in Section 7.1. Regardless of the glove type, if suitable surface-treating agents or polymer coatings are used as secondary materials to help users wear and remove gloves more easily, they are required to conform to the JIS T 0993-1: 2012. Moreover, when compounding agents, such as vulcanization accelerators and anti-aging agents, or coloring agents are used, they must be harmless to living bodies. Indeed, some people may suffer delayed allergic reactions to certain rubber compounding agents and need gloves coated with other compounding agents. Materials used as surface treatment agents must be harmless to living bodies and must be indicated if necessary. In addition, the JIS for single-use surgical, dental, and examination rubber gloves specify that the materials must be bioabsorbable if they are to be used as surface treatment agents.

For single-use surgical rubber gloves, their biological safety must be evaluated according to the JIS T 0993-1: 2012 (Table 3). The biological safety of water-soluble proteins, of which amounts in the gloves are specified for securing the quality of single-use dental and examination rubber gloves, must be evaluated as well. At the purchaser's request, marketing authorization holders must provide data that show compliance with biological safety standards. In the future, chemical safety may be specified for the limits of leached substances, such as water-soluble proteins, allergenic proteins, residual chemicals, and endotoxins. The measurement methods of

TABLE 7.4

List of Standards Cited in the Japanese Industrial Standards (JIS) for Medical and Dental Grade Gloves

Citation Standards	Standard Name	JIS T 9107: 2018 Single-Use Sterile Surgical Rubber Gloves—Specification	JIS T 9113: 2018 Single-Use Dental Rubber Gloves	JIS T 9114: 2018 Single-Use Dental PVC Gloves	JIS T 9115: 2018 Single-Use Examination Rubber Gloves	JIS T 9116: 2018 Single-Use Examination PVC Gloves
ISO 10282: 2014	Single-use sterile rubber surgical gloves—specification	○				
ISO 11193-1: 2008 and Amendment 1: 2012	Single-use medical examination gloves—Part 1: Specification for gloves made from rubber latex or rubber solution		○		○	
ISO 11193-2: 2006	Single-use medical examination gloves—Part 2: Specification for gloves made from poly(vinyl chloride)			○		○
ISO 21171: 2006	Medical gloves: Determination of removable surface powder	○	○	○	○	○
JIS K 6250: 2006	Rubber: General procedures for preparing and conditioning test pieces for physical test methods	○	○	○	○	○
JIS K 6251: 2017	Rubber, vulcanized or thermoplastic—Determination of tensile stress-strain properties	○	○	○	○	○
JIS K 6257: 2010	Rubber, vulcanized or thermoplastic—Determination of heat aging properties	○	○	○	○	○

(Continued)

TABLE 7.4 (CONTINUED)

List of Standards Cited in the Japanese Industrial Standards (JIS) for Medical and Dental Grade Gloves

Citation Standards	Standard Name	JIS T 9107: 2018 Single-Use Sterile Surgical Rubber Gloves—Specification	JIS T 9113: 2018 Single-Use Dental Rubber Gloves	JIS T 9114: 2018 Single-Use Dental PVC Gloves	JIS T 9115: 2018 Single-Use Examination Rubber Gloves	JIS T 9116: 2018 Single-Use Examination PVC Gloves
JIS T 0307: 2004	Medical devices—Symbols to be used with medical device labels, labelling and information to be supplied	○	○	○	○	○
JIS T 0993-1: 2012	Biological evaluation of medical devices—Part 1: Evaluation and testing within a risk management process	○	○	○	○	○
JIS Z 9015-1: 2006	Sampling procedures for inspection by attributes—Part 1: Sampling schemes indexed by acceptance quality limit (AQL) for lot-by-lot inspection	○	○	○	○	○
Reference standards						
ISO 12243	Medical gloves made from natural rubber latex—Determination of water-extractable protein using the modified Lowry method	○	○		○	
JIS T 9010	Safest methods relevant to biological safety of rubber products	○	○		○	

(Continued)

TABLE 7.4 (CONTINUED)

List of Standards Cited in the Japanese Industrial Standards (JIS) for Medical and Dental Grade Gloves

Citation Standards	Standard Name	JIS T 9107: 2018 Single-Use Sterile Surgical Rubber Gloves—Specification	JIS T 9113: 2018 Single-Use Dental Rubber Gloves	JIS T 9114: 2018 Single-Use Dental PVC Gloves	JIS T 9115: 2018 Single-Use Examination Rubber Gloves	JIS T 9116: 2018 Single-Use Examination PVC Gloves
JIS T 0806-1: 2015	Sterilization of healthcare products—Radiation—Part 1: Requirements for development, validation, and routine control of a sterilization process for medical devices	O	O	O	O	O
JIS T 0806-2: 2014	Sterilization of healthcare products—Radiation—Part 2: Establishing the sterilization dose	O	O	O	O	
JIS T 0806-3: 2010	Sterilization of healthcare products—Radiation—Part 3: Guidance on dosimetric aspects	O	O	O	O	

water-soluble proteins are described in the JIS T 9010,[17] Section 3.6 "Water-soluble proteins," and International Organization for Standardization (ISO)12243.[18]

7.5.3   Nominal, Nominal Numbers, and Dimensions

There are ten types of single-use surgical rubber gloves, in which types 5–9.5 (intervals of 0.5) are defined as "nominal," and the width of the palm part, minimum total length, and minimum thickness are specified as the dimensions. There are another five types, including SS, S, M, L, and LL, which are defined as "nominal" for other gloves. The items regarding the dimensions are only for single-use surgical rubber gloves. The "nominal number" is designated for single-use dental rubber and vinyl gloves.

7.5.4   Quality

Regardless of their type, a visual inspection and inspection of water tightness using the pinhole test are required to assess glove quality. The acceptable level of residual powder on the finished product is ≤2 mg per glove. The minimum values of tensile strength and elongation at breaking point before and after accelerated aging are specified for the acceptable performance levels of each glove (Table 7.5). Table 7.6 shows the inspection levels and acceptable quality levels for the dimensions (width, total length, and thickness), water tightness, and tensile strength and elongation at the breaking point.

7.5.5   Other Items

Thermoplastic elastomers (single-use surgical, dental, and examination rubber gloves), PVC resins, and plasticizers (single-use dental and examination vinyl gloves) are defined using relevant standards. The methods of sampling and selection of the test pieces for each test and the implementation methods of dimension measurement and each test are also specified in the standards. The water tightness test (pinhole test) is described in detail in Annex A (normative) of all five standards. In addition, items relating to sterilization treatment, packaging, and indications are described, and a table showing the comparisons between the JIS and corresponding international standards is included in Annex JA (reference) of the standards as well.[12–16]

7.6   QUALITY MANAGEMENT SYSTEM FOR GLOVES AS MEDICAL DEVICES

Marketing authorization holders of medical devices, including medical and dental gloves, needs to establish a quality management system (QMS) for manufacturing process management and quality assurance.

A QMS manages and supervises manufacturing processes to ensure the quality of products by specifying the company's rules and procedures. QMS applies to all processes, from quality assessment at the time of acceptance of raw materials to the

TABLE 7.5

Tensile Properties and the Test Methods Established by the Japanese Industrial Standards (JIS) for Medical and Dental Grade Gloves

JIS No.	JIS T 9107: 2018			JIS T 9113: 2018			JIS T 9114: 2018		JIS T 9115: 2018			JIS T 9116: 2018	
JIS Name	Single-Use Sterile Surgical Rubber Gloves—Specification			Single-Use Dental Rubber Gloves			Single-Use Dental PVC Gloves		Single-Use Examination Rubber Gloves			Single-Use PVC Gloves for Dentistry	
Test Items/Performance, Conditions, and Methods	Type 1 Performance	Type 2 Performance	Conditions/Methods	Type 1 Performance	Type 2 Performance	Conditions/Methods	Performance	Conditions/Methods	Type 1 Performance	Type 2 Performance	Conditions/Methods	Performance	Conditions/Methods
Before accelerated aging													
Tensile strength at breaking point (Mpa)	≥12.5	≥9.0	JIS K 6250: 2006	≥21	≥15	JIS K 6250: 2006ᵇ	≥8	JIS K 6250: 2006ᶜ	≥21	≥15	JIS K 6250: 2006ᵇ	≥8	JIS K 6250: 2006ᶜ
Elongation at breaking point (%)	≥700 / ≤3.0	≥600 / ≥2.0	JIS K 6251: 2017	≥700	≥500	JIS K 6251: 2017ᵇ	≥350	JIS K 6251: 2017ᶜ	≥700	≥500	JIS K 6251: 2017ᵇ	≥300	JIS K 6251: 2017ᶜ
After accelerated aging													
Tensile strength at breaking point (Mpa)	≥9.5	≥9.0	JIS K 6250: 2006	≥16	≥11	JIS K 6250: 2006	≥8	JIS K 6250: 2006	≥16	≥11	JIS K 6250: 2006	≥8	JIS K 6250: 2006
Elongation at breaking point (%)	≥550	≥500	JIS K 6251: 2017	≥500	≥450	JIS K 6251: 2017	≥350	JIS K 6251: 2017	≥500	≥450	JIS K 6251: 2017	≥300	JIS K 6251: 2017
			JIS K 6257: 2010ᵃ			JIS K 6257: 2010ᵃ		JIS K 6257: 2010ᵈ			JIS K 6257: 2010ᵃ		JIS K 6257: 2010ᵈ

ᵃ 70°C±2°C, 168 h±2 h.
ᵇ Tensile speed 500 mm/min.
ᶜ Tensile speed 200 mm/min.
ᵈ 70°C±2°C, 72 h±2 h.

TABLE 7.6

Properties and the Test Methods Established by the Japanese Industrial Standards (JIS) for Medical and Dental Grade Gloves

JIS No.	JIS T 9107: 2018		JIS T 9113: 2018		JIS T 9114: 2018		JIS T 9115: 2018		JIS T 9116: 2018	
JIS Name	Single-Use Sterile Surgical Rubber Gloves—Specification		Single-Use Dental Rubber Gloves		Single-Use Dental PVC Gloves		Single-Use Examination Rubber Gloves		Single-Use Examination PVC Gloves	
Item/ Inspection Level/ Acceptable Quality Level	Testing Level	Acceptable Quality Level	Testing Level	Acceptable Quality Level	Testing Level	Acceptable Quality Level	Testing Level	Acceptable Quality Level	Testing Level	Acceptable Quality Level
Dimensions (width, total length, and thickness)	S-2	4.0	S-2	4.0	S-2	4.0	S-2	4.0	S-2	4.0
Water tightness (pinhole)	G-1	1.5	G-1	2.5	G-1	2.5	G-1	2.5	G-1	2.5
Tensile strength and elongation at breaking point*	S-2	4.0	S-2	4.0	S-2	4.0	S-2	4.0	S-2	4.0

* Before and after accelerated aging.

release of final products. Specifically, a QMS is necessary to ensure a certain level of product quality by establishing an organizational system and various rules to be observed in the manufacturing process and compliance with them as a company. Therefore, marketing authorization holders are required to undergo a compliance inspection to confirm compliance with the requirements of the "Ministerial Ordinance on Standards for Manufacturing Control and Quality Control for Medical Devices and In-Vitro Diagnostic Reagents (QMS Ministerial Ordinance)" (December 17, 2004; MHLW Ministerial Ordinance No. 169) before obtaining approval or certification for their products.[19] QMS compliance inspections of products to be approved and certified are conducted by the PMDA and registered certification bodies, respectively. In addition, marketing authorization holders are required to undergo a QMS compliance inspection of the product every five years after obtaining approval or certification.

In association with the revision of the Pharmaceutical Affairs Act and the QMS Ordinance in 2014,[6] employees of the manufacturing site and marketing authorization holder are required to work on the establishment of the QMS. The current QMS Ministerial Ordinance is a standard consisting of six chapters on the organization, documentation, and operation processes. The contents of ISO 13485: 2003 ("Medical devices: QMS—Requirements for regulatory purposes"), an international standard developed by the ISO, are included in chapter 2 of the current QMS Ministerial Ordinance. However, it should be noted that the QMS requirements in Japan are not identical to those of the ISO standards, since the sections in this chapter describe additional requirements that are specific to our country. The QMS compliance inspection is conducted for each product group in association with the revision of the QMS Ministerial Ordinance. Accordingly, the QMS compliance inspection can be omitted when manufacturing processes, for which QMS compliance has been confirmed, are used for new products belonging to the previously approved product group at the time of approval or certification. Thus, the system was rationalized. "The Ministerial Ordinance on Standards for System for Operations of Manufacturing Control and Quality Control for Medical Devices or In-Vitro Diagnostics (Ministerial Ordinance on QMS System)" (Aug 6, 2014: Ministerial Ordinance No. 94 of MHLW), which specifies a system for the operation of the QMS Ministerial Ordinance by marketing authorization holders, was also newly issued. Compliance with the Ministerial Ordinance for QMS System became a requirement for all marketing authorization holders of medical devices, irrespective of their classification, and it was decided that inspections and reviews should be conducted by the division in charge in each prefecture. Currently, the QMS Ministerial Ordinance has been revised in 2021, of which Chapter 2 includes the contents of ISO 13485:2016, and enforced from 2022.

In Japan, surgical rubber gloves used in medical and dental fields are classified as Class 2 medical devices and are certified product items; thus, certification standards for marketing have been established. These certification standards require that the QMS established by the marketing authorization holder complies with the QMS Ministerial Ordinance, and therefore, it must undergo a QMS compliance inspection.

For Class 1 medical devices, only the products designated by the Minister of Health, Labour, and Welfare in the notification are subjected to QMS compliance inspection. Because rubber gloves for examination are not subject to the relevant notification, they do not need to undergo QMS compliance inspection at the time of notification; however, the establishment of a QMS is essential to ensure the quality of medical devices. It should be noted that when these gloves are manufactured and marketed through the sterilization process, QMS compliance inspection is required even for Class 1 products.

7.7 INSURANCE REIMBURSEMENT SYSTEM FOR MEDICAL DEVICES

The sales prices of medical devices depend on insurance and distribution systems; therefore, the situation differs by country and region. There are two types of medical devices sold under the Japanese insurance system: products in which the reimbursement prices are determined as part of the "technical fees" of doctors and other healthcare practitioners and "special treatment medical materials," in which the reimbursement prices are determined individually. Based on this framework, marketing authorization holders of medical devices set list prices and determine the selling price by negotiating with hospitals. The MHLW revises the reimbursement prices every two years based on the results of a market price survey.

The reimbursement prices of expensive implanted devices, such as pacemakers, implantable defibrillators, and stents, are individually determined as special treatment medical materials. Medical devices can also be applied to the C category, in which new reimbursement prices are determined because of their high novelty. However, many of these devices are usually classified into existing categories of medical devices with similar functions for which reimbursement prices have already been fixed in the current system. Thus, it is difficult for medical devices to achieve high reimbursement prices only because of their novelty. In contrast, the prices of drugs are examined for each new drug and determined with additional premiums to those of existing drugs, which differs largely from the system used for medical devices.

7.8 INFECTION CONTROL AND GLOVE USE

The major academic societies on infectious diseases in Japan are the Japanese Society for Infectious Diseases and the Japanese Society for Infection Control and Prevention. The former was established in 1926 and has 10,985 members as of February 2019, with medical doctors accounting for 80% of the members and focusing on infectious disease treatment. They established an infectious disease specialist certification system in 1998 and certified 1,500 specialists.[20] The latter was established in 1986 and has 9,500 members as of April 2019. It consists of various medical professionals such as medical doctors, nurses, pharmacists, and clinical laboratory engineers and is an academic society that focuses on nosocomial and environmental infection control. In 1990, Japan's first nosocomial infection control guideline, the "Hospital Infection Prevention Guideline," was published, and in 2001, the "Hospital Infection Control Manual" was published to conduct research and promote education on infection control. The Society established the ISO/TC304 National Deliberation Committee in 2018 to facilitate international cooperation. [21]

Regarding the use of gloves in infection control, the US CDC published the Standard Precautions Guidelines for the first time in 1987 and issued the Isolation Precautions Guidelines in 2007.[22,23] The WHO also stated in the 2004 Practical Guidelines for Infection Control in Health Care Facilities that medical and dental gloves are the basic PPE for infection prevention, and the WHO's standard precautions include the presence or absence of infectious diseases. Regardless, it is essential to protect healthcare workers from infections caused by infectious agents, blood, and bodily substances.[3]

In Japan, with the enforcement of the partial amendment of the Medical Law in April 2007, the managers of hospitals, clinics, and midwifery centers are responsible for ensuring medical safety, such as nosocomial infection control; thus, a committee on nosocomial infection control has been established. Staff members such as facility managers, nursing departments, pharmaceutical departments, testing departments, and doctors specializing in infection control should be assigned as members of the committee and meetings should be held monthly, and facilities should be held. Administrators have been encouraged to organize an infection control team (ICT) to carry out daily activities related to nosocomial infection control.[24] Because of the revision of medical fees in the 2006 fiscal year, if no nosocomial infection prevention measures are implemented, the calculation of the basic hospitalization fee will not be permitted, and the facility standard for adding medical safety measures must be the assignment of a full-time nosocomial infection manager. In-hospital infection control has been promoted in medical institutions nationwide.[25] In 2011, "In-hospital measures at medical institutions" were issued, and details of nosocomial infection measures were described.[4] Among them, the following statements were issued to thoroughly implement standard precautions: "All moist biomaterials should be treated as infectious. Wear new gloves when touching moist biomaterials, mucous membranes, and wounds." In addition, wearing gloves as a preventive measure for each infection route was described.[4] Since 2006, due to the ICT, infection control certified nurse system,[26] placement of full-time infection control doctors, and dissemination of infectious disease control knowledge measures against infection control have definitely improved in terms of legal compliance in Japanese medical facilities.

As of February 2021, the third wave of the COVID-19 pandemic hit Japan, and a state of emergency was declared in ten cities. As the demand for PPE increases in the medical field, the need for the domestic production of PPE is recognized again in Japan.

7.9 GLOVE-RELATED ALLERGY AND PRODUCT SELECTION

As of the end of 2018, the supply of powdered medical gloves was banned in Japan.[27] According to MHLW statistics, the number of surgical gloves sold in Japan in 2019 was 68 million pairs made of natural rubber (powder-free) and 32 million pairs made of nonnatural rubber (synthetic rubber), while the number of examination gloves sold

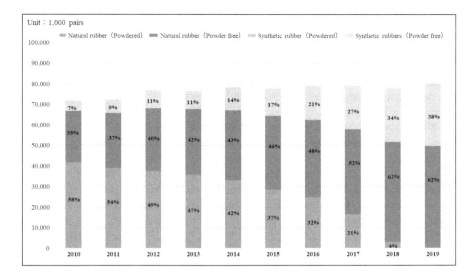

FIGURE 7.3 Domestic sales volumes of surgical gloves in Japan (2010–2019). Adapted from Japanese Nursing Association. Infection Control Certified Nurse System.[29]

was 338 million pairs made of natural rubber (powder-free) and 3,553 million made of nonnatural rubber (synthetic rubber).[28] Five companies belonging to the Japan Glove Manufacturers Association supplied 80% of the surgical rubber gloves sold in Japan. Looking at the number of sales from 2010 to 2019 by type, in 2010, 58% of all gloves were natural rubber gloves with powder, 35% were powder-free natural rubber gloves, and 7% were synthetic rubber gloves; whereas in 2019, 62% were powder-free natural rubber gloves and 38% were synthetic rubber gloves (Figure 7.3).[29] In recent years, the number of gloves made of synthetic rubber has been increasing, even for surgery, and 91% of gloves for inspection/examination are made of synthetic rubber. [28]

Allergies related to medical and dental gloves include latex allergy (LA), which is a type I (immediate-type) allergy, and type IV (delayed-type) allergy due to rubber-related chemicals.[30,31]

In Japan, in 1992, Shono et al. reported the first LA case with household NRL gloves that occurred in a housewife with atopic dermatitis.[32] Since then, the number of patients has increased, and multiple cases of anaphylaxis have been reported. Therefore, in 1996, the "Japanese Society of Latex Allergy" was established to perform case studies and epidemiological surveys and develop countermeasures. In 1999, the MHLW established guidelines for labeling medical NRL products,[33] and, at the end of 2018, it was decided that all medical gloves, including NRL, would be powder-free.[27]

In Japan, as a result of the 2003 LA epidemiological survey of 1512 healthcare workers (HCWs) at Fujita Health University Hospital, which was confirmed by a questionnaire survey and prick test, 3.3% (44 people) of workers were affected by LA.[34] In 2000, all NRL gloves in the hospital were made powder-free, and the HCWs with LA solely wore synthetic rubber gloves for both surgery and examination to avoid NRL contact in other situations. All 16 HCWs who were able to follow up continued to work, and latex-specific IgE antibodies were found to have decreased in 80% of them.[35] Since 2001, no HCWs have newly developed LA.

In the last five years, except for only one 19-year-old female nursing student with contact urticaria due to NRL gloves, no HCWs who have experienced anaphylaxis from NRL gloves have been reported. However, several cases of anaphylaxis due to LA have recently been reported in the medical field.[36–38] Since medical gloves have become powder-free, it is expected that there will be almost no new occurrences of LA among HCWs. However, LA measures for already sensitized individuals in healthcare settings, especially pediatric patients who have undergone frequent surgery, will continue to be an important and basic issue of medical safety.

The definitive diagnosis of LA is based on clinical symptoms and a prick test using NRL rubber glove extracts. Hevein b 6.02 is the main antigen of NRL gloves, and the Hev b 6.02-specific IgE antibody test, which has been covered by insurance since 2016, is now a useful test for LA diagnosis.[39] Hevein is included in class I chitinases of chestnut, avocado, and banana and is the responsible antigen that cross-reacts with these fruits and causes latex-fruit syndromes.[40]

Conversely, both medical NRL and synthetic rubber gloves, such as nitrile rubber, are treated with chemical substances such as vulcanization accelerators and anti-aging agents; if these residual contents are high, delayed-type allergies may develop.[30] When such a chemical comes into contact with the skin of an individual who has been sensitized again, it can cause symptoms such as erythema, infiltration, and vesicles with itching. In other words, allergic contact dermatitis occurs. A patch test with rubber-related chemicals conducted with the Japanese baseline series on 1,360 patients showed positive rates of 6.3%, 4.3%, 1.3%, 1.3%, and 1.0% to carba mix, thiuram mix, black rubber mix, mercapto mix, and mercaptobenzo-thiazole, respectively. It has been noted that the positive rate of carba mix containing 1,3-diphenyl guanidine is also high.[41]

The Japanese Society of LA, which was established in 1996, created the "LA Safety Measures Guidelines" in 2006,[42] and in the same year, a commentary with illustrations and photographs of "All about LA" was published in accordance with the guidelines.[43] A second edition of the guidelines was published in 2009,[44] the third edition in 2013,[28] and the fourth edition in 2018.[30] From the third edition, it has become a guideline, "including delayed allergies caused by chemical substances," such as latex-free medical equipment and synthetic rubber gloves that do not contain vulcanization accelerators.[30,45]

REFERENCES

1. Japanese Government. 2021. Population and population pyramid. Statistics of Japan. e-Stat. https://dashboard.e-stat.go.jp/en/ (in Japanese).
2. Emergo by UL Global Headquarters. 2021. JAPAN – Overview of medical device industry and healthcare statistics. https://www.emergobyul.com/jp/resources/market -japan (in Japanese).

3. WHO. 2004. Practical guidelines for infection control in health care facilities. SEARO Regional Publication No.41: 10–15.
4. MHLW. 2011. Nosocomial infections in medical institutions, etc. Medical Administration Directive 0617 No. 1 (in Japanese).
5. Hamann, C.P., Rogers, P.A., and Sullivan, K.M. 2005. Japanese regulations and standards for medical and dental grade gloves. In *Protective Gloves for Occupational Use*, 2nd ed., Boman, A., Estlander, T., Wahlberg, J.E., and Maibach, H.I., Eds. Washington, DC: CRC Press, 43–69.
6. Act No. 145. 1960. Act on securing quality, efficacy, and safety of pharmaceuticals, medical devices. Available at: https://www.mhlw.go.jp/web/t_doc?dataId=81004000&dataType=0&pageNo=1 (in Japanese).
7. MHLW. 2014. The ministerial ordinance on standards for system for operations of manufacturing control and quality control for medical devices or in vitro diagnostic agents. MHLW Ordinance No. 94. Available at: https://www.mhlw.go.jp/web/t_doc?dataId=81ab4198&dataType=0&pageNo=1 (in Japanese).
8. MHLW. 2004. The ministerial ordinance on standards for post-marketing safety control for drugs, quasi-drugs, cosmetics, medical devices, and regenerative medical products. MHLW Ordinance No. 135. Available at: https://www.mhlw.go.jp/web/t_doc?dataId=81aa6391&dataType=0&pageNo=1 (in Japanese).
9. MHLW. 2005. The standards for medical devices defined by the Minister of Health, Labour and Welfare in accordance with the provision of article 41, paragraph 3 of the act for ensuring the quality, efficacy, and safety of drugs and medical devices. MHLW Notification No. 122. Available at: https://www.mhlw.go.jp/web/t_doc?dataId=81004000&dataType=0 (in Japanese).
10. MHLW. 2005. The notification on certification standards, no. 112. Available at: https://www.mhlw.go.jp/web/t_doc_keyword?keyword=112&dataId=81aa6906&dataType=0&pageNo=1&mode=0 (in Japanese).
11. MHLW. 2004. MHLW notification no. 298. Available at: https://www.hapi.or.jp/documentation/yakuji/pdf/620.pdf (in Japanese).
12. Japanese Standards Association and Japan Globe Manufactures Association. 2018. JIS T 9107:2018. Single-use sterile rubber surgical gloves – specification. Japanese Standards Association, Tokyo, Japan, 1–16.
13. Japanese Standards Association and Japan Globe Manufactures Association. 2018. JIS T 9113:2018. Single-use rubber gloves for dentistry. Japanese Standards Association, Tokyo, Japan, 1–16.
14. Japanese Standards Association and Japan Globe Manufactures Association. 2018. JIS T 9114:2018. Single-use polyvinyl chloride gloves for dentistry. Japanese Standards Association, Tokyo, Japan, 1–14.
15. Japanese Standards Association and Japan Globe Manufactures Association. 2018. JIS T 9115:2018. Single-use rubber examination gloves. Japanese Standards Association, Tokyo, Japan, 1–16.
16. Japanese Standards Association and Japan Globe Manufactures Association. 2018. JIS T 9116:2018. Single-use polyvinyl chloride gloves for dentistry. Japanese Standards Association, Tokyo, Japan, 1–14.
17. Japanese Standards Association and Japan Globe Manufactures Association. 2020. JIS T 9010:1999. JIS T 9010:1999. Test methods relevant to biological safety of rubber products. Japanese Standards Association, Tokyo, Japan, 1–40.
18. Japanese Standards Association and Japan Globe Manufactures Association. 2003. ISO 12243:2003. Medical gloves made from natural rubber latex -- Determination of water-extractable protein using the modified Lowry method. Japanese Standards Association, Tokyo, Japan, 1–17.

19. MHLW. 2004. Ministerial ordinance on standards for manufacturing control and quality control for medical devices and in-vitro diagnostic reagents (QMS Ministerial Ordinance). Ministerial Ordinance No. 169. Available at: https://www.mhlw.go.jp/web /t_doc?dataId=81aa6618&dataType=0&pageNo=1 (in Japanese).

20. Tateda, K. 2019. Message from the president of the Japanese Society for Infectious Diseases. Available at: https://www.kansensho.or.jp/modules/about/index.php?content _id=2 (in Japanese).

21. Yoshida, M. 2019. Message from the president of the Japanese Society for Infection Prevention and Control. Available at: http://www.kankyokansen.org/modules/english/ index.php?content_id=1 (in Japanese).

22. CDC. 2003. Recommendations for prevention of HIV transmission in health-care settings. *MMWR* 1987 (6 Suppl. 2S), 3S–18S.

23. Siegel, J.D., Rhinehart, E., Jackson, M., and Chiarello, L. 2007. CDC. The Healthcare Infection Control Practices Advisory Committee. Guideline for isolation precautions: Preventing transmission of infectious agents in healthcare settings. 48–51. Available at: https://www.cdc.gov/infectioncontrol/pdf/guidelines/isolation-guidelines-H.pdf.

24. MHLW. 2007. Regarding the partial enforcement of the Medical Care Act, etc. to establish a system to provide high-quality medical care. Medical Administration Instruction No. 0330010 (in Japanese).

25. MHLW. 2006. Regarding facility standards for basic medical fees and the handling of procedures related to their notification. Nihon Medical No. 0306002. Available at: https://nintei.nurse.or.jp/nursing/qualification/kansencn (in Japanese).

26. MHLW. 2016. Handling of medical gloves with powder. Yakusei Anshin No. 1227 No. 1. Available at: https://www.pmda.go.jp/files/000215576.pdf (in Japanese).

27. MHLW. 2020. Production / import / shipment / inventory quantity by general name of medical equipment. Reiwa 1st year Pharmaceutical Affairs Industry Production Dynamics Statistics Annual Report Statistical Table, Table 16. https://www.mhlw.go.jp /topics/yakuji/2019/nenpo/toukeihyou.html (in Japanese).

28. Japan Glove Industry Association. 2021. Surgical gloves domestic sales volumes 2010– 2019 statistical data. Unpublished.

29. Japanese Nursing Association. 2021. Infection control certified nurse system. Available at: https://nintei.nurse.or.jp/nursing/qualification/probation_guide_cns.

30. Japanese Society of Latex Allergy: Latex Allergy Safety Measures Guideline Development Committee. 2018. *Latex Allergy Safety Measures Guidelines 2018-Including Delayed-Type Allergies Due to Chemical Substances*. Tokyo: Kyowa Kikaku Ltd. (in Japanese).

31. Kevin, K.J., and Sussman, G. 2017. Latex allergy: Where are we now and how did we get there? *J Allergy Clin Immunol Pract* 5:1212–1216.

32. Shono, M., and Maruyama, R. 1993. Contact urticaria from latex. *Jpn. J. Dermatoallergol* 1:37–43 (in Japanese).

33. Pharmacovigilance Bureau, Ministry of Health and Welfare, Japan. 1999. About natural rubber allergy, Pharmacovigilance Information No 153, 2. Available at: https://www.pmda .go.jp/safety/info-services/drugs/calling-attention/safety-info/0088.html#6 (in Japanese).

34. Kano, H., Yagami, A., Suzuki, K., Akita, H., Akamatsu, H., Matsunaga, K., and Ono, Y. 2014. Survey of awareness and current state of latex allergy among all health care workers at a university hospital. *Arerugi* 56:659–668 (in Japanese).

35. Yagami, A., Suzuki, K., Kano, H., and Matsunaga, K. 2006. Follow-up study of latex-allergic health care workers in Japan. *Allergol Int* 55:321–327.

36. Sugimoto, M., Ono, A., Yada, K., Mori, H., Ishibashi, H., and Kagami, S. 2018. Manifestation of intraoperative anaphylactic shock along with latex allergy: a pediatric case report. *J Med Invest* 65:292–295.

37. Shibuya, N., Ishizuka, M., Nagata, H., Iwasaki, Y., Takagi, K., Aoki, T., and Kubota, K. 2016. A case of anaphylactic shock due to latex allergy in a patient undergoing elective laparoscopy-assisted sigmoidectomy for sigmoid colon volvulus. *Nihon Gekakei Rengo Gakkaishi* 41:75–81 (in Japanese).

38. Mihara, Y., Suzuki, M., Kimura, H., Akasu, G., Hamada, N., and Shinozaki, K. 2015. Intraoperative anaphylactic shock caused by latex allergy potentially due to sensitization to a tattoo-a case report. *J Jpn Surg Assoc* 76:1801–1806 (in Japanese).

39. Yagami, A., Suzuki, K., Saito, H., and Matsunaga, K. 2009. Hev b 6.02 is the most important allergen in health care workers sensitized occupationally by natural rubber latex gloves. *Allergol Int* 58:347–355.

40. Yagami, T. 2002. Allergies to cross-reactive plant proteins. Latex-fruit syndrome is comparable with pollen-food allergy syndrome. *Int Arch Allergy Immunol* 128:271–279.

41. Matsunaga, K. 2019. Algorithm for contact dermatitis diagnosis. In *Contact Dermatitis and Patch Test*, K. Matsunaga, Ed. Tokyo: Gakken Medical Shujunsha Co., Ltd., 40–48 (in Japanese).

42. Japanese Society of Latex Allergy: Latex Allergy Safety Measures Guideline Development Committee. 2006. *Latex Allergy Safety Measures Guidelines 2006.* Tokyo: Japan Latex Allergy Study Group.

43. Matsunaga, K. 2006. *All about Latex Allergy.* Tokyo: Shujunsha Ltd. (in Japanese).

44. Japanese Society of Latex Allergy: Latex Allergy Safety Measures Guideline Development Committee. 2009. *Latex Allergy Safety Measures Guidelines 2009.* Japan Latex Allergy Study Group Latex Allergy Safety Measures Guideline Development Committee. 2009. Latex Allergy Safety Measures Guidelines 2009, T Tokyo: Kyowa Kikaku Ltd. (in Japanese).

45. Japanese Society of Latex Allergy: Latex Allergy Safety Measures Guideline Development Committee. 2013. *Latex Allergy Safety Measures Guidelines 2013-Including Delayed-Type Allergies Due to Chemical Substances.* Tokyo: Kyowa Kikaku Ltd. (in Japanese).

8 Australian Standards for Protective Gloves

D.L. McGeachie and R.L. Nixon

CONTENTS

8.1 INTRODUCTION

After the industrial revolution, occupational injuries resulted in significant morbidity and mortality among workers. By the end of the nineteenth century, the merits of standardization were recognized and became a national priority. In 1922, the Australian Commonwealth Engineering Standards Association was founded, and today this company is known as Standards Australia International Limited. It was a founding member of the International Organisation for Standardisation (ISO), established in 1947, and in 1950 received a Royal Charter to develop standards of national interest.[1]

The first generalized "all occupation" document relating to glove standards in Australia was "*AS Z4 – Specification for Industrial Leather Gloves and Mittens*," released in 1952. Since the humble beginnings of *AS Z4*, the Australian and New Zealand standards on occupational protective gloves have evolved into AS/NZS 2161, which comprises ten individual components maintained by three discrete steering committees:

Part 1.   Selection, use, and maintenance[2]
Part 2.   General requirements and test methods[3]
Part 3.   Protection against mechanical risks[4]
Part 4.   Protection against thermal risks (heat and fire)[5]
Part 5.   Protection against cold[6]
Part 6.   Protective gloves for structural firefighting—laboratory test methods and performance requirements[7]
Part 7.   Protection against cuts and stabs by hand knives[8–10]
Part 8.   Protection against ionizing radiation and radioactive contamination[11]
Part 9.   Method of measurement and evaluation of the vibration transmissibility of gloves at the palm of the hand[12]
Part 10.   Protective gloves against chemicals and micro-organisms[13–15]

DOI: 10.1201/9781003126874-10

There are three additional occupation-specific glove standards. Dating back as far as 1939, Australia developed the standard "Rubber Gloves for Electrical Purposes," today known as *IEC 60903:2020*.[16] The last three decades have seen specific standards developed for single-use medical examination gloves and sterile surgical gloves.[17–19]

8.2 DEVELOPMENT OF AUSTRALIAN STANDARDS

The process of development of standards in Australia is based on three internationally recognized principles: openness and transparency of the process, consensus, and balance of representation.[20] These principles are upheld by the six-stage process required for the development, revision, or amendment of any Australian standard. The six stages are defined as project proposal, project kick-off, drafting, public comment, ballot, and publication.[21] Approved proposals are allocated to a technical committee, which then divides into working groups to provide the technical content required for the drafting of the standard. Once drafted, the publication is open to the public for comment for nine weeks; all comments are considered by the technical committee.[21] Once a final draft is prepared, the technical committee members must vote and reach a consensus. Once consensus is reached, the standard is ready for publication.[22] However, in Australia, standards do not equate to mandatory adoption and are a guideline or recommended benchmark only. Australian legislation however can reference a specific standard, which then does make it mandatory.[23]

8.3 ALIGNING WITH INTERNATIONAL STANDARDS

Australian standards are continually undergoing review or updating to ensure that they remain relevant and up to date with changing technology. Where possible Australian standards aim to be aligned with or are an identical adoption of the corresponding international standard (see Table 8.1).[24] Currently two standards are withdrawn from the AS/NZS 2161 series: AS/NZS 2161.5 and AS/NZS 2161.9. Both of these standards are aged, and their international reciprocal had been updated; therefore the content was not current. The joint technical committee meetings in February or March 2021 will likely result in identical adoptions of EN 511:2006 and ISO 10819:2013 (R2018), respectively.

The most significant disparity between European standards and those of Australia and New Zealand 2161 series is that validation of a manufacturer's claimed EN-performance ratings for medium and high-risk applications is mandated by the European Union (EU) "notified testing bodies" under the personal protective equipment (PPE) directives. Australia and New Zealand have no legislative requirements to compel manufacturers to submit their products for testing and certification by accredited testing authorities.[2] This technically creates a loophole for manufacturers/suppliers of safety gloves where EN-performance claims can be made without independent proof of compliance. However, except for North America, most PPE manufacturers around the world have adopted the EN standards inclusive of EN pictograms and performance numbers on their products. The majority of these

TABLE 8.1

Occupational Protective Gloves Standards—AS/NZS vs European/International

AS/NZS	Description	Committee	EN/ISO	Comparison
2161.1:2016; First published as AS Z4—1952	Selection, use, and maintenance	SF/23	N/A	N/A
2161.2:2020; First published as AS Z4—1952	General requirements and test methods	SF-053	EN ISO 21420:2020 Previously EN 420:2003	Identical
2161.3:2020; First published as AS Z4—1952	Protection against mechanical risks	SF-053	EN 388:2016+A1:2018	Identical
2161.4:1999 (R2016); First published as AS Z4—1952	Protection against thermal risks (heat and fire)	SF/23	EN 407:1994	Identical
2161.5:1998; WITHDRAWN 26/11/2020	Protection against cold	SF-023	EN 511:1994 EN 511:2006 (current)	Identical
2161.6:2014; Originated as AS 2161.6(int)—2001	Protective gloves for structural firefighting: Laboratory test methods and performance requirements	SF-049	ISO 15383:2001	Based on but not equivalent
2161.7; Originated as part of NZSR 9:1965 and NZS 1988:1965	Protection against cuts and stabs by hand knives			
2161.7.1:1998 (R2016)	Chainmail gloves and arm guards	SF/23	EN 1082-1:1997	Identical
2161.7.2:2005 (R2017)	Gloves and arm guards made of material other than chainmail	SF/23	ISO 13999-2:2003	Identical
2161.7.3:2005 (R2017)	Impact cut test for fabric, leather, and other materials	SF/23	ISO 13999-3:2002	Identical
2161.8:2002 (R2016)	Protection against ionizing radiation and radioactive contamination	SF/23	EN 421:1994	Identical

(Continued)

TABLE 8.1 (CONTINUED)
Occupational Protective Gloves Standards—AS/NZS vs European/International

AS/NZS	Description	Committee	EN/ISO	Comparison
2161.9:2002; WITHDRAWN 26/11/2020	Method of measurement and evaluation of the vibration transmissibility of gloves at the palm of the hand	SF-053	ISO 10819:1996 (withdrawn) ISO 10819:2013 (R2018)	Identical
2161.10	Protective gloves against chemicals and micro-organisms			
2161.10.1:2005 (R2016)	Part 1: Terminology and performance requirements	SF-023	BS EN 374-1:2003	Identical
2161.10.2:2005 (R2016)	Part 2: Determination of resistance to penetration	SF-023	BS EN 374-2:2003	Identical
2161.10.3:2005 (R2016)	Part 3: Determination of resistance to permeation by chemicals	SF-023	BS EN 374-3:2003	Identical
4011	Single-use medical examination gloves			
4011.1:2014	Part 1: Specification for gloves made from rubber latex or rubber solution	HE-013	ISO 11193-1:2008	Modified
4011.2:2014	Part 2: Specification for gloves made from poly(vinyl chloride)	HE-013	ISO 11193-2:2006	Modified
4179:2014	Single-use sterile rubber surgical gloves— specification	HE-013	ISO 10282:2014	Modified
IEC 60903:2020; Originated at AS C87—1939	Live working— Electrical insulating gloves	EL-004	IEC 60903 ed. 3.0	Identical

Notes: Joint technical committee SF/23=occupational protective gloves; Joint technical committee SF-053=protective clothing; Joint technical committee SF-049=firefighters PPE; Joint technical committee HE-013=surgical apparel; and Joint technical committee EL-004=electrical accessories.

manufacturing companies have their performance ratings validated by independent testing authorities. It is not guaranteed that manufacturers consistently follow these procedures for products marketed outside of the EU; however, it would be uneconomical for a company to have different procedures in place for the same products. If there is any doubt about performance, in Australia, glove companies can perform their testing and issue their compliance statements.[2]

REFERENCES

1. Standards Australia. 2020. *About us – Our history.* Available from: https://www.standards.org.au/about/our-history [Accessed 29/12/2020].
2. Standards Australia. 2016. *Occupational protective gloves. Part 1: Selection, use and maintenance.* AS/NZS 2161.1:2016, viewed 13 Jan 2021, retrieved from SAI Global database.
3. Standards Australia. 2020. *Occupational protective gloves. Part 2: General requirements and test methods.* AS/NZS 2161.2:2020, viewed 13 Jan 2021, retrieved from SAI Global database.
4. Standards Australia. 2020. *Occupational protective gloves. Part 3: Protection against mechanical risks.* AS/NZS 2161.3:2020, viewed 13 Jan 2021, retrieved from SAI Global database.
5. Standards Australia. 2016. *Occupational protective gloves. Part 4: Protection against thermal risks (heat and fire).* AS/NZS 2161.4:1999 (R2016), viewed 13 Jan 2021, retrieved from SAI Global database.
6. Standards Australia. 1998. *Occupational protective gloves. Part 5: Protection against cold.* AS/NZS 2161.5:1998, viewed 13 Jan 2021, retrieved from SAI Global database.
7. Standards Australia. 2014. *Occupational protective gloves. Part 6: Protective gloves for structural firefighting - Laboratory test methods and performance requirements.* AS/NZS 2161.6:2014, viewed 13 Jan 2021, retrieved from SAI Global database.
8. Standards Australia. 2016. *Occupational protective gloves. Part 7.1: Protection against cuts and stabs by hand knives - Chainmail gloves and arm guards.* AS/NZS 2161.7.1:1998(R2016), viewed 13 Jan 2021, retrieved from SAI Global database.
9. Standards Australia. 2017. *Occupational protective gloves. Part 7.2: Protection against cuts and stabs by hand knives - Gloves and arm guards made of material other than chainmail.* AS/NZS 2161.7.2:2005(R2017), viewed 13 Jan 2021, retrieved from SAI Global database.
10. Standards Australia. 2017. *Occupational protective gloves. Part 7.3: Protection against cuts and stabs by hand knives - Impact cut test for fabric, leather and other materials.* AS/NZS 2161.7.3:2005 (R2017), viewed 13 Jan 2021, retrieved from SAI Global database.
11. Standards Australia. 2016. *Occupational protective gloves. Part 8: Protection against ionizing radiation and radioactive contamination.* AS/NZS 2161.8:2002 (R2016), viewed 13 Jan 2021, retrieved from SAI Global database.
12. Standards Australia. 2002. *Occupational protective gloves. Part 9: Method of measurement and evaluation of the vibration transmissibility of gloves at the palm of the hand.* AS/NZS 2161.9:2002, viewed 13 Jan 2021, retrieved from SAI Global database.
13. Standards Australia. 2016. *Occupational protective gloves. Part 10.1: Protective gloves against chemicals and micro-organisms - Terminology and performance requirements.* AS/NZS 2161.10.1:2005(R2016), viewed 13 Jan 2021, retrieved from SAI Global database.

14. Standards Australia. 2016. *Occupational protective gloves. Part 10.2: Protective gloves against chemicals and micro-organisms - Determination of resistance to penetration.* AS/NZS 2161.10.2:2005(R2016), viewed 13 Jan 2021, retrieved from SAI Global database.
15. Standards Australia. 2016. *Occupational protective gloves. Part 10.3: Protective gloves against chemicals and micro-organisms - Determination of resistance to permeation by chemicals.* AS/NZS 2161.10.3:2005(R2016), viewed 13 Jan 2021, retrieved from SAI Global database.
16. Standards Australia. 2020. *Live working – Electrical insulating gloves.* IEC 60903:2020, viewed 13 Jan 2021, retrieved from SAI Global database.
17. Standards Australia. 2014. *Single use medical examination gloves. Part 1: Specification for gloves made from rubber latex or rubber solution.* AS/NZS 4011.1:2014, viewed 13 Jan 2021, retrieved from SAI Global database.
18. Standards Australia. 2014. *Single use medical examination gloves. Part 2: Specification for gloves made from poly(vinyl chloride).* AS/NZS 4011.2:2014, viewed 13 Jan 2021, retrieved from SAI Global database.
19. Standards Australia. 2014. *Single-use sterile rubber surgical gloves – specification.* AS/NZS 4179:2014, viewed 13 Jan 2021, retrieved from SAI Global database.
20. Standards Australia. 2020. *Standards development SG-002: Structure and operation of standardisation committees.* Version 4.2. p1–19. Available from: https://www.standards.org.au/getmedia/00a7a293-b416-4bb5-81f7-79e9a6cf2107/SG-002-Structure-and-Operation-of-Standardisation-Committees.pdf.aspx [Accessed 29/12/2020].
21. Standards Australia. 2020. *Standards development, our process.* Available from: https://www.standards.org.au/standards-development/developing-standards/process [Accessed 29/12/2020].
22. Standards Australia. 2019. *Standards development SG-001: Preparing standards.* Version 4.15. p1–13. Available from: https://www.standards.org.au/getmedia/8067250b-e8c3-4db5-a661-e1df043e6b3d/SG-001-Preparing-Standards.pdf.aspx   [Accessed 29/12/2020].
23. Standards Australia. 2019. *Standards development SG-003: Standards and other publications.* Version 1.11. p1–23. Available from: https://www.standards.org.au/getmedia/d9da035d-2fbc-4417-98c1-aa9e85ef625d/SG-003-Standards-and-Other-Publications.pdf.aspx [Accessed 29/12/2020].
24. Standards Australia. 2016. *Standards development SG-007: Adoption of international standards.* Version 1.7, p1–8. Available from: https://www.standards.org.au/getmedia/98dfe8c9-4d35-4b14-bcf3-1bfef35e935f/SG-007-Adoption-of-International-Standards.pdf.aspx [Accessed 29/12/2020].

9 Regulations and Standards for Protective Gloves for Occupational Use in Croatia

M. Bubaš and S. Ljubojevic Hadzavdic

CONTENTS

9.1 INTRODUCTION

An occupational disease is a disease that is proven to be a consequence of harmful effects in the work process and/or the work environment, or a disease that is known to be a consequence of harmful effects related to the work process and/or work environment, and the intensity of harm and the duration of exposure to that harm is at a level known to cause damage to health.[1] Occupational skin diseases are among the most common occupational diseases in Europe with an estimated annual incidence of 0.5–1 cases per 1,000 employees,[2] although this number could be higher, given a large number of unrecognized and unreported cases. The most common occupational skin disease is contact dermatitis, which includes allergic and irritant contact dermatitis and contact urticaria. Underlying their occurrence, physical and chemical hazards disrupt the skin barrier as well as hypersensitivity reactions to chemical hazards in the workplace. Occupational skin diseases are therefore more common in occupations characterized by working with allergens and irritants, among which cleaners,[3] hairdressers and beauticians,[4] health workers,[5] food preparation workers,[6] and construction and metal-working workers are the most common.[7] In these occupations, occupational skin diseases are a significant cause of reduced quality of life, absence from work, as well as temporary or permanent reduction of working ability.

According to the data from the Register of Occupational Diseases of the Occupational Medicine Service of the Croatian Institute of Public Health from 2008–2020, there were a total of 1,078 proven occupational diseases.[8] Occupational

DOI: 10.1201/9781003126874-11

diseases caused by asbestos are excluded from the overall analysis, since they are kept in a special register, and these are mainly retirees who have initiated the procedure of recognizing an occupational disease to use their rights from the special ordinance. In these 12 years, 85 of the 1,078 cases were occupational skin diseases.[8] This means that occupational skin diseases make up to 8% of the total number of all recognized occupational diseases.[8] Of the 85 occupational skin diseases, 69 were allergic contact dermatitis, 15 were irritant contact dermatitis, and 1 was unspecified contact dermatitis.[8] Most cases of occupational skin diseases are found in manufacturing, craftwork, healthcare, and construction. People who are employed in crafts, production, and services employed in trade occupations, such as technicians and associates, are the most affected.[8] Occupational skin diseases in the Republic of Croatia (RH) account for 8% of the total number of all occupational diseases,[8] while in 2001 occupational skin diseases in Europe accounted for 11.2% of the total number of all occupational diseases.[9] The rate of patients suffering from occupational skin diseases in the Republic of Croatia is 2.31 per 100,000 workers, and in the European Union 5.5 per 100,000 workers.[10,11] In the Republic of Croatia, contact allergic dermatitis accounts for 81% of all occupational skin diseases, and irritant contact dermatitis for 18%.[8] Research in Northern Bavaria has shown that 4.5 workers per 10,000 employees suffer from irritant contact dermatitis and 4.1 workers per 10,000 employees from allergic contact dermatitis.[12] The reasons why few occupational diseases are reported in the Republic of Croatia include (1) harmful working conditions, (2) poor use of proper personal protective equipment or inadequate selection of protective gloves, and (3) fear of losing employment. Workers, employers, and safety experts lack information and knowledge about the harmful effects of working conditions on the skin. The number of cases of reported irritative dermatitis tends to improve if the worker cares for his or her hands, uses proper personal protective equipment, and reduces exposure to irritants. To prevent allergic contact dermatitis, it is necessary to avoid exposure to allergens, because once the worker is sensitized, even the slightest exposure leads to the appearance of dermatitis.

9.2   GLOVE STANDARDS

Personal protective equipment (PPE) for hand protection, to the greatest extent, refers to gloves made of different materials and for different purposes. A glove is defined as an item of PPE that protects the hand or any part of the hand from hazards (EN 420). The basic European standard, accepted in the Republic of Croatia, is HRN EN 420: 2011 (EN 420: 2003—"Protective Gloves—General Requirements and Test Methods").[13]

Protective gloves primarily protect workers from injuries at work (scratches, cuts, stings, bruises, burns) and occupational skin diseases (contact irritant dermatitis, contact allergic dermatitis, phototoxic dermatitis, photoallergic dermatitis, contact urticaria syndrome). According to the standard HRN EN 420: 2011 (EN 420: 2003), gloves must meet certain criteria (in terms of ergonomics, safety, size, finger dexterity), should be marked with an appropriate pictogram (Figure 9.1), and have enclosed instructions for use and maintenance. In accordance with Regulation (EU) 2016/425

Pictogram	The meaning of protection
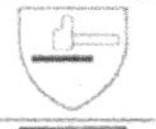	Mechanical protection
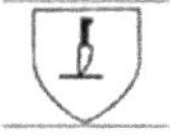	Mechanical protection
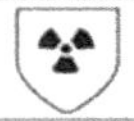	Protection against ionizing radiation
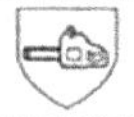	Chainsaw protection
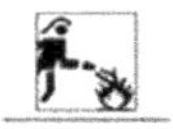	Protection in firefighting
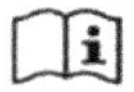	Instruction manual
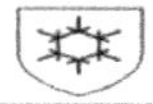	Cold protection
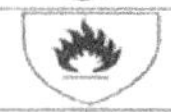	Heat and fire protection
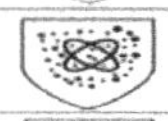	Protection against radioactive contamination
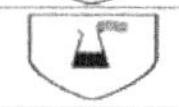	Chemical protection
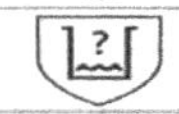	Protection against microorganisms

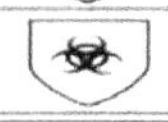

FIGURE 9.1 Pictograms for protective gloves (adopted in Croatia as part of the HRN EN standards system). Each pictogram is closely aligned with the HRN EN standard. Displayed with the permission of the Croatian Institute of Public Health, formerly Croatian Institute for Health Protection and Safety at Work. Adapted from: https://www.iso.org/obp/ui#iso:pub:PUB400001:en.

of the European Parliament and of the Council from March 9, 2016, on personal protective equipment and repealing Council Directive 89/686/EEC of December 21, 1989, on the approximation of the laws of the Member States relating to personal protective equipment,[14] there are three categories of personal protective equipment, and therefore three categories of protective gloves, according to the risk:

- Category I—covers only minimal risks (e.g., surface mechanical injuries, contact with mild cleaners or prolonged contact with water, contact with hot surfaces whose temperature does not exceed 50°C, etc.)
- Category II—covers risks not listed in categories I and III
- Category III—covers risks that can cause very serious consequences or permanent health consequences (e.g., contact with substances and mixtures dangerous to health, harmful biological agents)

Depending on the danger or harmfulness, protective gloves are roughly divided into those that (1) protect against mechanical, chemical, and biological hazards, (2) protect against thermal hazards, (3) protect against electric shock and high voltage, (4) protect against harmful radiation, and (5) protect against vibration.[15,16]

Protective gloves that *protect against mechanical hazards* must comply with the standard HRN EN 388: 2019 (EN 388: 2016 + A1: 2018)—Gloves for Protection Against Mechanical Hazards,[17] and the resistance to wear, tear, puncture, cutting, and punching is tested. They can be recognized by the hammer symbols on the pictogram. Examples are gloves made of a combination of polyamide and polyurethane, and they are often used for assembly work where it is necessary to preserve fine motor skills, or gloves made of a combination of kevlar and latex are used for cutting metal, handling sharp edges, etc.

Gloves for the *protection against chemical and biological hazards* must comply with the standards HRN EN 374-1: 2016 (EN 374-1: 2016) Gloves for Protection Against Hazardous Chemicals and Microorganisms—Part 1: Terminology and Requirements for Chemical Risk Properties,[18] HRN EN 374-2: 2015 (EN 374-2: 2014)—Gloves for Protection Against Dangerous Chemicals and Microorganisms—Part 2: Determination of Resistance to Leakage,[19] and HRN EN 374-3: 2003 Gloves for Protection Against Chemicals and Microorganisms—Part 3: Determination of Resistance to Absorption of Chemicals.[20] When gloves are used for protection against hazardous chemicals, it is necessary to select those listed in the safety data sheet obligatory for each chemical that is produced or placed on the market of the Republic of Croatia.

Gloves for the *protection against thermal hazards* must comply with the standard HRN EN 407: 2005 (EN 407: 2004)—Gloves for the Protection Against Thermal Risks (heat and/or fire),[21] and must have a mark for resistance to conduction, convection, and radiation.

Cold protection gloves must comply with the standard HRN EN 511: 2007 (EN 511: 2006)—Cold Protection Gloves,[22] and must be marked with cold resistance by convection, conduction, and waterproofness. Cryogenic gloves are used to protect hands and arms at extremely low temperatures.

Gloves for the electricians are made of latex of different thicknesses (depending on the operating voltage for which they are applied) and must comply with the standard IEC 60903: 2002 + Corr.:2003, MOD; EN 60903: 2003 Undervoltage Work—Gloves Made of Insulating Material.[23]

Gloves that reduce harmful radiation to hands must comply with the standard HRN EN 421: 2010 (EN 421: 2010)—Gloves for Protection Against Ionizing Radiation and Radioactive Contamination.[24] These gloves contain a certain amount of lead, so they are also known as lead rubber gloves.

Anti-vibration gloves reduce vibrations transmitted to the hands and arms and must comply with the standard HRN EN ISO 10819: 2013 Mechanical Vibrations and Shocks—Hand Vibrations—Method of Measuring and Evaluating the Transmission of Gloves to the Palm of the Hand.[25] However, there are different views on the effectiveness of these gloves. Namely, there are significant differences in the damping properties of individual types of anti-vibration gloves, so for the selection of proper gloves, it is necessary to carry out preliminary measurements of their damping properties.[26]

9.3   USE OF LATEX GLOVES

Unfortunately, even today many health professionals still use latex gloves. The usage of latex gloves among the Croatian population arose during the COVID-19 pandemic due to a shortage of PPE. Although the usage of latex gloves is still frequent, we rarely see a positive patch and/or prick reaction to latex. However, in a cross-sectional study conducted in one Croatian dermatovenerology clinic, 7% of the subjects (dentists, assistants, technicians, and students) were allergic to latex and 4.8% rubber additives.[27] Skin lesions appeared significantly more frequently in the group with longer work experience and hand washing and in subjects with a history of atopies (atopic dermatitis, allergic rhinitis, allergic conjunctivitis, and others).[27]

9.4   OUTREACH ACTIVITIES IN CROATIA

The Occupational Medicine Service of the Croatian Institute of Public Health (the legal successor of the Croatian Institute for Health Protection and Safety at Work) has been holding the seminar "Hands Are Your Most Important Tool" since 2012.[28] The seminar is intended for occupational safety experts, occupational medicine, and sports specialists, employers, and employers' representatives and workers' commissioners. The seminar aims to acquaint participants with the health risks for hands and skin, informing them about the importance of using protective gloves at work and education and assistance in choosing and using protective gloves according to the requirements of the work process. So far, 715 participants have been educated through the seminar (*the population of Croatia is around 4 million people*).

To choose a proper glove for a specific exposure, testing of glove performance is standardized in several international standards that are used in Croatia as well. These standards measure the permeation of chemicals and leakage through imperfect membranes. There are no ideal gloves, and no type of glove can give ideal protection; however, selection must meet requirements of the type of the hazard and duration of exposure according to the job and risk assessment. It is necessary to obtain information on current standards, the nature of the hazard, the acceptable level of exposure to hazards, quality requirements, performance data, and the nature of dermatologic adverse effects caused by protective gloves.

REFERENCES

1. Croatian Employment Service. 2021. Act on the list of occupational diseases (Official Gazette 162/98, 107/07). Available at: https://www.hzz.hr/en/about-ces/legal-basis/ (accessed February 1, 2021).
2. Diepgen, T.L. 2003. Occupational skin-disease data in Europe. *Int Arch Occup Environ Health* 76(5):331–8.
3. Mirabelli, M.C., Vizcaya, D., Martí Margarit, A., Antó, J.M., Arjona, L., Barreiro, E., Orriols, R., Gimenez-Arnau, A., and Zock, J.P. 2012. Occupational risk factors for hand dermatitis among professional cleaners in Spain. *Contact Dermatitis* 66(4):188–96.
4. Leino, T., Tuomi, K., Paakkulainen, H., and Klockars, M. 1999. Health reasons for leaving the profession as determined among Finnish hairdressers in 1980–1995. *Int Arch Occup Environ Health* 72(1):56–9.

5. Szepietowski, J., and Salomon, J. 2005. Hand dermatitis: A problem commonly affecting nurses. *Rocz Akad Med Bialymst* 50(1) Supplement 1:46–8.
6. Teo, S., Teik-Jin Goon, A., Siang, L.H., Lin, G.S., and Koh, D. 2009. Occupational dermatoses in restaurant, catering and fast-food outlets in Singapore. *Occup Med (Lond)* 59(7):466–71.
7. Bock, M., Schmidt, A., Bruckner, T., and Diepgen, T.L. 2003. Occupational skin disease in the construction industry. *Br J Dermatol* 149:1165–71.
8. Croatian Institute Of Public Health. 2021. Department of Occupational Health: Register of occupational diseases. Available at: http://www.hzzzsr.hr/wp-content/uploads/2021/05/Registar-profesionalnih-bolesti-za-2020.pdf (accessed February 4, 2021).
9. Karjalainen, A., and Niederlaender, E. 2004. Occupational diseases in Europe in 2001. European Occupational Diseases Statistics (EODS) Eurostat. Available at: https://ec.europa.eu/eurostat/documents/3433488/5316393/KS-NK-04-015-EN.PDF/05b3b108-3589-4044-aba2-63e2403f6e0a (accessed February 4, 2021).
10. Bogadi-Šare, A., Bubaš, M., Kerner, I., Macan, J., Pejnović, N., Skroza, D., and Turk, R. 2014. *Approach to Occupational Skin Diseases in Occupational Medicine.* Zagreb, Croatia: Institut za medicinska istraživanja i medicinu rada [Institute for Medical Research and Occupational Health].
11. European Agency for Safety and Health at Work. 2008. Occupational skin diseases and dermal exposure in the European Union (EU-25): Policy and practice overview. Brussels, Belgium: European Agency for Safety and Health at Work. Available at: https://data.europa.eu/doi/10.2802/15493 (accessed February 4, 2021).
12. Dickel, H., Kuss, O., Schmidt, A., Kretz, J., and Diepgen, T.L. 2002. Importance of irritant contact dermatitis in occupational skin disease. *Am J Clin Dermatol* 3(4): 283–9.
13. CEN (European Standard). 2011. HRN EN 420:2011 (EN 420:2003) – Zaštitne rukavice – Opći zahtjevi i ispitne metode [Protective gloves – General requirements and test methods]. Available at: https://repozitorij.hzn.hr/norm/HRN+EN+420%3A2011 (accessed February 4, 2021).
14. European Union (EU). Uredba (EU) 2016/425 Europskog parlamenta i Vijeća od 9. 2016. ožujka 2016. o osobnoj zaštitnoj opremi i o stavljanju izvan snage Direktive Vijeća 89/686/EEZ Uredba (EU) 2016/425 Europskog parlamenta i Vijeća od 9. ožujka 2016. o osobnoj zaštitnoj opremi i o stavljanju izvan snage Direktive Vijeća 89/686/ EEZ (accessed February 4, 2021).
15. Pejnović, N. 2010. Rukavice za zaštitu od opasnosti i štetnosti pri radu [Croatian Institute for Health Protection and Safety at Work]. *Zbornik radova 3. međunarodno stručno-znanstvenog skupa Zaštita na radu i zaštita zdravlja, Veleučilište u Karlovcu, 95–101.* Karlovac: Veleučilište u Karlovcu.
16. Kirin, S. 2017. Zaštitne rukavice kao važan faktor u zaštitu ruku [Protective gloves as an important factor in hand protection]. Zbornik radova XI međunarodne naučne konferencije o proizvodnom inženjerstvu, Univerzitet u Bihaću – Tehnički fakultet. Available at: https://tfb.ba/repozitorij/2/RIM/RIM2017/118-Snje%C5%BEana%20Kirin-ZA %C5%A0TITNE%20RUKAVICE%20KAO%20VA%C5%BDAN%20FAKTOR%20U %20ZA%C5%A0TITU%20RUKU.pdf (accessed February 4, 2021).
17. CEN (European Standard). 2018. HRN EN 388:2019 (EN 388:2016+A1:2018) – Rukavice za zaštitu od mehaničkih rizika [Protective gloves against mechanical risks]. Available at: http://31.45.242.218/HZN/Todb.nsf/wFrameset2?OpenFrameSet&Frame =Down&Src=%2FHZN%2FTodb.nsf%2F66011c0bda2bd4dfc1256cf300764c2d%2Fc 9589d0e60cde18bc125823300502d8e%3FOpenDocument%26AutoFramed (accessed February 4, 2021).

18. CEN (European Standard). 2016. HRN EN 374-1:2016 (EN 374-1:2016) Rukavice za zaštitu od opasnih kemikalija i mikroorganizama -1.dio: Nazivlje i zahtjevi za svojstva za kemijske rizike [Gloves for protection against dangerous chemicals and micro-organisms – Part 1: Terminology and performance requirements for micro-organism risks]. Available at: https://www.ejendals.com/globalassets/inriver/resources/uis_836_a4.pdf (accessed February 4, 2021)

19. CEN (European Standard). 2014. HRN EN 374-2:2015 (EN 374-2:2014) – Rukavice za zaštitu od opasnih kemikalija i mikroorganizama – 2.dio: Određivanje otpornosti na propuštanje [Gloves for protection against dangerous chemicals and micro-organisms – Part 2: Determination of resistance to leakage]. Available at: https://repozitorij.hzn.hr /norm/HRN+EN+374-2%3A2015 (accessed February 4, 2021).

20. CEN (European Standard). 2003. HRN EN 374-3:2003 (EN 374-3:2003) Rukavice za zaštitu od kemikalija i mikroorganizama – 3. dio: Određivanje otpornosti na upijanje kemikalija [Gloves for protection against chemicals and micro-organisms. Part 3: Determination of resistance to chemical absorption]. Available at: https://repozitorij .hzn.hr/norm/HRN+EN+374-3%3A2003 (accessed February 4, 2021).

21. CEN (European Standard). 2004. HRN EN 407:2005 (EN 407:2004) – Rukavice za zaštitu od toplinskih rizika (topline i/ili vatre) [Protective gloves and other equipment for the protection of hands against thermal risks (heat and/or fire)]. Available at: https:// repozitorij.hzn.hr/norm/HRN+EN+407%3A2005 (accessed February 4, 2021).

22. CEN (European Standard). 2006. HRN EN 511:2007 (EN 511:2006) – Rukavice za zaštitu od hladnoće [Gloves for protection against cold]. Available at: http://31.45.242.218/ HZN/Todb.nsf/wFrameset2?OpenFrameSet&Frame=Down&Src=%2FHZN%2FTodb .nsf%2F66011c0bda2bd4dfc1256cf300764c2d%2F2db7345fa809a96ec12570a40 03d1b56%3FOpenDocument%26AutoFramed (accessed February 4, 2021).

23. CEN (European Standard). 2003. IEC 60903:2002 + Corr.:2003, MOD; EN 60903:2003 – Rad pod naponom – Rukavice od izolacijskog materijala [Live working – Gloves of insulating material].

24. CEN (European Standard). 2010. HRN EN 421:2010 (EN 421:2010) – Rukavice za zaštitu od ionizirajućeg zračenja i radioaktivne kontaminacije [Gloves for protection against ionizing radiation and radioactive contamination]. Available at: http://31.45.242.218/ HZN/Todb.nsf/wFrameset2?OpenFrameSet&Frame=Down&Src=%2FHZN%2FTodb .nsf%2F66011c0bda2bd4dfc1256cf300764c2d%2Ff5d84c524c607f64c125709f0 04ac877%3FOpenDocument%26AutoFramed (accessed February 4, 2021).

25. CEN (European Standard). 2013. HRN EN ISO 10819:2013 Mehaničke vibracije i udari – Vibracije ruke – Metoda mjerenja i vrednovanje prenosa vibracija rukavica na dlan ruke [Mechanical vibration and shock – Hand vibration – Method for measuring and evaluating the transmission of glove vibration to the palm of the hand]. Available at: https:// repozitorij.hzn.hr/norm/HRN+EN+ISO+10819%3A2013 (accessed February 4, 2021).

26. Goglia, V., Žgela, J., and Đukić, I. 2008. Učinkovitost antivibracijskih rukavica: II dio [Effectiveness of anti-vibration gloves: Part II]. *Šumarski list* 5–6:239–44.

27. Japundžić, I., Vodanović, M., and Lugović-Mihić, L. 2018. An analysis of skin prick tests to latex and patch tests to rubber additives and other causative factors among dental professionals and students with contact dermatoses. *Int Arch Allergy Immunol* 177(3):238–44.

28. Croatian Institute of Public Health. 2021. Your hands are your most important tool. Available at: https://www.hzzzsr.hr/index.php/tecajevi-seminari-i-skupovi/hzzzsr/ strucni-seminari/ruke-su-vas-najvazniji-alat/ (accessed February 9, 2021).

10 Testing of Protective Effect against Liquid Chemicals

R.N. Phalen

CONTENTS

10.1 TERMS AND DEFINITIONS

Even if there are regulations with demands on the use and/or proven efficacy of protective gloves, they do not cover all possible situations that can arise. However, there are several methods for testing the resistance to chemicals of polymeric materials used in chemical protective clothing and gloves. First, a few definitions:

> *Degradation* is defined as a deleterious change in one or more physical properties of a protective clothing material due to contact with a chemical.[1]
>
> *Permeation* is usually defined as the process by which a chemical migrates through the protective clothing material on a molecular level. The permeation process involves three stages: (1) sorption of molecules of the chemical into the outside surface of the material, (2) diffusion of the sorbed molecules through the material, and (3) desorption of the molecules from the inside surface of the material into the collecting medium.[1–3]

DOI: 10.1201/9781003126874-12

Penetration is usually defined as the flow of a chemical through closures, porous materials, seams, pinholes, or other imperfections in a protective clothing material on a nonmolecular level.[1]

Protective clothing material is defined as any material or combination of materials used in an item of clothing to isolate parts of the body from direct contact with a potentially hazardous chemical.[1]

Protective glove material is defined as any material or combination of material used in a glove to isolate the hands and arms from direct contact with a chemical and/or microorganism.[2]

And acronyms:

ASTM: American Society for Testing and Materials (now ASTM International)
CEN: Comité Européen de Normalisation
CEN/TC 162: CEN/Technical Committee 162: Protective Clothing; this committee has 12 working groups (WG), including WG 8: Protective Gloves
EN: European Standard (E), Norme Européene (F), and Europäische Norm (G)
ISO: International Organization for Standardization
prEN: draft European Standard

10.2 DEGRADATION TESTING

The immersion test was one of the first tests used by the manufacturers to describe the chemical resistance of protective gloves. Pieces of glove materials were immersed in the different chemicals for some time and then visibly inspected and rated according to resistance, for example, as excellent, good, fair, or not recommended. The results can be misleading as more than one surface of the material is exposed to the chemical, the outside, inside, and cross sections. This is a problem especially when testing supported gloves.

The ability of the material to resist degradation by chemicals was earlier a commonly used method to evaluate the protective effect.[4] Before the first edition of this book, several drafts of an ASTM test method for evaluation of protective clothing materials for resistance to degradation by liquid chemicals have been written. The test cell used is the ASTM permeation test cell, where the collecting side has been modified and only the outer surface of the glove is exposed to the chemical. The property measured is weight change after exposure to the chemical. The degradation test method still needed some modifications before it can be a standard test method but can be used in the screening procedure when developing new polymeric materials for protective gloves or clothing.[5–7]

Currently, three standards can be used to evaluate the degradation of protective clothing materials: ASTM D 471, ANSI/ISEA 105, and EN 374-4.[8–10] In these testing strategies, the chemical is either immersed or put in contact with one side of the material. The exposure time and temperature can vary, as can the evaluation of degradation, e.g., changes in weight, thickness, volume, tensile properties, or other physical characteristics such as color or shape. Even though the results can indicate chemical incompatibility and/or potential for failure, they may not be well associated with the product's barrier properties under conditions of use. They are more an indication of chemical incompatibility and potential for degradation following exposure to the chemical.

ASTM D 471,[8] *Standard Test Method for Rubber Property—Effect of Liquids*, is designed to evaluate changes in mass, volume, dimension, or tensile properties associated with immersion or surface contact of a test specimen with a chemical at a set temperature and time. It can be used with rubber-like elastomers and coated fabrics.

ANSI/ISEA 105,[9] *American National Standard for Hand Protection Classification*, is related more to the evaluation of the puncture resistance of chemical protective gloves; however, the results can be used to indicate chemical incompatibility or degradation. It evaluates changes in puncture resistance and provides a rating scale from zero to nine. The change in puncture resistance, a tensile property, can be an indication of molecular changes within the elastomer and chemical action on the glove material.

The 2019 revision of EN 374-4,[10] *Protective gloves against dangerous chemicals and micro-organisms—Part 4: Determination of resistance to degradation by chemicals*, is similar to ANSI/ISEA 105 except it does not provide a rating scale. The exposure time is 60 min, and degradation is expressed as a percent change in applied force. A nonmandatory finger-immersion test for weight change is also included. All results are reported as a percent change, and there is no pass or fail.

Overall, a standardized rating system has yet to be developed and adopted for degradation. Several such conventions have been proposed for changes in weight, surface area, and tensile properties (Table 10.1).[11,12] Some of these have been used by glove manufacturers to provide useful information on degradation to customers.

10.3 PERMEATION TESTING

During the last several decades, standardization work has resulted in several standards for permeation testing that are in use.[2,3, 13–20]

The first standard test method (ASTM F 739) was developed in the United States, subsequently promulgated by ASTM in 1981, and updated in 1985, 1991, 1999, 2007, 2012, and 2020.[1,13,16] In Europe, a standard was established by CEN concerning protective gloves against chemicals and microorganisms.[2,3,17,18] These standards have been accepted and adopted in other parts of the world.[19] Subsequently, an

---

TABLE 10.1

Examples of Degradation Ranking Based on Changes in Glove Surface Area, Weight, and Tensile Property

Degradation Ranking	Observed Surface Area Change[12]	Observed Weight Change[11,12]	Observed Tensile Change[11]
Excellent	<5%	<10%	<20%
Good	<10%	<20%	<40%
Fair	<15%	<30%	<60%
Poor	<25%	<50%	<80%
Not Recommended	>25%	>50%	>80%

international ISO standard was developed.[20] The standards have served as a foundation for efforts to create a reasonable system of rules and demands, which together with good knowledge of work and exposure situations will be the basis for the selection and use of protective gloves at work with hazardous chemicals.

10.3.1 KEY PARAMETERS

The principle of permeation testing is a flow-through system where a two-compartment permeation cell of standard dimensions is used. The test specimen acts as a barrier between the first compartment of the cell, which contains the test chemical, and the second compartment through which a stream of the collecting medium (gas or liquid) is passed for the collection of diffused molecules of the test chemical or its component chemicals for analysis. The outside of the glove or clothing material is in continuous contact with the test chemical in excess and with the collecting medium on the other (inner) side. The resistance is determined by measuring the breakthrough time and the permeation rate of the chemical through the test material. The definitions of the key parameters, including those current and older parameters available in the literature, are provided below.[14–16]

Current Parameters

Breakthrough detection time (BDT), the elapsed time, usually in minutes, measured from the start of the test to the sampling time that immediately precedes the sampling time at which the test chemical is first detected. The BDT can be dependent on detector sensitivity.

Cumulative permeation (CP, $\mu g/cm^2$), the total mass of a chemical that permeates a defined surface area of a material over a specified time. Generally, this is for the duration of the permeation test and represents the total mass collected upon completion of the test.

Minimum detectable mass permeated, the smallest mass of permeant that is detectable with the complete permeation test system.

Minimum detectable permeation rate (MDR), the lowest rate of permeation that is measurable with the complete permeation test system.

Normalized breakthrough time (NBT, min), the time, in minutes, at which the permeation rate reaches $0.1 \mu g/cm^2/min$ (ASTM F 739-20 or ISO 6529:2016) or $1 \mu g/cm^2/min$ (EN 374-1:2016/A1:2018 and EN 16523-1:2015+A1:2018).

Standardized BT (SBT, min), the elapsed time when a permeation rate of $0.1 sg/cm^2/min$ (ASTM F 739-20) is reached.

Steady-state permeation (SSPR), a state that is reached when the permeation rate becomes virtually constant; measured as mass/unit time/unit area ($\mu g/min/cm^2$) (see Figure 10.1).

Older Parameters

Breakthrough time (BT, min), the elapsed time between the initial application of a test chemical to the appropriate surface of the material and its subsequent presence on the other side of the material measured as described in the standards. The BT can be dependent on detector sensitivity.

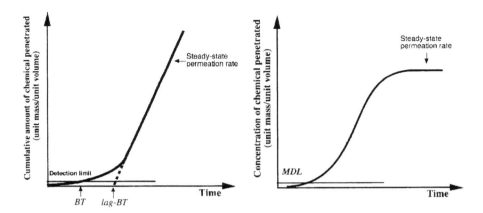

FIGURE 10.1 Permeation of chemicals through test specimen: (left) cumulative amount of chemical permeating vs. time (closed-loop system), (right) concentration in collecting medium vs. time (open-loop system). BT=measured breakthrough time; lag BT=cumulative breakthrough time; MDL=minimum detectable level (concentration). Source: Mellström, G.A., Carlsson, B., and Boman, A. 1994. Testing protective effect against liquid chemicals, in *Protective Gloves for Occupational Use*, Mellström, G.A., Wahlberg, J.E., and Maibach, H.I., Eds. Boca Raton, FL: CRC Press.[23]

Normalized breakthrough detection time (NBDT), used in ASTM F 739 and defined as the time, in minutes, at which the permeation rate reaches 0.1 µg/cm²/min.

Normalized BT, the breakthrough time in minutes divided by the material thickness in mm; the normalized breakthrough has sometimes been used in investigation reports and makes it possible to directly compare test results between glove materials independent of the thickness.[21,22]

Permeation rate (PR), the mass of test chemical permeating the material per unit time per unit area (µg/min/cm²) (see Figure 10.1).

Time-lag breakthrough (lag-BT), sometimes called cumulative, is the extrapolation of the steady-state permeation portion of the cumulative permeation curve to the time axis (Figure 10.1),[18,23] given in minutes.

Because all the standardized test methods in use are similar to ASTM F 739, this standard is the focus of the following discussion.

10.3.2 STANDARD TEST METHODS

Although following a standard test method, the permeation testing can be performed in different ways, as the protocols stated in the standard test methods may vary. For permeation testing of chemicals, there are three standard test methods: the ASTM F 739-20,[15] the EN ISO 6529:2016, and the EN 374-1:2016/A1:2018 with corresponding EN 16523-1:2015+A1:2018.[16] There are both differences and similarities between the test methods as evident in their designations.

ASTM F 739: Standard Test Method for Permeation of Liquids and Gases Through Protective Clothing Materials Under Conditions of Continuous Contact.

ASTM F 1383: Standard Test Method for Resistance of Protective Clothing Materials to Permeation by Liquids or Gases Under Conditions of Intermittent Contact.[24]

EN 374-1: Protective Gloves against Chemicals and Micro-organisms. Part 3: Determination of Resistance to Permeation by Chemicals.

EN 16523: Determination of material resistance to permeation by chemicals. Permeation by potentially hazardous liquid chemicals under conditions of continuous contact.

ISO 6529: Protective clothing—Protection against chemicals—Determination of resistance of protective clothing materials to permeation by liquids and gases.

The purpose of EN 374-1, with corresponding EN 16523, is for the determination of the permeation of protective *gloves* by *solid or liquid chemicals*, whereas for ISO it is the determination of protective *clothing* by *liquid and gaseous chemicals*, and ASTM F 739 and ASTM 1383 adds *chemical gases* under conditions of continuous contact vs. intermittent contact.

Variables in permeation testing that are of importance for the results are the nature of the collecting medium, the flow rate of the collecting medium, the volume of the collecting chamber, whether the system is open or closed, the temperature, the exposed area of the sample, the sampling mode and frequency, the method of analysis, etc.[16,25–32]

The *collecting medium* can be an inert gas, such as dried air, nitrogen, helium, or a liquid. The liquid used as a collecting medium must be proved not to influence the resistance of the test material. Water is the most commonly used liquid medium. The test chemical shall be freely soluble in the collecting gas or liquid.

The *flow system* can either be an open-loop or closed-loop flow-through system (Figure 10.2). In a closed-loop system, the possibility of saturation should be considered.

Sampling mode and frequency—the assessment of the permeating chemical in the system can be continuous or time-scheduled sampling, depending on the analytical technique and equipment used.

The *temperature* should be the most relevant to the use of the material; maintaining it constantly during the testing $\pm 1^\circ$C at the appropriate temperature is crucial.

The *analytical system* shall have sensitivity for the test chemical of 0.1 µg/min/cm^2 minimum detectable permeation rate (MDR).[2,3,15,16]

Calculations and expressions of results—the calculation of the results is well described in the test methods, as well as the expression of the results.

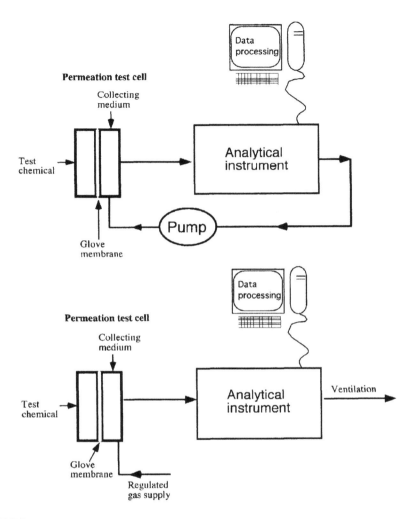

FIGURE 10.2   Flow system: Closed-loop system (top) and open-loop system (bottom).

10.3.3 PERMEATION TEST CELLS

The standard ASTM test cell is a glass (2 in. diameter), chemical permeation cell available from Pesce Lab Sales (Kennett Square, PA). A smaller version of the ASTM test cell (1 in. diameter) is also available. The exposed membrane is in a vertical position. The inlet and outlet of the collecting medium are situated almost at right angles to each other, with the inlet directed toward the test membrane (Figure 10.2). In the ASTM F 739 standard, it is possible to use alternative test cells provided that they have been found equivalent to the standard reference cell (2 in. cell). Standard practice for the determination of equivalency of optional chemical permeation test cells to that of the ASTM cell has been developed but requires further modification.[33]

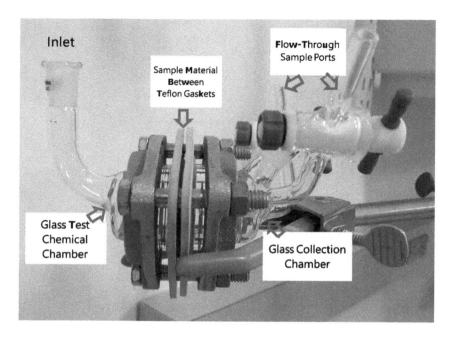

FIGURE 10.3   ASTM-type chemical permeation cell showing the glass chemical challenge chamber and inlet, sample interface where the material is placed between two Teflon gaskets, and the glass collection chamber with flow-through ports for continuous sampling.

The original ISO test cell was a stainless steel permeation cell. The internal dimensions of the collecting compartment and its piping are critical to the performance of the test. A photograph of the ASTM permeation test cell can be seen in Figure 10.3, and specifications are presented in Table 10.2.

The standard EN 374-1 and EN 16523 are equivalent to the ASTM standard test.[16] This standard is also adopted elsewhere.[19]

10.3.4   FACTORS INFLUENCING THE PERMEATION TEST RESULTS

Permeation is described as a molecular process by which chemicals are first adsorbed on the surface of the material, diffused through the material along a concentration

TABLE 10.2
ASTM F 739 Test Cell Specifications

Specification	2-Inch Test Cell	1-Inch Test Cell
Volume of collecting medium	100 mL	15 mL
Exposed area	20.3 cm^2	5.3 cm^2
Position of exposed area	Vertical	Vertical
Ratio: area/volume	0.203	0.353
Alternative test cell allowed	Yes	Yes

gradient, and desorbed from the other surface of the material.[13] The mathematical theory of diffusion is based on Fick's first law and can be expressed as:

$$P = -D\delta C / \delta x \qquad (10.1)$$

where

P = rate of transfer per unit area
C = concentration
x = distance within the material, e.g., thickness of the material
D = the diffusion coefficient, a proportionality constant that may be a function of chemical concentration.[32,34]

The diffusion coefficient, however, is usually treated as a constant. The theoretical, mathematical model for the permeation process resulting in differential equations for the total amount of the chemical permeating per unit area at a time and for the permeation rate of the chemical as a function of time per unit area of the material have been described and discussed by Schwope et al.[32] They pointed out that the detection of BT, which was defined as the time t at which the concentration of the chemical is detected in the collecting side of a permeation test cell, is dependent on the material thickness, the sensitivity of the analytical equipment, and the cell size. Theoretical and experimental approaches have been taken to identify the parameters that have a crucial influence on the detection of the breakthrough time by Billing and Bentz.[34] Five different kinds (A to E) of permeation rate vs. time behavior due to interaction between chemical and glove material have been described by Nelson et al.[35] The most typical pattern is the A-type, where the permeation rate stabilizes at a "steady state" level. In the B-type, the permeation behavior is due to structural modification of the material specimen by the test chemical, resulting in a change, instead of stabilization, of the permeation rate, which gradually increases or decreases. In the C-type, a sudden, very large increase in permeation rate occurs. The D-type of behavior, with an initial high rate that decreases slowly and eventually stabilizes during the exposure time, occurs when there is moderate to heavy swelling of the material. The E-type occurs when there is a high degree of swelling, resulting in a continuous increase in permeation rate with intermittent levels of steady-state.[35] The manner and extent of the effect of chemical interaction with the glove material can sometimes be hard to distinguish from the influence of different test conditions on the permeation test results.

The importance of how to present and evaluate test data and test conditions in a way that gives valuable information to the consumer has been discussed by both Jamke and Kairys.[36,37] They have pointed out that the most important variables to evaluate include the detector sensitivity, sampling method, system flow rate, surface of the sample, and the test system (open or closed) used.

From the formula given for calculating permeation rate in an open-loop system, it can easily be seen that the cell size, exposed area, and flow rate of the collecting medium in the test cell will influence test results, the steady-state permeation rate, and the breakthrough time.[32]

$$P = (C \cdot F)/A \qquad (10.2)$$

where
   P = steady-state permeation rate (SSPR) sg/cm²/min
   C = concentration of the chemical, sg/L
   F = flow rate of the collecting medium, L/min
   A = exposed area, cm²

The flow rate through the collecting medium compartment can also be expressed as volume changes per minute (vol/min).

Measurement of the concentration of the permeated chemical in the collecting medium is dependent on the *detector sensitivity*. A higher concentration is needed for a less-sensitive detector. The breakthrough time will increase when the minimum detectable level increases. For the same glove material tested with different analytical equipment, different BT can be reported. In EN ISO 6529, the *minimum detection limit* (MDPR) is specified as 0.1 µg/cm²/min; in EN 374-1, it is 1 µg/cm²/min, and thus the BT is the time when PR equals MDR (Figure 10.4). In ASTM F 739, the detection limits are specified to 0.1 µg/cm²/min. The term normalized breakthrough time (NBT) is the time at which the permeation rate reaches 0.1 µg/cm²/min.

The concentration in the collecting medium is also dependent on the *sampling method*. The measurement can be either continuous or performed by sampling according to a time schedule. When the sampling frequency decreases from, e.g., every second minute to every 5 or 10 min, the BT will increase. Continuous measurement gives shorter BT values compared to measurement by sampling.[37]

The ratio between the surface area and the volume of the collecting chamber also influences the concentration of the chemical in the collecting medium. A larger

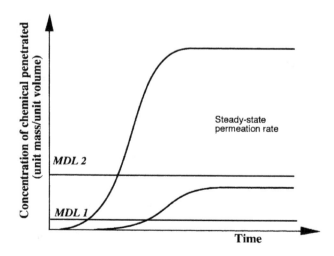

FIGURE 10.4 Effect of system detection limit in an open-loop system. Breakthrough time for materials with different permeability.

amount of chemical will be permeating through a larger surface area than through a smaller area per unit time into the same volume (closed-loop system) or volume changes/min (open-loop system) of collection medium, and the BT will decrease (become shorter) as the MDR will be reached faster.[32,37]

In an open system, the flow rate will influence the concentration, as well as the measured BT and PR. At an increasing flow rate, the measured BT values will increase (become longer) due to the dilution of the chemical in the collecting medium. This is not the case in a closed system where the MDR will be reached more rapidly, resulting in a shorter reported BT. In a closed system, the possibility of saturation in the collection medium can influence the measured SSPR value.[37]

10.3.5 Evaluation of Test Results

During the development of the standards, there have been several comparative investigations performed to evaluate different parameters influencing the outcome of the tests. The parameters that were studied are (1) flow rate and mixing, (2) cell size and design, (3) open- or closed-loop system, (4) temperature, and (5) thickness and formulation of the test material. The results from these studies are summarized by Mellström[23] and were considered in the development of the standard test methods. This work with a critical assessment of the influence of various parameters has since been further expanded.[38–40]

More recently, Gao et al.,[41] with the National Institute for Occupational Safety and Health (NIOSH), developed Permeation Calculator, a Windows-based and macOS computer program for permeation testing data analysis. The goal was to provide an automated decision-making process for the calculation of permeation parameters, which could be used with ASTM F 739, ASTM D 6978, and ISO 6529 standards. This includes calculations for the BDT, NBT, SBT, SSPR, cumulative permeation (CP) mass at a given elapsed time, and elapsed time at a given cumulative permeation mass for either closed-loop or open-loop permeation tests. The Permeation Calculator software is freely available from NIOSH, as DHHS (NIOSH) Publication Number 2007-143C (https://www.cdc.gov/niosh/). In 2010, ASTM adopted the Permeation Calculator under ASTM F 2815, *Standard practice for chemical permeation through protective clothing materials: testing data analysis by use of a computer program.* ASTM reapproved it in 2014.

10.3.6 Intermittent Contact Permeation Testing

In real working situations with hazardous chemicals, splashes or intermittent contact occurs more often than continuous contact. The ASTM F 739 Standard Test Method involves constant contact usually during 3–4 h, and this could be considered unusually severe for gloves used for protection in cases of accidental splashes or intermittent contact with smaller volumes of chemicals. Man et al.[42] have performed a comparative permeation study of liquid contact by liquid splashes and vapor influence on the BT. They compared liquid contact for 3 h, intermittent exposure every 15 and 30 min until breakthrough, and a single initial splash. The ASTM procedure was slightly modified, and for the intermittent liquid contact, the test cell was tilted through the vertical until the test material was horizontal, which allowed a small amount (1–2 mL) of the chemical to contact and completely cover the material for a period of 2 s. The test cell was then returned to its original position. Two distinct modes of behavior were observed. In the first, a more prolonged or concentrated liquid contact resulted in a shorter BT, as expected. In the second mode, the breakthrough times of the pure liquid and all splash conditions were essentially the same and it was the case when the surface was wetted by the liquid and retained in constant contact with the glove material. It was also observed that some of the test chemicals showed one mode of behavior with one material and another mode of behavior with a second material.[42]

This work has been the basis for the development of a modification of permeation testing resulting in the ASTM F 1383 *Standard Test Method for Resistance of Protective Clothing Materials to Permeation by Liquids or Gases Under Conditions of Intermittent Contact*.[24]

10.3.7 PROTECTION INDEX

In the standard EN 374-1, *Part 1: Terminology and Performance Requirements*, each combination of gloves/test chemicals should be classified according to the BT results and given a protection index.[43] See Table 10.3. This kind of classification can probably facilitate the selection of protective gloves for a certain working situation, but it should be remembered that chemical permeation test data are not the only criteria to be taken into account in the selection process.[44–46] The more recent changes in 2016 separated gloves into three classifications (Type A, Type B, and Type C) based on a set of required minimum BT performance levels and the number of chemicals tested from a list of 18 representative chemicals.[43] As a result, glove products are labeled with a pictogram showing the classification Type A, B, or C, as well as identifiers for each of the chemicals used in testing the glove. Examples of the 18 test chemicals include methanol as a primary alcohol, formaldehyde as an aldehyde, diethylamine as an amine, nitric acid 65% as an oxidizing inorganic mineral acid, and ammonium hydroxide 25% as an organic base.

TABLE 10.3

Classification of Protective Gloves from Chemical Permeation Test Results (EN 374-1)

Protective Index	Measured Breakthrough Time
Class 1	>10 min
Class 2	>30 min
Class 3	>60 min
Class 4	>120 min
Class 5	>240 min
Class 6	>480 min

10.3.8 MODIFIED PERMEATION TESTING

The described standard test methods and test cells are useful in most cases of permeation testing, but in some situations modifications are used. For example, when testing highly toxic substances such as pesticides, smaller test cells are preferred to avoid handling large quantities of test chemicals. It can be the same kind of permeation cell that is used for studies of percutaneous absorption *in vitro*.[47] When chemicals with low water solubility or low volatility are to be tested, other collecting media must be used. Solvent mixtures or aqueous solutions with surface-active agents added can sometimes be used if proved not to affect the glove material.[48,49] For low volatile pesticide formulations, solid silicon rubber sheets have been used as collecting media in a modified ASTM test cell by Ehntholt et al.[50,51] Pinette et al.[52] compared an intermittent collection procedure as an alternative to the solid collection method for nonvolatile water-soluble chemicals. They found that the splash-collecting procedure had advantages over the solid-collecting method regarding the surface contact and adsorption efficiency. They concluded that a method is needed for testing the permeation of water-soluble chemicals having low volatility, but today there is no general procedure available.[52]

Spence describes a sample trapping system to concentrate low volatile compounds in the sample of the collecting medium to avoid the risk of saturation of the gas in the collecting compartment.[53] Lara et al.[54] used a modified version of the ASTM F 739 permeation cell in a horizontal position in tests with dynamite gel preparations.

More recently, several whole-glove permeation methods have used robotic hands, pneumatic systems, and other methods to simulate hand movement and in-use conditions (e.g., elevated temperature during use). These are not standardized methods and are well beyond the scope of this chapter; however, Banaee and Que Hee[55] provide an extensive 2020 review on the topic. This review includes the various effects on permeation associated with temperature, glove decontamination with reuse, simulated movement, double gloving, and mixtures. Some of these concepts are covered in other chapters of this book.

10.4 PENETRATION TESTING

Penetration testing is used to determine the flow of liquids through gloves and protective clothing materials on a nonmolecular level. It can be used to investigate the penetration of chemicals and/or microorganisms through porous materials, seams, closures, pinholes, and other imperfections in the glove material. Standard penetration test methods are used as quality control testing for freedom from holes in gloves (leakage test). There is one ASTM standard test method and one EN standard method for penetration testing of protective gloves and protective clothing materials for resistance to liquid chemicals. There is also one EN standard draft for a leakage test of medical gloves for single use:

ASTM F 903 Standard Test Method for Resistance of Materials Used in Protective Clothing to Penetration by Liquids.[56]

EN 374-2 Protective Gloves against Chemicals and Micro-organisms. Part 2: Determination of Resistance to Penetration (two alternative methods are presented, the air leak test and the water leak test).[57]

EN 455-1 Medical Gloves for Single Use. Part 1: Requirement and Testing for Freedom from Holes.[58]

The water leak test in EN 374-2 is almost equal to that described in EN 455-1, with only a minor difference between the fill tubs that should be attached to the glove. In the test, 1,000 mL water shall be added to the glove and then immediately examined for water leaks. If the glove does not leak immediately, a second observation shall be made after another 2 min. If no leak can be observed, the unit passes. In the air leak test (EN 374-2), the glove is attached to a circular fixing mandrel and inflated underwater at room temperature with air to given gauge pressure. The mandrel shall be rated in order to examine the whole glove surface for the emergence of air bubbles.

The two EN standard test methods can be used for standard quality control testing, as the whole glove is used. They also have the same requirements concerning the sampling procedure for inspection, with reference to the ISO 2859-1: *Sampling Procedure for Inspections by Attributes*.[48, 59] Three inspection levels determine the relationship between the lot or batch size and the sample size. The AQL (acceptable quality level) is a designated value of defects per hundred units that the consumer indicates will be accepted most of the time by the acceptance sampling procedure to be used. If more than a given number of the tested gloves fails (AQL), the lot/or batch shall be rejected. The standard quality control testing and virus penetration are discussed in more detail in Chapter 11.

In the ASTM F 903 standard test method, a circular specimen of the glove is mounted in a penetration test cell, then charged with a challenge liquid under defined pressure. The glove specimen is observed after 5 min in atmospheric pressure and then after 10 min at 13.8 kPa. The appearance of a drop of liquid indicates failure. This method is used to investigate the penetration of chemicals through glove materials, closures, and seams connecting gloves to protective suits.[60]

There are several standardized leakage test methods designed for medical gloves, that is, surgical gloves and examination gloves of rubber or plastic. Six of these, three developed by ASTM and three by the Department of Defense, were evaluated in a laboratory test by Carey et al.,[61] who found that all tests had inherent limitations. The US Food and Drug Administration also has a regulation on *Patient examination gloves and surgeons' gloves; sample plans and test method for leakage defects; adulteration* (21 CFR Section 800.20), which details sampling strategies and assigned AQLs.[62] The ability of water leak tests for medical gloves to detect gloves with potential for virus penetration has been studied by Kotilainen et al.[63–65] Extreme variability in vinyl glove quality but less in latex glove was observed, but gloves that passed a 1,000-mL water challenge are unlikely to allow the passage of small viruses. Phalen and Wong[66] also found inherent limitations of the 1,000-mL water leak test in detecting holes (0.15 ± 0.05 mm) capable of passing a virus. They developed a modified method that standardized the volume of water (up to 2 L) to reliably detect known holes in the glove brands and lots they tested. About 22%

of the medical grade gloves required extra water volume to reliably detect holes, especially in the fingers. In some cases, Douglas et al.[67] compared standard leak test methods for medical gloves. The testing was done by air inflation, chemical fill, and water fill methods. The methods varied in reproducibility, and the chemical fill method detected the highest portion of pinholes.[67]

Standard quality control testing is discussed in detail in Chapter 11.

10.5   CONCLUSIONS

The protective effect of gloves against chemicals depends on the following factors:

- Material quality and formulation
- Material thickness

The protective effect can be evaluated by the following:

- Degradation testing (screening)
- Permeation testing (resistance)
- Penetration testing (leakage)

A standard test method is a method designed for laboratory testing in a standardized way and is not supposed to represent all conditions likely to be found in working situations.

The test data should be restricted to the comparison of the glove materials mainly on a relative basis.

The permeation test results depend to a certain extent on the test conditions such as:

- Test cell and design
- Collecting medium, volume, and/or flow rate
- System mode (open or closed loop)
- Continuous or sampling measurement
- Sensitivity of the analytical equipment/system
- Test temperature
- Testing personnel (educated and well trained)

The permeation and penetration test data, together with results from mechanical tests and other factors, must be evaluated in the selection process of the most suitable protective glove for different kinds of working situations.[68] The risk assessments of exposure to hazardous agents and the application of test data in the selection process are discussed in more detail in separate chapters in this book.

REFERENCES

1. ASTM. 1985. *ASTM F 739–85: Standard Test Method: Resistance of Protective Clothing Materials to Permeation by Liquids or Gases. Annual Book of ASTM Standards.* Philadelphia, PA: American Society for Testing and Materials, 426.

2. CEN (European Standard). 1992. *EN 374–1: Protective Gloves against Chemicals and Micro-Organisms. Part 1: Terminology and Performance Requirements*. Brussels: Comité Européen de Normalisation (CEN/TC 162), April.

3. CEN (European Standard). 1992. *EN 374–3: Protective Gloves against Chemicals and Micro-Organisms. Part 3: Determination of Resistance to Permeations to Chemicals*. Brussels: Comité Européen de Normalisation (CEN/TC 162), April.

4. Stampfer, J.F., Beckman, R.J., and Berardinelli, S.P. 1988. Using immersion test data to screen chemical protective clothing. *Am Ind Hyg Assoc J* 49:579.

5. Schwope, A.D., Carroll, T.R., Huang, R., and Royer, M.D. 1988. Test kit for field evaluation of the chemical resistance of protective clothing, in *Performance of Protective Clothing: Second Symposium*, ASTM STP 989, Mansdorf, S.Z., Sager, R., and Nielsen, A.P., Eds. Philadelphia, PA: American Society for Testing and Materials, 314.

6. Henry, N.W., III. 1987. A critical evaluation of protective clothing test methods, in *Proceedings from Second Scandinavian Symposium on Protective Clothing against Chemicals and Other Health Risks*, 7–8 Nov. 1986, *Arbete & Hälsa* 1987:12, Mellström, G., and Carlsson, B., Eds. Stockholm: National Board of Occupational Safety and Health, 65.

7. Berardinelli, S., and Roder, M. 1986. Chemical protective clothing field evaluation methods, in *Performance of Protective Clothing: First Symposium*, ASTM STP 900, Barker, R.L., and Coletta, G.C., Eds. Philadelphia, PA: American Society for Testing and Materials, 250.

8. ASTM International. 2012. *ASTM D 471–12: Standard Test Method for Rubber Property—Effect of Liquids*. Philadelphia, PA: ASTM International.

9. ANSI. 2016. *ANSI/ISEA 105-2016: American National Standard for Hand Protection Classification*. Washington, DC: American National Standards Institute (ANSI).

10. CEN (European Standard). 2019. *EN ISO 374-4:2019: Protective Gloves against Dangerous Chemicals and Micro-Organisms - Part 4: Determination of Resistance to Degradation by Chemicals*. Brussels: Comité Européen de Normalisation.

11. Henry III, W.H., and Stull, J.O. 2003. Test methods and standards, in *Chemical Protective Clothing*, Anna, D.H., Ed. Fairfax, VA: AIHA Press, 188–189.

12. Steele, K.M., Pelham, T., and Phalen, R.N. 2017. Evaluating polymer degradation with complex mixtures using a simplified surface area method. *J Occup Environ Hyg* 14(9):720–726. DOI: 10.1080/15459624.2017.1322208.

13. ASTM. 1981. *ASTM F 739–81: Test for Resistance of Protective Clothing Materials to Permeation by Hazardous Liquid Chemicals, Annual Book of ASTM Standards*. Philadelphia, PA: American Society for Testing and Materials, 1.

14. ASTM. 2003. *ASTM F 739–99a: Standard Test Method: Resistance of Protective Clothing Materials to Permeation by Liquids or Gases under Continuous Conditions, Annual Book of ASTM Standards*. Philadelphia, PA: American Society for Testing and Materials.

15. ASTM International. 2020. *ASTM F 739–20: Standard Test Method for Permeation of Liquids and Gases through Protective Clothing Materials under Conditions of Continuous Contact*. Philadelphia, PA: ASTM International.

16. Banaee, S., and Que Hee, S.S. 2019. Glove permeation of chemicals: The state of the art of current practice, Part 1: Basics and the permeation standards. *J Occup Environ Hyg* 16(12):827–839. DOI: 10.1080/15459624.2019.

17. CEN (European Standard). 1992. *EN 374–2: Protective Gloves against Chemicals and Micro-Organisms. Part 2: Determination of Resistance to Penetration*. Brussels: Comité Européen de Normalisation (CEN/TC 162), April.

18. CEN (European Standard). 1992. *EN 374–3: Protective Gloves against Chemicals and Micro-Organisms. Part 3: Determination of Resistance to Permeation by Chemicals*. Brussels: Comité Européen de Normalisation (CEN/TC 162), April.

19. Australian Standards. 2003. *Committee SF-203 — Current Publications: Occupational Protective Gloves.* Sydney, NSW: Standards Australia International Ltd.
20. ISO (Standard). 2001. *ISO 6529.2001: Protective Clothing — Protection against Liquid Chemicals — Determination of Resistance of Air-Impermeable Materials to Permeation by Liquids.* Geneva: International Organization for Standardization (ISO), TC94/SC13, 1.
21. Berardinelli, S.P., and Hall, R. 1985. Site-specific whole glove chemical permeation. *Am Ind Hyg Assoc J* 46:60.
22. Vahdat, N. 1987. Permeation of polymeric materials by toluene. *Am Ind Hyg Assoc J* 48:155.
23. Mellström, G.A., Carlsson, B., and Boman, A. 1994. Testing protective effect against liquid chemicals, in *Protective Gloves for Occupational Use*, Mellström, G.A., Wahlberg, J.E., and Maibach, H.I., Eds. Boca Raton, FL: CRC Press, pp. 53–77.
24. ASTM International. 2020. *ASTM F 1383–20: Standard Test Method: Resistance of Protective Clothing Materials to Permeation by Liquids or Gases Under Conditions of Intermittent Contact.* Philadelphia, PA: American Society for Testing and Materials.
25. Berardinelli, S.P., and Moyer, E.S. 1988. Chemical protective clothing breakthrough time: Comparison of several test systems. *Am Ind Hyg Assoc J* 49:89.
26. Berardinelli, S.P., Mickelsen, P., and Roder, M.M. 1983. Chemical protective clothing: A comparison of chemical permeation test cells and direct-reading instruments. *Am Ind Hyg Assoc J* 44:886.
27. Berardinelli, S.P., Rusczek, R.A., and Mickelsen, R.L. 1987. A portable chemical protective clothing test method: Application at a chemical plant. *Am Ind Hyg Assoc J* 48:804.
28. Jencen, D.A., and Hardy, J.K. 1988. Method for the evaluation of the permeation characteristics of protective glove materials. *Am Ind Hyg Assoc J* 49:293.
29. Henry, N.W., III. 1988. Comparative evaluation of a smaller version of the ASTM permeation test cell versus the standard cell, in *Performance of Protective Clothing: Second Symposium*, ASTM STP 989, Mansdorf, S.Z., Sager, R., and Nielsen, A.P., Eds. Philadelphia, PA: American Society for Testing and Materials, 236.
30. Moody, R.P., and Ritter, L. 1990. Pesticide glove permeation analysis: Comparison of the ASTM F 739 test method with an automatic flow-through reverse-phase liquid chromatography procedure. *Am Ind Hyg Assoc J* 51:79.
31. Schwope, A.D., Costas, P.P., Mond, C.M., Nolen, R.L., Conoley, M., Garcia, D.B., Walters, D.B., and Prokopetz, A.T. 1988. Gloves for protection from aqueous formaldehyde: Permeation resistance and human factors analysis. *Appl Am Ind Hyg* 111:6.
32. Schwope, A.D., Goydan, R., Reid, R.C., and Krishnamurthy, S. 1988. State-of-the-art review of permeation testing and the interpretation of its results. *Am Ind Hyg Assoc J* 49:557.
33. Patton, G.L., Conoley, M., and Keith, L.H. 1988. Problems in determining permeation cell equivalency, in *Performance of Protective Clothing: Second Symposium*, ASTM STP 989, Mansdorf, S.Z., Sager, R., and Nielsen, A.P., Eds. Philadelphia, PA: American Society for Testing and Materials, 243.
34. Billing, C.B., and Bentz, A.P. 1988. Effect of temperature, material thickness and experimental apparatus on the permeation measurement, in *Performance of Protective Clothing: Second Symposium*, ASTM STP 989, Mansdorf, S.Z., Sager, R., and Nielsen, A.P., Eds. Philadelphia, PA: American Society for Testing and Materials, 226.
35. Nelson, G.O., Lum, B.B., Carlson, G.J., Wong, C.M., and Johnson, J.S. 1981. Glove permeation by organic solvents. *Am Ind Hyg Assoc J* 42:217.
36. Jamke, R.A. 1989. Understanding and using chemical permeation data in the selection of chemical protective clothing, in *Chemical Protective Clothing Performance in Chemical Emergency Response*, ASTM STP 1037, Perkins, J.L., and Stull, J.O., Eds. Philadelphia, PA: American Society for Testing and Materials, 11.

37. Kairys, C.J. 1989. MDPR — The need for minimum detectable permeation rate requirement in permeation testing of chemical protective clothing, in *Chemical Protective Clothing Performance in Chemical Emergency Response*, ASTM STP 1037, Perkins, J.L., and Stull, J.O., Eds. Philadelphia, PA: American Society for Testing and Materials, 265.
38. Zellers, E.T., and Sulewski, R. 1993. Modeling the temperature dependence of *N*-methyl-pyrrolidone permeation through butyl- and natural-rubber gloves. *Am Ind Hyg Assoc J* 54:465.
39. Anna, D.H., Zellers, E.T., and Sulewski, R. 1998. ASTM F 739 method for testing the permeation resistance of protective clothing materials: Critical analysis with proposed changes in procedure and test-cell design. *Am Ind Hyg Assoc J* 59:547.
40. Mäkelä, E.A., Vainiotalo, S., and Peltonen, K. 2003. Permeation of 70% isopropyl alcohol through surgical gloves: Comparison of the standard methods ASTM F 739 and EN 374. *Ann Occup Hyg* 47:305.
41. Gao, P., Weise, T., and Tomasovic, B. 2009. Development of a computer program for permeation testing data analysis. *J Occup Environ Hyg* 6(6):363–373. DOI: 10.1080/15459620902864973.
42. Man, V.L., Bastecki, V., Vandal, G., and Bentz, A. 1987. Permeation of protective clothing materials: Comparison of liquid contact, liquid splashes and vapors on breakthrough times. *Am Ind Hyg Assoc J* 48:551.
43. CEN (European Standard). 2016. *EN 374–1: Protective Gloves against Chemicals and Micro-Organisms. Part 1: Terminology and Performance Requirements*. Brussels: Comité Européen de Normalisation (CEN/TC 162).
44. Perkins, J.L. 1988. Chemical protective clothing: I. Selection and use. *Appl Ind Hyg* 2:222.
45. Mellström, G.A. 1991. Protective gloves of polymeric materials: Experimental permeation testing and clinical study of side effects. *Acta Derm Venereol Suppl (Stockh)* 163:1–54. PMID: 1771997.
46. Leinster, P., Bonsall, J.L., Evans, M.J., and Lewis, S.J. 1990. The application of test data in the selection and use of the gloves against chemicals. *Ann Occup Hyg* 34:85.
47. Colligan, S.A., and Horstman, S.W. 1990. Permeation of cancer chemotherapeutic drug through glove materials under static and flexed conditions. *Appl Occup Environ Hyg* 5(12):848.
48. Que Hee, S.S. 1989. Permeation of some pesticidal formulations through glove materials, in *Chemical Protective Clothing Performance in Chemical Emergency Response*, ASTM STP 1037, Perkins, J.L., and Stull, J.O., Eds. Philadelphia, PA: American Society for Testing and Materials, 157.
49. Ehntholt, D.J., Cerundolo, D.L., Bodek, I., Schwope, A.D., Royer, M.D., and Nielsen, A.P. 1990. A test method for the evaluation of protective glove materials used in agricultural pesticide operations. *Am Ind Hyg Assoc J* 51:462.
50. Ehntholt, D.J., Almeida, R.F., Beltis, K.J., Cerundolo, D.L., Schwope, A.D., Whelan, R.H., Royer, M.D., and Nielsen, A.P. 1988. Test method development and evaluation of protective clothing items used in agricultural pesticide operations, in *Performance of Protective Clothing: Second Symposium*, ASTM STP 989, Mansdorf, S.Z., Sager, R., and Nielsen, A.P., Eds. Philadelphia, PA: American Society for Testing and Materials, 727.
51. Ehntholt, D.J., Bodek, I., Valentine, J.R., Schwope, A.D., Royer, M.D., Frank, U., and Nielsen, A.P. 1989. The effects of solvent type and concentration on the permeation of pesticide formulations through chemical materials protective glove, in *Chemical Protective Clothing Performance in Chemical Emergency Response*, ASTM STP 1037, Perkins, J.L., and Stull, J.O., Eds. Philadelphia, PA: American Society for Testing and Materials, 146.

52. Pinette, M.F.S., Stull, J.O., Dodgen, C.R., and Morley, M.G. 1992. A preliminary study of an intermittent collection procedure as an alternative permeation method for nonvolatile, water soluble chemicals, in *Performance of Protective Clothing: Fourth Volume*, ASTM STP 1133, McBriarty, J.P., and Henry, W.N., Eds. Philadelphia, PA: American Society for Testing and Materials, 339.

53. Spence, M.W. 1988. An analytical technique for permeation testing of compounds with low volatility and water solubility, in *Performance of Protective Clothing: Second Symposium*, ASTM STP 989, Mansdorf, S.Z., Sager, R., and Nielsen, A.P., Eds. Philadelphia, PA: American Society for Testing and Materials, 277.

54. Lara, J., and Drolet, D. 1992. Testing the resistance of protective clothing materials to nitroglycerin and ethylene glycol dinitrate, in *Performance of Protective Clothing: Fourth Volume*, ASTM STP 1133, McBriarty, J.P., and Henry, W.N., Eds. Philadelphia, PA: American Society for Testing and Materials, 153.

55. Banaee, S., and Que Hee, S.S. 2020. Glove permeation of chemicals: The state of the art of current practice—Part 2. Research emphases on high boiling point compounds and simulating the donned glove environment. *J Occup Environ Hyg* 17(4):135–164. DOI: 10.1080/15459624.2020.1721509.

56. ASTM International. 2018. *ASTM F 903–18: Standard Test Method for Resistance of Materials Used in Protective Clothing to Penetration by Liquids*. Philadelphia, PA: ASTM International.

57. CEN (European Standard). 2019. *EN 374-2:2019: Protective Gloves against Dangerous Chemicals and Micro-Organisms. Part 2: Determination of Resistance to Penetration*. Brussels: Comité Européen de Normalisation (CEN/TC 162).

58. CEN (European Standard). 2020. *EN 455-1:2020: Medical Gloves for Single Use - Part 1: Requirement and Testing for Freedom from Holes*. Brussels: Comité Européen de Normalisation (CEN/TC 205/WG 3).

59. ISO (International Standard). 2019. *ISO 2859-1:1999(en): Sampling Procedures for Inspection by Attributes — Part 1: Sampling Schemes Indexed by Acceptance Quality Limit (AQL) for Lot-by-Lot Inspection*. Geneva: International Organization for Standardization (ISO).

60. Berardinelli, S.P., and Cottingham, L. 1986. Evaluation of chemical protective garment seams and closures for resistance to liquid penetration, in *Performance of Protective Clothing: First Symposium*, ASTM STP 900, Barker, R.L., and Coletta, G.C., Eds. Philadelphia, PA: American Society for Testing and Materials, 263.

61. Carey, R., Herman, W., Herman, B., and Casamento, J. 1989. A laboratory evaluation of standard leakage tests for surgical and examination gloves. *J Clin Eng* 14:133.

62. U.S. Food and Drug Administration. 2021. 21CFR800.20: Patient examination gloves and surgeons' gloves; sample plans and test method for leakage defects; adulteration. https://www.accessdata.fda.gov/scripts/cdrh/cfdocs/cfcfr/cfrsearch.cfm?fr=800.20.

63. Kotilainen, H.R., Brinker, J.P., Avato, J.L., and Gantz, N.M. 1989. Latex and vinyl examination gloves. Quality control procedures and implications for health care workers. *Arch Intern Med* 149:2749.

64. Kotilainen, H.R., Avato, J.L., and Gantz, N.M. 1990. Latex and vinyl nonsterile examination gloves: Status report on laboratory evaluation of defects by physical and biological methods. *Appl Environ Microbiol* 56:1627.

65. Kotilainen, H.R., Cyr, W.H., Truscott, W., Nelson, M.G., Routson, L.B., and Lytle, C.D. 1992. Ability of 1000 mL water leak test for medical gloves to detect gloves with potential for virus penetration, in *Performance of Protective Clothing: Fourth Volume*, ASTM STP 1133, McBriarty, J.P., and Henry, W.N., Eds. Philadelphia, PA: American Society for Testing and Materials, 38.

66. Douglas, A.A., Neufeld, P.D., and Wong, R.K.W. 1992. An interlaboratory comparison of standard test methods for medical gloves, in *Performance of Protective Clothing: Fourth Volume*, ASTM STP 1133, McBriarty, J.P., and Henry, W.N., Eds. Philadelphia, PA: American Society for Testing and Materials, 99.

67. Phalen, R.N., and Wong, W.K. 2011. Integrity of disposable nitrile exam gloves exposed to simulated movement. *J Occup Environ Hyg* 8(5):289–299. DOI: 10.1080/15459624.2011.569285.

68. Stull, J.O., White, D.F., and Greimel, T.C. 1992. A comparison of the liquid penetration test with other chemical resistance tests and its application in determining the performance of protective clothing, in *Performance of Protective Clothing: Fourth Volume*, ASTM STP 1133, McBriarty, J.P., and Henry, W.N., Eds. Philadelphia, PA: American Society for Testing and Materials, 123.

11 Standard Quality Control Testing, Virus Penetration, and Glove Durability

R.N. Phalen and Y.K. Hamidi

CONTENTS

DOI: 10.1201/9781003126874-13

11.1   INTRODUCTION

Concerns and research about the quality of medical gloves originally arose from the possibility of transmission of a deadly disease: acquired immune deficiency syndrome (AIDS). Because of the AIDS epidemic, research studies on barrier protection for the healthcare worker have continued, focused on barrier effectiveness to the human immunodeficiency virus (HIV), the suspected etiological agent of AIDS. These studies have also provided data relevant to the possible transmission of other viral diseases, such as hepatitis B (HBV), hepatitis C (HCV), herpes simplex (HSV), and more recently Ebola or Ebola Virus Disease (EVD).

The original practice of wearing gloves for surgery started to reduce postoperative infections among surgical patients. The use of gloves has expanded outside the surgical suite and is now considered a primary precaution for protection by healthcare workers, emergency medical technicians, first responders, and laboratory workers. The primary concern is the integrity of the glove as a barrier to the transmission of infectious agents, especially viruses. Passage of viruses through gloves may occur when defects, e.g., pinholes or tears, are present. This passage is called penetration. On the other hand, permeation—where a substance might migrate or diffuse through intact material—is unlikely for viruses unless the glove has been degraded. The term *penetration*, as described above, is used throughout this chapter. The word *leakage* is defined as the passage of any challenge fluid through the glove and could result from penetration or permeation.

This chapter concerns the tests for medical glove integrity and the relevance of these tests in assuring continued barrier effectiveness against virus transmission. Since the first two editions of this chapter,[1,2] numerous studies have addressed perforation, puncture resistance, and other properties influencing the integrity of gloves during use. Many of the findings described in this chapter are based on standard tests for glove integrity or slight variations of those tests.

11.2   STANDARD TESTS FOR GLOVE INTEGRITY

11.2.1   THE 1000 ML WATER LEAK TEST

The US Food and Drug Administration (FDA) utilizes a quality assurance test known as the "1000 mL water leak test" to evaluate the barrier integrity of patient examination gloves and surgeons' gloves. Last amended in 2017, the protocol for this test is described in Title 21 Code of Federal Regulations (21 CFR) Part 800.20.[3] The American Society for Testing and Materials (now ASTM International) Standard D 5151, *Standard Test Method for Detection of Holes in Medical Gloves*, implements this test.[4] Any visually detectable water on the outside of the glove, i.e., a leak before or after a 2-min observation time, is considered a failure. Because this is a "pass–fail" test, it has not been subjected to the usual inter-laboratory and intra-laboratory analysis for precision or bias. However, previous research discussed in the first edition of this chapter indicated that, compared to other conventional leak tests, the 1000 mL water leak gave the best combination of utility and performance. The water leak test is intended to provide a measure of manufacturing quality.

The FDA collects samples from the manufactured lots of gloves and tests them according to the size of the lot, using a statistical sampling scheme also described in 21 CFR 800.20. The amended final rule, published in the December 19, 2006, *Federal Register* and effective December 19, 2008, identified a more stringent and appropriate acceptable quality level (AQL) at 1.5 for surgeons' gloves and 2.5 for patient examination gloves.[3] The prior AQLs were 2.5 for surgeons' gloves and 4.0 for patient examination gloves. For regulatory purposes, the FDA refers to this as the adulteration level. The manufacturer collects random samples from lots of medical gloves and performs the 1000 mL water leak test in accordance with FDA's sampling inspection plans, which have been derived from the tables in International Standards Organization (ISO) 2859-1:1999, *Sampling Procedures and Tables for Inspection by Attributes.*[5] FDA uses single sampling for lots of up to 1200 gloves and multiple sampling for lots of greater than 1200 gloves, where the term *lot* means a collection of gloves from which a sample is to be drawn and inspected. It may differ from a collection of gloves designated as a lot for other purposes, e.g., production or shipment.

Glove lots that are tested and rejected when using the 1000 mL water leak test and the AQLs specified in the final rule are considered adulterated and subject to regulatory action, such as refusal of imported gloves at the port of entry or seizure of domestic gloves. The actual sampling plans (sample size and accept/reject numbers) are shown in Tables 11.1 and 11.2. Note that sampling and testing may cease when a lot is determined to be violative, i.e., rejected.

The European Union has an equivalent 1000 mL water leak test for single-use medical gloves: EN-455-1, *Medical gloves for single use—Part 1: Requirements and testing for freedom from holes.*[6] The standard references ISO 2859-1 for sampling and the established AQL is 1.5.

11.2.2 Virus Leak Tests

The first edition of this chapter discussed testing for glove defects with viruses. Important properties of the viruses were also discussed. The consensus seems to have been reached that using the Phi-X174 bacteriophage in a leak test offers a good combination of utility and performance. The bacteriophage has an average diameter of 27 nm, which approaches molecular dimensions.[1] For example, a dextran of molecular weight 1 million also has a similar diameter but could change shape under shear during flow. Hemoglobin is about 6 nm in diameter. It is believed that the use of test particles smaller than Phi-X174 would result in an assessment of glove permeation rather than defects, pores, or microscopic tears. Assessment of glove permeation is discussed elsewhere in this book.

A viral penetration test for elastomeric materials using the Phi-X174 bacteriophage as a surrogate for HBV, HBV, and HIV is implemented in ASTM F 1671.[7] The method is based on the use of the ASTM F 903 penetration test cell, which is used for measuring the resistance of chemical protective clothing materials to penetration by liquids. A screening test, ASTM F 1670 that evaluates penetration of synthetic blood using the same test cell, is recommended. This test has several desirable features: the surface tension of the test viral suspension is controlled, a specific transmembrane

TABLE 11.1

Sampling Scheme for Lots of Surgeons' Gloves Where the Accepted Quality Level (AQL) Is 1.5

Lot Size	Sample	Sample Size	Number Examined	Number Accept	Number Defective Reject
>35,000	1st	125	125	1	7
	2nd	125	250	4	10
	3rd	125	375	8	13
	4th	125	500	12	17
	5th	125	625	17	20
	6th	125	750	21	23
	7th	125	875	25	26
10,001–35,000	1st	80	80	0	5
	2nd	80	160	3	8
	3rd	80	240	6	10
	4th	80	320	8	13
	5th	80	400	11	15
	6th	80	480	14	17
	7th	80	560	18	19
3,201–10,000	1st	50	50	0	4
	2nd	50	100	1	6
	3rd	50	150	3	8
	4th	50	200	5	10
	5th	50	250	7	11
	6th	50	300	10	12
	7th	50	350	13	14
1,201–3,200	1st	32	32	-	4
	2nd	32	64	1	5
	3rd	32	96	2	6
	4th	32	128	3	7
	5th	32	160	5	8
	6th	32	192	7	9
	7th	32	224	9	10
501–1200	Single	80	80	3	4
281–500	Single	50	50	2	3
91–280	Single	32	32	1	2
8—90	Single	20	8	0	1

(*Source:* 21 CFR 800.20)

pressure is applied to induce flow, there is a quantitative pass/fail criterion, and the test has been subjected to interlaboratory evaluation. Unfortunately, unlike the 1000 mL water leak test, it does not test the whole glove, and it has been shown to give false negatives in the case of micron-sized tears that are not necessarily open. The false negatives of this standard test method are mostly due to the flat, open-mesh

TABLE 11.2
Sampling Scheme for Lots of Patient Examination Gloves Where the Accepted Quality Level (AQL) Is 4.0

Lot Size	Sample	Sample Size	Number Examined	Number Accept	Number Defective Reject
>35,000	1st	125	125	2	9
	2nd	125	250	7	14
	3rd	125	375	13	19
	4th	125	500	19	25
	5th	125	625	25	29
	6th	125	750	31	33
	7th	125	875	37	38
10,001–35,000	1st	80	80	1	7
	2nd	80	160	4	10
	3rd	80	240	8	13
	4th	80	320	12	17
	5th	80	400	17	20
	6th	80	480	21	23
	7th	80	560	25	26
3201–10,000	1st	50	50	0	5
	2nd	50	100	3	8
	3rd	50	150	6	10
	4th	50	200	8	13
	5th	50	250	11	15
	6th	50	300	14	17
	7th	50	350	18	19
1201–3200	1st	32	32	0	4
	2nd	32	64	1	6
	3rd	32	96	3	8
	4th	32	128	5	10
	5th	32	160	7	11
	6th	32	192	10	12
	7th	32	224	13	14
501–1200	Single	80	80	5	6
281–500	Single	50	50	3	4
151–280	Single	32	32	2	3
51—150	Single	20	20	1	2
5—50	Single	5	5	0	1

(*Source:* 21 CFR 800.20)

retaining screen that prevents expansion of the test specimen. Kisielewski et al.[8] demonstrated that replacing the flat retainer with a rigid screen having a nearly hemispherical dome, which allows for controlled expansion of the specimen, significantly enhances the detection of tear defects in materials that pass the same test when a flat retaining screen is used.

11.2.3 PUNCTURE RESISTANCE

Users have noticed visible punctures or needle sticks that could compromise barrier effectiveness. The puncture resistance of various glove materials is described later. There is a standard method, ASTM F 1342, *Standard Test Method for Protective Clothing Material Resistance to Puncture*, for determining the puncture resistance of protective articles.[9] The method measures the force and displacement necessary to create a puncture using a rounded or blunt probe: Probe A is conical, Probe B rounded, and Probe C is spherical. In principle, the work (energy) necessary to create a puncture can be determined for a given material. It can test various parts of a glove and could be used for a relative ranking of glove materials. However, Nguyen et al.[10] showed that the puncture by the probes used in these tests is different from those made by medical needles. A more recent addition in 2010, and revised in 2019, was ASTM F 2878,[11] *Standard Test Method for Protective Clothing Material Resistance to Hypodermic Needle Puncture*, which uses 21-gauge, 25-gauge, or 28-gauge hypodermic needles. The test method still does not take into account all conditions of use that could affect puncture resistance, such as the stiffness of the backing materials or tension on the test specimen.

As previously mentioned, these ASTM standard test methods are limited in their ability to rank the performance of glove materials. In 1999, the American National Standards Institute/International Safety Equipment Association (ANSI/ISEA) established ANSI/ISEA 105 (last updated in 2016),[12] *American National Standard for Hand Protection Classification*, which establishes puncture resistance performance levels based on forces measured using standardized puncture tests. For hypodermic needles, the standard refers to ASTM F 2878 needle puncture testing using a 25-gauge needle. For blunt probe testing, the standard references the use of an EN 388 puncture probe and testing method. A performance ranking scale from 0 (minimal) to 5 (highest) is provided, based on the resulting puncture force. Products can be tested, labeled, and marketed to customers based on these relative performance levels.

The ANSI/ISEA 105 standard establishes performance levels for mechanical protection (e.g., cut, puncture, and abrasion resistance), chemical protection (e.g., permeation and degradation resistance), heat and flame protection (e.g., ignition and conductive heat resistance), vibration reduction, and dexterity. Chapter 6 discusses ANSI/ISEA 105 in more detail.

11.2.4 BREAKING STRENGTH

Strength at break might be considered irrelevant to barrier effectiveness. However, Lytle and Routson,[13] describe a situation involving some latex gloves that had breaking strengths below specification. Water seeped through the latex over large areas of the gloves, and the virus also passed through. Breaking strength is included in specifications for most protective gloves[14–17] and will screen out *grossly* inferior products. ASTM D 412 is a standard methodology and has been subjected to inter-laboratory evaluation.[18] It does have the limitation that the entire glove is not tested, and it does not predict glove durability. The European Union has a similar standard that includes a breaking strength test to be performed after simulated aging: EN 455-2, *Medical gloves for single use—Part 2: Requirements and testing for physical properties*.[19] It also references EN 455-4 for aging and shelf-life requirements.

11.2.5 TEAR STRENGTH

Another standard that can be applied for testing medical gloves is ASTM D 624.[20] This test method is used to measure the tear strength of vulcanized rubbers and thermoplastic elastomers. This standard is not necessarily relevant to barrier effectiveness and does have the limitation of not testing the entire glove. However, it does give a better idea of glove resistance to tearing. Less resistance implies microscopic tears are more likely to enlarge, which could seriously compromise barrier integrity.

11.3 INTEGRITY STUDIES OF NEW AND USED GLOVES

11.3.1 LEAK TESTS ON USED GLOVES

Multiple authors have studied the barrier integrity of gloves either after simulated use in a laboratory or after actual use in a clinical or laboratory setting. Earlier research has focused on comparisons between latex and nonlatex gloves, as problems with latex allergy have led users to seek gloves made from materials other than latex. Vinyl gloves have been available for many years, but nonsterile vinyl gloves are a less effective barrier than latex when assessed after use.[21–27] The studies mentioned in this section represent a cross section of earlier studies and those currently available in the published literature. This section begins with those studies in which barrier integrity was assessed using the 1000 mL water leak test, followed by those in which barrier integrity was assessed using viral penetration testing.

11.3.1.1 Testing with 1000 mL of Water

11.3.1.1.1 Earlier Studies

Douglas et al.[28] studied differences in water leakage rates and tensile properties among both new and used gloves from a hospital clinic. Three brands of latex and three brands of vinyl gloves were included in the study. All gloves were nonsterile except for one brand of vinyl gloves. For used gloves, the nonsterile vinyl gloves behaved as expected from the previous work mentioned above: Leakage rates from the 1000 mL water fill test averaged 26% for the nonsterile vinyl gloves and 8% for the latex gloves. However, because water leakage rates for the sterile vinyl gloves averaged only 3%, the authors concluded that "barrier durability" is not a sole function of glove material. The authors further concluded that leakage testing of new gloves was not a valid predictor of leakage during use since leakage rates for all gloves tested were found to be in the range of 2% or less. As for tensile testing, the most significant result was that one brand of latex gloves exhibited a significant increase in tensile strength and elongation after use, with the authors surmising continued vulcanization of the rubber as the cause.

Newsom et al.[29] compared leakage rates among latex and neoprene (chloroprene) gloves after surgical use. The authors found no significant difference in leakage rates between latex and neoprene gloves (roughly 10% for both types) using the 1000 mL water leak test. It was noted, however, that while 14 of 37 "punctures" (ruptures, tears, holes) in the neoprene gloves became obvious to the wearer during use, only 3 of 31 punctures were noted when latex gloves were worn. Upon laboratory examination, the neoprene punctures were generally noted to be larger than those in latex, but puncture size was not quantified. The tendency for tears to propagate more easily in punctured neoprene than latex, and thus be more readily apparent to the user, was further evident in the fact that 8 of 330 neoprene gloves were rejected before use (and excluded from the study) due to tearing upon donning. No latex gloves were excluded from the study for this reason. The authors suggest that a gentler donning process ought to be employed by users of neoprene gloves.

Rego and Roley[30] evaluated the barrier integrity of latex, vinyl, and nitrile gloves using the 1000 mL water leak test for both new gloves and gloves subjected to a simulated clinical use protocol. A total of 2000 gloves were tested: 100 new and 100 used, for each of 10 varieties of gloves. The authors found that after simulated use, latex and nitrile leakage rates were not significantly different from each other (0–4% for latex and 1–3% for nitrile), nor were they significantly different from those of new gloves (0–5% for latex and 3% for nitrile). Leakage rates for vinyl gloves ranged from 1% to 12% for new gloves and 12% to 61% after simulated use. These authors also concluded, as did Douglas et al.[28] that studies on new gloves are not predictive of barrier durability during use.

Muto et al.[31] used the 1000 mL water leak test to evaluate the barrier integrity of more than 3700 gloves comprising multiple varieties: sterile surgical gloves, nonsterile examination gloves, and sterile "procedure" gloves, made from latex with either high or low water-soluble protein content, or vinyl, nitrile, and neoprene materials. Water leak testing was performed on both new gloves and gloves that had been subjected to a simulated use protocol. The authors concluded that leakage rates were greater for examination gloves than for surgical gloves, as well as greater for used gloves than for new gloves. In addition, leakage rates for the high-protein-content latex surgical gloves were generally lower than those for all other types of gloves, especially after simulated use.

Korniewicz et al.[32] evaluated more than 5500 latex, nitrile, vinyl, and "copolymer" examination gloves for barrier integrity using the 1000 mL water leak test. Half of the gloves were new or "unstressed," while the other half had been "stressed" according to a simulated clinical use protocol. The average leakage rates for each material (encompassing several brands per material and also adjusting for stress level) were as follows: nitrile 1.3%; latex 2.2%; vinyl 8.2%; and copolymer

8.2%. The authors, therefore, concluded that nitrile examination gloves are a suitable alternative to latex but that vinyl and copolymer gloves provide less effective barrier protection.

11.3.1.1.2 Recent Studies

The literature is replete with articles using the 1000 mL water leak test to evaluate the integrity of surgical gloves used during surgical procedures, as well as for disposable medical gloves used by healthcare workers. The following more recent studies have been selected to highlight some of the newer findings concerning the time of use, glove thickness, and glove fit.

Tlili et al.[33] evaluated the integrity of surgical gloves used by 49 participants working in three different surgical units. All gloves were NRL (i.e., latex) of two different brands and thicknesses. They used the EN 455-1 1000 mL water leak test and found an overall leak failure rate of 16.5%. There were differences in perforations among the surgical specialties, with urology higher than general or maxillofacial, and additionally, the length of use was found to be associated with glove perforation. Surgeries that exceeded 90 min resulted in a significantly higher percentage of perforations (36 out of 156; 23.1%) than those procedures taking less time (11 out of 128; 8.6%). In a similar study by de Oliveira and Gama,[34] surgeries that exceeded 150 min resulted in significantly higher glove perforations than those procedures taking less time. Elce et al.[35] found that equine surgeries lasting more than 60 min were about 2.5 times more likely to result in a glove perforation than those requiring less time. Sayin et al.[36] similarly found that an operation time of greater than 60 min increased the risk of glove perforation by about 12.8 times with abdominal surgeries. Thus, the duration of use, as well as frequency of replacement, can be seen as an important factor associated with glove perforations.

Tlili et al.[33] also found that the glove brand was a factor associated with a significantly higher perforation rate. Brand A exhibited a significantly higher percentage of perforations (45 out of 238; 18.9%) than brand B (2 out of 46; 4.3%). The difference in thickness was 0.22 mm (brand A) versus 0.18 mm (brand B), which was a nominal difference and the thicker glove did not perform better. Han et al.[37] also reported that thicker surgical gloves did not offer an additional protective effect over conventional gloves. This is an indication that the glove formulation may be a more important factor in its resistance to perforation.

Zare et al.[38] evaluated the post-use integrity of different fitting (e.g., fit, tight, and loose) disposable medical gloves worn by 45 healthcare workers. The subjects were midwives in a maternity ward, with hand sizes (breadth) ranging from 6.5 (80–85 mm) to 8 (99–105 mm), and they reported using the gloves 5.5 ± 2 h per day. The researchers used the EN 455-1 1000 mL water leak test and found there were significant differences in leak failures with ill-fitted gloves. The leak failures were 20% for well-fit gloves, 35% for loose-fitting gloves, and 38% for tight-fitting gloves. They concluded that wearing the wrong-sized gloves can affect glove integrity, resulting in higher perforations. This study shows the importance of ensuring workers are properly trained on the selection of properly sized gloves, as well as ensuring an adequate selection of different glove sizes is made available to workers.

11.3.1.2   Testing with a Modified Water Leak Test

Phalen and Wong[39] developed a modified water leak test, which standardized the amount of water volume (up to 2.5 L) to reliably detect small 30-gauge needle holes (0.15 ± 0.05 mm) in the finger, thumb, and palm regions of disposable medical gloves. The method also used a restrictive 3-inch coupling over the cuff region of the glove, which served to increase water pressure and the sensitivity of the test. The rationale was based on that of Kotilainen et al.,[40] indicating the inability of the 1000 mL water leak test in reliably detecting holes made by a 30-gauge needle, as well as the passage of a virus through these holes. The researchers also performed a prescreening test and determined that the 1000 mL water leak test was unable to reliably detect holes made by a 21-gauge needle, especially in the fingers and thumb. The main objective was to evaluate the effect of simulated hand movement on the integrity of disposable nitrile gloves. Although simulated hand movement was not determined to significantly affect glove integrity, approximately 81.7% of leak failures were detected in the fingers and thumb. Thus, the modified water leak test detected small holes capable of passing a virus and in terminal regions of the glove, which may otherwise go undetected using the standard 1000 mL water leak test.

The modified water leak test was later used to evaluate the leak failure rates of two dissimilar types of disposable nitrile gloves (i.e., six cleanroom gloves and five low-modulus gloves).[41] The standardized water volume for the low-modulus gloves was 1 L and no additional water was required. However, for the cleanroom gloves, up to 2 L of water was required to reliably detect holes made by a 30-gauge needle. Half of the cleanroom gloves required more than 1 L of water. A logistic regression analysis indicated that the cleanroom gloves were about three times more likely to have a leak failure than the low-modulus gloves. Furthermore, gloves with a higher modulus (e.g., a maximum modulus ≥ 4 MPa) were about 3.7 times more likely to have a leak failure. Gloves with a higher area density (≥ 11 g/cm^2) were about 3.9 times more likely to have a leak failure.

Shless et al.[42] used the modified water leak test to evaluate the integrity of disposable NRL (powdered and non-powdered) and nitrile exam gloves exposed to repeated disinfection with an alcohol-based hand rub, dilute bleach solution, and soap and water. The study was conducted in response to the shortages of gloves during the COVID-19 pandemic and to evaluate the US Centers for Disease Control and Prevention recommendations for extended glove use. The standardized water volumes ranged from 1 L to 2.5 L, with the NRL gloves requiring more water on average. Similar to Phalen and Wong,[39] they found that a majority of the leak failures were in the finger regions. About 69% of the leak failures were in the fingers and interdigital webs of the fingers, whereas 24% of the total failures were in the palm region of the gloves.

Overall, one main advantage of this modified water leak test is that it can detect smaller holes with the potential to pass a virus in the whole glove, as compared to the ASTM F 1671 viral penetration test that tests only a swatch of material. The increased ability to detect small holes or defects can also increase the sensitivity over the traditional 1000 mL water leak test. One limitation is that these results are not easily comparable to studies relying on the FDA, ASTM D 5151, or EN 455-1 1000 mL water leak tests.

A recently developed leak test method using vacuum pressure to draw measured volumes of water through glove pieces and whole gloves is also available in the literature.[43] The method uses a Frazier air permeability tester and has the capability of measuring the flow rates through holes or tears in the material.

11.3.1.3 Testing with Viruses

The small bacteriophage Phi-X174 has proved to be very useful in testing barriers for their ability to stop viral penetration. The virus can be grown to very high titers and is safe to use, even on the open benchtop, without the protection of a safety cabinet. The assay is relatively inexpensive and can be performed in a few hours. Detection limits are very sensitive, with only a few viruses leading to a positive assay. Penetration studies have been done using uniform holes of varying sizes drilled by laser beams. These studies, summarized in Lytle et al.,[1] showed that virus penetration through a small hole can be described by the Poiseuille equation, which has been used to describe fluid flow through pipes. The rate of virus flowing through a hole varies as a function of the hole diameter to the fourth power and varies inversely with the length of the hole. This means that holes of small diameter and long length can effectively stop viral penetration because of the length of time it takes for the fluid to pass through that hole. It is very important to know that viral penetration depends on the flow of the fluid in which the virus is suspended and not on the size of the virus. Therefore, arguments that viruses are orders of magnitude smaller than holes in gloves (or condoms) are specious, as viruses do not act alone. They are suspended in fluid, and it is the flow of fluid that determines viral penetration.

Previous viral penetration studies have included gloves made of synthetic elastomers as many healthcare workers have switched from latex gloves to synthetic products because of latex sensitivity. Several studies of latex and nonlatex gloves have been published. Hamann and Nelson[44] tested synthetic, nonlatex, nonvinyl, thermoplastic elastomer (TPE) gloves and found them to be as good, if not better, as latex gloves. In addition, the authors also summarized more than a dozen studies on glove barrier studies. They reviewed the major conclusions from these studies, which are listed below:

1. Latex gloves are better barriers than vinyl gloves.
2. Surgical gloves perform better than examination gloves.
3. Choice of glove manufacturer may be more critical than the choice of glove material.
4. Leakage rates increase with increased time of use and with more stressful activities.
5. The performance of gloves can be decreased by exposure to humidity, heat, mechanical stress, ultraviolet light, and ozone. Therefore, the packaging of gloves is very important.

Two other studies compared powdered latex vs. nonpowdered latex gloves. Edlich et al.[45] examined two brands of latex examination gloves, three brands of nitrile gloves, and one brand of polyvinyl examination gloves. The gloves were filled with

300 mL of sterile buffer and were suspended in a flask of medium containing Phi-X174 bacteriophage (1600 mL at 10^6 viruses per mL). This study found no virus penetration in any of the brands of gloves. In contrast, Calhoun et al.[46] found considerable penetration of virus through powder-free latex gloves but no penetration in powdered gloves. In these experiments, the bacteriophage was inside the gloves, and the gloves were put in direct contact with agar plates that had been prepared with a lawn of *Escherichia coli* bacteria, the host for the bacteriophage. The difference in results may have been due to testing different brands or more likely due to the increased sensitivity of the Calhoun study to detect penetration of viruses.

All of the early virus studies on medical gloves tested only fingers or a small part of the gloves. ASTM has tried for many years to develop a test that would examine the entire surface area of the glove for virus penetration.[47] A draft standard under development parallels the work of Nelson et al.[48] Nelson et al. describe the procedures, which involved a suspension of entire gloves, filled with a sterile medium, immersed into a bath of medium with Phi-X174 bacteriophage. The gloves were agitated, and fluid samples were removed from their insides to determine if any virus had passed from the outside to the inside of the glove. Two different assays were made. A quantitative assay, in which aliquots of fluid from the inside were plated on agar plates with a lawn of *E. coli*, could determine how many viruses penetrated the glove barrier. A more sensitive assay involved adding the host bacterium, *E. coli*, to the aliquot. If the virus were present, it would use the host, multiply, and the entire aliquot would be cleared of bacteria, as the virus would lyse its host and clear the bacterial solution. This qualitative assay is very sensitive and would give the industry and public health community an assay for testing the entire surface area of the glove.

Broyles et al.[49] added polymerase chain reaction (PCR) analysis to the conventional plating assays.[48] PCR offers advantages in speed, automation, and use of less sample volume (about 1% of the volume required for plate counting). The use of Phi-X174 DNA in a PCR assay is nearly as sensitive as counting viral plaques on a lawn of host *E. coli* bacteria. The use of PCR technology can be done in real-time analysis and could be very useful to manufacturers or quality control laboratories. The researchers found that glove powder did not interfere with the PCR assay, probably due to the dilution of powder in the 300 mL of collection fluid, in contrast to another report.[49] Another report claimed that glove powder did interfere with the PCR assay.[50] More virus was detected by PCR analysis for synthetic gloves than for latex examination gloves, and the researchers attribute this finding to a phenomenon that has been termed *resealing*, or the retraction of latex around a hole once the puncturing object has been removed.

O'Connell et al.[51] evaluated three protocols for the direct examination of the viral penetration of nonlatex surgical and patient examination gloves. In two of the methods, the gloves were filled with and suspended within the nutrient broth solution, with test vessel agitation. The Phi-X174 bacteriophage was added to either the inside or outside of the glove. The third method did not involve agitation and the bacteriophage was added inside the glove. The methods involving the placement of the bacteriophage inside the glove provided greater sensitivity. With the introduction of two stress protocols, one a puncture with an 18-gauge needle and the other a donned manipulation of items, significant differences between the three methods were observed. It was presumed that the introduction of defects was necessary to observe these differences among the methods, as well as with the glove brands tested. Overall, placing bacteriophage inside the gloves provided a more sensitive means of detecting the passage of bacteriophage through a glove.

11.3.2 LEAK TESTS ON PUNCTURED GLOVES

Puncture (perforation) of protective gloves continues to be of concern. Rates of perforation for various types of medical procedures and surgeries continue to be studied,[52–55] and vary from a few percent to about 50% of gloves that were used. As expected, the likelihood of puncture increases with the duration of use. The existence of nonvisible punctures is often determined by the water leak test, as it is the quickest and most convenient test.

11.3.2.1 Results from 1000 mL Water Leak Tests

Some studies have attempted to produce positive controls by puncturing gloves with hypodermic needles of various sizes. These studies indicated that the water leak test becomes less effective as smaller-sized needles were used.[56,57] A puncture by a needle produces a crack or tear whose width is much, much narrower than its length.[8] Such a defect seriously challenges leak tests as discussed above. For example, ASTM F 1671 does not reliably detect micron-sized tears even when a transmembrane pressure of 2 psi (~140 cm water) is applied unless the tears are allowed to open.

Phalen and Wong[39] evaluated the morphology of holes made in a slightly inflated disposable nitrile glove with a 30-gauge needle. The holes were crescent-shaped and approximately 0.15 ± 0.05 mm in length. They also noted that the needle punctures were consistent with those glove defects observed with leak failures during normal testing. Most of the glove defects were long, slender slits in the glove material. This may be one reason why the developed 1000 mL water leak tests, based on earlier studies with uniform holes,[1] show discrepancies with the ability to detect smaller holes in glove materials. Sufficient pressure may be required to open the holes and allow water to flow through them. In addition, the surface tension of water may be an additional factor affecting the detection of holes with water leak testing methods.

11.3.2.2 Results from Virus Tests

Viral penetration through punctures introduced by acupuncture needles was discussed in the previous edition of this chapter. Limited studies at that time suggested that the water leak test was as sensitive as viral penetration. Subsequently, a few more studies have employed Phi-X174 in a whole-glove test where punctures by hypodermic needles were introduced as positive controls. Calhoun et al.[46] found that for powdered gloves virus leakage was not reliably detected for needle gauges above 25 (smaller diameters). Hamann and Nelson[44] examined, as described above, latex and elastomer nonpowdered gloves. Controls were produced by puncturing gloves with a 26-gauge needle. Transmission of the virus through the control punctures was not reliably detected by the quantitative method, but the qualitative (with biological amplification) assay gave positive results for all controls. This may be because the test volume of 200–300 mL decreases the transported virus concentration too much. The results of the modified ASTM F 1671 test also suggest that opening cracks would be very effective. Agitation may help do this, but a pressure difference between the inside and outside of the glove would also help. In the published whole-gloves studies it is difficult to tell what this pressure difference might have been.

As previously discussed, O'Connell et al.[51] found that placing bacteriophage inside the gloves provided a more sensitive means of detecting the passage of bacteriophage through a glove, whereas the addition of agitation did not significantly increase sensitivity.

The significance of these studies is difficult to assess. It would seem that perforation rates might be underestimated by the 1000 mL water leak test because some micron-sized tears are not detected. As discussed by Lytle and Routson,[13] in a previous publication, the risk associated with the passage of a few virus particles depends on the infectivity of the virus, the concentration, and the route of exposure. Virus leak tests are not nearly as rapid as the water leak test and are more resource-intensive. One possible solution could be the further development of a modified water leak test designed to reliably detect holes capable of passing a virus, as previously discussed.[39-42] The addition of a surfactant to reduce surface tension may also be worth investigating.

11.3.3 STUDIES OF PUNCTURE RESISTANCE

Several approaches to the problem of reducing glove puncture or perforation have been advocated: selection of puncture-resistant gloves, use of double gloves, and/or glove liners. Assessment of the effectiveness of these approaches involves a determination of glove resistance to sharps, i.e., puncture resistance. Puncture resistance could be used as part of a glove rating system or comparison in the selection of gloves and/or liners. For example, the previously discussed ANSI/ISEA 105 standard provides such a rating system. Additionally, the National Fire Protection Association (NFPA) published standard NFPA 1999 that offers a requirement for gloves that indicates a minimum requirement for puncture resistance when tested according to ASTM F 1342.[58]

11.3.3.1 Earlier Studies

A previous study looked at the puncture resistance of three latex gloves, of varying thickness, and a nitrile glove using the ASTM F 1342-specified test probe and also an 18-gauge hypodermic needle.[59] The ASTM F 1342 test probe had a diameter of 0.08 in., or 2.03 mm, while an 18-gauge hypodermic needle had a diameter of 1.27 mm. Hence, one might expect the tear length and work involved to differ for the two probes. Other test conditions were the same for both probes. Ten punctures by each probe were made for each glove. The force required to puncture the glove using the hypodermic needle was significantly lower, less than one-half, than for the standard probe. When the hypodermic needle was used, the nitrile glove required the most force for perforation. As might be expected, the two thicker latex gloves required more force than the thinnest one.

Subsequent studies evaluated orthopedic and examination gloves.[60–62] Measurements were made using the same ASTM F 1342 standard probe. These studies confirmed that among gloves of the same material type, the thicker gloves gave more penetration resistance. The material from which the glove was made also influenced the penetration resistance; the studies referenced above found nitrile to offer more resistance. The force needed to puncture gloves varied by a factor of 2. Fisher et al.[62] measured the puncture resistance of double gloves made of latex and other elastomers. With one exception, puncture resistance increased for double gloves compared to single ones. A study by Leslie et al.[63] evaluated liners and finger guards using taper point and cutting-edge surgical needles to penetrate the sample. Cutting edge needles required less force and work for penetration than did the comparably sized taper point needles. The standard test may give the same relative rankings of glove penetration resistance as would a probe more comparable to surgical instruments, but the comparison is quite limited and requires additional evaluation.

An interesting attempt to measure the resistance to cuts exhibited by latex gloves and various liners was made by Salkin et al.[64] Glove fingers were mounted on a phantom (a hot dog) finger that formed an electrical circuit with cutting instruments. A serrated knife and scalpel, both loaded at 0 and 1 kg, were oscillated at 1–20 Hz to simulate surgical cutting. The cutting time to breakthrough, measured by loss of electrical resistance, was recorded. This can be considered the time to abrade through the entire glove thickness with a sharp abrader. All times, which showed considerable variation, were less than 1 min, which is extremely short relative to use time. In use, accidental punctures would be more likely than intentional cuts. A nick, which is a cut that does not go through the material, might be more representative of an abrasive scuff produced by a knurled medical instrument.

From the studies above, it seems quite clear that tests of the penetration resistance of gloves will require well-defined probes that are clinically relevant. Resistance to nicking, more generally abrasion resistance, will also require better-defined tests that are clinically appropriate. Although tedious, both puncture and abrasion resistance tests can probably be made on most portions of the whole glove.

11.3.3.2   Recent Studies

Patel et al.[65] evaluated the puncture resistance of NRL and nitrile examination gloves using an adapted version of the ASTM F 1342 method. A 0.8 mm diameter 316 stainless steel puncture probe and a 0.45 mm injection needle (dental) were used in place of the standard probes. The index and middle finger regions were also evaluated in this modified test method. With the 0.8 mm puncture probe, the nitrile gloves had a significantly higher puncture resistance as compared to the NRL gloves. However, with the 0.45 mm injection needle, the NRL gloves had a significantly higher puncture resistance. Other findings included that puncture resistance increased with simulated aging and the index and middle finger regions had higher puncture resistance than other regions of the gloves.

As previously mentioned, Nguyen et al.[10] showed that the punctures by the probes used in the ASTM F 1342 standardized test are different from those made by medical needles. For rounded probes, the puncture occurs instantly at maximum load, whereas for needles penetration is gradual through the sample, reaches a maximum, and then diminishes slightly before plateauing. They concluded that puncture by rounded probes is controlled by a local deformation or failure strain, whereas, for medical needles, the puncture process involves crack growth and fracture energy dissipation. Further research by Nguyen and Vu-Khanh,[66] as related to ASTM F 1342, is available.

11.4   BARRIER (GLOVE) DURABILITY

11.4.1   MATERIAL FATIGUE

11.4.1.1   Earlier Studies

During use, gloves are repeatedly flexed through the motions of the fingers and hands. Testing of fatigue resistance of whole specimens is not practical for geometries as complex as that of gloves. Circular samples that are clamped at the circumference are amenable. Colligan and Horstman[67] recognized this and studied the permeation of chemotherapeutic drugs under static and flexed conditions. They used a version of a Franz diffusion cell, modified to permit flexing to "simulate occupational use." The O-ring-clamped circular specimens were bidirectionally flexed, with air, at a frequency of 0.267 Hz. They found the effect of flexing on permeation depended strongly on the quality of the glove. Surgical gloves were much more resistant than exam gloves.

Among the pioneers of this approach were Sinnott et al.[68] They were concerned with the effect of surface roughness on the fatigue life of membranes used in cardioplasty/cardiac valve replacement, and their material of choice was one of the polyether urethane ureas (Biomer®). To accommodate their circular specimens—solution cast from molds with fixed surface finishes—they constructed a constant-force apparatus that used air to pressurize a horizontally mounted specimen from below. The apparatus was driven by a cardiac-cycle-simulating program at a frequency of 1.833 Hz and peak pressure of 210 mmHg. The top surface of the specimen was covered by a given depth of deionized water.

Although Sinnott et al.[68] were reporting on work in progress, their early results are relevant to efforts that are currently underway. They had started specimens ($n = 3$) of each of the four surface finishes. They reported one specimen (with a 2-μ-inch finish) failed before two million elapsed cycles, while the others in that group remained intact. However, all specimens with a 250-μ-inch finish had failed between 30,000 and 40,000 cycles. The authors speculated that the higher stress concentrations associated with the rougher surface cause microcrack nucleation to progress faster and result in shortened fatigue lifetimes. Sinnott et al. conducted concurrent tensile testing with standard dog–bone specimens but did not see a difference in stress vs. strain curves among the four surface finishes. They concluded that their results supported earlier reports,[69] that material surface integrity has a significantly greater impact on test sensitivity under cyclic loading than it does on outcomes from monotonic loading. The authors summarized their preliminary results as documenting that the fatigue life of thin, flexing membranes will decrease as the order of surface roughness increases.

Other findings have implications for the design and conduct of cyclic fatigue tests, especially in terms of the correctness of simulating actual clinical tasks. Powell et al.[70] were concerned about the impact of glove fit on the progression of transient hand discomfort to a cumulative trauma disorder (CTD). Their experimental design was to have dental hygienists ($n = 176$) successively don an appropriately sized ambidextrous glove and have the first-to-the-fourth interknuckle distance measured while simulating prehensile grasp of an instrument; then repeat the procedure with a fitted glove. Although the Powell et al. results do not lead to a position about cyclic fatigue of glove material per se, their results contribute to a better understanding of the difference in relative risk of crack nucleation (or propagation) between ambidextrous and fitted examination gloves. Their compressive force calculations suggest that the ambidextrous gloves impose a 32.7% additional load onto the material area of concern as compared to their paired, fitted counterparts. They found that the percent elongation across the knuckles of an ambidextrous glove—with the hand in prehension—was 32.9% greater than that measured across a fitted glove ($\alpha > 0.9999$).

Another method used[71] was designed to provide very early detection of catastrophic structural changes in glove barriers rather than changes in steady-state permeability. Such changes would be caused by fatigue fracture(s) in the glove material due to repeated flexing. A modified permeation cell was used in which a circular section cut from a glove formed a membrane separating two chambers filled with electrolyte solutions. The membrane was repeatedly flexed at 0.1 Hz by applying varying air pressure to the top chamber. Assuming isotropic deformation, the peak linear strain was about 22%, comparable to Powell's findings. The introduction of electrodes into the chambers allowed the membrane capacitance and conductance to be measured continuously during the flex (fatigue) cycle. The addition of sodium ion to the upper chamber and a sodium ion electrode to the lower chamber allowed the sodium permeability to be monitored. Following detection of a catastrophic change after approximately 600 cycles (about 2 h), the membrane was examined by optical and electron microscopy to monitor for the onset of the material defects.

Scanning electron microscopy (SEM) provided evidence for the actual nature of the porous structure. Custom mounting of the glove material in both its original and extended state allowed these observations: Upon extension, the nature of the connecting fibrillar structure becomes visible. In nonfatigued glove material, the fibrils are intact, whereas in the fatigued glove material, fibrillar breakage, etc., was observed.[71] Thus, the rapid onset of glove rupture can be explained by a classic fatigue mechanism where the glove material behaves normally until the accumulation of fatigue cycles (and stress) leads to a porous structure, crazing, formation of cracks and holes, and finally catastrophic rupture. In the extended state, the pores may exceed the diameter of viruses of concern. However, the flow needed for virus transport through the barrier (see Section 11.3) would be quite different from flow through a "hole."

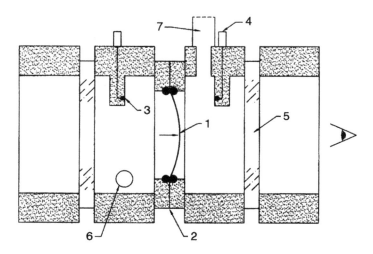

FIGURE 11.1 Principal test cell components of a biaxial fatigue apparatus: 1, membrane (slightly displaced); 2, specimen holder/O-rings; 3, electrode; 4, electrode connector; 5, optical window; 6, fluid inlet (to pump); 7, fluid reservoir.

Based on lessons learned from Dillon and Schroeder's experience,[71] a new generation of biaxial fatigue apparatus was designed and constructed.[72] In these newer investigations,[73] natural rubber latex gloves were acquired from a single manufacturer in three surface treatments: powdered (PD), powder-free with a polymeric coating (PF), and powder-free chlorinated (CL). Concerning conditioning, the gloves were left in an as-received condition; oven-aged at 50% relative humidity (RH) for 7 days at 70°C; and aged at 50% RH for 14 days at 70°C.

Oversized, circular specimens were sampled from the gloves' dorsum or palm. The nonconducting (to direct current) sample was clamped in a vertical position between two chambers later filled with a dilute aqueous salt solution held to 37°C (Figure 11.1). Electrodes were placed in each chamber (and connected to a lock-in amplifier). The electrodes served as both a source of a sinusoidally varying alternating current excitation voltage and as a phase-sensitive detector of current output from the cell. A displacement volume-controlling cam-and-race assembly, driven by a tunable-frequency motor set at a frequency of 0.8 Hz, delivered liquid into and out of one chamber. The other chamber was passively restored from a reservoir. At initial (and maximal) displacement, the membrane underwent a strain of approximately 35% in each direction. The onset of membrane failure was confirmed by recording a predefined slope change in transmembrane capacitance. The count of elapsed cycles corresponding to that failure event is recorded as the lifetime. Data were right-censored, in that failure events that occurred beyond 12,000 cycles were not recorded. Lifetime data were analyzed using the exact log-rank method, with appropriate significance-level adjustment for multiple comparisons.

After biaxial fatigue as described above, barrier integrity was also challenged with live viral preparations using ASTM Test Method F 1671.[7] ASTM F 1671 was modified to follow the rationale of Lytle and Baker,[74] and incorporated a hemispherical retaining screen,[8] to replicate the peak strain induced in the test specimen during the biaxial fatigue regime.

Viral passage tests of unflexed specimens indicated that even aging did not degrade barrier integrity to viruses for any of the glove conditions. More than half (53%) of the flexed specimens maintained integrity after 12,000 bidirectional cycles. The unaged PD and PF glove samples exhibited significantly longer fatigue lifetimes than the unaged CL samples. Survival times for the aged CL gloves were significantly longer than those for the unaged CL specimens, presumably due to aging-induced changes in the viscoelasticity of the treated material. In contrast, there was no statistical difference between the aged and unaged PD gloves, and the aged PF specimens showed only a marginally greater fatigue life than those unaged.

With flexed specimens, the occurrence of the electrical signature (change in slope of the capacitance signal) generally predicted viral passage, suggesting that the "signature" was a valid indicator of the breach of barrier integrity. The electrical means of detecting membrane dielectric loss may be equivalent to detecting a cylindrical hole <1.5 μm in diameter. Irreversible deformation is a confounding factor in interpreting glove durability based on this particular methodology: fixed peak-volume displacement (Figure 11.2). The increase in surface area, from the creep of the material early in its deformation history, leads to a progressive reduction in the stress in the sample as the cycling continues. This renders the approach unsuitable for determining the fatigue lifetimes of materials such as aged chlorinated latex.

The newer investigations have provided evidence that studies of latex glove specimens can detect differences in the durability of gloves across formulations and surface treatments/modifications. Using a phase-sensitive current detection method,[72,73] it has been shown that pore formation down to effective sizes less than viral diameters can be monitored and detected. This approach provides an alternative to using

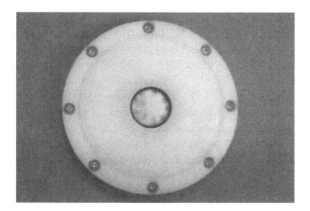

FIGURE 11.2 Glove specimen, clamped in a fixed peak-volume displacement holder, removed after a short cycling interval. "Dimpling" of specimen demonstrates an increase in the unstressed area after creep.

bioassay techniques that require extremely careful containment and sterility assurance; it offers the further benefit of near-real-time detection of integrity breaches.

Because of the excessive creep exhibited by latex subjected to some conditioning treatments, those samples underwent a monotonically decreasing stress as they were flexed, which led to a misleading prolongation of their test lifetimes. One solution to this dilemma would be to switch to a test methodology where the applied force can be servo-controlled to provide a dynamically adjusted, constant peak-force regiment.

However, after reviewing the above results, it became apparent that more than one stand-alone test is needed to assess glove durability. The results of earlier workers who relied solely on monotonic, uniaxial tensile testing of coupons cut from gloves have not shown the sensitivity to detect durability differences in glove material formulations or conditioning, that biaxial fatigue methodologies have demonstrated. Yet, as in the work of Schwerin et al.,[73] one cannot assume that fixed-peak displacement fatigue testing gives consistent results across all glove materials and conditioning (i.e., aging) regiments. Phua[69] had observed that material surface integrity has a significantly greater impact on test sensitivity under cyclic loading than under monotonic loading. Sinnot et al.[68] had concluded that the fatigue life of membranes will decrease as the order of surface finish increases. This reasoning suggests that the next attempts at characterization of glove materials, and/or their conditioning, should focus on tribologic properties—friction, lubrication, or wear—because they are associated directly with modification of a material's surface finish.

11.4.1.2   Recent Studies

A few studies have used a robotic hand to simulate repetitive hand movements and stretching of the gloved hands under conditions of chemical exposure to nonvolatile components. Phalen and Que Hee[75] developed a moving robotic hand to assess whole-glove permeation and penetration. They evaluated the system with disposable nitrile gloves for protection against the pesticide captan. An available Yaeger Innovative Products Corp. (Miami, FL) robotic hand was modified to conform with 50th percentile male reference dimensions and to facilitate glove donning and doffing. An inner nylon fabric glove was used to evaluate both chemical permeation and possible penetration. A water leak test was performed afterward to confirm penetration. Of the three disposable nitrile gloves tested, one brand catastrophically failed with exposure to movement. The failures occurred at the dorsal and ventral knuckle regions of the glove, where maximum stretching was observed. Analysis of chemical permeation was more involved and less conclusive, but the method showed promise for evaluating penetration, especially when followed up by water leak testing.

Similar studies with a robotic hand have been used to assess the effect of simulated hand movement on the permeation of low-volatile solvents such as cyclohexanol[76] and limonene.[77]

Phalen and Wong[78] developed a pneumatic system to simulate the bidirectional stretching of a donned glove on a human hand. Bidirectional stretching of gloved hands was measured using a novel ink stamp method, in which tape was used to capture the changes in length and width of the ink stamps with hand extension and flexion. Using the same method, air inflation was then optimized (0.10 in water gauge) to replicate the bidirectional stretching of the gloves donned by humans. A pneumatic controller (Geocontrol Pro, Geotech, Denver, Colo.) was used to inflate and deflate up to eight gloves at a time. The inflation and deflation cycle was 30 s and included a 5 s static time between stages. In a 2 h period, 240 inflation and deflation cycles were performed and the gloves were in continual movement for more than 80% of the time. Thirty brands of disposable nitrile gloves were evaluated out-of-box (controls) and under conditions of simulated movement. A modified water leak test was used to evaluate glove integrity.[39] Overall, simulated glove movement was not found to significantly increase leak failures.

The pneumatic system was also used to evaluate the effect of simulated hand movement on the chemical permeation of ethanol through various disposable gloves, including nitrile, NRL, and vinyl.[39,79]

The robotic hand and pneumatic systems show some promise in evaluating whole-glove mechanical fatigue and glove durability. Future research should focus on comparing results with those obtained in clinical or occupational settings.

11.4.2 TRIBOLOGIC STUDIES

Gloves are manipulated as users perform routine tasks such as twisting a capped needle onto a syringe or turning a knob on a piece of equipment, likely causing abrasion and eventually failure of the glove material. Roberts and Brackley[80,81] demonstrated the frictional properties of medical gloves. In their work, they documented the friction coefficients of various gloves under dry and wet conditions. Under dry conditions, gloves treated with powders, chlorination, and hydrogel coating demonstrated lower friction coefficients, while under wet conditions the gap between the various glove types reduced noticeably. Also, the friction rose noticeably as the glove surfaces wore away. When measuring the friction of a glove sample, a wavy glass plate was continuously rubbed against the glove material. By doing so, glove durability (abrasion resistance) was assessed. Of the various glove types (untreated, starch powdered, chlorinated, and hydrogel coated) studied, Roberts and Brackley observed that the hydrogel-coated gloves were more durable.

To further evaluate the abrasion resistance of medical gloves, a unique abrasion apparatus was designed.[82] The apparatus consisted of a smooth stainless steel abrading bar that exerted cyclic abrasion on the glove material, which was clamped down on top of a rubber spacer and a burlap cloth underlayment (Figure 11.3). Enough weight was added to the abrading bar to provide a load of 4 lb on the specimen. The glove material specimen was submerged in a water bath maintained at 37°C as a DC gear motor linearly stroked the abrading bar against the glove material specimen at a frequency of 1.0 Hz (60 cycles/min). Roughly, 1 in.^{2} of glove material was abraded on the glove in this process.

Glove specimens were cut from the dorsal section of the gloves. Five different glove materials were tested: one brand natural rubber latex, three brands neoprene, one brand nitrile, one brand styrene-ethylene/butylenes-styrene block copolymer (SEBS), and one brand vinyl. All except the vinyl were surgical gloves. Gloves were abraded until visual failure was reached. Visible holes/tears were usually less than

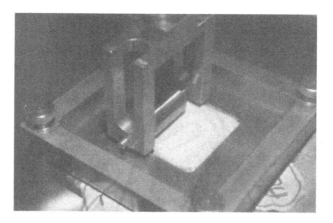

FIGURE 11.3   Glove specimen in place with abrading bar.

1 mm in diameter/width. Afterward, the specimens were subjected to either a water leak or viral penetration test to verify that the glove failure was more just than surface abrasion.

Significant differences in abrasion lifetimes were detected, thereby confirming that abrasion resistance is dependent on glove material and not necessarily on the thickness of the material itself. The nitrile gloves endured an average of 6871 cycles, SEBS 1102 cycles, latex lifetime of neoprene gloves can vary among brands. One brand was divided into two test samples, with the first lasting an average of 12,158 cycles while the second was more than 14,000 cycles. Two other brands of neoprene had lifetimes of 6609 and 917 cycles, respectively. Thus, it is evident that variations in manufacturing processes may have a significant effect on the abrasion resistance of glove materials.

Under extreme abrasion conditions, e.g., forceful contact with a surface having a noticeable degree of roughness, tearing of glove material may occur. Tear testing was performed on samples taken from the same glove lots as those used in the abrasion study.[82] Glove specimens were cut at a 90° angle into samples using Die C of ASTM D 624, then torn on a universal testing machine. We found that latex exhibited the highest tear strength while the vinyl tear strength was significantly lower than the four other materials tested.

Looking at both the abrasion and tear testing results we concluded that glove performance should be measured by a battery of tests. Ideally, the performance of the whole glove should be assessed. One approach under development by Kerr et al.[83] inserts a phantom hand into the glove, which is put into a beaker filled with abrasive material and the beaker placed on a shaker table. After shaking for a period of time the glove is subjected to the 1000 mL water leak test.

Kerr et al.[84] evaluated the durability of medical exam gloves using the hand phantom with artificial fingernails. The container with a gloved hand phantom was shaken using a reciprocating shaker table for 5 min in one direction and 5 min following a 90° rotation of the container. They compared this to a simulated clinical method, which consisted of manipulating various medical devices for 12 min. A water leak test was used to compare the results for gloves tested under each method. No significant differences in failure rates between the glove durability method (hand phantom) and simulated clinical method were observed. The patterns of leak failures were also similar between the two methods, showing failures in the finger, thumb, knuckle, upper palm (knuckle), and lower palm regions. In addition, they found that the durability of gloves varied, especially based on the glove type. Vinyl gloves were the least durable. Nitrile and chloroprene gloves performed similar to latex gloves.

Further studies are ongoing to analyze in more detail the correlation between flex-fatigue and abrasion.[85] Glove specimens are exposed to abrasion according to the methodology of Walsh et al.[82] for various numbers of abrasive cycles and then are placed in the flex-fatigue test cell following the methodologies of Long et al.[72] and Schwerin et al.[73] The proposed concept is to produce a comparison of the effects of varying the amount of abrasive wear on the lifetimes of samples that subsequently undergo flex-fatigue.

A number of recent studies have evaluated the coefficient of friction of gloves against various skin equivalents, as it relates to reducing surface friction (e.g., coatings and lubricants) and facilitating donning.[86–88]

11.4.3   OTHER FACTORS THAT INFLUENCE INTEGRITY

The integrity and durability of latex can be compromised by several other agents or conditions of use. Latex condoms (and by implication, latex gloves) can be affected by storage conditions, i.e., exposure to ozone, humidity, heat, or light. Studies in Indonesia[89] showed that latex condoms, packaged in plastic wrappers and "stored under tropic conditions for approximately 42 months" performed appreciably less well than unaged condoms in the ISO air burst test. Walsh et al.[90] studied the high-temperature, 70°C, aging of latex gloves for periods up to 21 days. Chlorination of latex gloves, a process often used to render gloves powder-free, can lessen the ability of gloves to retain their tensile strength after a 70°C aging. The heat resistance of latex, defined as retaining 100% elongation after two years of exposure, would be 60–70°C.[91] However, the Walsh study suggests that the durability of chlorinated gloves is questionable after exposure to extremely high temperatures. Another accelerated aging study involved measuring creep using a constant force comparable to that of hand gripping.[92] Measurements were made at five different temperatures above room temperature to study methods of estimating a shelf life. White et al.[93] reported that oil-based lubricants (and, possibly, hand creams) deteriorate latex. Ozone is also reported to deteriorate latex,[94] and precautions (antioxidants) are needed to prevent the deterioration induced during γ-irradiation sterilization of surgical gloves.

These results are corroborated by Das and Schroeder,[95] who studied the shelf life of natural rubber latex examination gloves based on creep behavior. Gloves were aged various times at several fixed temperatures and 25% RH. Creep testing was performed by applying a 50-kPa stress on finger samples of the aged and unaged glove. The researchers reported an acute drop in glove durability and shelf life with increasing temperature. For example, increasing the storage temperature merely by

10°C, from 15°C to 25°C, was found to decrease chlorinated glove shelf life from 49 years to 14 years. The shelf life would drop further to 59 months at 35°C and reach 20 months at 45°C.

11.5 CONCLUSIONS

A battery of tests should be used to evaluate the barrier integrity of new and used gloves. Some of the standardized tests, like the 1000 mL water leak test, are suited for quality control (QC); others may be used to check or confirm the QC tests. Leak tests using the virus Phi-X174 could be made more sensitive by employing biological amplification. Most studies show that properly manufactured new gloves provide considerable protection although some types are better than others. Hence, attention has turned to glove integrity during use (durability) and various means of reducing induced barrier breaches such as punctures. Methodologies for assessing glove durability, for example, by measuring abrasion and fatigue resistance of whole gloves, are still under development. A few studies have looked at the effect of temperature aging on glove properties, but the effect of long-term storage conditions on barrier integrity still needs to be assessed.

REFERENCES

1. Lytle, C.D., Cry, W.H., Carey, R.F., Shombert, D.G., Herman, B.A., Dillon, J.G., Schroeder, L.W., Bushar, H.F., and Kotilainen, H.J.R. 1994. Standard quality control testing and virus penetration, in *Protective Gloves for Occupational Use*, Mellstrom, G.A., Wahlberg, J.E., and Maibach, H.I., Eds. Boca Raton, FL: CRC Press, chap. 9.
2. Schroeder, L.W., Walsh, D.L., Schwerin, M.R., Richardson, D.C., Kisielewski, R.W., and Cyr, W.H. 2003. Standard quality control testing and virus penetration, in *Protective Gloves for Occupational Use*, 2nd edition, Boman, A., Estlander, T., Wahlberg, J.E., and Maibach, H.I., Eds. Boca Raton, FL: CRC Press, chap. 8.
3. Code of Federal Regulations. 2017. *21 CFR 800.20: Patient Examination Gloves and Surgical Gloves; Sample Plans and Test Method for Leakage Defects; Adulteration.* Washington, DC: U.S. Government Printing Office.
4. ASTM International. 2019. *ASTM D 5151–19: Standard Test Method for Detection of Holes in Medical Gloves.* Philadelphia, PA: ASTM International.
5. ISO (International Standard). 1999. *Sampling Procedures for Inspection by Attributes, ISO 2859-1:1999.* Geneva, Switzerland: International Organization for Standardization (ISO).
6. CEN (European Standard). 2020. *EN 455-1:2020: Medical Gloves for Single Use - Part 1: Requirements and Testing for Freedom from Holes.* Brussels: Comité Européen De Normalisation (CEN).
7. ASTM International. 2013. *ASTM F1671/F1671M-13: Standard Test Method for Resistance of Materials Used in Protective Clothing to Penetration by Blood-Borne Pathogens Using Phi-X174 Bacteriophage Penetration as a Test System.* Philadelphia, PA: ASTM International. DOI: 10.1520/F1671_F1671M-13.
8. Kisielewski, R.W., Rouston, L.B., Chaput, M.P., and Lytle, C.D. 2000. Modification of ASTM F 1671–97a: Resistance of materials to penetration by blood-borne pathogens, for use with elastomeric materials. *J Testing Eval* 28(2):136.

9. ASTM International. 2013. *ASTM F1342/F1342M-05(2013)e1: Standard Test Method for Protective Clothing Material Resistance to Puncture*. Philadelphia, PA: ASTM International. DOI: 10.1520/F1342_F1342M-05R13E01.

10. Nguyen, C.T., Vu-Khanh, T., Dolez, P.I., and Lara, J. 2009. Puncture of elastomer membranes by medical needles. Part I: Mechanisms. *Int J Fract* 155:75–81. DOI: 10.1007/s10704-009-9326-7.

11. ASTM International. 2019. *ASTM F2878-19: Standard Test Method for Protective Clothing Material Resistance to Hypodermic Needle Puncture*. Philadelphia, PA: ASTM International. DOI: 10.1520/F2878-19.

12. ANSI. 2016. *ANSI/ISEA 105-2016: American National Standard for Hand Protection Classification*. Washington, DC: American National Standards Institute (ANSI).

13. Lytle, C.D., and Routson, L.B. 1999. Lack of latex porosity: A review of virus barrier tests. *J Rubber Res* 2(1):29.

14. ASTM International. 2019. *ASTM D 3577–19: Standard Specification for Rubber Surgical Gloves*. Philadelphia, PA: ASTM International. DOI: 10.1520/D3577-19.

15. ASTM International. 2019. *ASTM D 3578–19: Standard Specification for Rubber Examination Gloves*. Philadelphia, PA: ASTM International. DOI: 10.1520/D3578-19.

16. ASTM International. 2019. *ASTM D 6319–19: Standard Specification for Nitrile Examination Gloves for Medical Application*. Philadelphia, PA: ASTM International. DOI: 10.1520/D6319-19.

17. ASTM International. 2019. *ASTM D 5250–19: Standard Specification for Poly(Vinyl Chloride) Gloves for Medical Application*. Philadelphia, PA: ASTM International. DOI: 10.1520/D5250-19.

18. ASTM International. 2021. *ASTM D 412–16R21: Standard Test Methods for Vulcanized Rubber and Thermoplastic Elastomers—Tension*. Philadelphia, PA: ASTM International. DOI: 10.1520/D0412-16R21.

19. CEN (European Standard). 2015. *EN 455-2:2015: Medical Gloves for Single Use - Part 2: Requirements and Testing for Physical Properties*. Brussels: Comité Européen De Normalisation (CEN).

20. ASTM International. 2020. *ASTM D 624-00(2020): Standard Test Method for Tear Strength of Conventional Vulcanized Rubber and Thermoplastic Elastomers*. Philadelphia, PA: ASTM International. DOI: 10.1520/D0624-00R20.

21. Kotilainen, H.R., Brinker, J.P., Avato, J.L., and Gantz, N.M. 1989. Evaluation of latex and vinyl examination gloves: Quality control procedures and implications for healthcare workers. *Arch Intern Med* 149:2749.

22. Brown, J.W., and Blackwell, H. 1990. Putting on gloves in the fight against AIDS. *Med Lab Observ* 22:1.

23. Klein, R.C., Party, E., and Gershey, E.L. 1990. Virus penetration of examination gloves. *Biotechniques* 9:196.

24. Korniewicz, D.M., Kirwin, M., Cresci, K., and Larson, E. 1993. Leakage of latex and vinyl exam gloves in high and low risk clinical settings. *Am Ind Hyg Assoc J* 54:22.

25. Kerr, L.N., Boivin, W.S., Chaput, M.P., Hamilton, S.L., Mailhot, S.A., O'Malley, L.G., and Teixeira, J.C. 2002. The effect of simulated clinical use on vinyl and latex exam glove durability. *J Testing Eval* 30(5):415.

26. Olsen, R.J., Lynch, P., Coyle, M.B., Cummings, J., Bokete, T., and Stamm, W.E. 1993. Examination gloves as barriers to hand contamination in clinical practice. *J Am Med Assoc* 270:350.

27. Korniewicz, D.M., Kirwin, M., Cresci, K., Sing, T., Choo, T.E., Wool, M., and Larson, E. 1994. Barrier protection with examination gloves: Double versus single. *Am J Infect Control* 22:12.

28. Douglas, A., Simon, T.R., and Goddard, M. 1997. Barrier durability of latex and vinyl medical gloves in clinical settings. *Am Ind Hyg Assoc J* 58:672.

29. Newsom, S.W.B., Smith, M.O., and Shaw, P. 1998. A randomised trial of the durability of non-allergenic latex-free surgical gloves versus latex gloves. *Ann R Coll Surg Engl* 80:288.

30. Rego, A., and Roley, L. 1999. In-use barrier integrity of gloves: Latex and nitrile superior to vinyl. *Am J Infect Control* 27:405.

31. Muto, C.A., Sistrom, M.G., Strain, B.A., and Farr, B.M. 2000. Glove leakage rates as a function of latex content and brand. *Arch Surg* 135:982.

32. Korniewicz, D.M., El-Masri, M., Broyles, J.M., Martin, C.D., and O'Connell, K.P. 2002. Performance of latex and nonlatex medical examination gloves during simulated use. *Am J Infect Control* 30:133.

33. Tlili, M.A., Belgacem, A., Sridi, H., Akouri, M., Aouicha, W., Soussi, S., Dabbebi, F., and Ben Dhiab, M. 2018. Evaluation of surgical glove integrity and factors associated with glove defect. *Am J Infect Control* 46(1):30–33. DOI: 10.1016/j.ajic.2017.07.016.

34. de Oliveira, A.C., and Gama, C.S. 2014. Evaluation of surgical glove integrity during surgery in a Brazilian teaching hospital. *Am J Infect Control* 42(10):1093–1096. DOI: 10.1016/j.ajic.2014.06.021.

35. Elce, Y.A., Laverty, S., Almeida da Silveira, E., Piat, P., Trencart, P., Ruzickova, P., and Reardon, R.J. 2016. Frequency of undetected glove perforation and associated risk factors in equine surgery. *Vet Surg* 45(8):1066–1070. DOI: 10.1111/vsu.12562.

36. Sayın, S., Yılmaz, E., and Baydur, H. 2019. Rate of glove perforation in open abdominal surgery and the associated risk factors. *Surg Infect (Larchmt)* 20(4):286–291. DOI: 10.1089/sur.2018.229.

37. Han, C.D., Kim, J., Moon, S.H., Lee, B.H., Kwon, H.M., and Park, K.K. 2013. A randomized prospective study of glove perforation in orthopaedic surgery: Is a thick glove more effective? *J Arthroplasty* 28(10):1878–1881. DOI: 10.1016/j.arth.2013.05.007.

38. Zare, A., Choobineh, A., Jahangiri, M., Seif, M., and Dehghani, F. 2021. Does size affect the rate of perforation? A cross-sectional study of medical gloves. *Ann Work Expo Health* 65(7):854–861. DOI: 10.1093/annweh/wxab007.

39. Phalen, R.N., and Wong, W.K. 2011. Integrity of disposable nitrile exam gloves exposed to simulated movement. *J Occup Environ Hyg* 8(5):289–299. DOI: 10.1080/15459624.2011.569285.

40. Kotilainen, H.R., Cy, W.H., Truscott, W., Gantz, N.M., Routson, L.B., and Lytle, C.D. 1992. Ability of 1000 ml water leak test for medical gloves to detect gloves with potential for virus penetration. In *Performance of Protective Clothing*, McBriarty, J.P., and Henry, N.W., vol. 4, Eds. Philadelphia, PA: American Society for Testing and Materials, 38–49.

41. Phalen, R.N., and Wong, W.K. 2012. Tensile properties and integrity of clean room and low-modulus disposable nitrile gloves: A comparison of two dissimilar glove types. *Ann Occup Hyg* 56(4):450–457. DOI: 10.1093/annhyg/mer116.

42. Shless, J., Crider, Y., Pitchik, H., Qazi, A., Styczynski, A., LeMesurier, R., Haik, D., Kwong, L., LeBoa, C., Bhattacharya, A., Hamidi, Y., and Phalen, R. 2021. Evaluation of the effects of repeated disinfection on medical exam gloves: Part 1. Changes in physical integrity. *J Occup Environ Hyg* 13:1–11. DOI: 10.1080/15459624.2021.2015072.

43. Mathews, A., and Que Hee, S.S. 2016. Quantitative leak test for microholes and microtears in whole gloves and glove pieces. *Polym Test* 54:244–249. DOI: 10.1016/j.polymertesting.2016.07.018.

44. Hamann, C.P., and Nelson, J.R. 1993. Permeability of latex and thermoplastic elastomer gloves to the bacteriophage XI74. *J Infect Control* 21:289–296.

45. Edlich, R.F., Suber, F., Neal, J.G., Jackson, E.M., and Williams, F.M. 1999. Integrity of powder-free examination glove to bacteriophage penetration. *J Biomed Mater Res* 48:755–758.

46. Calhoun, A.J., Rodrick, G.E., and Brown, F.H. 2002. Integrity of powdered and powder-free latex examination gloves. *J Public Health Dent* 62:170–172.

47. Smith, S. 2004. Updates coming for protective clothing standards: The ASTM committee F-23 on protective clothing is creating new standards for radiological, biological, physical, thermal and chemical hazards.*EHS Today*, May 12, 2004. https://www.ehstoday.com/ppe/protective-clothing/article/21908137/updates-coming-for-protective-clothing-standards

48. Nelson, J.R., Roming, T.A., and Bennett, J.K. 1999. A whole-glove method for the evaluation of surgical gloves as barriers to viruses. *Am J Contact Dermatitis* 10:183–189.

49. Broyles, J.M., O'Connell, K.P., and Korniewicz, D.M. 2002. PCR-based method for detecting viral penetration of medical exam gloves. *J Clin Microbiol* 40:2725–2728.

50. de Lomas, J.F., Sunzeri, F.J., and Buisch, M.P. 1992. False-negative results by polymerase chain reaction due to contamination by glove powder. *Transfusion* 32:83.

51. O'Connell, K.P., El-Masri, M., Broyles, J.B., and Korniewicz, D.M. 2004. Testing for viral penetration of non-latex surgical and examination gloves: A comparison of three methods. *Clin Microbiol Infect* 10(4):322–326. DOI: 10.1111/j.1198-743X.2004.00848.x.

52. Newsom, S.W.B., Smith, M.O., and Shaw, P. 1998. A randomized trial of the durability of non-allergenic latex-free surgical gloves versus latex gloves. *Ann R Coll Surg Engl* 80:288.

53. Driever, R., Beie, M., Schmitz, E., Holland, M., Knapp, M., Reifschneider, H.J., Hofmann, F., and Vetter, H.O. 2001. Surgical glove perforation in cardiac surgery. *Thorac Cardiovasc Surg* 49(60):328.

54. Eklund, A.M., Ojajärvi, J., Laitinen, K., Valtonen, M., and Werkkala, K.A. 2001. Glove punctures and postoperative skin flora of hands in cardiac surgery. *Ann Thorac Surg* 74(1):149.

55. Aarnio, P., and Laine, T. 2001. Glove perforation rate in vascular surgery-a comparison between single and double gloving. *Vasa* 30(2):122.

56. Sohn, R.L., Murray, M.T., Franko, A., Hwang, P.K., Dulchavsky, S.A., and Grimm, M.J. 2000. Detection of surgical glove integrity. *Am Surg* 66(3):302.

57. Miller, K.M., and Leonard, A. 1993. Unsuspected glove perforation during ophthalmic surgery. *Arch Ophthalmol* 111:186.

58. NFPA. 2018. *NFPA 1999: Standard on Protective Clothing and Ensembles for Emergency Medical Operations.* Quincy, MA: National Fire Protection Association (NFPA).

59. Jackson, E.M., Wenger, M.D., Neal, J.G., Thacker, J.G., and Edlich, R.F. 1998. Inadequate standard for glove puncture resistance; allows production of gloves with limited puncture resistance. *J Emerg Med* 16(30):461.

60. Jackson, E.M., Neal, J.G., Williams, F.M., Stern, C.A., Suber, F., Thacker, J.G., and Edlich, R.F. 1999. Biomechanical performance of orthopedic gloves. *J Biomed Mater Res (Appl Biomater)* 48:193.

61. Jackson, E.M., Williams, F.M., Neal, J.G., Suber, F., Thacker, J.G., and Edlich, R.F. 1999. Biomechanical performance of examination gloves. *J Biomed Mater Res (Appl Biomater)* 48:572.

62. Fisher, M.D., Reddy, V.R., Williams, F.M., Lin, K.Y., Thacker, J.G., and Edlich, R.F. 1999. Biomechanical performance of powder-free examination gloves. *J Emerg Med* 17(6):1011.

63. Leslie, L.F., Woods, J.A., Thacker, J.G., Morgan, R.F., McGregor, W., and Edlich, R.F. 1998. Needle puncture resistance of surgical gloves, finger guards, and glove liners. *J Biomed Mater Res (Appl Biomater)* 33(1):41.

64. Salkin, J.A., Stuchin, S.A., Kummer, F.J., and Reininger, R. 1995. The effectiveness of cut-proof glove liners; cut and puncture resistance, dexterity, and sensibility. *Orthopedics* 18(11):1067.

65. Patel, H., Fleming, G., and Burke, F. 2004. Puncture resistance and stiffness of nitrile and latex dental examination gloves. *Br Dent J* 196:695–700. DOI: 10.1038/sj.bdj.48113 53.

66. Nguyen, C.T., Dolez, P.I., Vu-Khanh, T., Gauvin, C., and Lara, J. 2010. Resistance of protective gloves materials to puncture by medical needles. *J ASTM Int* 7(5):1–16. DOI: 10.1520/JAI102923.

67. Colligan, S.A., and Horstman, S.A. 1990. Permeation of cancer chemotherapeutic drugs through glove materials under static and flexed conditions. *Appl Occup Environ Hyg* 5:848.

68. Sinnott, M.M., Hoeppner, D.W., Romney, E., and Dew, P.A. 1989. Effects of surface integrity on the fatigue life of thin flexing membranes. *ASAIO Trans* 35:687–690.

69. Phua, S.K., Castillo, E., Anderson, J.M., and Hiltner, A. 1987. Biodegradation of a polyurethane *in vitro*. *J Biomed Mater Res* 21:231–246.

70. Powell, B.J., Winkley, G.P., Brown, J.O., and Etersque, S. 1994. Evaluating the fit of ambidextrous and fitted gloves: Implications for hand discomfort. *J Am Dent Assoc* 125:1235–1242.

71. Dillon, J.G., and Schroeder, L.W. 1997. Permeability and material characteristics of vulcanized latex film during and following cyclic fatigue in a saline environment. *J Appl Polym Sci* 64:553–566.

72. Long, M.C., Kisielewski, R.W., Richardson, D.C., and Schroeder, L.W. 2001. An experimental technique for determining biaxial fatigue lifetimes in biomedical elastomers. *Int J Fatigue* 23:911–916.

73. Schwerin, M.R., Walsh, D.L., Coleman, R.D., Kisielewski, R.W., Kotz, R.M., Routson, L.B., and David Lytle, C.. 2002. Biaxial flex-fatigue and viral penetration of natural rubber latex gloves before and after artificial aging. *J Biomed Mater Res (Appl Biomater)* 63B:739–745.

74. Lytle, C.D., and Baker, K.H. 1999. Ability of a viral penetration test (ASTM F1671-95) to detect small holes. *J Testing Eval* 27:231–233.

75. Phalen, R.N., and Que Hee, S.S. 2008. A moving robotic hand system for whole-glove permeation and penetration: Captan and nitrile gloves. *J Occup Environ Hyg* 5(4):258–270. DOI: 10.1080/15459620801934786.

76. Mathews, A.R., and Que Hee, S.S. 2017. Whole glove permeation of cyclohexanol through disposable nitrile gloves on a dextrous robot hand: Fist clenching vs. nonclenching. *J Occup Environ Hyg* 14(4):252–257. DOI: 10.1080/15459624.2016.1250006.

77. Banaee, S., and Que Hee, S.S. 2017. Permeation of limonene through disposable nitrile gloves using a dextrous robot hand. *J Occup Health* 59(2):131–138. DOI: 10.1539/joh.16-0179-OA.

78. Phalen, R.N., and Wong, W.K. 2011. Integrity of disposable nitrile exam gloves exposed to simulated movement. *J Occup Environ Hyg* 8(5):289–299. DOI: 10.1080/15459624.2011.569285.

79. Phalen, R.N., Le, T., and Wong, W.K. 2014. Changes in chemical permeation of disposable latex, nitrile, and vinyl gloves exposed to simulated movement. *J Occup Environ Hyg* 11(11):716–721. DOI: 10.1080/15459624.2014.908259.

80. Roberts, A.D., and Brackley, C.A. 1992. Friction of surgeons' gloves. *J Phys D Appl Phys* 25:A28–A32.

81. Roberts, A.D., and Brackley, C.A. 1996. Comfort and frictional properties of dental gloves. *J Dent* 24:339–343.
82. Walsh, D.L., Schwerin, M.R., Kisielewski, R.W., Kotz, R.M., Chaput, M.P., Varney, G.W., and To, T.M. 2004. Abrasion resistance of medical glove materials. *J Biomed Mater Res (Appl Biomater)* 68B:81–87.
83. Chaput, M.P., Teixeira, J.C., Boivin, W.S., Kerr, L.N., Mailhot, S.A., and O'Malley, L.G. 2003. A method for the assessment of the durability of medical gloves. *J Testing Eval* 31(6):472–478.
84. Kerr, L.N., Chaput, M.P., Cash, L.D., O'Malley, L.G., Sarhrani, E.M., Teixeira, J.C., Boivin, W.S., and Mailhot, S.A. 2004. Assessment of the durability of medical examination gloves. *J Occup Environ Hyg* 1(9):607–612. DOI: 10.1080/15459620490491803.
85. Schwerin, M.R., and Richardson, D.C. 2004. *Abrasion Occuring during Emergency Response Can Hasten Loss of Glove Integrity*. Washington, DC: FDA Science Forum, Sigma Xi Poster Session, May 18–19.
86. Manhart, J., Hausberger, A., Maroh, B., Holzner, A., Schaller, R., Kern, W., and Schlögl, S. 2019. Tribological characteristics of medical gloves in contact with human skin and skin equivalents. *Polym Test* 82:106318. DOI: 10.1016/j.polymertesting.2019.106318.
87. Preece, D., Ng, T.H., Tong, H.K., Roger Lewis, R., and Carré, M.J. 2021. The effects of chlorination, thickness, and moisture on glove donning efficiency. *Ergonomics* 64(9):1205–1216. DOI: 10.1080/00140139.2021.1907452.
88. Preece, D., Lewis, R., and Carré, M.J. 2021. A critical review of the assessment of medical gloves. *Tribol Mat Surf Inter* 15(1):10–19. DOI: 10.1080/17515831.2020.173061.
89. Free, M.J., Hutchings, J., Lubis, F., and Natakusumah, R. 1986. An assessment of burst strength distribution data for monitoring quality of condom stocks in developing countries. *Contraceptions* 33:285.
90. Walsh, D.L., Chwirut, D.J., and Kotz, R.M. 1999. Environmental degradation of natural rubber latex gloves; the effects of elevated temperature on tensile strength. *J Testing Eval* 27(6):396.
91. Hofmann, W. 1989. *Rubber Technology Handbook*. Munich: Hansen, 29.
92. Das, S.S., and Schroeder, L.W. 2002. Shelf life of medical gloves-an indispensable protective device-accelerated temperature aging, in *Biomedical Engineering Recent Developments*, Vossoughi, J., Ed. Washington, DC: Medical and Engineering Publishers, 225.
93. White, N., Taylor, K., Lyszkowski, A., Tullett, J., and Morris, C. 1988. Dangers of lubricants used with condoms. *Nature* 335:19.
94. Baker, R.F., Sherwin, R.P., Bernstein, G.S., Nakamura, R.M., Voeller, B., and Coulson, A.H. 1988. Precautions when lightning strikes during the monsoon. The effect of ozone on condoms. *J Am Med Assoc* 260:1404.
95. Das, S.S., and Schroeder, L.W. 2008. Estimation of shelf life of natural rubber latex exam-gloves based on creep behavior. *J Biomed Mater Res* 85B(2):398–408. DOI: 10.1002/jbm.b.30958.

12 In Vivo Testing of the Protective Effect of Gloves

N. Hamnerius, C. Svedman,
M. Bruze, and O. Bergendorff

CONTENTS

12.1 INTRODUCTION

The use of efficient protective gloves is of crucial importance in workplaces where hazardous chemicals are handled. Such workplaces include those within the chemical industry and the plastic industry, as well as in environments such as dental practices, hairdressing, and beauty salons.

A major task in occupational dermatology is to provide advice regarding how to avoid or protect the patient against allergens found in the work environment. The dermatologist can provide the patient with important information and advice regarding the correct use of gloves. Gloves can be used for protection from skin exposures with regard to both systemic uptake and localized effect on the skin. The exposure can be an infectious agent, a cancerogenic substance, a substance with a teratogenic effect, a corrosive or irritant substance that causes a chemical burn or irritant contact dermatitis, or a potential contact allergen. In this chapter, the testing of the protective effect of gloves, mainly regarding contact allergens or potential sensitizers, is described.

This chapter aims to give a brief review of *in vitro* and *in vivo* testing of gloves and focus on an *in vivo* model that has been developed for testing different glove materials against hazardous materials while making it possible to a certain extent to mimic the workplace conditions.

DOI: 10.1201/9781003126874-14

The skin protection from a glove depends on several factors such as the barrier function of the glove, whether or not the material is affected by the substance during use, and whether the glove is reusable. The period for which the glove will be stored, how the glove is stored before use, and how long the glove is used are other factors that might influence the protective effect of the glove. Testing of the material used for gloves and the glove itself can be performed in different ways. The choice of protective material can be based on data from technical testing of polymeric membranes or on *in vivo* evaluation of the protective effect.[1,2] The importance of standardized test methods and performance requirements for protective gloves has been recognized for a long time. National and international standards have therefore been developed to achieve reproducible results in testing glove performance and properties and are described in greater detail in Chapters 11, 13, and 14.

In vitro degradation, permeation (resistance), and penetration (leakage) tests are used to assess the protective effect of gloves against different chemicals (Chapter 10). The information achieved is usually the basis for the choice of protective equipment. *In vitro* permeation testing is based on a flow-through system where a two-compartment permeation cell of standard dimension is used. The test chemical is placed in one of the compartments. A collecting medium is flowed through the other compartment and analyzed chemically at time intervals. The result reflects the degree of diffusion of the chemical through the glove material; a key parameter is the breakthrough time, i.e., the elapsed time between the initial application of the test chemical to the glove surface and its subsequent presence on the other side of the material. The permeation rate describes the mass of a test chemical permeating the glove material per unit time per unit area, i.e., $mg/min/cm^2$. The *in vitro* methods for testing can also be adapted to simulate the strain from the movement of the glove.[2–5] However, *in vitro* methods have their limitations: neither the interaction between the glove and the skin, such as the effect of occlusion or possible chemical interaction, nor the possible metabolism of the substance is taken into consideration. The effect of the working situation is another factor that is not taken into consideration.[6] *In vivo* evaluation is thus needed to supplement the *in vitro* testing of available protective materials.

12.2   *IN VIVO* TESTING OF GLOVES

In vivo testing can be performed in animals or humans. It is important to know if a relationship exists between *in vitro* and *in vivo* testing, as well as the nature of the relationship, to reduce *in vivo* testing, which is time-consuming and must consider ethical aspects. Often, however, because of the different factors that influence the use of gloves in real life, *in vivo* testing is to be preferred.

Animal testing can be performed in guinea pigs,[7,8] where a glass ring with the attached glove material under investigation is glued to the shaved skin area to be exposed. In the ring, on the glove, the chemical is applied, and the penetration and the systemic uptake can be measured by blood samples. An exposure time is decided, and blood samples are drawn regularly. The test setup can be enhanced to simulate the clinical situation by stripping the skin of the back of the guinea pig, thus simulating a broken skin barrier.[7,8] The animal model comes closer to the clinical situation, as different biological factors such as the effect of occlusion and a broken skin barrier can be taken into account, and the effect of different time intervals for exposure can be calculated. This method measures penetration and absorption to the blood; what happens in the epidermis/dermis; or whether the substance partly stays in the interstitial room is not possible to measure. Furthermore, the model does not take into consideration the possible significance of various factors in the work situation for the penetration and absorption of chemical substances. To study the biologically significant response, i.e., evaluation of irritant reaction, contact urticaria, or allergic contact dermatitis, data obtained from human experiments, preferably in the work situation, are needed.

12.2.1 PATCH TESTING WITH ALLERGEN AND GLOVE

Patch testing with the actual allergen applied onto pieces of gloves is one way to test the glove material in humans and illustrate the protective effect of the glove. This has been performed in various studies showing the protective effect of gloves from, for example, photographic chemicals, epoxy system components, glyceryl monothioglycolate, diallyl disulfide, methylisothiazolinone, and (meth)acrylates.[9-15]

This method can be used when no data on penetration or permeation are available or when detection and quantification of the substance the glove should protect from are difficult.[16,17] The test is performed in sensitized individuals and can easily be performed in the clinic when the patient comes for a patch test for suspected work dermatitis. When a patient with hand dermatitis is tested for different materials in the workplace and a sensitizer is found, the protective gloves at work are usually also tested. In this setting, it is very easy to perform the testing of the glove's protective function by testing the allergen with the glove between the substance and the back of the patient. As a positive control, the substance is tested without the glove material, and as a negative control the glove material alone.[16] When this test method is used, diluted chemicals are usually applied,[9,12] with an application time under occlusion of two days. However, to mimic the everyday exposure, the patient's own products can be tested, and the exposure time can be adapted to the history of the patient.[15]

12.2.2 USE OF AN OPEN CHAMBER SYSTEM

In industry, different chemicals are handled, different protective gloves are used, and the skin of the persons handling the chemical and using the gloves will be in different conditions; furthermore, routines for handling the chemicals and gloves will differ. The dermatologist should be able to give the patient and also the industry/workplace advice on how to ensure primary and secondary prevention. The optimal testing system should thus be possible to use in clinical practice. The testing should imitate the practical use of the glove, should be safe for the patient, and should provide data of benefit for the individual patient.

To enable testing of the protective efficacy of the glove material against hazardous materials, a model using an open chamber system has been developed.[6] The model has been evaluated in studies testing with (meth) acrylates[18–20] and hair colors.[21,22] In these studies, dental bonding products containing 2-hydroxyethyl methacrylate (2-HEMA), (meth) acrylate-containing nail-building gels, and p-phenylenediamine-containing hair-coloring cream have been used for testing different protective gloves. Some of the results are shown in Table 12.1. Table 12.1 illustrates well the time aspect: a glove might have a good protective effect when used during a very limited time, and then the effect might quickly deteriorate. Furthermore, Table 12.1 illustrates variation not only between gloves of different materials but also between gloves made of the same material. This model enables an *in vivo* testing in humans with negligible risks and where such factors as skin temperature, occlusion, and humidity may be taken into consideration.

12.2.2.1 Testing Device

Open circular stainless steel chambers, 12 mm height, 12 mm inner diameter, are used. These chambers virtually exclude chemical reactions between the chemical and the device. The test chambers are placed in numbers of three in a 1-mm-thick, transparent, and slightly flexible acrylic plate (Figures 12.1 and 12.2). Eight glove materials can be tested simultaneously. Then the glove material is fixed to the chambers with a nickel-free clip. Thus, the glove material will constitute the bottom of the chamber and the contact surface with the skin. It is of great importance that the fixation of the glove to the chamber is performed with great care, as there is a risk of damaging the glove material. The testing device is washable and thus reusable.

12.2.2.2 Method

The patient is placed in a comfortable position, preferably supine, since the test area should be kept horizontal throughout the procedure. The test plates are taped to the skin by use of hypoallergenic tape (e.g., Scanpor, Norgeplaster, and Norway). The best areas for testing are the back and the volar aspect of the forearm. To enable blind reading, the test procedure and reading can be performed by different persons.

After the glove material has been attached to the chamber, a standardized volume of the product/chemical, preferably 50 µl in liquid form, as used commercially, is applied to the bottom of the chambers. This amount ensures that the bottom of the chamber is covered in excess, as the level of the applied liquid in the chamber is approximately 0.4 mm high. Preferably, the test concentration of a product to which the patient is exposed should be chosen. Three different exposure times for each glove can be chosen to mimic the possible exposure to the product in practical use. For control, it is recommended to apply the test product/chemical into a chamber without the glove as a positive control test and into another chamber with a glove with known excellent protection ("best possible protection"), or test with chambers with the glove without applying the test product/chemical (negative controls). The exposure time is preferably chosen according to how the chemical is handled in the industry where the patient works.[10–12,15,20–22] For dental acrylates, exposure times of 7.5, 15, 30, and 60 min have been used after field studies at different workplaces.[6,18,19] If positive controls are used, the testing time at these sites might have to be shortened to limit the

TABLE 12.1

Study with Open Exposure Test Using PPD-Containing Hair Dye and Different Gloves Recommended for Hair-Dyeing in Eight PPD Allergic Subjects, a–g

Tested Glove (Thickness mm)	Exposure Time (min)	Subject						
		a	b	c	d	e	f	g
No glove[1]	60	+++	+++	+++	+++	+++	++	+++
Glove with best possible protection [2]	60	–	–	–	–	–	–	–
Nitrile (0.035)	15	–	–	–	–	–	–	–
	30	–	–	–	–	–	–	–
	60	–	–	–	–	–	–	–
Nitrile (0.040)	15	–	–	–	–	–	–	–
	30	–	–	–	–	–	–	–
	60	–	–	–	–	–	–	–
Natural rubber (0.038)	15	–	–	–	–	–	++	+++
	30	–	–	++	–	++	+	+++
	60	–	–	+++	+++	+++	+	+++
Polyvinylchloride (0.034)	15	–	–	–	–	(+)	+	–
	30	–	–	–	–	++	+	++
	60	–	(+)	+++	+++	+++	+	++
Polyvinylchloride (0.037)	15	–	–	–	–	–	+	–
	30	–	–	++	–	(+)	+	++
	60	–	+++	+++	++	+++	++	++
Polyethylene (0.029)	15	–	–	–	–	–	–	++
	30	–	–	–	–	+	+	++
	60	–	–	–	++	++	+	++
Patch test reactivity to PPD[3] (% in petrolatum)		1.0	0.1	0.01	0.01	0.01	0.01	0.01

[1] Test with hair dye preparation *as is* in test chamber without a glove.

[2] Test with hair dye preparation *as is* in the test chamber with a polyethylene/ethylene vinyl alcohol/polyethylene glove.

[3] p-Phenylenediamine.

The hair dye was prepared by mixing the coloring cream containing PPD, with the developer cream containing hydrogen peroxide 3% at equal parts. The initial PPD concentration in the final testing product was 0.9%. The exposure times used simulated the exposure of hairdressers. The reactivity of the subject, the exposure time, and the glove material will decide the test results (read as the strongest reaction on D4/D7). The subject's reactivity was tested in the study with dilution series of PPD (dilution series of PPD in acetone:1.0%, 0.1%, 0.01%, 0.001%, and 0.0001%). The lowest concentration the subject reacted to is presented. Table modified after Antelmi et al. Are gloves sufficiently protective when hairdressers are exposed to permanent hair dyes? An *in vivo* study.[21] One patient from the original study is excluded since no reaction occurred to the tested hair dye as such.

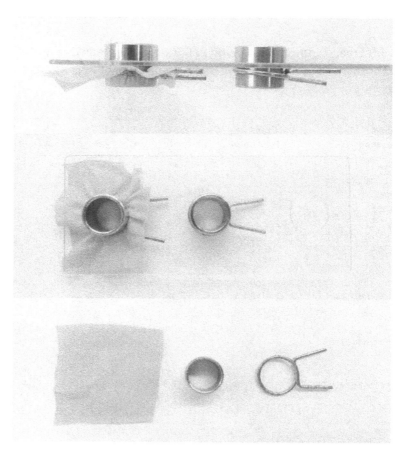

FIGURE 12.1 Two test chambers fixed in a test plate, from the side and from above, respectively. The glove material is fixed to the chambers by metal clips and thus constitutes the bottom of the chambers.

eczematous response. After testing, the chambers are removed. The chamber should leave a ring-shaped impression on the skin to ensure that the contact between the back and the glove has been sufficient. The test positions are then marked with a pen (Figure 12.3). Depending on the test design, the test surface can then be washed or left unwashed after testing. The positive control area can also, depending on the study design, be washed (e.g., with soap and water) or wiped immediately after testing. This procedure can also be used to study the efficacy of different ways to clean exposed skin.

A dilution series of the chemical tested can be performed with traditional patch testing to measure the reactivity of the individual. This is preferably done on the lateral aspect of the upper arm. The reactions are read according to ICDRG standards,[23,24] on days 3 and 7 after testing. Additionally, the test reactions can be

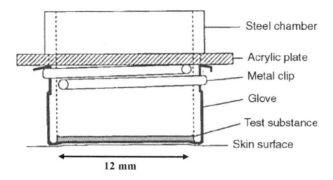

FIGURE 12.2 Cross-sectional drawing of test chamber.

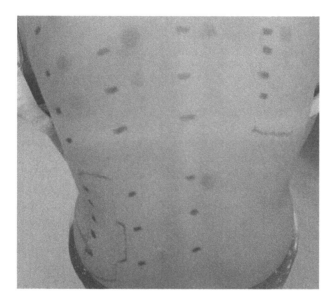

FIGURE 12.3 Subject sensitized to paraphenylenediamine being exposed to protective gloves and hair dye at different exposure times: 15, 30, and 60 minutes. Reading at day 3.

photo-documented and noninvasive techniques, such as laser Doppler perfusion imaging,[25,26] evaporimetry,[27,28] and thermography,[29] can be used for multiparameter assessment of reactions.

12.2.2.3 Evaluation

This testing procedure is easy to use and without side effects for the patient; the only discomfort for the patient is the eczematous response when a sufficient number of molecules have entered through the glove material, reached the patient´s skin, and caused a localized reaction similar to that seen in patch testing. The method has been evaluated using acrylates,[18–20] and hair dyes,[21,22] and has been found to discriminate well between the protection of different gloves. The fact that different application times can be used for each glove enables the observation of a possible dose–time relationship. The choice of application time should be based on the exposure time seen in the actual work environment. The positive test reactions observed are usually + and ++ reactions. A few +++ reactions have been seen but no exceptionally strong ones. The total testing of the patient takes approximately 30 min in preparation, to which are then added the maximal exposure time and the two test reading occasions, 15 min each.

The test system is best suited for testing thin elastic gloves. If thicker glove material is to be tested, a slight modification of the way the glove is attached to the chamber should be performed. A major use of the test method is to investigate the protective capacity of gloves against a contact sensitizer, as a discrete substance or when present in a product, to get results that can be used for general recommendations within a group such as dental personnel and hairdressers.[18,19,21,22] The limiting factor might be the recruitment of a sufficient number of hypersensitive individuals to enable comparisons between gloves based on statistical calculations.[21,22] Furthermore, the method does not allow for a proper evaluation if the movement of the glove material could influence the protective effect. There are, however, several advantages: the technique is easy to use and thus possible to use in the clinical practice and for the individual patient as the testing takes into consideration the exposure conditions at the worksite and the degree of reactivity to the product/sensitizer tested. The patient can be informed immediately of which glove(s) gives the best protection, and thus recommendations for the workplace can be given. It enables measurement of reactivity, and the method allows for *in vivo* factors such as skin–glove contact, skin temperature, and humidity to be taken into consideration. The test method may also be adapted to testing gloves against substances/products causing contact urticaria, corrosive substances, and chemical irritants. For a test of protection against corrosive substances and chemical irritants, the recruitment of subjects will be easier as the subject does not need to be sensitized. This testing can start with low concentrations to prevent a chemical burn if a glove material fails to prevent penetrations of a corrosive chemical. The system is quite easy to adjust according to needs. Changes might be required if the chemical tested is very volatile; the chamber then needs to be closed. Nonliquid products can also be tested, either by grinding the product or by solubilizing it. The latter, however, means taking a step away from imitating the exposure to the product/chemical in the workplace. Thicker glove materials, as well as products with longer breakthrough times, can be tested. In these tests, longer exposure times are needed, which is often inconvenient to the patient. This inconvenience can be reduced by starting exposure to the glove material before application onto the back of the patient. As opposed to *in vitro* testing alone, this procedure does still include an *in vivo* component. This modified testing procedure can also be used to test reusable gloves.

The *in vivo* glove test model is a good supplement to *in vitro* permeation testing and can give new valuable data on maximum protection time for different gloves in practical use. As it is easy to use, this testing procedure can be done in different workplaces with the chemicals used there and thus be of great preventive importance in the investigation of various work situations where it would otherwise be difficult to give good advice regarding the use of gloves. This concerns the chemical and plastic industry as well as many other worksites where hazardous chemicals are used. Optimally, protective gloves can also mean that already sensitized individuals might be able to stay at work, which is of great benefit not only to the individual but also to the community.

REFERENCES

1. Banaee, S., and Hee, S. S. Q. 2019. Glove permeation of chemicals: The state of the art of current practice, Part 1: Basics and the permeation standards. *Journal of Occupational and Environmental Hygiene* 16 (12):827–839. DOI: 10.1080/15459624.2019.1678754.
2. Banaee, S., and Hee, S. S. Q. 2020. Glove permeation of chemicals: The state of the art of current practice-Part 2. Research emphases on high boiling point compounds and simulating the donned glove environment. *Journal of Occupational and Environmental Hygiene* 17 (4):135–164. DOI: 10.1080/15459624.2020.1721509.
3. Phalen, R. N., Thi, L., and Wong, W. K. 2014. Changes in chemical permeation of disposable latex, nitrile, and vinyl gloves exposed to simulated movement. *Journal of Occupational and Environmental Hygiene* 11 (11):716–721. DOI: 10.1080/15459624.2014.908259.
4. Phalen, R. N., and Wong, W. K. 2015. Polymer properties associated with chemical permeation performance of disposable nitrile rubber gloves. *Journal of Applied Polymer Science* 132 (6):1–11. DOI: 10.1002/app.41449.
5. Mathews, A. R., and Hee, S. S. Q. 2017. Whole glove permeation of cyclohexanol through disposable nitrile gloves on a dextrous robot hand: Fist clenching vs. non-clenching. *Journal of Occupational and Environmental Hygiene* 14 (4):252–257. DOI: 10.1080/15459624.2016.1250006.
6. Andersson, T., and Bruze, M. 1999. In vivo testing of the protective efficacy of gloves against allergen-containing products using an open chamber system. *Contact Dermatitis* 41 (5):260–263. DOI: 10.1111/j.1600-0536.1999.tb06157.x.
7. Boman, A., and Mellström, G.A. 1989. Percutaneous absorption of 3 organic solvents in the guinea pig (IV). Effect of protective gloves. *Contact Dermatitis* 21:260–266.
8. Boman, A. S., and Mellström, G. A. 1994. Percutaneous absorption studies in animals. In *Protective Gloves for Occupational Use*, edited by G. A. Mellström, J. E. Wahlberg, and H. I. Maibach, 91–106. Boca Raton, FL: CRC Press.
9. Liden, C. 1984. Occupational dermatoses at a film laboratory. *Contact Dermatitis* 10 (2):77–87. DOI: 10.1111/j.1600-0536.1984.tb00340.x.
10. Jolanki, R., Estlander, T., and Kanerva, L. 1987. Contact allergy to an epoxy reactive diluent-1,4-butanediol diglycidyl ether. *Contact Dermatitis* 16 (2):87–92. DOI: 10.1111/j.1600-0536.1987.tb01385.x.
11. McClain, D. C., and Storrs, F. J. 1992. Protective effect of both barrier cream and a polyethylene laminate glove against epoxy resin, glyceryl monothioglycolate, Frullania, and Tansy. *American Journal of Contact Dermatitis* 3:201.

12. Rietschel, R. L., Huggins, R., Levy, N., and Pruitt, P. M. 1984. In vivo and in vitro testing of gloves for protection against uv-curable acrylate resin systems. *Contact Dermatitis* 11 (5):279–282. DOI: 10.1111/j.1600-0536.1984.tb01009.x.

13. Moyle, M., Frowen, K., and Nixon, R. 2004. Use of gloves in protection from diallyl disulphide allergy. *The Australasian Journal of Dermatology* 45 (4):223–225. DOI: 10.1111/j.1440-0960.2004.00102.x.

14. Espasandin-Arias, M., and Goossens, A. 2014. Natural rubber gloves might not protect against skin penetration of methylisothiazolinone. *Contact Dermatitis* 70 (4):249–251. DOI: 10.1111/cod.12221.

15. Morgado, F., Batista, M., and Goncalo, M. 2019. Short exposures and glove protection against (meth)acrylates in nail beauticians-Thoughts on a rising concern. *Contact Dermatitis* 81 (1):62–63. DOI: 10.1111/cod.13222.

16. Mellström, G. 1991. Protective gloves of polymeric materials - experimental permeation testing and clinical-study of side-effects. *Acta Dermato-Venereologica Suppl (Stockh)* 163:1–54.

17. Liden, C., and Wrangsjö, K. 1994. Protective effect of gloves illustrated by patch testing- practical aspects. In *Protective Gloves for Occupational Use*, edited by G. Mellstrom, J. E. Wahlberg, and H. I. Maibach, 207–212. Boca Raton, FL: CRC Press.

18. Andersson, T., Bruze, M., and Björkner, B. 1999. In vivo testing of the protection of gloves against acrylates in dentin-bonding systems on patients with known contact allergy to acrylates. *Contact Dermatitis* 41 (5):254–259. DOI: 10.1111/j.1600-0536.1999.tb06156.x.

19. Andersson, T., Bruze, M., Gruvberger, B., and Björkner, B. 2000. In vivo testing of the protection provided by non-latex gloves against a 2-hydroxyethyl methacrylate-containing acetone-based dentin-bonding product. *Acta Dermato-Venereologica* 80 (6):435–437.

20. Ursberg, A. M., Bergendorff, O., Thorsson, A. C., and Isaksson, M. 2016. Is there a good in vivo method to show whether gloves are sufficiently protective when a nail technician is exposed to (meth)acrylates? An in vivo pilot study. *Contact Dermatitis* 75 (1):62–65. DOI: 10.1111/cod.12573.

21. Antelmi, A., Young. E., Svedman, C., Zimerson, E., Engfeldt, M., Foti, C., and Bruze, M. 2015. Are gloves sufficiently protective when hairdressers are exposed to permanent hair dyes? An in vivo study. *Contact Dermatitis* 72 (4):229–236. DOI: 10.1111/cod.12320.

22. Antelmi, A., Bruze, M., Zimerson, E., Engfeldt, M., Foti, C., and Svedman, C. 2019. In vivo evaluation of the protective capacity of different gloves against hair dyes. *International Journal of Occupational and Environmental Medicine* 1 (1):19–32. DOI: 10.14302/issn.2690-0904.ijoe-19-2985.

23. Fregert, S. 1981. *Manual of Contact Dermatitis*. 2nd ed. Copenhagen: Munksgaard.

24. Johansen, J. D., Aalto-Korte, K., Agner, T., Andersen, K. E., Bircher, A., Bruze, M., Cannavo, A., Giménez-Arnau, A., Gonçalo, M., Goossens, A., John, S.M., Lidén, C., Lindberg, M., Mahler, V., Matura, M., Rustemeyer, T., Serup, J., Spiewak, R., Thyssen, J.P., Vigan, M., White, I.R., Wilkinson, M., and Uter, W. 2015. European Society of Contact Dermatitis guideline for diagnostic patch testing - recommendations on best practice. *Contact Dermatitis* 73 (4):195–221. DOI: 10.1111/cod.12432.

25. Wardell, K., Andersson, T., and Anderson, C. 1996. Analysis of laser Doppler perfusion images of experimental irritant skin reactions. *Skin Research and Technology* 2 (4):149–157. DOI: 10.1111/j.1600-0846.1996.tb00142.x.

26. Svedman, C., Cherry, G. W., Strigini, E., and Ryan, T. J.. 1998. Laser Doppler imaging of skin microcirculation. *Acta Dermato-Venereologica* 78 (2):114–118.

27. Nilsson, G. E. 1977. On the measurement of evaporative water loss, methods and clinical applications. Thesis, Linköping University, Sweden.

28. Serup, J., and Staberg, B. 1987. Differentiation of allergic and irritant reactions by trans-epidermal water-loss. *Contact Dermatitis* 16 (3):129–132. DOI: 10.1111/j.1600-0536.1987.tb01404.x.

29. Anzengruber, F., Alotaibi, F., Kaufmann, L. S., Ghosh, A., Oswald, M. R., Maul, J.-T., Meier, B., French, L. E., Bonmarin, M., and Navarini, A. A. 2019. Thermography: High sensitivity and specificity diagnosing contact dermatitis in patch testing. *Allergology International* 68 (2):254–258. DOI: 10.1016/j.alit.2018.12.001.

Section III

Glove Sensitivity and Effects on Skin

13 Irritation and Contact Dermatitis from Protective Gloves
An Overview

S. Levitt and H.I. Maibach

CONTENTS

13.1 INTRODUCTION

The beneficial value of using protective gloves varies, but for most people, the advantages outweigh the disadvantages. Side effects on the skin of users' hands and forearms unfortunately are not uncommon. In a Japanese questionnaire investigation,[1] among 792 housewives, 456 used gloves, and, of these, 61 (13%) reported skin troubles. In some cases, the adverse effects are so severe that users have to abandon these excellent prophylactic devices.

In any single case, it is hard to predict the interaction and relative importance of exposure to chemicals and products, a preexisting hand dermatosis with or without impaired barrier function, the glove materials, and the occlusive effect of the gloves.

Protective gloves should be used for contact with toxic or irritant substances, allergens, or infectious material. Although it is widely accepted that gloves protect against irritants,[2] allergens, and microbial agents, there are concerns that occlusive gloves themselves are a substantial factor in the promotion of occupational irritant hand dermatitis (OIHD) if not used properly.

DOI: 10.1201/9781003126874-16

TABLE 13.1

Side Effects on the Skin When Using Protective Gloves: An Overview

Side Effects	Discussed in Chapter(s)
Allergic contact dermatitis from ingredients/components in gloves made of rubber or plastic[3,4]	14
Contact urticaria from latex gloves	16 and 17
Glove dermatitis—other reactions: irritation (glove powders, occlusion, maceration, etc.), other urticaria, chemical leukoderma, endotoxins, ethylene oxide	18

Some common and more or less well-defined side effects are presented in Table 13.1. Allergic contact dermatitis (CD) from glove materials, contact urticaria (CU), and glove dermatitis of other types are reviewed in detail in Chapters 14, 16, 17, and 18. However, there remain patients in whom no specific skin disease can be diagnosed despite the extensive and detailed examination procedures described in these chapters and Chapter 15.

This chapter presents the examination and management of those cases where a specific cause or a defined skin disease—according to Table 13.1—has been excluded.

13.2   HISTORY

A careful history is essential for disclosing atopy/atopic hand eczema, hyperhidrosis/pompholyx, psoriasis, tinea, dermographism, or any other hand dermatoses that might be worsened by the occlusive effect of the gloves. Were gloves first used due to a preexisting skin disease, a general recommendation from a supervisor, or on the patient's own initiative?

13.3   SYMPTOMS AND SIGNS

The patient's usual report of itching, burning, redness, edema, fissuring, and scaling is of minor value when deciding whether the complaints are glove related. The location of these symptoms on the back of the hands and fingers, with a sharp cut-off dermatitis at the wrists, suggests that the condition is glove related.[5] Glove materials will rarely cause side effects on the volar aspects of the hands, solely. The distribution, then, will be of some help with the diagnosis, while the morphology of the lesions may mimic several other hand dermatoses.

Some patients referred to us were diagnosed as having scabies, pustulosis palmaris, or hand psoriasis and had incorrectly blamed the gloves they had used. Differential diagnoses are discussed in Chapters 14, 16, 17, and 18.

13.4   EXPOSURE CONDITIONS

The relative contribution of the following factors must be considered:

- The glove materials (with and without linings): rubber, plastic, leather, textile, wire cloth, metal mesh, or different combinations of these. Each type has its own area of use and pattern of skin side effects.
- What chemicals and products were handled? Are any of these known to be irritants, allergens, and/or permeable through glove materials? (See Chapters 10–12). Once the penetrants are inside the gloves, their harmful effects are enhanced by occlusion, humidity, and skin temperature. Some solvents and tensides (e.g., soap) can also act as extractants and vehicles and bring ingredients of glove materials to the skin surface, thereby facilitating the induction of irritation and allergy.
- Were the gloves accidentally contaminated through their openings? Such contamination might give rise to high concentrations of a chemical or product inside the glove and—if undetected—cause skin irritation augmented by occlusion.
- Were the gloves used during the entire exposure period?
- Have barrier creams or moisturizers been applied before or after glove-wearing and thereby influenced skin irritation?[6] Experimental studies have demonstrated that occlusion from gloves can cause irritation and impaired barrier function, quantified by bioengineering techniques.[7,8–10] Occlusion also seems to increase irritation, in particular on compromised skin. This irritation can be reduced by applying moisturizers.[11,12]
- Were there periods of exposure with unprotected hands—at work, at home, or in leisure time? Patients might wrongly blame the gloves they have used.
- How often were the gloves changed? Were new pairs used regularly, or were the contaminated gloves cleaned and reused? After removal of the gloves, the diffusion of chemicals through the glove membrane will continue and the chemicals will be trapped—unless the gloves are cleaned. On the following day, the threshold of the irritancy of a particular agent might have been reached and the subject will experience subjective and objective signs of skin irritation.
- Has a recent change taken place in brands of gloves (batch-to-batch variation)?
- Were any other people affected simultaneously after using gloves from the same supplier or delivery?

One new phenomenon that became common during the COVID-19 pandemic is double gloving, which appears to increase the frequency of dermatologic side effects, such as irritation and latex allergy.[13] The increase of skin damage as the consequence of greater PPE use and increased hand hygiene has been a consequence of COVID-19 handling. This practice of double gloving is only recommended for surgical procedures that carry a high risk of disrupting the integrity of the glove. A questionnaire-based study suggested that 88.5% of skin reactions on the hands are associated with the use of latex gloves.[14] Some adverse effects of glove use: latex allergy; reaction to talcum powder in the gloves; excessive dryness and pruritus (associated with irritant dermatitis) may be aggravated by occlusion, which may lead to sweating and/or over-hydration.[13] These effects may increase the permeability to sanitizers or detergents, creating a vicious cycle plus aggravation of hand dermatitis. A peculiar pattern of hand dermatitis has been recognized, characterized by erythema and fine scaling on the palms and web spaces. This may be attributed to the depletion of surface lipids, resulting in deeper penetration of detergents, and progressive damage of skin lay-ers is a major pathogenic mechanism. Irritant contact dermatitis is more commonly found with iodophors, chlorhexidine, chloroxylenol, triclosan, and alcohol-based products.

13.5   SKIN IRRITATION—STRATEGY FOR EXAMINATION AND SUGGESTED INVESTIGATIONS

The tests necessary for confirming the diagnoses of contact allergy and contact urti-caria are discussed in Chapters 14, 16, and 17. It is essential to detect these cases early to initiate the appropriate prophylactic approach and then in follow-up consul-tations to check the course and outcome.

Some of the side effects described in Chapter 18 cannot be verified by any objec-tive tests or analyses—the diagnoses are then based essentially on exclusion criteria.

The situation for skin irritation is similar—there is no confirmative test or analy-sis, and the diagnosis cannot be settled until other alternatives have been excluded. Some common causes of skin irritation in glove users are summarized in Table 13.2.

13.5.1   PROVOCATION TESTS

Patients are asked to bring all suspected gloves to the clinic, and provocation tests with the whole intact glove on moistened skin are carried out under supervision. In

---

TABLE 13.2
Some Common Causes of Skin Irritation in Glove Users

- Occlusion, sweating, and maceration
- Enhanced penetration of irritants from remaining detergents and skin care products due to the occlusion
- Agents that have penetrated the glove membranes from the outside (environmental exposure)
- Contamination of the inside by accidental entrance through the glove opening
- Agents/materials emanating from the glove itself
- Agents/materials remaining from the glove manufacturing process
- Agents remaining from the glove washing procedure—detergents and moisture
- Glove powders, barrier creams, moisturizers, ethylene oxide, etc. are discussed in Chapter 18
- Friction from the seams of leather and textile gloves[15]

some cases, 1–3 h of exposure is insufficient for eliciting symptoms or rashes; the test must be repeated on subsequent days.

13.5.2 PATCH TESTS WITH PIECES OF GLOVE

Patch tests with pieces of gloves have probably already been carried out when looking for contact allergy (see Chapter 14) and for contact urticaria (see Chapter 17). When a patient reacts only to such pieces but not to the rubber allergens in the standard series, this may indicate glove-related skin irritation. However, hundreds of rubber chemicals are known, and the standard patch test series contains the most important allergens among these.

Simultaneous patch tests are recommended with new (unused) and used (i.e., contaminated) glove pieces (with the inside as well as the outside glove surface toward the skin). The results should then be compared. A reaction only to the used glove membrane indicates that the reactivity might be related to factors other than the glove itself.

Rubber glove-induced skin symptoms have been prevalent among healthcare workers (HCWs). HCWs ($n = 1,584$) were evaluated using a written questionnaire, and 295 respondents with glove-induced skin symptoms were tested.[4] The study exhibited that 10.5% of patients exhibited positive patch tests for rubber-related allergens. The most positive readings were obtained from the Thiuram mix and Carba mix. Of the 295 cases, 93.2% were contact dermatitis, 4.4% contact urticaria, and 2.4% CD associated with CU. The majority of skin complaints of latex gloves are related to skin irritation rather than an allergy.

The immediate allergy to latex and the delayed allergy to rubber chemicals suggest that the healthcare workers with glove-related dermatoses should undergo both skin prick test and patch test to detect type IV hypersensitivity to rubber chemicals and type I hypersensitivity to latex.

13.5.3 WORKPLACE VISITS

If the tests discussed above fail to reproduce the symptoms and signs of irritation, a workplace visit is recommended. In some cases, the riddle is solved during such a visit, and the gloves are found not to be the culprit.

The prevalence of latex allergy has been high (17%) among groups at risk of occupational dermatitis, such as healthcare workers. A questionnaire was administered to 140 participants to analyze the effects of latex gloves in the workplace.[3] Irritant dermatitis was found in 40.7% of cases. One hundred and twenty-one healthcare workers (81.2%) used bleach and water to clean their hands. None of the participants indicated any allergy to latex prior to the study. The risk factors of atopic dermatitis and irritant dermatitis were found. The correlation between irritant dermatitis and frequent use of bleach and water suggests that these practices should be eradicated since it plays an important role in the development of contact urticaria and anaphylactic reactions.

Irritant contact dermatitis of the hands is a significant occupational problem. Management primarily involves cessation of exposure to hazardous substances. If used correctly, protective gloves can reduce or eliminate exposure of the hands to hazardous substances. If not, protective gloves can cause or worsen irritant contact dermatitis of the hands by increasing exposure of the hands to hazardous chemicals. Glove failure can occur by penetration, permeation, or contamination. By understanding the mechanisms of glove failure, clinicians can make more appropriate recommendations for the selection and use of protective gloves in the workplace.

A study was conducted to explore the problems of adverse skin reactions among healthcare workers (HCW) who have been using PPE, specifically latex gloves, for a long period.[14] The study was conducted by the distribution of questionnaires to HCWs to collect data on the duration of PPE use, as well as adverse skin reactions caused by use. Among 61 HCWs who regularly used latex gloves, 54 (88.5%) reported adverse skin reactions, including dry skin (55.7%), itching (31.2%), rash (23.0%), and chapped skin (21.3%). For an average of 3.5 months, latex gloves were used for an average of 10 hours. No one reported the use of plastic gloves and cloth gloves to cause adverse skin reactions. The most common adverse reactions to wearing latex gloves in this study were dry skin, itching, and rash. Three proposed reasons why these reactions occur: Immunoglobulin E-mediated hypersensitivity to latex; latex allergy and irritant contact dermatitis, which arises from repeated handwashing with soap and detergent; and not completely drying the hands before doffing gloves. If the symptoms of irritant contact dermatitis cannot be resolved, latex allergy testing is necessary, and latex gloves should be avoided.

13.6 SUMMARY AND CONCLUSION

Skin irritation cannot be diagnosed by any specific test: a "diagnosis of exclusion" (Table 13.3) is required. It is essential to diagnose contact allergy, contact urticaria, and other types of glove dermatitis (see Chapters 14, 16, 17, and 18) as these are preventable.

To support the diagnosis of skin irritation, we recommend provocation tests with whole gloves, patch tests with pieces of the glove, and workplace visits, especially in those cases where contact allergy, contact urticaria, etc., have been ruled out.

The World Health Organization (WHO) encourages healthcare workers to wear protective gloves for patient care during the COVID-19 pandemic. Medical gloves are made of different polymers, including NRL (latex), nitrile, PVC (vinyl), polyurethane, and neoprene (chloroprene). In general, both NRL and nitrile gloves are more durable

---

TABLE 13.3
Skin Irritation from Glove Use: A Diagnosis of Exclusion

- Exclude contact allergy and contact urticaria (according to the criteria presented in Chapters 14, 16, and 17)
- Exclude other types of glove dermatitis (presented in Chapter 18)
- Supervised provocation tests at the clinic, using suspected gloves
- Patch tests with used and unused glove pieces; both inside and outside of the glove

---

and provide better protection. However, adverse skin reactions are reported with the use of all types of gloves,[16,17] which should be considered. Recommendations for the prevention of irritant reactions to gloves include washing hands after glove removal with mild soap and drying thoroughly, not using hand creams or lotion while latex glove use, not wearing gloves on wet hands, using a cotton inner liner if prolonged exposure exists, treating underlying hand eczema, and powder-free glove use.

REFERENCES

1. Aoyama, M., Sugiura, K., Fujise, H., and Naruse, M. 1982. On use of gloves in the home and their influence upon skin irritation. *Nagoya Med* 27:65.
2. Bauer, A., Rönsch, H., Elsner, P., Dittmar, D., Bennett, C., Schuttelaar, M., Lukács, J., John, S.M., and Williams, H.C. 2018. Interventions for preventing occupational irritant hand dermatitis. *Cochrane Database Syst Rev* 4(4):CD004414.
3. Ly, F., Mbaye, I., Wone, I., Gaye-Fall, C., Sow, M.L., Ndiaye, B., and Mahé, A. 2006. Allergie aux gants en latex chez les professionnels de la santé à Dakar [Allergy to latex gloves among healthcare workers in Dakar]. *Ann Dermatol Venereol* 133(12):971–974.
4. Nettis, E., Assennato, G., Ferrannini, A., and Tursi, A. 2002. Type I allergy to natural rubber latex and type IV allergy to rubber chemicals in health care workers with glove-related skin symptoms. *Clin Exper Aller: J Br Soc Aller Clin Immunol* 32(3):441–447.
5. Fisher, A.A. 1985. Management of dermatitis due to surgical gloves. *J Dermatol Surg Oncol* 11:628.
6. Wigger-Alberti, W., and Eisner, P. 1998. Do barrier creams prevent or provoke contact dermatitis? *Am J Contact Dermatitis* 9:100.
7. Graves, C.J., Edwards, C., and Marks, R. 1995. The effects of protective occlusive gloves on stratum corneum barrier properties. *Contact Dermatitis* 33:183.
8. Ramsing, D.W., and Agner, T. 1996. Effect of glove occlusion on human skin. I. Short-term experimental exposure. *Contact Dermatitis* 34:1.
9. Ramsing, D.W., and Agner, T. 1996. Effect of glove occlusion on human skin. II. Long-term experimental exposure. *Contact Dermatitis* 34:258.
10. Zhai, H., and Maibach, H.I. 2001. Skin occlusion and irritant and allergic contact dermatitis: An overview. *Contact Dermatitis* 44:201.
11. Held, E., and Lund Jorgensen, L. 1999. The combined use of moisturizers and occlusive gloves: An experimental study. *Am J Contact Dermatitis* 10:146.
12. Zhai, H., Schmidt, R., Levin, C., Klotz, A., and Maibach, H.I. 2002. Prevention and therapeutic effects of a model emulsion on glove-induced irritation and dry skin in man. *Dermatol Beruf Umwelt* 50:134.
13. Anedda, J., Ferreli, C., Rongioletti, F., and Atzori, L. 2020. Changing gears: Medical gloves in the era of coronavirus disease 2019 pandemic. *Clin Dermatol* 38(6):734–736.
14. Hu, K., Fan, J., Li, X., Gou, X., Li, X., and Zhou, X. 2020. The adverse skin reactions of health care workers using personal protective equipment for COVID-19. *Medicine* 99(24):e20603. DOI: 10.1097/MD.0000000000020603.
15. Estlander, T., and Jolanki, R. 1988. How to protect the hands. *Dermatol Clin* 6:105.
16. Tabary, M., Araghi, F., Nasiri, S., and Dadkhahfar, S. 2021. Dealing with skin reactions to gloves during the COVID-19 pandemic. *Infect Control Hosp Epidemiol* 42(2):247–248.
17. Kwon, S., Campbell, L.S., and Zirwas, M.J. 2006. Role of protective gloves in the causation and treatment of occupational irritant contact dermatitis. *J Am Acad Dermatol* 55(5):891–896.

14 Allergic Contact Dermatitis from Rubber and Plastic Gloves

S. Levitt and H.I. Maibach

CONTENTS

14.1 INTRODUCTION

Protective gloves made of polymeric rubber and plastic materials are important, although they are only secondary safeguards against factors hazardous to the hands. Gloves can be used to protect the hands from chemical, physical, mechanical, and biological hazards. In work situations where advanced technical solutions are not possible or available, then proper use is essential for hand protection. It may be the only way to protect the hands against hazards or even modify their effects. Apart from hand protection, gloves may be used to protect the product being manufactured from the worker's hands or to protect patients from microbes on the hands of the personnel.

Although gloves are chosen to give the best possible protection against hazards, their use entails many problems, including irritation (dirt, occlusion, friction, maceration, dermographism), development of allergy to glove materials, absorption or penetration of chemicals, worsening of preexisting dermatoses, becoming caught in moving or revolving parts of machinery, endotoxin, and ethylene oxide reactions,

DOI: 10.1201/9781003126874-17

and chemical leukoderma. The development of allergy, especially to rubber materials and other possible agents in gloves, is probably the most harmful side effect of polymer gloves.[1–6]

Once developed, allergy is generally permanent, and clinical signs and symptoms, e.g., dermatoses, recur when a sensitized person comes into contact with a specific allergen. Two forms of allergic reactions to polymer gloves are known: delayed (type IV allergy) and immediate (type I allergy). Glove allergy usually involves one of the two types of reactions, but occasionally both coincide. In a study of 143 patients with type I allergy to natural rubber latex (NRL), 18 also had a type IV allergy to rubber chemicals.[7] Sensitization to both rubber and plastic glove materials, one after another, is also possible. Most of the reported cases of type IV allergy to rubber gloves are due to gloves made of NRL, and cases due to synthetic materials are few. Reports usually describe allergy to neoprene gloves,[4,5,8,9] but sensitization to other materials, e.g., nitrile rubber, is also possible.[8] Gloves made of NRL are the chief cause of type I allergy, but also latex-free nitrile gloves,[10] and gloves made of mixtures of synthetic rubber and NRL have been reported to cause type I sensitization and contact urticaria.[11,12] NRL gloves are also the major contributor to latex aeroallergens in operating rooms.[13,14]

Plastic gloves usually cause allergic contact dermatitis as a result of the development of type IV allergy in response to glove materials. Type I reactions to plastic materials are rare. A case of contact urticaria from polyethylene gloves and another case caused by vinyl-chloride slip-guard in cotton gloves have been reported.[15,16]

14.2 FREQUENCY OF ALLERGIC CONTACT DERMATITIS DUE TO GLOVES

14.2.1 RUBBER GLOVES

Rubber gloves have long been the main source of occupational and non-occupational allergy to rubber;[1–5,17–20] 40%–70% of all occupationally induced type IV rubber allergy cases have been reported to be caused by rubber gloves.[2–5,21,22] Previously, the figures for gloves as causes of occupational rubber allergy have been even higher when housewives were included in the occupational groups.[23,24]

Based on the information obtained from the Finnish Register of Occupational Diseases (FROD; 1997–1999), rubber chemicals were the most important cause of occupational allergic eczema in the entire country, explaining 22% of 1020 cases. NRL was, after animal epithelia, the second most common cause of contact urticaria and protein contact dermatitis, causing 23% of 475 cases. Almost all cases were due to NRL gloves. In women, NRL and rubber chemicals were the most important of the chemical causative factors. They caused 17% of all women's chemically induced occupational contact dermatoses, whereas they were in men only the fourth most common cause, responsible for 9% of the cases.[25] Rubber gloves were considered to be the most common source of type IV allergy to rubber chemicals, causing more than 50% of the cases. When all occupations are considered, roughly 70% of the rubber glove allergy cases are due to a delayed-type reaction and 30% to an immediate-type reaction.[5,26] It has been suggested that type I allergy to NRL could be more important than type IV allergy to rubber chemicals in occupations where gloves are used for long periods every day, e.g., in hospitals, dental care, and laboratory work.[20,27–30] The study on Finnish dental nurses confirmed that acrylics and rubber gloves were the most common cause of their occupational allergic dermatoses. Type I sensitization to NRL materials was, however, not more common than type IV allergy but almost as common as type IV sensitization.[31]

14.2.2 Plastic Gloves

Completely cured plastic materials are not generally considered sensitizers, and polyvinyl chloride (PVC), polyethylene or polyethylene (PE), polyvinyl acetate (PVAc), polyvinyl alcohol, and other materials used in plastic gloves rarely cause allergic contact dermatitis. The use of plastic materials for personal protective equipment has become common since the 1950s, but in most countries, plastic gloves are possibly less used than rubber gloves. One reason for this may still be that the users find plastic gloves less comfortable because they are not always as soft and pliable as rubber gloves and do not completely follow the contours of the hands. Accordingly, most reports on allergic contact eczema from plastic gloves are based on only one or a few cases.[5] In a German study, 31 patients investigated from 1969 to 1984 were sensitized from the use of rubber or vinyl gloves; 10% of them were allergic to vinyl gloves.[32] Similar results were obtained in a Finnish study: 5 (7%) of 68 patients were sensitized due to the use of PVC gloves.[2] Since then, only three definite cases of vinyl glove allergy have been diagnosed at the Finnish Institute of Occupational Health (FIOH).[33,34] In a Japanese questionnaire study, however, 31 (51%) of 61 women who had developed contact dermatitis from using household gloves linked their skin symptoms with the use of vinyl gloves and 26 (43%) with rubber gloves. Irritation was suggested as the cause of the vinyl glove dermatitis, not an allergy to the material itself.[35]

14.3 SENSITIZERS

14.3.1 Rubber Gloves

Rubber and plastic gloves are usually manufactured by automated processes, of which the dipping method is the most common. The primary ingredient in rubber gloves is rubber polymer, blended with various additives, including vulcanizing agents, accelerators, antioxidants, pigments, fillers, and oils (Table 14.1). Rubber polymer can be a natural product made from the milky liquid (natural latex) of the rubber tree, or it can be manufactured synthetically. Whether a rubber glove is called natural (NRL) or synthetic depends on the origin of the polymer used in its production. Neoprene and nitrile rubbers are synthetic polymers used in glove production. Blending NRL with neoprene or nitrile rubbers is common in order to combine the favorable properties of both materials.

Additives, usually accelerators such as thiurams, dithiocarbamates, and benzothiazoles, and antioxidants are usually responsible for type IV glove alle

TABLE 14.1

Sensitizers in Rubber Gloves

Main

    Accelerators

        Thiurams

        Dithiocarbamates

        Benzothiazoles

        Thioureas

Other

    Antioxidants

        p-Phenylenediamine derivative

        Phenol derivatives

    Vulcanizers

    Colorants

        Organic pigments

        Disperse dyes

    Preservatives

        Isothiazolinones

    Antistatic agents

        Cetylpyridinium chloride

Potential

    Donning powders

    Fragrances

Questionable

    Vulcanizing retarders

        Cyclohexylthiophthalimide

rgy.[2–5,18,19,21,36] Thiurams have most commonly been responsible for the reactions due to rubber gloves—the frequencies ranging previously from 54% to 80%. Dipentamethylenethiuram disulfide (PTD), tetraethylthiuram disulfide, and tetramethylthiuram monosulfide and disulfide have variably been the most frequent reactors among the thiurams, possible reflecting variations in the glove materials in different countries. According to recent studies, thiurams are still the leading allergens in occupational rubber glove allergy despite that many rubber glove manufacturers have replaced thiurams with dithiocarbamates or mercaptobenzothiazole and its derivatives.[36,37] In a study of the Information Network of Departments of Dermatology (IVDK) in Germany concerning rubber glove allergy,[36] thiurams (16.2% of the reactions) were by far the most frequent rubber allergens in these patients. According to the authors, one possible explanation may be that in many hospitals huge numbers of inexpensive NRL gloves are used, and it cannot be excluded that these gloves still contain thiurams. Of the thiurams, TEDT was the leading allergen, inducing 10.3% of the positive patch test reactions, whereas 3.9% of the patients reacted to dithiocarbamates, mostly to zinc diethyldithiocarbamate (ZDEC). Only 5 of the 1377 tested patients reacted to zinc dibutyldithiocarbamate

(ZDBC). Concomitant sensitization to thiurams and dithiocarbamates was common. Analysis of cross-reactions between thiurams and dithiocarbamates confirms the clinical experience that individuals sensitized to thiurams may tolerate gloves with dithiocarbamates for a certain length of time, but that patients with contact allergy to dithiocarbamates never tolerate thiuram-containing rubber gloves.[18] Because these two groups of related chemicals often occur simultaneously in NRL, concomitant sensitization cannot be completely excluded. Mercaptobenzothiazole (MBT) and its derivatives caused 2.9% of the positive reactions. The derivatives morpholinylmer-captobenzothiazole (MOR), N-cyclohexyl-2-benzothiazylsulfenamide (CBS), and dibenzothiazyl disulfide (MBTS) can also be used as accelerators. A chemical analy-sis of 11 NRL gloves revealed CBS in some gloves.[38] In addition, a commercial grade of MBT can be contaminated with CBS.[39] In the mentioned German study, MOR elicited an even greater number of positive reactions than MBT. In a Danish study of glove-allergic patients, PTD was the most frequent reactor on patch testing, followed by zinc dimethyldithiocarbamate, ZDEC, zinc MBT, and MBT.[40,41]

Ethyl isothiocyanate (EITC) and butyl isothiocyanate (BITC) are possible caus-ative chemicals responsible for nitrile rubber glove-induced allergic contact derma-titis.[42] The patient exhibited positive patch test reactions to nitrile rubber gloves, in addition to dithiocarbonate mix and thiuram mix. Chemical analysis revealed that EITC and BITC, which might have been produced from dithiocarbamate-type accelerators (DTCs) or thiuram-type accelerators (thiurams) during the vulcaniza-tion process, were present in the nitrile rubber gloves that the patient used at her workplace, as was ZDBC. No other DTCs or thiurams were detected. Patch testing of the detected materials produced positive reactions to EITC and BITC, but not to ZDBC. The patient was diagnosed with allergic contact dermatitis due to the EITC and BITC present in nitrile rubber gloves and suggested that alkyl isothiocyanate might also have played a causative role. It is recommended that nitrile rubber gloves should be produced without using vulcanization accelerators.

Other potential type IV sensitizers include thiourea and phenol derivatives, diphenylguanidine (DPG), mercaptobenzimidazole, quinoline derivatives, antioxi-dants, preservatives, antistatic agents, glove powder ingredients, as well as fragran ces.[3,4,18,19,43,44] Reports on sensitization to thiourea compounds (e.g., diphenylthiourea [DPTU]) from rubber gloves are few and involve mostly gloves made of neoprene rubber, which may also contain DPG.[3,4,8,9,45] Thioureas, classified as moderate sensi-tizers, can be found in hypoallergenic surgical gloves. They are efficient accelerators in the vulcanization of neoprene rubber. In addition to gloves, neoprene is widely used in orthopedic braces, wet suits and other diving accessories, sports shoes and clothing, protective goggles, weather stripping, and adhesives.[45] In a study of IVDK and the German Contact Dermatitis Research Group,[36] thioureas (DPTU, dibutyl-thiourea) and DPG caused only a few positive patch test reactions.

Guanidine is a rubber accelerator and a common contact allergen found among healthcare workers. A study conducted in a Belgium hospital performed patch test-ing to highlight the role of 1,3-diphenylguanidine (DPG) as the culprit allergen in contact hand dermatitis to synthetic rubber gloves.[46] Patch test data was collected from healthcare workers who developed contact hand dermatitis after wearing rubber gloves and reacted positively to glove samples and rubber additives. The study demonstrated that 86% reacted positively to DPG, 84% reacted positively to "carba mix" (containing diphenylguanidine [DPG], zinc dibutyldithiocarbamate [ZDBC], and zinc diethyldithiocarbamate [ZDEC]), and 30% reacted positively to thiuram mix. DPG was the most commonly identified allergen, far ahead of thiurams, which had previously been described as the most sensitizing accelerator. The use of DPG-free gloves is recommended.[46,47]

Patch tests were performed with the guanidine accelerator, triphenylguanidine (TPG), to detect the presence of the molecule.[47] TPG, an accelerator not previously reported as being present in rubber gloves, was found in the glove extracts. Patch testing with TPG suggested that contact allergic reactions in patients with hand dermatitis was caused by rubber gloves. In this case, a rubber accelerator previously not reported as a possible contact allergen was found in surgical glove extracts.

Antioxidants are less frequent sensitizers.[3,36] Allergy from gloves to N-isopropyl-V-phenyl paraphenylenediamine has been reported,[3,4,17,18,48] although paraphenylenediamine (PPDA) derivatives are seldom used in rubber gloves, except in black- or dark-colored industrial gloves. Phenol derivatives are rare sensitizers in rubber gloves.[3,4,18,49] In the 1990s high sensitization rates (2.9%–4.6%) to N-(cyclohexylthio) phthalimide (CTP), a prevulcanization inhibitor, have also been reported, but the relevance of the reactions has remained unknown.[50,51] In a study of the IVDK and the German Contact Dermatitis Research Group,[51] the analysis of the 1936 patients' data showed that among CTP-allergic patients there were more patients with occupational dermatitis, hand dermatitis, face dermatitis, and suspected glove allergy. About 20% of these patients had medical occupations. Nearly half also had a contact allergy to other rubber chemicals. According to one manufacturer, CTP is used only in the production of solid rubber, not for medical applications, including gloves, or in consumer goods, e.g., shoe soles and rubber bands. In addition, several rubber glove manufacturers have stated that they would not use CTP.[50,51]

Dihydroxydiphenyl (DOD) and monobenzyl ether of hydroquinone (monobenzone) have at least previously been used in the manufacture of rubber gloves. A case of allergy caused by DOD in neoprene gloves has been reported.[52] It was also the cause of glove dermatitis in four surgeons and a nurse.[53] Two glove-allergic patients in the FIOH also reacted to DOD in the 1980s.[3] In 1991–2000 not one of 159 rubber-allergic patients reacted to DOD; 3 reacted to monobenzone.[50] The chemical has also been reported as a cause of occupational rubber glove-induced leukoderma.[6] Nowadays DOD and monobenzone are not included in even extensive rubber chemical patch test series, and thus they are excluded from the statistics of rubber chemical sensitivity. As a result, manufacturers may draw a false conclusion and consider them non-sensitizers.

More recently, a FIOH report on skin sensitization related to different occupations has become available, which will be of value to manufacturers, end-users of the products, dermatologists, and occupational health professionals.[54]

Organic pigments, used in both rubber and plastic materials, may be leachable and induce sensitization.[55] Cetylpyridinium chloride (CPC), a quaternary ammonium compound, has also been reported as the cause of sensitization to surgical rubber gloves.[56,57] Since 1992, rubber polymer itself has increasingly been listed among the possible causes of delayed allergy to rubber.[58–63] The allergy frequencies to NRL have varied from 1.2% to 6% in various studies. Five centers of the British Contact Dermatitis Group conducted a prospective study on the prevalence of type IV sensitivity to NRL.[63] Altogether, 2738 consecutive patients were patch tested with ammonia-preserved NRL solution; 27 (1%) had an allergic reaction to NRL. Positive patch test reactions to NRL may be caused by thiurams or dithiocarbamates, added as stabilizers or accelerators to NRL test solution, or by benzisothiazolin-3-one, added as a preservative. Therefore, in this study, prick and patch testing was performed with ammonia-preserved NRL, which did not contain additives, except ammonia. Of these 27 patients, 14 also had a positive prick test or specific Immunoglobulin E (IgE) to NRL, 19 (70%) were atopic, and 13 (48%) had hand eczema. Thus, type IV sensitization to NRL can be a problem for a proportion of hand eczema patients. Concomitant type I allergy to NRL is also common in these patients.

In Germany, sensitization to thiurams has been much more common than to DPG, but this can be because DPG is overlooked as a relevant allergen in healthcare workers. Four patients presented from different regions in Germany were diagnosed with occupational allergic contact dermatitis of the hands.[41] They had worn sterile DPG-containing polyisoprene surgical gloves from the same glove manufacturer at work. The manufacturer disclosed that the gloves contain DPG and have a CPC inner coating. Other studies have reported that DPG is a relevant allergen in sterile polyisoprene gloves. In the four cases, occupational allergic contact dermatitis of the hands was diagnosed and the surgical gloves were replaced by alternative gloves free of DPG or CPC. Three of the patients continued their occupation with markedly improved skin conditions. A follow-up was not available for the fourth patient. To conclude, DPG and CPC should be patch tested in healthcare workers with suspected allergic contact dermatitis who use sterile surgical gloves. Moreover, DPG-free and CPC-free gloves should be encouraged, and product labeling of glove constituents should be enforced.[41]

Apart from additives known to induce contact sensitization, the number of rubber additives used in the manufacture of rubber products is much greater, and many other additives, which may prove to be sensitizers, are possibly used in the manufacture of gloves.

Apart from glove ingredients, glove powder can also be the cause of glove dermatitis. A case of sensitization to glove powder has been reported, but the allergen was not specified.[44] Preservatives (e.g., sorbic acid, isothiazolin-3-one derivatives) and epichlorohydrin are potential sensitizers found in glove powders,[21] as well as fragrances used occasionally in both rubber and plastic gloves.[64]

14.3.2 PLASTIC GLOVES

Most allergy problems arise from the use of PVC gloves. PVC is made by polymerization of vinyl chloride monomer, a plastic material softened by heating or adding plasticizers. When a small amount (<5%) of plasticizers is added, the product hardens. When the amount of plasticizers is 30%–50%, the product becomes soft. A vinyl glove material may, for example, contain about 50% PVC and 50% additives.

These include plasticizers, stabilizers, ultraviolet (UV) absorbers, fungicides, bactericides, flame retardants, and colorants.[43,65] Although plastic materials are generally considered non-sensitizers, some additives may be leachable and cause contact sensitization.[1,55] PVC itself is probably not a sensitizer. In most reported cases of allergy to plastic gloves, the actual sensitizer in the material has remained undetermined.[2,32,66–70] The commonly used patch test series of plastics and glues contain some potential allergens in PVC materials, and the ingredients of the suspected glove materials are seldom available for testing. This is possibly the most important reason for the specific allergen to be detected only in exceptional cases.

Contact allergy to polyvinylchloride (PVC) gloves have been seldomly reported. However, a study conducted a test on patients who had positive patch test reactions to PVC gloves. The study obtained a collection of PVC raw materials from industrial producers and suppliers—isocyanates and isocyanate prepolymers, plastics, and glue series.[71] Nine PVC glove samples for triphenyl phosphate and its derivatives were analyzed. Two patients reacted to a technical PVC antioxidant and triphenyl phosphite (TPP), one of its components. Contact allergy to TPP was prominent in one patient and the main cause of hand dermatitis. The other patient had other contact allergies that explained the symptoms. Three patients reacted to the PVC gloves; however, a specific allergen was not identified. It was determined that six of the PVC glove samples contained TPP at 0.004%–0.099%. During storage, TPP transforms into triphenyl phosphate. Overall, TPP represents a new allergen detected in high concentrations in PVC gloves.[71]

Sensitization to an epoxy resin used as a plasticizer has been reported by Fregert and Rorsman.[72] Epoxy resins can be used as plasticizers and stabilizers in PVC (e.g., gloves), PVAc plastics, and neoprene.[73] A patient at the FIOH having allergic contact dermatitis from the use of certain PVC gloves of household type reacted on patch testing repeatedly to her gloves and bisphenol A. Interestingly, one of five previous patients sensitized from their plastic gloves had been sensitized from the use of PVC household gloves of the same brand but was not allergic to bisphenol A.[2] Since then two other patients, after using disposable PVC gloves, reacted to their glove materials and bisphenol A. Chemical analyses of the glove materials revealed bisphenol A, which was probably the cause of their hand dermatitis.[33,34] On further follow-up, one of these three patients, a female dentist who primarily had worn PVC gloves started to use NRL gloves after becoming sensitized to bisphenol A. In less than a half year her dermatitis renewed and she was found to be sensitized to dithiocarbamates used in the production of these NRL gloves, kindly provided by the manufacturer for patch testing. The dentist continued her work and used disposable nitrile gloves with polyethylene gloves under them.[74]

Epoxy resin monomers are strong skin sensitizers known to cause occupational allergic contact dermatitis. Diglycidyl ethers of bisphenol A and F (DGEBA and DGEBF) are widely used as components in epoxy resin products. Alternative compounds have been designed, synthesized, and assessed for sensitizing potency using in vivo murine local lymph node assay. Studies have shown that the allergenic effects of diglycidyl ethers of bisphenol F (DGEBF) depend on the absence of oxygen in the side chain of the molecule, known as the "terminal epoxide groups."[75] Thus, an epoxy resin that lacks oxygen in the side chain was considered promising and was synthesized. As predicted, the sensitizing potency was reduced by a factor of ten with the removal of the oxygen molecule. The technical properties of the newly synthesized polymer were not considered sufficient. Developing an alternative epoxy material is a delicate balance between allergenic activity and polymerization properties. The use of improved epoxy resin monomers with less skin sensitizing effects is one way to address contact allergy to epoxy resin.[76]

Plasticizers were possibly the cause of one patient's dermatitis when five patients were sensitized to their PVC gloves.[2] The patient reacted to tricresyl phosphate and triphenyl phosphate, known to be used as plasticizers in PVC. Other potential plasticizer sensitizers include phthalates, e.g., dibutyl and dioctyl phthalate, syn. di(ethylhexyl) phthalate (DOP), di(2-n-butyl) phthalate, butyl benzyl phthalate, and di-n-butyl maleate.[43,65] No cases of type IV allergy from plastic gloves due to phthalates have been reported, but the possibility of a type I allergy should be kept in mind. In a case of contact urticaria reported from the use of PE gloves, chemical analyses of the glove material revealed three fractions, which on scratch testing induced positive whealing reactions confirming type I sensitization. The fractions contained octadecanoic acid methyl ester, 2,6-di-tert-butylphenol, DOP, cis-13-docosenoic acid amide (Erucamide), and octadecyl 3-(3,5)-di-tert-butyl-4-hydroxyphenyl propionate (Irganox 1076). Interestingly, the patient's elder brother had previously suffered from contact urticaria syndrome caused by DOP in a vinyl- chloride slip-guard in cotton gloves.[15,16]

In addition, colorants may cause PVC glove dermatitis. The colorant Irgalite Orange F2G (CI Pigment Orange 34) was the actual sensitizer in one of the five above-mentioned patients.[2] There may also be other potential sensitizers in plastic gloves. The distinction between the terms *synthetic rubber* and *plastic polymers* is somewhat artificial. Therefore, the manufacturers and distributors of gloves may sometimes call a certain material a plastic, whereas others may designate the same material as synthetic rubber. On the other hand, some of the same chemicals can be used in both plastics and rubbers, e.g., certain thiourea derivatives.[9,43,77]

Acrylates and methacrylates are a large group of chemically reactive monomers that are polymerized into acrylic plastics. They have a broad application in glues, adhesives, coatings, and various plastic materials prevalent in dentistry and nail technician occupations. Dermatology and Allergology Units of the University Hospital of Bari investigated frequent sensitizing acrylates and assessed the role of 2-hydroxyethyl methacrylate (2-HEMA) as a screening allergen.[78] From January 2013 to December 2014, 217 patients with a history of allergic contact dermatitis (ACD) were patch tested with an extended series of acrylates. 2-HEMA was detected in 100% of sensitized patients to acrylates.

14.4   CLINICAL ASPECTS

14.4.1   PREDISPOSING FACTORS

Development of type IV allergy to polymer gloves is influenced by factors, such as the quality of the polymers, the amounts and types of substances in the polymer mixtures, the bioavailability of additives in gloves, duration of contact with the skin, quality of the materials handled with gloves, the temperature of the work environment, sweating, and health state of the skin of the hands.[4,5,40]

The use of rubber gloves involves more risk of sensitization than the use of plastic gloves, as rubber usually contains more potent and more leachable additives than plastic. There are great differences in the materials of rubber gloves despite the same nominal quality. The composition of gloves varies from one manufacturer to another because different chemicals in different states of purity and different amounts are used for the same purposes, e.g., as accelerators and antioxidants.[1,4,5,79] Accordingly, patients allergic to certain dithiocarbamate compounds have, on patch testing, tested positive for some gloves containing that particular dithiocarbamate, while remaining negative for some others although they contain the same chemical.[80] Long-standing daily use of rubber gloves, simultaneous exposure of hands to chemical or mechanical irritants, or wet work seems to constitute the most important risk of developing an allergy to glove materials.[5] Based on the information obtained from the FROD, women are at higher risk of developing an allergy to rubber chemicals and NRL than men. Women wear rubber (and plastic gloves) at work more often than men because they are also more often employed in jobs that require hand protection, and the use of gloves is also common in households.[5,25,32,80] However, allergy to gloves, both type I and IV, is also common in male workers who regularly use rubber gloves.[5,19,32,81–87] In addition to housework, risk occupations include work in medical and dental health services (surgeons, gynecologists, obstetricians, orthopedists, midwives, nurses, instrument caretakers, dentists, dental nurses), hospital and other cleaners, hairdressers, kitchen workers or workers in the food industry, farmers, and industrial workers, e.g., masons and construction workers.

It is not completely known how additives are leached from vulcanized rubber products, but perspiration and high temperature may promote the release of these agents from products, and thus enhance the development of allergy. Degradation of rubber by heat, friction, and ozone may also contribute to the development of sensitization.[5,80] Experimental studies in conditions simulating the normal use of gloves have even proved the release of additives from gloves. At the same time, some degradation of the released chemicals has been found to take place.[80]

Allergens easily penetrate the skin if it is macerated or inflamed. Irritant dermatitis or allergic contact dermatitis from other causes often precedes sensitization to rubber gloves. Often, the use of gloves has been started only after the appearance of skin irritation or hand eczema.[1,2,4] From clinical experience, it is also known that sensitivity to the rubber may complicate other types of dermatoses, e.g., psoriasis and atopic eczema of the hands.

Chemicals coming into contact with the glove materials may also promote the development of allergy to glove ingredients. Organic solvents can extract allergenic compounds from glove materials and carry them inside the glove.[40,88,89] Some other chemicals, e.g., bleaching agents, can transform the structure of a chemical in rubber products so that it becomes allergenic.[90] Surgeons may treat the thumb, index, and middle fingers of their surgical gloves with sodium hypochlorite to produce good

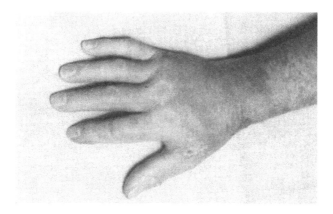

FIGURE 14.1   Typical appearance of rubber glove dermatitis

traction of the material,[91] at the same time possibly increasing the risk to be sensitized to the material.

14.4.2   LOCATION AND APPEARANCE OF DERMATITIS

Polymer gloves typically cause skin signs and symptoms corresponding to glove contours, on dorsal hands, but sometimes also on the palms near the thumbs, on both sides of the wrists, and on the forearms. The border of dermatitis on the midarm, corresponding to the upper border of the glove, is often abrupt. Dermatitis may first appear as a few small papules on the fingers and then extend to the whole dorsal hand. The symptoms may include swelling, intense redness, vesicles or even blisters, scaling or rhagades, itching, and a stinging or burning sensation depending on the stage and duration of dermatitis (Figure 14.1). Another typical manifestation is diffuse or patchy eczema on the dorsal hands and the forearms, not extending over the whole glove area. Forearms, the face, and also larger areas may be involved in more severe rubber glove dermatitis. Sometimes the face can be more affected than the hands (Figure 14.2). When rubber allergy superimposes other types of dermatoses, the appearance may not differ much from that of the prevailing dermatosis. Sensitization of glove material may also be the cause of the worsening of a patient's dermatosis when a rubber-allergic patient is treated locally, and the nurse wears rubber gloves.[4,43,77,92] Rare manifestations connected with rubber allergy include localized leukoderma, purpuric, lichenoid, and erythema-multiforme-like dermatoses. The lesions may be located on the back of the hands and forearms related to the use of gloves.[93] Depigmented lesions occur rarely nowadays.[94]

14.5   DIAGNOSIS AND DIFFERENTIAL DIAGNOSIS

The possibility of glove allergy should be suspected in cases in which even careful wearing of rubber or plastic (PVC) gloves with or without separate inner gloves

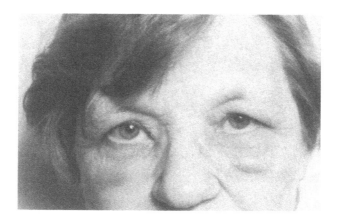

FIGURE 14.2   Allergy to rubber gloves appearing as eyelid edema

seems to be of no use. Wearing thin cotton gloves does not always prevent the development of an allergy, as the additives released from the gloves may easily penetrate
the fabric and reach the skin. The possibility of glove dermatitis should also be kept
in mind in cases where skin problems from contact with other rubber objects have
been encountered.[43] Also, the occasional use of gloves made of polymeric materials,
although not considered important by the patient, should be borne in mind, especially in the cases of dermatoses other than contact eczema.[92]

Investigations should include patch testing with pieces of rubber and plastic glove
materials, using the 48-h occlusion time. A longer occlusion time has been considered necessary, especially when thin gloves like an examination or surgical gloves
are tested.[77] However, a longer occlusion time also increases the risk of false-positive
reactions. Testing with solid materials always includes a risk of false-positive irritant
reactions, but retesting and control tests on non-exposed persons, as well as experience in reading tests,[4,5] may help to distinguish irritant reactions from allergic ones.
Tests with ultrasonic bath extracts of glove materials may sometimes help to detect
the sensitizer in the materials.[95] The best results have been obtained by testing glove
pieces in a drop of water.

Further testing with a standard series, e.g., the European series (Chemotechnique
Diagnostics Ab, Mahno, Sweden) is needed to confirm allergy to rubber. The series
contains rubber mixes, a thiuram mix, black rubber mix, and carba mix (CM), and
MBT, which detect most cases of rubber glove allergy.[5,96] Especially the thiuram
mix has been shown to be a good detector of glove allergy.[43,82,96] It has also been suggested that in cases of rubber glove allergy it is not important to know which specific
thiuram compound is the sensitizer, because all thiuram-containing gloves must be
avoided.[96] However, as far as carba mix is concerned, it does not seem to be a reliable
diagnostic tool except for patients who are not allergic to its components.[97] The three
single components of the mix, i.e., ZDEC, ZDBC, and DPG, have therefore been
recommended to be tested separately from the beginning.[97] Testing MBT instead of
mercapto mix increases the sensitivity of the test because, in addition to detecting

allergy to MBT, it reveals allergies to CBS, MBTS, or MOR with the same sensitivity as mercapto mix. In the living epidermis CBS, MBTS, and MOR are converted into MBT.[38]

Carba mix contains 1,3-diphenylguanidine (DPG), an allergen that is not often tested separately. A study conducted by the North American Contact Dermatitis Group performed patch tests in contact allergic dermatitis patients to determine allergies to either DPG or CM.[98] A total of 10,457 patients participated: 5.8% had allergic reactions to either CM or DPG, 31.1% had a reaction to DPG only, and 21% had reactions to both DPG and CM. Overall, 39.4% of CM-allergic patients reacted to DPG, and 59.7% of DPG-allergic patients reacted to CM. The researchers concluded that patch testing to CM will miss 25%–40% of positive reactions to DPG and that further studies need to include DPG in the baseline assessment for contact allergens.[98]

The standard series contains no thiourea compounds, but some are included in a specific rubber series, e.g., Chemotechnique Diagnostics Ab. Cross-reactivity occurs between thiourea compounds, but not always,[9,99] so each thiourea compound needs to be tested separately. A thiourea mix (Chemotechnique) has been taken into the standard series by some groups. In cases where testing with a standard series and/or glove pieces gives an uncertain result, further testing with a rubber additive series, e.g., Chemotechnique, which contains 24 chemicals, may increase the accuracy of patch testing and help to find alternative materials for patients having a specific rubber additive allergy.

Possible sensitization to rubber polymers themselves, as well as glove powders, should also be ruled out.[21,53,100] The authors also recommend that NRL (preserved solely with ammonia) should be included in a rubber series for screening those patients with hand dermatitis who are users of NRL gloves. The fragrances used to deodorize the materials may also be the cause of glove allergy.

A series of plastics and glues containing, e.g., tricresyl phosphate, bisphenol A, and phthalates such as DOP,[4,66] may help in cases where PVC or PE gloves are suspected. Patch testing with all actual components of polymer gloves would give the best and most reliable results[2,100] and would also give more information on the allergenic compounds found in gloves.

Investigations should also include tests to detect type I allergy to polymeric glove materials and glove powders (prick tests, determinations of latex-specific IgE antibodies in serum, e.g., RAST, and challenges with suspected gloves). See also Chapters 13 and 14.

14.6   PREVENTION OF GLOVE DERMATITIS

Preventive aspects should be considered carefully.[1,4,5,101–104] A detailed job analysis should be done; all materials to be handled with the gloves should always be checked to see whether the material is suitable for the job in question. Also, the demands of the user should be taken into account before the gloves are selected.

New directives and regulations covering the use and safety requirements of protective gloves have come into force in Europe. It is necessary to obtain information on quality requirements and performance data on protective gloves, as well as on the acceptable level of exposure to hazards, and problems in glove usage before gloves are selected, purchased, or used.[79,105]

In Europe, gloves intended to protect the user are considered personal protective equipment (PPE) and covered by the Personal Protective Equipment Directive 89/686/ EEC. Gloves that are intended for medical purposes are covered by the Council Directive 93/42/EEC concerning medical devices. The European Committee for Standardization (CEN) is responsible for establishing the necessary new standards for Europe. A survey of the US rules, regulations, and standards concerning protective gloves for occupational use has been presented by Henry.[106]

The glove usage should be started at the same time as the handling of hazardous materials, but gloves made of polymeric materials should not be used needlessly, e.g., during cleaning jobs in which no liquids are handled. The gloves should be for personal use, and the condition of the gloves should be the user's responsibility. Workers with long-lasting dermatitis should be referred to a dermatological examination including appropriate skin testings.[1,104]

Only gloves with European conformity (CE) markings should be used at work, at least in the countries of the European Union. Since July 1, 1995, only PPE with CE markings can be distributed inside the European Economic Area. This mark guarantees that the product fulfills the essential requirements of directive 89/686/EEC. It also implies that all PPE (categories II to III), except those that are meant against minimal risk only (category I), must be type-examined by a notified body before the CE mark can be affixed on the PPE. The Department of Physics at the FIOH is such a notified body. The user of the PPE is also entitled to receive information about the PPE, its classification as a PPE, and about the standardized tests it has passed, from the distributor of the PPE. This is especially important because glove packages no longer need to contain information on the glove material. Directive 89/656/EEC, however, obligates employers to make risk assessments and to define the suitability of gloves for each job, as well as to organize a system of glove maintenance and training for glove users.[4,5,105] There should, for example, be a specific place at every worksite where gloves can be left without any risk of becoming soiled or mechanically damaged.[107]

Persons allergic to rubber should use gloves made of plastic materials unless the sensitizers and the chemicals used in the manufacture of the alternative rubber material are known. Disposable rubber gloves free from thiuram accelerators are available on the market (see Chapter 16). Especially NRL gloves (of industrial or household types) are best suited for occasional use. Inner cotton or inner disposable PVC or PE gloves are recommended to be used with rubber gloves because the inner gloves increase the protection of gloves and decrease the risk of sensitization.[1,3,4,108] In addition, the material of at least disposable NRL gloves should be of low protein content.[109] Manufacturers and shops specified to distribute PPE, including gloves, can help sensitized persons to select suitable gloves. In some cases of rubber allergy, gloves made of synthetic rubber can be used with separate inner textile gloves, when exact information about the glove material is not known.

Separate textile gloves should always be worn under unlined gloves made of polymers when there are symptoms of skin irritation or dermatitis of the hands, or the hands sweat profusely. Inner gloves should be made of soft materials, e.g., cotton, viscose, polyamide, or wool. A moisturizer used underneath an occlusive glove may decrease irritation from exposure to detergent followed by the prolonged wearing of gloves, especially in some occupational settings including dentists and surgeons. A moisturizer used inside a glove may either protect against or facilitate transportation of allergens and irritants.[110] A moisturizer or protective cream may even increase the transfer of protein allergens.[111] In another study, an increase in allergic reactions was described in a group using a protective cream before donning gloves, but the difference was not statistically significant compared to those not using the cream.[112] On the other hand, a study indicated that applying a skin protection cream before donning gloves with a high content of latex protein decreased the frequency of positive skin responses in a wearing test from 47% to 30% in subjects reporting type I allergy to NRL gloves.[113] In our opinion, barrier creams should not be used under household or industrial NRL gloves. An industrial worker with initially healthy hands developed hand dermatitis from the production of plastic boats in 1 month after using a foamy barrier cream under his rubber gloves. At the FIOH on patch testing, he was positive for his glove material, three thiurams, a dithiocarbamate, and methyl dibromoglutaronitrile (probably from Euxyl K 400 used in the barrier foam).[114] The case suggests that skin protection creams may in some cases promote the uptake of allergens from the gloves, thus increasing the development of allergy to the glove material, and at the same time, the occlusive effect of the glove may also promote sensitization to ingredients of the creams.

An experimental study discovered that the use of alcoholic disinfectant prior to polyisoprene glove donning increased the amount of DPG recovered from the hands.[115] The study compared the amount of DPG left on hands after wearing gloves for 60 minutes between hands exposed and not exposed to alcohol disinfectant. The use of alcoholic disinfectant prior to polyisoprene glove donning increased the amount of DPG recovered from the hands. Of the DPG released from polyisoprene gloves into artificial sweat, almost 84% was released within 10 minutes.[115] The use of alcoholic disinfectant increased skin exposure to the rubber accelerator DPG, even within a short duration of time. DPG release was higher from investigated polyisoprene gloves than from nitrile gloves. The inside of these gloves released more DPG than the outside, which was suggested to be related to CPC, an antimicrobial agent in the coating of the inside of the polyisoprene glove.[41]

REFERENCES

1. Estlander, T., and Jolanki, R. 1988. How to protect the hands. *Dermatol Clin* 6:105.
2. Estlander, T. 1990. Occupational skin disease in Finland. Observations made during 1974 to 1988 at the Institute of Occupational Health, Helsinki. *Acta Derm Venereol* Suppl. 155:1–85.
3. Estlander, T., Jolanki, R., and Kanerva, L. 1994. Allergic contact dermatitis from rubber and plastic gloves, in *Protective Gloves for Occupational Use*, Mellström, G.A., Wahlberg, J.E., and Maibach, H.I., Eds. Boca Raton, FL: CRC Press, 221.
4. Estlander, T., Jolanki, R., and Kanerva, L. 1996. Rubber glove dermatitis: A significant occupational hazard prevention, in *Prevention of Contact Dermatitis*, Eisner, P., Lachapelle, J.M., Wahlberg, J.E., and Maibach, H.I., Eds. Basel: Karger, 170.

5. Estlander, T., Jolanki, R., and Kanerva, L. 2000. Disadvantages of gloves, in *Handbook of Occupational Dermatology*, Kanerva, L., Eisner, P., Wahlberg, J.E., and Maibach, H.I., Eds. Berlin: Springer, 426.

6. Wattanakrai, P., Miamoto, L., and Taylor, J.S. 2000. Occupational pigmentary disorders, in *Handbook of Occupational Dermatology*, Kanerva, L., Eisner, P., Wahlberg, J.E., and Maibach, H.I., Eds. Berlin: Springer, 280.

7. Nettis, E., Colanardi, M.C., Ferrannini, A., and Tursi, A. 2001. Sensitivity to rubber additives. *Allergy* 56:1018.

8. Estlander, T., Kanerva, L., and Jolanki, R. 1995. Rubber additive sensitization from synthetic rubber gloves and boots. *Allergologie* 18:470.

9. Kanerva, L., Estlander, T., and Jolanki, R. 1994. Occupational allergic contact dermatitis caused by thiourea compounds. *Contact Dermatitis* 31:242.

10. Brehler, R. 1996. Contact urticaria caused by latex-free nitrile gloves. *Contact Dermatitis* 34:296.

11. Heese, A., Peters, K.-P., and Hornstein, O.P. 1992. Anaphylactic reaction to unexpected latex in polychloroprene gloves. *Contact Dermatitis* 27:336.

12. Kwangsuktith, C.H., and Maibach, H.I. 1995. Contact urticaria from polyurethane-membrane hypoallergenic gloves. *Contact Dermatitis* 33:200.

13. Heilman, D.K., Jones, R.T., Swanson, M.C., and Yunginger, J.W. 1996. Prospective, controlled study showing that rubber gloves are the major contributor to latex aeroallergen levels in the operating room. *J Allergy Clin Immunol* 98:325.

14. Palosuo, T., Mäkinen-Kiljunen, S., Alenius, H., Reunala, T., Yip, E., and Turjanmaa, K. 1998. Measurement of natural rubber latex allergen levels in medical gloves by allergen specific IgE-ELISA inhibition, RAST inhibition, and skin prick test. *Allergy* 53:59.

15. Sugiura, K., Sugiura, M., Hayakawa, R., Shamoto, M., and Sasaki, K. 2000. Di(2-ethylhexyl)phthalate (DOP) in vinyl-chloride slip-guard of cotton gloves caused contact urticaria syndrome. *Environ Dermatol* 7:211.

16. Sugiura, K., Sugiura, M., Shiraki, R., Hayakawa, R., Shamoto, M., Sasaki, K., and Itoh, A. 2002. Contact urticaria due to polyethylene gloves. *Contact Dermatitis* 46:262.

17. Conde-Salazar, L., del-Río, E., Guimaraens, D., and González Domingo, A. 1993. Type IV allergy to rubber additives. A 10-year study of 686 cases. *J Am Acad Dermatol* 29:176.

18. Fuchs, T. 1995. *Gummi und Allergie*. Munich: Dustri.

19. Heese, A., Peters, K.-P., and Koch, H.U. 1995. Allergien gegen Latexhandschuhe. *Allergologie* 18:358.

20. de Groot, A., de Jong, N.W., Duijster, E., Gerth van Wijk, R., Vermeulen, A., van Toorenenbergen, A.W., Geursen, L., and van Joost, T. 1998. Prevalence of natural rubber latex allergy (type I and type IV) in laboratory workers in the Netherlands. *Contact Dermatitis* 38:159.

21. Heese, A., van Hintzenstern, J., Peters, K.P., Koch, H.U., and Hornstein, O.P. 1991. Allergic and irritant reactions to rubber gloves in medical health services. Spectrum, diagnostic approach, and therapy. *J Am Acad Dermatol* 25:831.

22. Wrangsjö, K., and Meding, B. 1994. Occupational allergy to rubber chemicals. A follow-up study. *Dermatosen* 42:184.

23. Romaguera, C., and Grimalt, F. 1980. Statistical and comparative study of 4600 patients tested in Barcelona (1973–1977). *Contact Dermatitis* 6:309.

24. Themido, R., and Menezes-Brandao, F. 1984. Contact allergy to thiurams. *Contact Dermatitis* 10:251.

25. Estlander, T., and Jolanki, R. 2003. Ammatti-ihotaudit ja sukupuoli [Occupational dermatoses and gender], in *Sukupuoli ja Terveys* [Gender and Health], Luoto, R., Viisainen, K., and Kulmala, K., Eds. Tampere: Vastapaino, 84.

26. Jolanki, R., Savela, A., Estlander, T., and Kanerva, L. 2001. Ihotaudit ammattitau-titilastojen mukaan [Skin diseases according to the occupational disease statistics]. *Työterveyslääkäri* 1:10.
27. Turjanmaa, K. 1994. Contact urticaria from latex gloves, in *Protective Gloves for Occupational Use*, Mellström, G.A., Wahlberg, J.E., and Maibach, H.I., Eds. Boca Raton, FL: CRC Press, 241.
28. Field, E.A. 1998. Atopy and other risk factors for UK dentists reporting an adverse reaction to latex gloves. *Contact Dermatitis* 38:132.
29. Jolanki, R., Savela, A., Estlander, T., and Kanerva, L. 1998. Ammatti-ihotautien aiheuttajat Suomessa 1990–96 [Causes of occupational skin diseases in Finland 1990–96]. *Suomen Lääkärilehti* [*Finnish Med. J.*] 53:409.
30. Jolanki, R., Estlander, T., Alanko, K., Savela, A., and Kanerva, L. 1998. Occupational contact urticaria or protein contact dermatitis from natural rubber latex by occupation. *JEADV* 1(Suppl. 2):207.
31. Alanko, K., Susitaival, P., Jolanki, R., and Kanerva, L. 2000. Occupational dermatoses in dental nurses, and prevention. *Contact Dermatitis* 42(Suppl. 2):10.
32. Frosch, P.J., Bom, C.M., and Schütz, R. 1987. Kontaktallergien auf Gummi-, Operations- und Vinylhandschuhe. *Hautarzt* 38:210.
33. Estlander, T., Jolanki, R., and Kanerva, L. 1999. Occupational allergy to bisphenol A. *Contact Dermatitis* 40:52.
34. Aalto-Korte, K., Alanko, K., Henriks-Eckerman, M.-J., Estlander, T., and Jolanki, R. 2004. Allergic contact dermatitis from bisphenol A in PVC gloves. *Contact Dermatitis* 49:202.
35. Naruse, M., and Iwama, M. 1992. Dermatitis from household vinyl gloves. *Bull Environ Contam Toxicol* 48:843.
36. Geier, J., Lessmann, H., Uter, W., and Schnuch, A. 2003. Occupational rubber glove allergy: Results of the Information Network of Departments of Dermatology (IVDK), 1995–2001. *Contact Dermatitis* 48:39.
37. Gibbon, K.L., McFadden, J.P., Rycroft, R.J., Ross, J.S., Chinn, S., and White, I.R. 2001. Changing frequency of thiuram allergy in health care workers with hand dermatitis. *Br J Dermatol* 144:347.
38. Hansson, C., and Agrup, G. 1993. Stability of 2-mercaptopbenzothiazole (MBT). *Contact Dermatitis* 28:29.
39. Jung, J.H., McLaughlin, J.L., Stannard, J., and Guin, J.D. 1988. Isolation, via activity-directed fractionation, of mercaptobenzothiazole and dibenzothiazyl disulfide, two allergens responsible for tennis shoe dermatitis. *Contact Dermatitis* 19:254.
40. Knudsen, B.B., Hametner, C., Seycek, O., Heese, A., and Koch, H.-U. 2000. Bioavailability of rubber accelerators in rubber gloves and patch test reactivity. *Derm Beruf Umwelt* 48:127.
41. Hansen, A., Buse, A.S., Wilke, A., Skudlik, C., John, S.M., and Brans, R. 2020. Sensitization to 1,3-diphenylguanidine: An underestimated problem in physicians and nurses using surgical gloves? *Contact Dermatitis* 84:207–208. DOI: 10.1111/cod.13713.
42. Iijima, S., Numata, M., and Sasaki, K. 2020. Allergic contact dermatitis with nitrile rubber gloves. *Arerugi [Allergy]* 69(8):669–677. DOI: 10.15036/arerugi.69.669.
43. Cronin, E. 1980. *Contact Dermatitis*. Edinburgh: Churchill Livingstone.
44. Milcovic-Kraus, S. 1992. Glove powder as a contact allergen. *Contact Dermatitis* 26:198.
45. McCleskey, P.E., and Swerlick, R.A. 2001. Clinical review: Thioureas and allergic contact dermatitis. *Cutis* 68:387.
46. Dejonckheere, G., Herman, A., and Baeck, M. 2019. Allergic contact dermatitis caused by synthetic rubber gloves in healthcare workers: Sensitization to 1,3-diphenylguani-dine is common. *Contact Dermatitis* 81(3):167–173. DOI: 10.1111/cod.13269.

47. Dahlin, J., Bergendorff, O., Vindenes, H.K., Hindsén, M., and Svedman, C. 2014. Triphenylguanidine, a new (old?) rubber accelerator detected in surgical gloves that may cause allergic contact dermatitis. *Contact Dermatitis* 71(4):242–246. DOI: 10.1111/cod.12276.

48. Foussereau, J., Tomb, R., and Cavelier, C. 1990. Allergic dermatitis from safety clothes and individual protective devices. *Dermatol Clin* 8:127.

49. Rich, P., Belozer, M.L., Norris, P., and Storrs, F.J. 1991. Allergic contact dermatitis to two antioxidants in latex gloves: 4,4´- thiobis(6-tert-butyl-meta-cresol) (Lowinox 44S36) and butylhydroxyanisole. *J Am Acad Dermatol* 24:37.

50. Kanerva, L., Estlander, T., and Jolanki, R. 1996. Allergic patch test reactions caused by rubber chemical cyclohexyl thiophthalimide. *Contact Dermatitis* 34:23.

51. Geier, J., Lessmann, H., Frosch, P.J., and Schnuch, A. 2003. Contact sensitization to *N*-(cyclohexyl thio)phthalimide, results of a multicenter study of the Information Network of Departments of Dermatology (IVDK) and the German Contact Dermatitis Research Group (DKG). *Contact Dermatitis* 48:1.

52. Masmoudi, M.L., and Lachapelle, J.M. 1987. Occupational dermatitis to dihydroxy-diphenyl and diphenylthiourea in neoprene gloves. *Contact Dermatitis* 16:290.

53. Polano, M.K. 1958. Ekzem durch Gummihandsschuhe. *Dermatologica* 116:105.

54. Grier, J., and Schubert, S. 2021. *Frequency of Skin Sensitization to Specific Substances and in Specific Occupational Groups.* Dortmund, Germany: Federal Institute for Occupational Safety and Health. DOI: 10.21934/baua:bericht20210122.

55. Jolanki, R., Kanerva, L., and Estlander, T. 1987. Organic pigments in plastics can cause allergic contact eczema. *Acta Derm Venereol Suppl.* 134:95.

56. Castelain, M., and Castelain, P.-Y. 1993. Allergic contact dermatitis from cetyl pyridinium chloride in latex gloves. *Contact Dermatitis* 28:118.

57. Steinkjer, B. 1998. Contact dermatitis from cetyl pyridinium chloride in latex surgical gloves. *Contact Dermatitis* 39:29.

58. Lezaun, A., Marcos, C., Martín, J.A., Quirce, S., and Díez Gómez, M.L. 1992. Contact dermatitis from natural latex. *Contact Dermatitis* 27:334.

59. Wyss, M., Elsner, P., Wüthrich, B., and Burg, G. 1993. Allergic contact dermatitis from natural latex without contact urticaria. *Contact Dermatitis* 28:154.

60. Häffner, A.C., Zepter, K., Elsner, P., and Burg, G. 1996. Isolated delayed-type hyper-sensitivity to latex rubber. *Contact Dermatitis* 35:247.

61. Placucci, F., Vincenzi, C., Ghedini, G., Piana, G., and Tosti, A. 1996. Coexistence of type I and type IV allergy to rubber latex. *Contact Dermatitis* 34:76.

62. Wilkinson, S.M., and Beck, M.H. 1996. Allergic dermatitis from latex rubber. *Br J Dermatol* 134:910.

63. Sommer, S., Wilkinson, S.M., Beck, M.H., English, J.S., Gawkrodger, D.J., and Green, C. 2002. Type IV hypersensitivity reactions to natural rubber latex: Results of a multi-center study. *Br J Dermatol* 146:114.

64. Menezes Brandao, F. 1990. Rubber dermatitis, in *Occupational Skin Disease*, 2nd ed., Adams, R.M., Ed. Philadelphia, PA: W.B. Saunders, 462.

65. Sugiura, K., Sugiura, M., Hayakawa, R., Shamoto, M., and Sasaki, K. 2002. A case of contact urticaria syndrome due to di(2-ethylhexyl)phthalate (DOP) in work clothes. *Contact Dermatitis* 46:13.

66. Templeton, H.J. 1950. Contact dermatitis from plastic mittens. *Arch Dermatol Syph* 61:854.

67. Morris, G.E. 1953. Vinyl plastics. *Arch Ind Hyg Occup Med* 8:535.

68. Guillet, M.H., Menard, G., and Guillet, G. 1991. Sensibilisation de contact aux gants en vinyl. *Ann Dermatol Venereol* 118:723.

69. Krasteva, M., Chefai, M., Dupoy, M., and Chabeau, G. 1992. Vinyl glove intolerance, in *Book of Abstracts*, 1st ed. Brussels: Congr. Eur. Soc. Contact Dermatitis, 8–10 October 1992, 73.
70. Monma, S., and Tsunoda, T. 1999. Two cases of contact dermatitis to polyvinyl chloride gloves. *Environ Dermatol* 6(Suppl. 1):84.
71. Suuronen, K., Pesonen, M., Henriks-Eckerman, M.L., and Aalto-Korte, K. 2013. Triphenyl phosphite, a new allergen in polyvinylchloride gloves. *Contact Dermatitis* 68(1):42–49. DOI: 10.1111/j.1600-0536.2012.02159.x.
72. Fregert, S., and Rorsman, H. 1963. Hypersensitivity to epoxy resins used as plasticizers and stabilizers in polyvinylchloride (PVC) resins. *Acta Dermatol Venereol* 43:10.
73. Fregert, S., and Rorsman, H. 1964. Allergens in epoxy resin. *Acta Allergol* 19:296.
74. Estlander, T., and Jolanki, R. 2003. Unpublished data.
75. Ponting, D.J., Ortega, M.A., Niklasson, I.B., Karlsson, I., Seifert, T., Stéen, J., Luthman, K., and Karlberg, A.T. 2019. Development of new epoxy resin monomers - A delicate balance between skin allergy and polymerization properties. *Chem Res Toxicol* 32(1):57–66. DOI: 10.1021/acs.chemrestox.8b00169.
76. O'Boyle, N.M., Niklasson, I.B., Tehrani-Bagha, A.R., Delaine, T., Holmberg, K., Luthman, K., and Karlberg, A.T. 2014. Epoxy resin monomers with reduced skin sensitizing potency. *Chem Res Toxicol* 27(6):1002–1010. DOI: 10.1021/tx5000624.
77. Taylor, J.S. 1986. Rubber, in *Contact Dermatitis*, 3rd ed., Fisher, A.A., Ed. Philadelphia, PA: Lea & Febiger, 603.
78. Romita, P., Foti, C., Masciopinto, L., Nettis, E., Di Leo, E., Calogiuri, G., Bonamonte, D., Angelini, G., Dipalma, G., Ballini, A., and Inchingolo, F. 2017. Allergic contact dermatitis to acrylates. *J Biol Regul Homeost Agents* 31(2):529–534.
79. Mellström, G.A., and Boman, A. 2000. Protective gloves, in *Handbook of Occupational Dermatology*, Kanerva, L., Eisner, P., Wahlberg, J.E., and Maibach, H.I., Eds. Berlin: Springer, 417.
80. Knudsen, B.B., Larsen, E., Egsgaard, H., and Menné, T. 1993. Release of thiurams and carbamates from rubber gloves. *Contact Dermatitis* 28:63.
81. Lammintausta, K., and Kalimo, K. 1985. Sensitivity to rubber. A study with rubber mixes and individual rubber chemicals. *Dermatosen* 33:204.
82. Themido, R., and Menezes-Brandao, F. 1984. Contact allergy to thiurams. *Contact Dermatitis* 10:251.
83. Maso, M.J., and Goldberg, D.J. 1990. Contact dermatoses from disposable glove use: A review. *J Am Acad Dermatol* 23:733.
84. Jacobsen, N., Aasenden, R., and Hensten-Pettersen, A. 1991. Occupational health complaints and adverse reactions perceived by personnel in public dentistry. *Community Dent Oral Epidemiol* 19:155.
85. Tarvainen, K., Jolanki, R., Forsman-Grönholm, L., Estlander, T., Pfäffli, P., Juntunen, J., and Kanerva, L. 1993. Exposure, skin protection and occupational skin disease among workers in the glass fibre-reinforced plastics industry. *Contact Dermatitis* 29:119.
86. Tarvainen, K. 1996. Occupational dermatoses from plastic composites based on polyester resins, epoxy resins and vinyl ester resins (thesis). *People and Work Research Reports 11*. Helsinki: Finnish Institute of Occupational Health.
87. Conde-Salazar, L., Gatica, M.E., Barco, L., Iglesias, C., Cuevas, M., and Valks, R. 2002. Latex allergy among construction workers. *Contact Dermatitis* 47:154.
88. Estlander, T., Kilpikari, I., and Eskolin, E. 1980. Polymeerikäsineen läpäisevyys ja sen valmistuksessa käytettävät kemikaalit [Permeability of polymer gloves and chemicals used in the manufacture of gloves]. *Suomen Lääkärilehti [Finnish Med. J.]* 35:800.

89. Williams, J.R. 1979. Permeation of glove materials by physiologically harmful chemicals. *Am Ind Hyg Assoc J* 40:877.

90. Jordan, W.P., and Bourlas, M.C. 1975. Allergic contact dermatitis to underwear elastic, chemically transformed by a laundry bleach. *Arch Dermatol* 111:593.

91. Guin, J.D. 1992. The doctor's surgical/examination gloves — Problems with and without them. *Int J Dermatol* 31:853.

92. Pagliaro, J.A., and Jones, S.K. 1999. Recurrent erythrodermic psoriasis in thiuram-allergic patient due to contact with nurses' rubber gloves. *Br J Dermatol* 140:567.

93. Conde-Salazar, L. 1990. Rubber dermatitis, clinical forms. *Dermatol Clin* 8:49.

94. Lu, C.Y., and Sun, C.C. 2001. Localized erythema-multiforme-like contact dermatitis from rubber gloves. *Contact Dermatitis* 45:311.

95. Braze, M., Trulsson, L., and Bendsöe, N. 1992. Patch testing with ultrasonic bath extracts. *Am J Contact Dermatitis* 3:133.

96. Holness, D.L., and Nethercott, J.R. 1997. Results of patch testing with a special series of rubber allergens. *Contact Dermatitis* 36:207.

97. Geier, J., and Gefeller, O. 1995. Sensitivity of patch tests with rubber mixes: Results of the information network of departments of dermatology from 1990 to 1993. *Am J Contact Dermatitis* 6:143.

98. Warshaw, E.M., Gupta, R., Dekoven, J.G., Fowler, J.F. Jr, Silverberg, J.I., Atwater, A.R., Taylor, J.S., Reeder, M.J., Maibach, H.I., Sasseville, D., Belsito, D.V., DeLeo, V.A., Pratt, M.D., Marks, J.G. Jr, Zug, K.A., and Zirwas, M.J. 2020. Patch testing to diphenylguanidine by the North American Contact Dermatitis Group (2013–2016). *Dermatitis* 31(6):350–358. DOI: 10.1097/DER.0000000000000629.

99. Roberts, J.L., and Hanifin, J.M. 1980. Contact allergy and cross reactivity to substituted thiourea compounds. *Contact Dermatitis* 6:138.

100. Wilkinson, S.M., and Burd, R. 1998. Latex: A cause of allergic contact eczema in users of natural rubber gloves. *J Am Acad Dermatol* 38:36.

101. Estlander, T., Jolanki, R., and Kanerva, L. 1997. Occupational allergic contact dermatitis from 2,3-epoxypropyl trimethyl ammonium chloride (EPTMAC) and Kathon LX in starch modification factory. *Contact Dermatitis* 36:191.

102. Estlander, T., Jolanki, R., and Kanerva, L. 2002. Protective gloves, in *Hand Eczema*, 2nd ed., Menné, T., and Maibach, H.I., Eds. Boca Raton, FL: CRC Press, 310.

103. Knudsen, B.B., and Turjanmaa, K. 2002. Hand eczema from rubber gloves, in *Hand Eczema*, 2nd ed., Menné, T., and Maibach, H.I., Eds. Boca Raton, FL: CRC Press, 275.

104. Agner, T., and Held, E. 2002. Skin protection programmes. *Contact Dermatitis* 46:253.

105. Mellström, G.A., and Boman, A.S. 1997. Protective gloves: Test results compiled in a database, in *The Work Place*, Vol. 1, Brune, D., Gerhardsson, G., Crockford, G.W., and D'Auria, D., Eds., Fundamentals of Health, Safety and Welfare, International Occupational Safety and Health Information Centre (CIS). Geneva: International Labour Office and Oslo: Scandinavian Science Publisher, 716.

106. Henry, N.W., III. 1994. Protective gloves for occupational use — U.S. rules, regulations and standards, in *Protective Gloves for Occupational Use*, Mellström, G.A., Wahlberg, J.E., and Maibach, H.I., Eds. Boca Raton, FL: CRC Press, 45.

107. Rycroft, R.J.G. 1986. Environmental factors of occupational dermatology. *Dermatosen* 34:157.

108. Mäkelä, E., Mäkelä, E.A., Väänänen, V., Alanko, K., Jolanki, R., Estlander, T., and Kanerva, L. 1999. Resistance of disposable gloves to permeation by 2-hydroxyethyl methacrylate and triethyleneglycol dimethacrylate. *J Occup Hygiene* 5:121.

109. Palosuo, T. 1997. Latex allergens. *Rev Fr Allergol* 37:1184.

110. Held, E., Mygind, K., Wolff, C., Gyntelberg, F., and Agner, T. 2002. Prevention of work related skin problems: An intervention study in wet work employees. *Occupational and Environmental Medicine* 59:556–561.
111. Beezhold, D.H., Kostyal, D.A., and Wieman, J. 1994. The transfer of protein allergens from latex gloves. A study of influencing factors. *AORN J* 59:605.
112. Baur, X., Chen, Z., Allmers, H., and Raulf-Heimsoth, M. 1998. Results of wearing test with two different latex gloves with and without skin protection cream. *Allergy* 53:441.
113. Allmers, H. 2001. Wearing test with 2 different types of latex gloves with and without the use of skin protection cream. *Contact Dermatitis* 4:30.
114. Estlander, T., and Jolanki, R. 2003. Unpublished data.
115. Hamnerius, N., Pontén, A., Björk, J., Persson, C., and Bergendorff, O. 2019. Skin exposure to the rubber accelerator diphenylguanidine in medical gloves-An experimental study. *Contact Dermatitis* 81(1):9–16. DOI: 10.1111/cod.13238.

GENERAL READING

Baran, R.L., and Maibach, H.I. 2017. Textbook of Cosmetic Dermatology (5th ed.). Boca Raton, FL: CRC Press, Taylor & Francis Group.
Bronaugh, R.L., and Maibach, H.I. 2002. Topical Absorption of Dermatological Products. Hoboken, NJ: CRC Press.
Chew, A., and Maibach, H.I. 2010. Irritant Dermatitis. Berlin: Springer.
Gimenez-Arnau, A.M., and Maibach, H.I. (Eds.). 2019. *Contact Urticaria Syndrome*. Cham, Switzerland: Springer.
Wilhelm, K., Zhai, H., and Maibach, H.I. 2012. Dermatotoxicology (8th ed). London: Informa Healthcare.

15 Clinical Testing of Occupational Glove Sensitivity

K.F. Mose and R. Bach

CONTENTS

15.1 INTRODUCTION

Occupational contact allergy/contact urticaria caused by gloves is prevalent in certain industries and occupations such as the construction industry, the mechanical industries, cleaning, housekeeping, hairdressing, and in particular the healthcare professions.[1] Protective gloves are used for preventing skin contact and also often to hinder aggravating exposure of damaged or inflamed skin, to a plethora of potentially allergenic and irritant substances. However, frequent use of gloves in itself may also contribute to the impairment of the skin barrier with increased penetration of irritants and subsequent development of irritant contact dermatitis,[2] in addition to exposure to glove allergens. Moreover, individuals with a history of atopy, and particularly those suffering from hand dermatitis, are liable to develop adverse reactions to gloves.[3,4] That gloves can cause intolerance reactions even in those not wearing them became particularly apparent with the contact urticaria syndrome caused by latex, but this may also occur with contact dermatitis.

In general, allergic reactions due to gloves are either contact dermatitis reactions (type IV), which may be exceptionally present with clinical features such as erythema multiforme,[5–7] leukoderma,[8] psoriasis köbnerizing contact dermatitis,[9] or contact urticaria reactions (type I); rubber gloves are much more often reported to be causes of contact allergic reactions than are plastic or leather gloves.[10–12] A wide range of different types of gloves based on material, e.g. latex, nitrile, neoprene, polyvinyl chloride (PVC), leather, and textile just to name a few, are commercially available. An attempt to list the numerous chemical components of these various glove types has been compiled in recent years.[13]

DOI: 10.1201/9781003126874-18

The allergens responsible for contact dermatitis to rubber gloves are generally chemicals added to or used during the glove manufacturing process. These include vulcanizing agents, accelerators, and antioxidants. Rubber accelerators constitute the major class of chemicals giving rise to glove allergy in patients. Among the group of accelerators, thiurams and carbamates are the most common glove allergens.[14] Other causal agents have also been reported: starch;[15] indeed, chemicals such as epichlorohydrin, sorbic acid, and even isothiazolinone derivatives may be present in such powders;[16] cetyl pyridinium chloride present on a glove's surface;[17,18] latex protein,[19,20] although an additive already present in the latex, may not always be ruled out as the causal factor;[21] and even a bacterial endotoxin in gamma radiation-treated gloves[22] and residual ethylene oxide.[23] In plastic gloves, different plasticizers, e.g. adipic polyesters in PVC gloves, are added to the plastic to either harden or soften them, and it has been documented that such compounds can cause allergic contact dermatitis.[24,25] Further, the addition of coloring agents (organic pigments), antioxidants (Bisphenol A), and different antimicrobials (formaldehyde and 1,2-benzisothiazolinone) during the production of plastic gloves have been reported to cause reactions,[26-31] while in leather gloves, chromium salts are the main sensitizers.[32,33]

Contact urticarial reactions and protein contact dermatitis are most often due to various raw foods and natural rubber latex (NRL) proteins (a polyurethane membrane offering no protection against the latter).[34,35] However, several authors have also considered cornstarch[36-41] (although it is mostly contaminated with latex protein) and certain rubber additives[16,42,43] to be the causal agents in the contact urticaria syndrome. Further, some authors reported on contact urticaria to nonrubber gloves as well, i.e. morpholinyl mercaptobenzothiazole in nitrile[44] and di-(2-ethylhexyl) phthalate in PVC gloves,[45] as well as to polyethylene gloves.[46] Urticarial reactions to chemicals need to be differentiated from dermographism.[47,48]

15.2 CONTACT URTICARIA FROM LATEX RUBBER

Over 10 years from January 2010 through December 2020, 2851 patients were tested for latex allergy at the Dept. of Dermatology, Odense University Hospital, Denmark, with prick test and/or RAST test (radio allergo-sorbent test), of which 277 patients with hand dermatitis were tested based on known exposure to latex products, including gloves, in the occupational setting. Six patients (~2.2%) of this workforce were diagnosed as suffering from contact urticarial reactions to latex. The occupations involved were healthcare professionals, cleaners, and kitchen workers. At first glance, this number appears very small. However, the prevalence rate of sensitization to latex among healthcare workers has been estimated between 2.7% and 11.4%, which is considerably higher compared to the estimates of between 1% and 1.37% for the general population.[49-51] Data on the prevalence of clinical NRL allergy in the general population suggest that latex allergy is on the decline.[52] The high prevalence among healthcare workers reflects the much higher degree of skin exposure to latex, in addition to inhalation of latex protein-coated glove powder.[51] Powder inhalation is also the main source of exposure to latex among workers in the latex production industry (i.e. another high-risk profession), resulting in respiratory symptoms, skin manifestations, eye irritation, and abnormal pulmonary function tests. But in contrast to healthcare workers, very few (between 0% and 1.5%) of the workers in the latex production industry developed a positive skin prick test reaction to latex extract.[53]

Due to the small number of patients suffering from occupational contact urticarial reactions to latex in our clinic, further profiling of this group of patients will not contribute to the overall understanding of associated conditions to latex allergy, including concomitant contact allergies, potentially accompanying extracutaneous symptoms, and fruit allergies. However, these pieces of information are highly relevant because awareness of these additional symptoms followed by proper diagnosis may contribute to an increased patient quality of life through avoidance and/or treatment. These aspects are therefore briefly outlined in the following:

- *Concomitant contact allergy*: A combined contact urticaria syndrome to latex and allergic contact dermatitis to rubber additives has been reported.[54,55]
- *Extracutaneous symptoms*: Rhinitis, conjunctivitis, and asthma are associated with latex allergy. Latex sensitized individuals may upon exposure to aerosolized latex proteins experience ocular itching and respiratory symptoms, including nasal congestion, sneezing, and rhinorrhea. Latex aeroallergen exposure can trigger asthma exacerbation with chest tightness, wheezing, coughing, and dyspnea.
- *Associated fruit allergies*: Latex allergy is associated with an allergy to fruit. It predominates in atopic individuals. Crossreactivity between latex and banana, avocado, chestnut, and kiwi fruit has been demonstrated. Some of the proteins in latex that cause latex allergy are also present in these fruits.[56–58]

All of our patients diagnosed as having latex sensitivity were administered prick tests with commercial latex glove extracts, which is the most appropriate method.[59] Specific IgEs were not sought in all patients; from the literature, we know that they cannot be found in all latex-sensitive subjects as diagnosed by prick testing[59–62] (see Ebo and Stevens[63] for a review on the subject).

15.3   ALLERGIC CONTACT DERMATITIS

From January 2010 through December 2020, 5414 patients were examined in our Contact Allergy Unit. The MOAHLFA-index percentages are as follows:

- Males: 34%
- Occupational dermatitis: 21%
- Atopy: 21%
- Hand dermatitis: 50%
- Leg ulcers/stasis dermatitis: 5%
- Facial dermatitis: 32%
- Age > 40 years: 60%

TABLE 15.1

The Distribution of Rubber Mix Allergens Found in 67 Cases of Occupational Contact Dermatitis

1.	Tetraethylthiuram disulphide (TETD)	35
2.	Tetramethylthiuram monosulphide (TMTM)	27
3.	Tetramethylthiuram disulphide (TMTD)	18
4.	Dipentamethylenthiuram disulfide	17
5.	Carba mix	10
6.	Diethyldithiocarbamate, Zinc	9
7.	1,3-Diphenylguanidine (DPG)	8
8.	Morpholinylmercaptobenzothiazole	6
9.	N-Cyclohexylbenzothiazyl sulphenamide	5
10.	Mercaptobenzothiazole (MBT)	5
11.	Cyclohexylthiophtalimide	4
12.	Dibenzothiazyl disulfide	4
13.	4,4-Diaminodiphenylmethane (MDA)	3
14.	Methenamine	1
15.	Zinc dibutyldithiocarbamate	1
16.	Diethylthio urea	1

Of them, 3152 (~58.2%) showed at least one positive patch test reaction, and 67 (1.2% of the total patient population tested) presented with clear glove-related, occupation-induced allergic contact dermatitis. Data on occupational allergic contact dermatitis to the three main groups of glove accelerators/rubber mix allergens (thiuram, carba, and mercapto compounds) among these 67 patients are shown in Table 15.1.

The mean age of these patients was 43 years; 45 (67.2%) were female and 22 (32.8%) were male. The occupations concerned are listed in Table 15.2.

Constituents of the thiuram mix were the most frequent positive rubber mix allergens observed in this patient population suffering from occupational glove allergy and are most often related to housework and the medical and paramedical professions. This is in agreement with the results of other studies (von Hintzenstern et al.[3] and Lammintausta and Kalimo[4]). Although thiuram mix and carba mix are most often associated,[64] the latter can be found without thiuram sensitivity.[65] In contrast to thiurams and carbamates, mercapto compounds can also be found in a wide variety of nonrubber products.[66] However, contact allergy to mercapto compounds is relatively uncommon, and an overall decline in the number of cases of allergic contact dermatitis caused by mercapto mix and mercaptobenzothiazole has been reported.[67-69] From our data, it is evident that the prevalence of occupational contact allergy to mercapto compounds among our group of patients is low compared to carba and thiuram contact allergy.

Twenty years ago, a newcomer in rubber-glove allergy N-(cyclohexylthio) phthalimide was reported. It was identified as a potential allergen in rubber

TABLE 15.2

Occupations Involved in Contact Allergy to Glove Dermatitis (N = 67)[a]

1.	Cleaning/kitchen work	15
2.	Nurses	7
3.	Agriculture/farming	6
4.	Construction worker	5
5.	Store employee	3
	Chiropractor/physiotherapist	3
	Metalwork/industrial painters/welder	3
	Production technician	3
6.	Veterinarian	2
	Midwife	2
	Social and health assistant	2
	Kindergarten teacher	2
	Painter	2
	Physician	2
7.	Florist	1
	Tattoo artist	1
	Home helper	1
	Cab driver	1
	Plastic worker	1
	Cafe owner	1
	Speech therapist	1
	Occupational therapist/healer	1
	Upholsterer	1
	Cosmetics, soap industry	1

[a] Some may, in addition to their job, perform household work.

materials including gloves,[70,71] albeit in contradiction to the information obtained from the manufacturers.[72] Although not the most prevalent rubber chemical in gloves in our occupational patient population, some reactions were found in healthcare professionals.

Of course, patients may also become sensitized upon contact with rubber gloves worn by medical professionals.[73]

15.4   PENETRATION OF CHEMICALS THROUGH GLOVES

Gloves do not always prevent contact dermatitis to the chemicals handled.[74] Indeed, glove-related dermatitis can also be caused by various chemicals penetrating through the gloves.[75] Examples are methylisothiazolinone (MI), [76] plant allergens,[77] para-phenylenediamine (PPD),[78] and glutaraldehyde.[79]

The chemicals found to be causes of occupational allergic contact dermatitis,[80] in relation to their penetration through gloves, are acrylate compounds in dental professionals,[81] ammonium thioglycolate in hairdressers,[82] acrylamide in a laboratory technician,[83] and an epoxysilane compound[84] in a patient who compounded polyurethane and silicone resins.

15.5   CONCLUSIONS

Analyses of our occupational data show that the prevalence of latex allergy among our occupational patient population is somewhat lower compared with the literature data on contact urticaria syndrome. Our data on occupational allergic contact dermatitis to thiurams as being the most prevalent cause of an allergy to gloves show concordance with the literature.

Obviously, a significant number of glove-related occupationally induced cases of contact urticaria and contact dermatitis could be substantially reduced if the presence of important allergens could be reduced or eliminated. This is particularly important as patients with glove dermatitis are predominantly young. For proteins, washing the gloves after molding, before they are dried, and steam sterilization, may decrease or even suppress immediate-type allergenicity.[85] With regard to additives such as thiuram derivatives and carbamates, the release of which can be measured, their presence should also be reduced to a minimum and, perhaps, even be restricted by law.[86] For people allergic to glove materials, allergen alternatives are available,[16,87,88] although apparently the labels placed on gloves cannot always be relied upon.[87] The glove manufacturing industry has through the years developed new glove manufacturing processes, e.g. low-protein natural rubber gloves, vulcanization accelerator-free gloves, and specific-purpose gloves containing antimicrobial agents and moisturizers.[89] Switching from conventional medical single-use rubber gloves to accelerator-free rubber gloves improves occupational hand eczema, and some patients may even become completely free of symptoms.[90]

When chemicals penetrate the gloves, the risk of sensitization, of course, is increased because of the occlusion effect. This belies the sense of security patients feel when they wear "protective" gloves. Hence, information about penetration rates and the development of suitably safe products are necessary for people who work with hazardous chemicals. Therefore, the risks should be analyzed, and the appropriate gloves should be selected.[91]

Guidance for patients with glove allergy is freely available through several websites providing information on allergens found in gloves and advisory information on the choice of gloves in relation to occupation. Different glove materials have been shown to provide varying degrees of protection to specific irritants and allergens.[75, 92, 93] Moreover, glove manufacturers have been making efforts to respond to specific requirements, improve the glove quality,[94] and provide information on the chemical agents used,[95] as well as on the specific allergens present in the gloves on the market.[96, 97]

REFERENCES

1. Fisher, A.A. 1991. Management of allergic contact dermatitis due to rubber gloves. *Cutis* 47:301.
2. Zhai, H., and Maibach, H.I. 2001. Skin occlusion and irritant and allergic contact dermatitis: An overview. *Contact Dermatitis* 44:201.
3. von Hintzenstern, J., Heese, A., Koch, H.U., Peters, K.P., and Hornstein, O.P. 1991. Frequency, spectrum and occupational relevance of type 4 allergens to rubber chemicals. *Contact Dermatitis* 24:244.
4. Lammintausta, K., and Kalimo, K. 1985. Sensitivity to rubber. Study with rubber mixes and individual rubber chemicals. *Dermatosen* 33:204.
5. Bourrain, J.L., Woodward, C., Dumas, V., et al. 1996. Natural rubber latex contact dermatitis with features of erythema multiforme. *Contact Dermatitis* 35:55.
6. Lu, C.-Y., and Sun, C.-C. 2001. Localized erythema-multiforme-like contact dermatitis from rubber gloves. *Contact Dermatitis* 45:311.
7. Leis-Dosil, V.M., Campos-Domínguez, M., Zamberk-Majlis, P.E., Suárez-Fernández, R.M., and Lázaro-Ochaita, P. 2006. Erythema multiforme-like eruption due to carbamates and thiurams. *Allergol Immunopathol* 34:121.
8. Taylor, J.S., Norris, M.J., and Evey, P. 2000. Contact leukoderma from industrial and surgical rubber gloves. *Contact Dermatitis* 42:64.
9. Hill, V.A., and Ostlere, L.S. 1998. Psoriasis of the hands köbnerizing in contact dermatitis. *Contact Dermatitis* 39:194.
10. Estlander, T., Jolanki, R., and Kanerva, L. 1986. Dermatitis and urticaria from rubber and plastic gloves. *Contact Dermatitis* 14:20.
11. Frosch, P.J., Bom, C.M., and Schütz, R. 1987. Kontaktallergien auf gummi-, operations, und vinylhandschuhe. *Hautarzt* 38:210.
12. Guillet, M.H., Menard, N., and Guillet, G. 1991. Sensibilisation de contact aux gants en vinyl. A propos d'un cas de polysensibilisation aux gants médicaux. *Ann Dermatol Vénéreol* 118:723.
13. Rose, R.F., Lyons, P., Horne, H., and Wilkinson, S.M. 2009. A review of the materials and allergens in protective gloves. *Contact Dermatitis* 61:129.
14. Geier J., Lessmann, H., Ute, W., and Schnuch, A. 2003. Occupational rubber glove allergy: Results of the Information Network of Departments of Dermatology (IVDK), 1995–2001. *Contact Dermatitis* 48:39.
15. Milkovic-Kraus, S. 1992. Glove powder as a contact allergen. *Contact Dermatitis* 26:198.
16. Heese, A., von Hintzenstern, J., Peters, K.-P., Koch, H.U., and Hornstein, O.P. 1991. Allergic and irritant reactions to rubber gloves in medical health services: Spectrum, diagnostic approach, and therapy. *J Am Acad Dermatol* 25:831.
17. Castelain, M., and Castelain, P.-Y. 1993. Allergic contact dermatitis from cetyl pyridinium chloride in latex gloves. *Contact Dermatitis* 28:118.
18. Steinkjer, B. 1998. Contact dermatitis from cetyl pyridinium chloride in latex surgical gloves. *Contact Dermatitis* 39:29.
19. Wyss, M., Eisner, P., Wüthrich, B., and Burg, G. 1992. Allergic contact dermatitis to natural latex. *J Am Acad Dermatol* 27(4):650.
20. Wilkinson, S.M., and Burd, R. 1998. Latex: A cause of allergic contact eczema in users of natural rubber gloves. *J Am Acad Dermatol* 38:36.
21. Heese, A. 1992. Allergic contact dermatitis to natural latex. *J Am Acad Dermatol* 27(4):651.
22. Shmunes, E., and Darby, T. 1984. Contact dermatitis due to endotoxin in irradiated latex gloves. *Contact Dermatitis* 10:240.

23. Royce, A., and Moore, K.S. 1955. Occupational dermatitis caused by ethylene oxide. *Br J Ind Med* 12:169.
24. Sowa, J., Kobayashi, H., Tsuruta, D., Sugawara, K., and Ishii, M. 2005. Allergic contact dermatitis due to adipic polyester in vinyl chloride gloves. *Contact Dermatitis* 53:243.
25. Ueno, M., Adachi, A., Horikawa, T., Inoue, N., Mori, A., and Sasaki, K. 2007. Allergic contact dermatitis caused by poly(adipic acid-co–1,2-propylene glycol) and di-(n-octyl) tin-bis(2-ethylhexylmaleate) in vinyl chloride gloves. *Contact Dermatitis* 57:349.
26. Matthieu, L., Godoi, A.F.L., Lambert, J., and van Grieken, R. 2004. Occupational allergic contact dermatitis from bisphenol A in vinyl gloves. *Contact Dermatitis* 49:281.
27. Aalto-Korte, K., Alanko, K., Henriks-Eckerman, M.L., Estlander, T., and Jolanki, R. 2003. Allergic contact dermatitis from bisphenol A in PVC gloves. *Contact Dermatitis* 49:202.
28. Aalto-Korte, K., Ackermann, L., Henriks-Eckerman, M.L., Välimaa, J., Reinikka-Railo, H., Leppänen, E., and Jolanki, R. 2007. 1,2-Benzisothiazolin–3-one in disposable polyvinyl chloride gloves for medical use. *Contact Dermatitis* 57:365.
29. Aalto-Korte, K., Alanko, K., Henriks-Eckerman, M.L., and Jolanki, R. 2006. Antimicrobial allergy from polyvinyl chloride gloves. *Arch Dermatol* 142:1326.
30. Ponten, A. 2006. Formaldehyde in reusable protective gloves. *Contact Dermatitis* 54:268.
31. Jolanki, R., Kanerva, L., and Estlander, T. 1987. Organic pigments in plastic can cause allergic contact dermatitis. *Acta Derm Venereol* 134:95.
32. Fregert, S., and Gruvberger, B. 1979. Chromium in industrial leather gloves. *Contact Dermatitis* 5:189.
33. Hansen, M.B., Rydin, S., Menne, T., and Johansen, J.D. 2002. Quantitative aspects of contact allergy to chromium and exposure to chrome-tanned leather. *Contact Dermatitis* 47:127.
34. Pesonen, M., Koskela, K., and Aalto-Korte, K. 2020. Contact urticaria and protein contact dermatitis in the Finnish register of occupational diseases in a period of 12 years. *Contact Dermatitis* 83:1.
35. Kwangsukstith, C., and Maibach, H.I. 1995. Contact urticaria from polyurethane-membrane hypoallergenic gloves. *Contact Dermatitis* 33:200.
36. van der Meeren, H.L.M., and van Erp, P.E.J. 1986. Life-threatening contact urticaria from glove powder. *Contact Dermatitis* 14:190.
37. Fisher, A.A. 1986. Contact urticaria due to cornstarch surgical glove powder. *Cutis* 38(5):307.
38. Assalve, D., Cicioni, C., Perno, P., and Lisi, P. 1988. Contact urticaria and anaphylactoid reaction from cornstarch surgical glove powder. *Contact Dermatitis* 19:61.
39. Liu, W., and Nixon, R.L. 2007. Corn contact urticaria in a nurse. *Australas J Dermatol* 48:130.
40. Fisher, A.A. 1987. Contact urticaria and anaphylactoid reaction due to corn starch surgical glove powder. *Contact Dermatitis* 16:224.
41. Crippa, M., and Pasolini, G. 1997. Allergic reactions due to glove-lubricant-powder in health care workers. *Int Arch Occup Environ Health* 70:399.
42. Geier, J., and Fuchs, T. 1990. Kontakturtikaria durch Gummihandschuhe. *Z Hautkr* 65(3):267.
43. Wrangsjö, K., Mellström, G., and Axelsson, G. 1986. Discomfort from rubber gloves indicating contact urticaria. *Contact Dermatitis* 15:79.
44. Brehler, R. 1996. Contact urticaria caused by latex-free nitrile gloves. *Contact Dermatitis* 34:296.

45. Sugiura, K., Sugiura, M., Hayakawa, R., and Sasaki, K. 2000. Di(2-ethylhexyl)phtalate (DOP) in the dotted polyvinyl-chloride grip of cotton gloves as a cause of contact urticaria syndrome. *Contact Dermatitis* 43:237.
46. Sugiura, K., Sigiura, M., Shiraki, R., Hayakawa, R., Shamoto, M., Sasaki, K., and Itoh, A. 2002. Contact urticaria due to polyethylene gloves. *Contact Dermatitis* 46:262.
47. Armstrong, D.K.B., Smith, H.R., and Rycroft R.J.G. 1999. Glove-related hand urticaria in the absence of type I latex allergy. *Contact Dermatitis* 41:42.
48. Thomson, K.F., and Wilkinson, S.M. 1999. Localized dermographism: A differential diagnosis of latex glove allergy. *Contact Dermatitis* 41:103.
49. Liss, G.M., and Sussman, G.L. 1999. Latex sensitization: Occupational versus general population prevalence rates. *Am J Ind Med* 35:196.
50. Meade, B.J., Weissman, D.N., and Beezhold, D.H. 2002. Latex allergy: Past and present. *Int Immunopharmacol* 2:225.
51. Caballero, M.L., and Quirce, S. 2015. Identification and practical management of latex allergy in occupational settings. *Expert Rev Clin Immunol* 11:977.
52. Blaabjerg, M.S.B., Andersen, K.E., Bindslev-Jensen, C., and Mortz, C.G. 2015. Decrease in the rate of sensitization and clinical allergy to natural rubber latex. *Contact Dermatitis* 73:21.
53. Moghtaderi, M., Farjadian, S., Momeni, Z., and Najib, K. 2012. Natural latex sensitization and respiratory function among workers in latex glove factories: A pilot study. *J Occup Environ Hyg* 9:183.
54. Turjanmaa, K. 1994. Contact urticaria from latex gloves, Chapter 17, in *Protective Gloves for Occupational Use*, Mellström, G.A., Wahlberg, J.E., and Maibach, H.I., Eds. Boca Raton, FL: CRC Press.
55. Görtz, J., and Goos, M. 1989. Immediate and late-type allergy to latex: Contact urticaria, asthma and contact dermatitis, in *Current Topics in Contact Dermatitis*, Frosch, P.J., Dooms-Goossens, A., Lachapelle, J.-M., Rycroft, R.J.G., and Scheper, R.J., Eds., Berlin: Springer-Verlag, 457.
56. Turjanmaa, K., Räsänen, L., Lehto, M.I., Mäkinen-Kiljunen, S., and Reunala, T. 1989. Basophil histamine release and lymphocyte proliferation tests in latex contact urticaria. *Allergy* 44:181.
57. M'Raihi, L.F., Charpin, D., Pons, A., Bongrand, P., and Vervloet, D. 1991. Cross-reactivity between latex and banana. *J Allergy Clin Immunol* 87:129.
58. Ceuppens, J.L., Van Dunne, P., and Dooms-Goossens, A. 1992. Severe food-induced anaphylaxis in patients with latex allergy. *Lancet* 339:493.
59. Turjanmaa, K., Reunala, T., and Räsänen, L. 1988. Comparison of diagnostic methods in latex surgical glove contact urticaria. *Contact Dermatitis* 19:241.
60. Wrangsjö, K., Wahlberg, J.E., and Axelsson, I.G.K. 1988. IgE-mediated allergy to natural rubber in 30 patients with contact urticaria. *Contact Dermatitis* 19:264.
61. Pecquet, C., Leynadier, F., and Dry, J. 1990. Contact urticaria and anaphylaxis to natural latex. *J Am Acad Dermatol* 22:631.
62. Jaeger, D., Kleinhans, D., Czuppon, A.B., and Baur, X. 1992. Latex-specific proteins causing immediate-type cutaneous, nasal, bronchial and systemic reactions. *J Allergy Clin Immunol* 89(3):759.
63. Ebo, D.G., and Stevens, W.J. 2002. IgE-mediated natural rubber latex allergy: An update. *Acta Clin Belg* 57:58–70.
64. Van Ketel, W.G., and Van den Berg, W.H.H.W. 1984. The problem of the sensitisation to dithiocarbamates in thiuram-allergic patients. *Dermatologica* 169:70.
65. Rademaker, M., and Forsyth, A. 1989. Carba mix: A useful indicator of rubber sensitivity, in *Current Topics in Contact Dermatitis*, Frosch, P.J., Dooms-Goossens, A., Lachapelle, J-M., Rycroft, R.J.G., and Scheper, R.J., Eds. Berlin: Springer-Verlag, 136.

66. Marks, J., and DeLeo, V., Eds. 1997. Standard allergens, in *Contact and Occupational Dermatology*, 2nd ed. St. Louis, MO: Mosby, 98–102.

67. Uter, W., Schnuch, A., Geier, J., and Frosch, P.J. 1989. Epidemiology of contact dermatitis: The information network of Departments of Dermatology (IVDK) in Germany. *Eur J Dermatol* 1:36–40.

68. Warburton, K.L., Urwin, R., Carder, M., Turner, S., Agius, R., and Wilkinson, S.M. 2015. UK rates of occupational skin disease attributed to rubber accelerators, 1996–2012. *Contact Dermatitis* 72:305.

69. North American Contact Dermatitis Group. 2005. *Interim Report 2003–2004*. Chicago, IL: North American Contact Dermatitis Group.

70. Kanerva, L., Estlander, T., and Jolanki, R. 1996. Allergic patch test reactions caused by the rubber chemical cyclohexyl thiophtalimide. *Contact Dermatitis* 34:23.

71. Huygens, S., Barbaud, A., and Goossens, A. 2001. Frequency and relevance of positive patch tests to cyclohexylthiophthalimide, a new rubber allergen. *Eur J Dermatol* 11:443.

72. Geier, J., Lessmann, H., Frosch, P.J., and Schnuch, A. 2003. Contact sensitization to N-(cyclohexy- lthio)phtalimide. *Contact Dermatitis* 48:1.

73. Goh, C.L. 1989. Contact allergy to surgeon's gloves in their patients. *Contact Dermatitis* 20:223.

74. Wigger-Alberti, W., and Eisner, P. 1998. Do barrier creams and gloves prevent or provoke contact dermatitis. *Am J Contact Dermatitis* 9:100.

75. Havmose, M., Thyssen, J.P., Zachariae, C., and Johansen, J.D. 2020. Use of protective gloves by hairdressers: A review of efficacy and potential adverse effects. *Contact Dermatitis* 83:75.

76. Espasandín-Arias, M., and Goossens, A. 2014. Natural rubber gloves might not protect against skin penetration of methylisothiazolinone. *Contact Dermatitis* 70:249.

77. Gonçalo, M., Mascarenhas, R., Vieira, R., and Figueiredo, A. 2004. Permeability of gloves to plant allergens. *Contact Dermatitis* 50:200.

78. Antelmi, A., Young, E., Svedman, C., Zimerson, E., Engfeldt, M., Foti, C., and Bruze, M. 2015. Are gloves sufficiently protective when hairdressers are exposed to permanent hair dyes? An in vivo study. *Contact Dermatitis* 72:229.

79. Lehman, P.A., Franz, T.J., and Guin, J.D. 1994. Penetration of glutaraldehyde through glove material: Tactylon versus natural rubber latex. *Contact Dermatitis* 30:176.

80. Dooms-Goossens, A.E. 1994. Clinical testing of occupation-related glove sensitivity, Chapter 12, in *Protective Gloves for Occupational Use*, Mellström, G.A., Wahlberg, J.E., and Maibach, H.I., Eds. Boca Raton, FL: CRC Press.

81. Prasad Hunasehally, R.Y., Hughes, T.M., and Stone, N.M. 2012. Atypical pattern of (meth)acrylate allergic contact dermatitis in dental professionals. *Br Dent J* 213:223.

82. Valks, R., Conde-Salazar, L., Malfeito, J., and Ledo, S. 2005. Contact dermatitis in hairdressers, 10 years later: Patch test results in 300 hairdressers (1994 to 2003) and comparison with previous study. *Dermatitis* 16:28.

83. Dooms-Goossens, A., Garmyn, M., and Degreef, H. 1991. Contact allergy to acrylamide. *Contact Dermatitis* 24:71.

84. Dooms-Goossens, A., Bruze, M., Buysse, L., Fregert, S., Gruvberger, B., and Stals, H. 1995. Contact allergy to allyl glycidyl ether present as an impurity in 3-glycidyloxypropyltrimethoxysilane, a fixing additive in silicone and polyurethane resins. *Contact Dermatitis* 33:17.

85. Leynadier, F., Tran Xuan, T., and Dry, J. 1991. Allergenicity suppression in natural latex surgical glove. *Allergy* 46:619.

86. Knudsen, B.B., Larsen, E., Egsgaard, H., and Menné, T. 1993. Release of thiuram and carbamates from rubber gloves. *Contact Dermatitis* 28:63.

87. Rich, P., Belozer, M.L., Norris, P., and Storrs, F.J. 1991. Allergic contact dermatitis to two antioxidants in latex gloves: 4,4′-thiobis (6-tert-butyl-meta-cresol) (Lowinox 44S36) and butylhydroxyanisole. Allergen alternatives for glove-allergic patients. *J Am Acad Dermatol* 24:37.
88. Lopushinsky, K.M., Gill, N., Shea, W.K., Elliott, J.F., Straube, S., and Dytoc, M.T. 2020. Making glove decision less of a white knuckling experience: A systematic review and inventory of glove accelerator contents. *J Cutan Med Surg* 24:386.
89. Crepy, M-N. 2016. Rubber: New allergens and preventive measures. *Eur J Dermatol* 26:523.
90. Crepy, M-N., Lecuen, J., Ratour-Bigot, C., Stocks, J., and Bensefa-Colas, L. 2018. Accelerator-free gloves as alternatives in cases of glove allergy in healthcare workers. *Contact Dermatitis* 78:28.
91. Cleenewerck, M.-B. 2010. Update on medical and surgical gloves. *Eur J Dermatol* 20:434.
92. Andersson, T., Bruze, M., and Björkner, B. 1999. *In vivo* testing of the protection of gloves against acrylates in dentin-bonding systems on patients with known contact allergy to acrylates. *Contact Dermatitis* 41:245.
93. Andersson, T., and Bruze, M. 1999. *In vivo* testing of the protective efficacy of gloves against allergen-containing products using an open chamber system. *Contact Dermatitis* 41:260.
94. Belleri, L., and Crippa, M. 2008. Old and new types of sanitary gloves: What has improved? *Med Lav* 99:80.
95. Fuchs, T. 1995. *Gummi und Allergie*. Munich: Dustri-Verlag Dr. Karl Feistle.
96. Geier, J. 2001. Internet-Liste mit Allergenen in Schutzhandschuhen (Aktuelles). *Dermatosen* 49:251.
97. Rose, R.F., Lyons, P., Horne, H., and Wilkinson S.M. 2009. A review of the materials and allergens in protective gloves. *Contact Dermatitis* 61:129.

16 Management of Natural Rubber Glove Sensitivity

A.M. Giménez-Arnau and A. Salman

CONTENTS

16.1 INTRODUCTION

Natural rubber latex (NRL) is a plant-derived substance, and owing to its excellent flexibility and mechanical and durability properties, it has been widely used in the manufacturing of various products including medical devices, gloves, car tires, clothes, and toys.[1]

Natural rubber gloves are generally used for protection purposes, e.g. from infections and various drug chemicals in healthcare work, from chemical hazards and disease transmission in the food industry. Despite those remarkable benefits, NRL gloves might be the primary cause of various medical conditions, particularly through allergic mechanisms.

DOI: 10.1201/9781003126874-19

Following the increased use of medical gloves during the HIV epidemic in the 1980s, an increase in allergic reactions to natural rubber latex gloves has been observed. Although the regulations and advances in manufacturing processes have decreased the prevalence, it continues to be a problem, particularly in groups at higher risk. Moreover, rubber additives used during manufacture are important causes of type IV hypersensitivity and allergic contact dermatitis. The accurate diagnosis and implementation of preventive measures are of great importance to avoid severe respiratory or skin involvement and increased time away from work. A vital part of the management of natural rubber glove sensitivity is the continuing education of the patients and increased awareness about the symptoms and ways to control the exposures.

In this chapter, the manufacturing processes of NRL gloves, possible allergens found in NRL gloves, related reactions, in vivo and in vitro diagnostic tests, and management of NRL glove sensitivity will be reviewed.

16.2   MANUFACTURING OF NRL GLOVES

Natural rubber latex, a polymer of isoprene (1,4-polyisoprene), is primarily derived from *Hevea brasiliensis*. The centrifugation of the milky fluid obtained from the Hevea trees results in separation into three phases called rubber phase, C-serum, and a bottom fraction (B-serum). Besides the other organic and inorganic ingredients, approximately 1.5% of the whole fluid is protein and all latex proteins are suspended in the C-serum fraction. Most of these proteins are eliminated during the manufacturing processes, and the allergic reactions to latex are attributed to the remaining portion of proteins, the residual extractable proteins (EPs). The amount of residual EPs depends on the quality of manufacturing processes as a significant portion can be washed out through different processing approaches.[1]

There are two types of raw Hevea latex from which natural rubber products are manufactured: liquid latex concentrate and solid dry rubber. The liquid latex concentrate is used in the production of NRL products, and its polyisoprene content is about 60%. The NRL gloves are preferred for providing a good barrier, elasticity, tactile sensitivity, and endurance.

Natural rubber is elastic between 15°C and 30°C. Below or above this range of temperature, it gets hard or soft, respectively. Several manufacturing processes are used to modify these characteristics, and various chemical compounds are added to NRL during these processes. Among those, polymerization, or vulcanization, comprises a reaction between polyisoprene polymers and sulfur to improve elasticity and reduce plasticity. Vulcanization is accelerated through the addition of different substances called accelerators and activators. Other added substances include antioxidants, stabilizers, blowing, and coloring agents. These substances can be associated with type IV hypersensitivity and allergic contact dermatitis.

Most of the type I hypersensitivity reactions to NRL gloves are associated with latex proteins. The amount of residual EPs is closely related to the allergenic potential of the products. It is highly variable (from <20 to >1000 mcg/g) and dependent on the quality of manufacturing processes.[2] An earlier study has compared the EP levels of gloves with different processing standards. The researchers also evaluated the allergic responses against extracts of these gloves. The study demonstrated that high EP levels were associated with positive skin prick test responses, while gloves with low EP levels were less likely to incite a positive response. The negative response rates were up to 100% using gloves with EP levels less than 100 mcg/g.[3] The relationship between EP levels and the allergenic potential of NRL gloves was supported in further studies.[4] Also, the medical gloves have been grouped into low and moderate-to-high allergenic depending on the levels of four NRL allergens (Hev b 1, 3, 5, and 6). A threshold value of 0.15 mcg/g showed high sensitivity and specificity in this approach.[5]

The efforts to reduce the EP levels in NRL gloves led to novel and effective processing methods including the use of low-protein latex, leaching, deproteinization, chlorination, and polymer coating.

During the manufacturing of powdered NRL gloves, the residual EPs are uptaken by the powder particles leading to the formation of aeroallergens during the use of gloves. In the case of proper manufacturing and thus low EP content, the risk of powder-related aeroallergen formation is lower.

16.3 NRL GLOVES-RELATED ALLERGENS AND REACTIONS

Natural rubber latex gloves contain various allergens that may cause different types of hypersensitivity reactions and clinical presentations. The clinical manifestations and the severity of the symptoms depend on the route and amount of exposure (skin or mucous membranes) and the host-related factors. In addition to immunologic mechanisms, mechanical and frictional effects caused by gloves may result in irritant reactions. The clinical and pathophysiologic characteristics of the NRL gloves-related reactions are summarized in Table 16.1.

16.3.1 Type I Hypersensitivity Reactions

Type I hypersensitivity or immediate-type reaction occurs in the presence of allergen-specific IgEs in sensitized individuals. The clinical presentation of contact urticaria syndrome may range from localized contact urticaria to generalized urticaria, wheezing, and anaphylaxis.

The primary allergens responsible for the immediate-type reactions are latex allergens. There are 15 latex allergens defined to date. The classification of latex allergens and their clinical importance are detailed in Table 16.2. Apart from the latex allergens, some NRL gloves may rarely contain cow's milk casein. This might cause a positive reaction to gloves in individuals sensitized to cow's milk and might be misinterpreted as latex allergy.[6]

16.3.2 Contact Urticaria Syndrome

Three subtypes of contact urticaria syndrome (CUS) exist: immunologic contact urticaria, non-immunologic contact urticaria, and contact urticaria of uncertain cause.

TABLE 16.1

Clinical Manifestations of Natural Rubber Glove Sensitivity

Clinical Presentation		Pathophysiology	Clinical Findings	Diagnostic Tests	Relevant Allergens
Allergic	Contact urticaria syndrome	Type I hypersensitivity	Localized wheals, generalized urticarial lesions, allergic rhinoconjunctivitis, asthma	Skin prick testing, scratch test, in vitro serologic tests, provocation tests	NRL proteins
	Protein contact dermatitis	Type I vs type I + IV hypersensitivity	Eczematous lesions on the site of contact with proteins	Skin prick testing, scratch test, in vitro serologic tests, provocation tests	NRL proteins
	Allergic contact dermatitis	Type IV hypersensitivity	Erythematous scaly patches with vesicles and papules, edema, hyperkeratosis and fissures in chronic cases, occasional dissemination of the lesions	Patch testing	Rubber additives
Irritant	Irritant contact dermatitis	Mechanical, frictional forces, non-immunologic	Erythematous scaly patches, fissures, hyperkeratosis, dry skin	(–)	None

The immunologic contact urticaria occurs through allergen-specific IgEs; thus, previous sensitization and re-exposure to allergens are prerequisites. It usually presents with a localized wheal formation at the site of contact with the allergen. The onset of the wheal is generally within 30 min following the exposure. It most commonly involves the hands, arms, and face.[7] The clinical presentation and severity depend on the dose and route of exposure.[8] NRL allergens are present on the glove surfaces and also in the cornstarch powder used in the powdered NRL gloves. Those allergens can be aerosolized and inhaled and might cause sensitization through contact with mucosal surfaces.[9,10]

The manifestations of CUS are categorized into four stages as follows: localized urticaria (stage 1), generalized urticaria (stage 2), allergic asthma and/or allergic

TABLE 16.2

The Characteristics of Allergens Found in the Natural Rubber Gloves Associated with Type I Hypersensitivity (World Health Organization and International Union of Immunological Societies (WHO/IUIS) Allergen Nomenclature Sub-committee, allergen.org)

Allergen	Biochemical Name	Molecular Weight (kDa)	Populations at Higher Risk	Other Features
Hev b 1	Rubber elongation factor	14	Patients with spina bifida	
Hev b 2	Beta-1,3-glucanase; glucan endo-1,3-beta-glucosidase, basic vacuolar isoform	35, 36.5, and 38		
Hev b 3	Small rubber particle protein (SRPP)	24	Patients with spina bifida	
Hev b 4	Lecithinase homologue; GDSL lipase/esterase family member	53–55	Healthcare Workers	
Hev b 5	Acidic protein, unknown function	16	Healthcare workers and patients with spina bifida	Cross-reactivity with kiwi
Hev b 6	Hevein precursor Hev b 6.01	20	Healthcare workers	Cross-reactivity with banana, avocado, chestnut (latex-fruit syndrome)
	Hevein Hev b 6.02	4.7		
	Win-like protein Hev b 6.03	14		
Hev b 7	Patatin-like protein	42		
Hev b 8	Profilin	15		Possible cross-reactivity with pollen profilins
Hev b 9	Enolase	51		
Hev b 10	Superoxide dismutase (Mn)	26		
Hev b 11	Class I chitinase	30		
Hev b 12	Non-specific lipid transfer protein type 1 (nsLTP1)	9		
Hev b 13	Esterase	42	Healthcare workers	
Hev b 14	Hevamine	30		
Hev b 15	Serine protease inhibitor	7.5		

rhinitis (stage 3), and anaphylaxis or anaphylactoid reactions (stage 4). Natural rubber latex is among the primary causes of immunologic CUS. The localized contact urticaria is the most common symptom in NRL-sensitized patients, whereas severe symptoms including anaphylaxis were reported in 13% of the patients.[11] In a study from Finland, 29% of 45 patients with NRL-induced CUS had concomitant occupational asthma and/or rhinitis.[12] In a recent study from Germany, the frequency of asthmatic symptoms (stage 3 CUS) was 25% in patients with CU related to any allergen. There were no cases of stage 4 CUS in the same study population.[13]

NRL-related CUS usually develops in an occupational setting. In Australia, 8.3% of the patients with an occupational skin disease were diagnosed with occupational contact urticaria, with the majority of them being NRL related.[7] This rate was 11% in Finland between 2005 and 2016.[14]

It is commonly associated with the use of medical/surgical gloves or cleaning gloves, as well.[15] In a study of 251 patients with occupational CUS, half of the cases were due to NRL, with a majority of those being healthcare workers (HCWs).[16] In Spain, sensitization to NRL and contact urticaria from NRL were more common in HCWs compared to non-HCWs. Nevertheless, NRL sensitivity was a significant problem also in food handlers, construction workers, painters, hairdressers, plastic products machine operators, and cleaners.[14,17] In addition to occupation, a history of atopy is also a risk factor for NRL-related CUS.[7,11] The use of gloves for more than 4 h per day and wet work also increase the risk for immediate-type reactions.[13,18] The presence of hand dermatitis is also associated with an increased risk of being sensitized to NRL, possibly due to increased allergen penetration because of a skin barrier defect.[11] Earlier studies have reported a decreasing prevalence of NRL sensitization and symptoms during the 2000s in Italy and France.[16,18] Another study from Denmark showed that the prevalence of NRL sensitization decreased from 6.1% (2002–2005) to 1.2% (2010–2013).[11] Although NRL was the third most common cause of CU in Finland between 1995 and 2011, only five cases were diagnosed after 2004.[12]

Protein contact dermatitis (PCD) presents with pruritic eczematous lesions. It usually involves the hands and the periungual areas. Despite a lack of understanding of the underlying mechanisms, a combination of type I and type IV hypersensitivity reactions to plant-/animal-derived proteins is suggested. Compared to CU, PCD is more likely to recur and cause more significant morbidity and increased sick leave.[19]

The homologies between NRL and fruit (banana, kiwi, avocado) proteins (i.e. Hev b 6 and endochitinases) are associated with the cross-reactivity and the so-called "latex-fruit syndrome."[8] In Denmark, 52% of the NRL-sensitized patients had reported a history of reaction related to oral intake of fruits or vegetables. The most common fruits were kiwi, banana, and avocado. Most of the food-related symptoms were mild, primarily oral allergy syndrome (85%). Of note, the patients with NRL-related clinical symptoms were more likely to have more severe food-related symptoms compared to those who had only positive prick test responses to NRL. The same study showed that 64% of the patients had positive prick reactions to both NRL and birch pollen.[11] This should be kept in mind as clinically non-relevant NRL sensitization might be associated with cross-reactivities.

16.3.3   Type IV Hypersensitivity Reactions

Contact dermatitis is an acute or chronic inflammatory skin reaction caused by exposure to an irritant and/or allergen substances. Two types of contact dermatitis exist
depending on the underlying pathomechanism: irritant contact dermatitis (ICD) and
allergic contact dermatitis (ACD).

Type IV hypersensitivity or delayed-type reactions to NRL gloves present with
ACD. The primary culprit allergens for ACD are rubber additives, and patch testing
is the gold standard in the diagnosis of ACD.

16.3.4   Allergic Contact Dermatitis

Allergic contact dermatitis is the immune-mediated form of contact dermatitis and
occurs in previously sensitized individuals. It requires a sensitization phase which
occurs during the initial exposure to the allergen and lasts for 10–14 days. Re-exposure
to the sensitizing substance leads to the development of papulovesicular lesions with
erythema over the site of contact with allergen within 24–48 h, which is called the
elicitation phase. Xerosis, fissures, and lichenification can be seen in chronic cases.

Unlike the ICD, the lesions of ACD tend to extend beyond the site of contact.
Pruritus is usually intense. The risk of NRL-related ACD is high in healthcare workers, hairdressers, cleaners, food handlers, food processing industry workers, and
construction workers.[20–22] A history of atopic dermatitis/atopy and a longer duration
of glove use are additional risk factors.[23,24] In Sweden, contact allergy to rubber
additives was significantly common in HCWs with hand eczema compared to HCWs
without hand eczema (6% vs 1%). Occupational contact allergy to rubber additives
was significantly related to sick leave in the same study population.[24] A study from
Italy has demonstrated an increased risk of sensitization to carbamates and thiurams in HCWs. Thiuram sensitivity was also associated with dermatitis in restaurant
workers, hairdressers, construction workers, and mechanics.[25]

Although latex proteins are very rarely reported to cause type IV hypersensitivity,[26]
it is suggested that the cases of type IV hypersensitivity to latex are actually caused
by the presence of rubber additives (i.e. thiurams and/or dithiocarbamates).[27] The
major allergens for the development of NRL gloves related to ACD are compounds
(i.e. accelerators and antioxidants) added during the manufacturing processes. The
allergens associated with NRL glove-related ACD are shown in Table 16.3.

Rubber accelerators are used to increase the resilience and strength of natural
rubber. They have been the most frequent cause of occupational ACD.[28,29] The rubber accelerators include thiurams, carbamates, guanidines, thioureas, and thiazoles.
Until the replacement with carbamates and thiazoles, thiurams were the most commonly identified rubber accelerator. In a study of 30 patients with glove-related
ACD, 80% of them tested positive with thiurams.[30] A study from Italy showed the
increasing role of carbamates by replacing thiurams during a 16-year-period between
1996 and 2012.[25] Data from 12 European countries also confirmed the increasing
prevalence of carba mix sensitization and a decline in contact allergy to thiuram
mix.[31] Another study of operating room staff presenting with glove-related symptoms, 14.6% of them had type IV allergy to rubber additives (the most common

TABLE 16.3

The Primary Type IV Hypersensitivity-Associated Allergens in the Natural Rubber Gloves

Functions	Allergen Groups	Allergens and Patch Test Materials	Potential Exposures Other Than Gloves
Accelerators	Thiazoles	Mercapto mix [N-cyclohexyl-2-benzothiazyl sulphenamide, dibenzothiazyl disulfide, 2-mercaptobenzothiazole (MBT), 2-(4-morpholinylmercapto) benzothiazol]	Condoms, rubber parts of shoes, hoses, tires
	Thiurams	Petrolatum tetramethylthiuram monosulfide (TMTM), tetramethylthiuram disulfide (TMTD), tetraethylthiuram disulfide (TETD), dipentamethylenethiuram disulfide (PTD) (included in thiuram mix)	Elastic bands, adhesives, medical devices, swimwear, tires, earphones, fungicides
	Dithiocarbamates	Zinc dibutyldithiocarbamate (ZBC), zinc diethyldithiocarbamate (ZDC) (included in carba mix)	Adhesives, condoms, medical devices, leather shoes, textile, tires
	Guanidines	1,3-Diphenylguanidine (included in carba mix)	Adhesives, condoms, medical devices, leather shoes, textile, tires
	Thioureas	N,N′-Dibutylthiourea, N,N′-diphenylthiourea (DPTU) (included in thiourea mix)	Adhesives, anticorrosives, elastic textile
	Amine aldehydes	–	
Antioxidants	Amines	Phenylenediamines (N-cyclohexyl-N-phenyl-4-phenylenediamine, N,N′-diphenyl-p-phenylenediamine (DPPD), N-isopropyl-N-phenyl-4-phenylenediamine [IPPD]) (included in black rubber mix), quinolines	Rubber products, cutting fluids
	Phenols	Hydroquinones, BHT (butylhydroxytoluene)	Foods, cosmetics, topical medications, paints
	Phosphites	–	

additive being tetramethyl thiuram monosulfide).[32] Of 3448 patients with occupational contact allergy with rubber gloves, 13% were sensitized to thiurams followed by dithiocarbamates (3.5%), mercaptobenzothiazoles (3%), and thioureas (0.4%).[33] Co-sensitization to thiurams and carbamates is very frequent.[34]

A recent study analyzing the accelerators used in 190 gloves has reported that the most frequently used accelerator is carbamates (90.5%) followed by thiurams (5.8%).[35] In Finland, despite a slow annual decrease from 2005 to 2016, rubber-related occupational ACD constituted the largest group (16.7%) among all ACD cases during the study period.[36] A similar trend was observed in Thailand, with a continuous decrease in patch test reactivity against rubber additives between 2006 and 2018 (from 23.1% in 2006–2008 to 8.6% in 2016–2018).[37]

Other possible allergens in NRL gloves associated with type IV hypersensitivity are antioxidants. They are added to the NRL products to decrease rubber degeneration by oxygen and/or ozone. They include amines, phenols, and phosphites.[38,39]

16.3.5 IRRITANT REACTIONS

16.3.5.1 Irritant Contact Dermatitis

ICD is the most common form of contact dermatitis and usually develops in occupational settings. It represents a non-specific, non-immunologic reaction of the skin to the irritant substances in the environment, e.g. water, detergents, solvents, oils, sweating, occlusion, and moisture caused by glove use.[40,41] Moist environment caused by the prolonged use of occlusive gloves for >2 h per day might disrupt the epidermal barrier and lead to the development of ICD.[40] The negative effect of rubber glove use for >6 h per day on the skin barrier has been demonstrated,[42] although the following studies failed to show a similar effect.[43]

ICD does not require a sensitization phase as in ACD. Endogenous factors such as atopy also contribute to the development of ICD. It may either present as an acute or a chronic reaction, depending on the strength of the irritant. Frequent and repeated exposure to mild irritants such as water and cleansers presents erythema, dryness, and hyperkeratosis, whereas strong irritants including acid or alkali substances cause an acute reaction presenting with edema, and erythema sometimes leading to necrosis. The lesions are usually confined to the site of contact with the irritants.[40,41] Nevertheless, the concurrence of ICD and ACD in the same patient is not uncommon and makes the diagnosis more complicated.

16.4 DIAGNOSTIC EVALUATION

16.4.1 HISTORY

A thorough medical history is essential in the diagnosis of NRL sensitivity. In a patient with suspected NRL glove sensitivity, the following aspects of the history should be asked in detail:[44–46]

- Duration and characteristics of the symptoms
- Relationship between the symptoms and the occupation

TABLE 16.4

Risk Factors for Natural Rubber Glove Sensitivity (Type I or IV)

Atopy (allergic rhinitis, asthma, atopic dermatitis, food allergy)

Healthcare occupation

Food handlers

Housekeepers

Hairdressers

Regular use of gloves at work

Repeated exposure to rubber products

History of cutaneous or systemic reaction to rubber

Personal history of:
- Multiple surgeries during childhood
- Spina bifida
- Myelomeningocele
- Urogenital anomalies

- Distribution of the lesions
- Presence of extracutaneous symptoms
- Temporal relationship between suspected materials and development of lesions
- Presence of personal or familial history of atopy
- Concomitant medications
- Presence of risk factors (Table 16.4)

16.4.2 DIAGNOSTIC TESTS

16.4.2.1 Type I Hypersensitivity

In addition to a thorough medical history, various in vivo and in vitro tests can be used in the diagnosis of CUS. A proposed algorithm suggests to start testing with an open application test, and if negative, occlusive application tests can be used. Those should be applied on normal skin; however, in case of a negative reaction on normal skin, the test can be repeated on slightly affected skin too. If the open application tests yield no positive reaction, the testing can be continued with invasive methods, which include prick testing, prick-by-prick testing, scratch tests, and intradermal testing.[47] Skin prick testing (SPT) has a high specificity in NRL sensitization and is usually used in combination with in vitro tests. The degree of SPT response highly correlates with the clinical severity of NRL-related symptoms.[48]

In addition to in vivo tests, in vitro diagnosis is also possible with the use of serum-specific IgE level measurement and Basophil activation tests. The clinical relevance of the positive in vitro tests should be carefully evaluated before making a diagnosis.[47] In vitro radioallergosorbent test (RAST) can be used to detect the presence of latex protein-specific IgEs in the serum. False-negative results might occur in up to 10% of the tests.[46,49] Specific IgE against Hev b 6.01 and Hev b 5 had the highest clinical correlation in a study.[50] In suspected NRL-related occupational asthma, the combined use of specific IgE levels against Hev b 5, 6.01, and 6.02 was the best predictor of bronchial response to NRL.[51]

Challenge tests also have an important role in the diagnosis. In patients with negative SPT and RAST responses but with a highly suggestive history of NRL sensitization, challenge tests can be performed. Caution is warranted during the challenge tests, especially in those with a history of anaphylaxis or severe asthma. Glove challenge, nasal challenge, and conjunctival challenge tests can confirm the diagnosis.[52] Although the inhalation challenges are the gold standard in the diagnosis of NRL-related asthma, it is uncommonly performed because the test is expensive, is time consuming, and might induce severe asthma episodes.[53] In a study of patients with NRL-related symptoms and negative prick and specific-IgE tests, the glove challenge and conjunctival challenge tests were positive in 2% and 18%, respectively.[11]

16.4.2.2   Type IV Hypersensitivity

Patch testing is the gold standard method in the diagnosis of delayed-type reactions or ACD. In a patient with suspected ACD caused by NRL gloves, the testing should include additional rubber series in addition to baseline series (Table 16.5). In a previous study, only 41% of the contact allergies could be detected with the baseline series, emphasizing the importance of individual patch testing in the management of NRL glove sensitivity.[24] The benefit of testing with additional rubber series in detecting more allergens was also supported by the data from European countries.[54] An earlier study has reported that 13% of the patients with NRL allergy showed positive patch test response to rubber accelerators, i.e. carbamates and thiurams.[11]

Pieces of gloves should also be tested "as is." Although identification of the exact allergen is not possible with this method, it is of great importance in determining a relationship between the material and contact allergy. Testing with both sides of the gloves is recommended, and before testing the pieces might be soaked in water, ethanol, or acetone to increase allergen penetration.[39]

16.5   MANAGEMENT

The lack of diagnosis and treatment of natural rubber glove sensitivity, particularly in occupational settings, can have serious consequences for the patients such as increased absenteeism, impaired career development and burden of symptoms, and life-threatening complications in case of type I hypersensitivity.[55]

The proper choice of the glove for patients with NRL sensitization requires close collaboration and communication between the physician, patient, employer, and glove industry. The user preferences including dexterity, flexibility, comfort, and fit should be taken into account to ensure the compliance of suggested products.[55]

16.5.1   EDUCATION AND AWARENESS

Continuing education of the patients is of major importance to ensure the effectiveness of treatment and preventive measures and thus avoid recurrences. Following

TABLE 16.5
Additional Rubber Allergen Series for Patch Testing

Suggested European Rubber Series[39]		Rubber Additive Series (*Chemotechnique MB Diagnostics AB*)	
	(all in pet.)	Tetramethylthiuram disulfide (TMTD)	1.0% pet
Tetramethylthiuram disulfide	1.0	Tetramethylthiuram monosulfide (TMTM)	1.0% pet
Tetramethylthiuram monosulfide	1.0	Tetraethylthiuram disulfide (TETD)	1.0% pet
Tetraethylthiuram disulfide (Disulfiram)	1.0	Dipentamethylenethiuram disulfide	1.0% pet
Dipentamethylenethiuram disulfide	1.0	N-cyclohexyl-N-phenyl-4-phenylenediamine	1.0% pet
Zinc dibutyldithiocarbamate	1.0	N,N'-diphenyl-p-phenylenediamine (DPPD)	1.0% pet
Zinc diethyldithiocarbamate	1.0	N-isopropyl-N-phenyl-4-phenylenediamine (IPPD)	0.1% pet
1,3-Diphenylguanidine	1.0	2-Mercaptobenzothiazole (MBT)	2.0% pet
2-Mercaptobenzothiazole	2.0	N-cyclohexyl-2-benzothiazolesulfenamide	1.0% pet
N-cyclohexyl-2-benzothiazyl sulfenamide	1.0	Dibenzothiazyl disulfide (MBTS)	1.0% pet
Dibenzothiazyl disulfide	1.0	2-(4-Morpholinylmercapto) benzothiazol (MOR)	1.0% pet
Morpholinylmercaptobenzothiazole	1.0	1,3-Diphenylguanidine	1.0% pet
Dibutylthiourea	1.0	Zinc diethyldithiocarbamate (ZDC)	1.0% pet
Diphenylthiourea	1.0	Zinc dibutyldithiocarbamate (ZBC)	1.0% pet
Diethylthiourea	1.0	N,N'-di-2-naphtyl-4-phenylenediamine (DBNPD)	1.0% pet
N-isopropyl-N-phenyl-4-phenylenediamine	0.1	N-phenyl-2-naphtylamine (PBN)	1.0% pet
N-cyclohexyl-N-phenyl-4-phenylenediamine	1.0	Methenamine	2.0% pet
N,N'-diphenyl-p-phenylenediamine	1.0	4,4'-Diaminodiphenylmethane (MDA)	0.5% pet
N,N'-di-2-naphthyl-4-phenylenediamine	1.0	N,N'-Diphenylthiourea (DPTU)	1.0% pet
Cyclohexyl thiophthalimide	0.5	Zinc dimethyldithiocarbamate (Ziram)	1.0% pet
Own gloves (both sides)	"as is"	2,2,4-Trimethyl-1,2-dihydroquinoline	1.0% pet
		N,N'-Diethylthiourea	1.0% pet
		N,N'-Dibutylthiourea	1.0% pet
		Dodecyl mercaptan	0.1% pet
		N-(cyclohexylthio) phthalimide	1.0% pet
		Thiourea	0.1% pet
		4,4'-Dithiodimorpholine	1.0% pet

the determination of the sensitivity and the culprit allergen, physicians can help to educate workers during follow-up visits and publish informational materials. The physicians can also help workers in obtaining material safety data sheets (MSDSs) and interpreting the ingredients. Educational activities, increasing awareness, and providing information on the allergens have been reported to increase the likelihood of success in NRL gloves associated with type I and type IV hypersensitivity.[56–59]

The MSDSs and product labels do not always reflect the possible changes in the ingredients during the manufacturing processes. This should be taken into account for properly counseling the patients.

16.5.2 Product Selection in Patients with Natural Rubber Glove Sensitivity

Individuals with type I hypersensitivity to NRL gloves should not use any NRL-containing gloves including semi-synthetic rubber gloves or coated NRL gloves as they might still release NRL allergens.[60] The use of low allergen NRL gloves instead of high allergen NRL gloves has been effective in reducing airborne NRL allergens and improving respiratory symptoms in sensitized patients.[56,61–64] However, NRL gloves labeled as low protein or hypoallergenic should also be avoided. Food and Drug Administration (FDA) strongly discourages labeling as "latex-free," "does not contain latex," or "does not contain natural rubber latex" in medical devices, as it might create a false sense of security in NRL-sensitized individuals. The labeling as "is not made with natural rubber latex" should be sought in case of NRL allergy.[65,66] Patients with type I hypersensitivity to NRL gloves should prefer fully synthetic rubber or thermoplastic elastomer gloves with or without powder.[55]

The primary prevention strategies consist of restricting the use of NRL gloves to specific scenarios (e.g. medical interventions requiring high tactile sensitivity) and replacing powdered NRL gloves with non-powder/non-NRL gloves.[67] In particular, the use of non-powdered gloves successfully helped to decrease the prevalence of NRL sensitization in previous studies.[61,68–72] The use of powder-free gloves by patients and their co-workers was also effective in reducing symptoms of NRL allergy and absenteeism in patients with NRL allergy.[11,73,74] Moreover, in Finland, NRL gloves with very low allergen content were successfully used by NRL-sensitized patients without any clinical symptoms.[75]

In the case of type IV hypersensitivity to NRL gloves, the use of nitrile or chloroprene gloves is not sufficient for prevention because these gloves may contain rubber accelerators or antioxidants, too. These patients should prefer gloves without any vulcanization process during manufacturing such as polyvinyl chloride (PVC) or polyurethane or styrene-based copolymer gloves.[55] A recently updated list of accelerator-free gloves was given in Table 16.6.

16.6 CONCLUSIONS

Despite a trend to decrease, type I and type IV hypersensitivity associated with NRL gloves continues to be an important cause of absenteeism in the workplace, morbidity, and rarely life-threatening reactions. Accurate diagnosis, determination of

TABLE 16.6
Accelerator-Free Gloves (Adapted from Reference [38])

Company	Type of Glove	Product Name
Ansell Healthcare LLC	Medical examination	Microflex Sensation Nitrile Exam
	Medical examination	Micro-Touch NitraFree Nitrile Exam
	Surgical gloves	GAMMEX Non-Latex Polyisoprene Surgical Glove
	Surgical gloves	GAMMEX Non-Latex Sensitive Synthetic Sensoprene Surgical Glove
Cardinal Health	Medical examination	Low Dermatitis Potential Nitrile Exam
CT International	Medical examination	FFNT Series FingerFlex Accelerator-Free Nitrile Exam Gloves
Dynarex Corporation	Medical examination	Tillotson True Advantage Nitrile Exam Gloves
Hourglass International	Medical examination	HandPRO FreeStyle1100 Nitrile Exam
Innovative Healthcare Corp.	Medical examination	Pulse® PURE™ Nitrile Exam Gloves—Series 178
Sempermed USA	Medical examination	SemperSure Nitrile Exam
SmartPractice	Medical examination	Reflection Sapphire Sensitive Nitrile PF Violet Blue
Medline Industries	Surgical gloves	DermAssure Green Powder-Free Neoprene Surgical Glove
Mölnlycke	Surgical gloves	Biogel NeoDerm Neoprene Surgical Glove
Allerderm	Household (cleaning, dishes)	Allerderm Heavy Duty Vinyl Gloves
Showa Group	Industrial use (chemical resistant)	N-Dex 9500 PF Nitrile
	Industrial use (chemical resistant)	7712 PVC
Honeywell	Industrial use (chemical resistant)	Honeywell North Silver Shield/4H Gloves

the culprit allergen, product selection, and prevention require close communication between the physician, patient, and glove industry. Wider availability of allergen-free glove alternatives along with the continuing education of the personnel will likely contribute to the decreasing trend of NRL glove sensitivity in the future.

REFERENCES

1. Yip, E., Cacioli, P. 2002. The manufacture of gloves from natural rubber latex. *J Allergy Clin Immunol* 110 Supplement:S3–14.
2. Yunginger, J.W., Jones, R.T., Fransway, A.F., Kelso, J.M., Warner, M.A., and Hunt, L.W. 1994. Extractable latex allergens and proteins in disposable medical gloves and other rubber products. *J Allergy Clin Immunol* 93:836–42.

3. Yip, E., Turjanmaa, K., Ng, K.P., Mok, K.L. 1994. Allergic responses and levels of extractable proteins in NR latex gloves and dry rubber products. *J Nat Rubb Res* 9:79–86.

4. Yip, E., Sussman, G.L. 2000. Allergenicity of latex gloves with reference to latex protein sensitive individuals in a Canadian population. *J Rubb Res* 3:129–41.

5. Palosuo, T., Reinikka-Railo, H., Kautiainen, H., Alenius, H., Kalkkinen, N., Kulomaa, M., Reunala, T., and Turjanmaa, K. 2007. Latex allergy: The sum quantity of four major allergens shows the allergenic potential of medical gloves. *Allergy Eur J Allergy Clin Immunol* 62:781–6.

6. Ylitalo, L., Mäkinen-Kiljunen, S., Turjanmaa, K., Palosuo, T., and Reunala, T. 1999. Cow's milk casein, a hidden allergen in natural rubber latex gloves. *J Allergy Clin Immunol* 104:177–80.

7. Williams, J.D.L., Lee, A.Y.L., Matheson, M.C., Frowen, K.E., Noonan, A.M., and Nixon, R.L. 2008. Occupational contact urticaria: Australian data. *Br J Dermatol* 159:125–31.

8. Amaro, C., Goossens, A. 2008. Immunological occupational contact urticaria and contact dermatitis from proteins: A review. *Contact Dermatitis* 58:67–75.

9. Charous, B.L., Schuenemann, P.J., Swanson, M.C. 2000. Passive dispersion of latex aeroallergen in a healthcare facility. *Ann Allergy Asthma Immunol* 85:285–90.

10. Swanson, M.C., Bubak, M.E., Hunt, L.W., Yunginger, J.W., Warner, M.A., and Reed, C.E. 1994. Quantification of occupational latex aeroallergens in a medical center. *J Allergy Clin Immunol* 94:445–51.

11. Blaabjerg, M.S.B., Andersen, K.E., Bindslev-Jensen, C., Mortz, C.G. 2015. Decrease in the rate of sensitization and clinical allergy to natural rubber latex. *Contact Dermatitis* 73:21–8.

12. Helaskoski, E., Suojalehto, H., Kuuliala, O., Aalto-Korte, K. 2017. Occupational contact urticaria and protein contact dermatitis: Causes and concomitant airway diseases. *Contact Dermatitis* 77:390–6.

13. Süß, H., Dölle-Bierke, S., Geier, J., Kreft, B., Oppel, E., Pföhler, C., Skudlik, C., Worm, M., and Mahler, V. 2019. Contact urticaria: Frequency, elicitors and cofactors in three cohorts (Information Network of Departments of Dermatology; Network of Anaphylaxis; and Department of Dermatology, University Hospital Erlangen, Germany). *Contact Dermatitis* 81:341–53.

14. Pesonen, M., Koskela, K., Aalto-Korte, K. 2020. Contact urticaria and protein contact dermatitis in the Finnish Register of Occupational Diseases in a period of 12 years. *Contact Dermatitis* 83:1–7.

15. Turjanmaa, K., Laurila, K., Makinen-Kiljunen, S., Reunala, T. 1988. Rubber contact urticaria. *Contact Dermatitis* 19:362–7.

16. Bensefa-Colas, L., Telle-Lamberton, M., Faye, S., Bourrain, J.L., Crépy, M.N., Lasfargues, G., Choudat, D., RNV3P members, and Momas, I. 2015. Occupational contact urticaria: Lessons from the French National Network for Occupational Disease Vigilance and Prevention (RNV3P). *Br J Dermatol* 173:1453–61.

17. Valks, R., Conde-Salazar, L., Cuevas, M. 2004. Allergic contact urticaria from natural rubber latex in healthcare and non-healthcare workers. *Contact Dermatitis* 50:222–4.

18. Larese, F.F., Bochdanovits, L., Capuzzo, C., Cerchi, R., and Rui, F. 2014. Ten years incidence of natural rubber latex sensitization and symptoms in a prospective cohort of health care workers using non-powdered latex gloves 2000–2009. *Int Arch Occup Environ Health* 87:463–9.

19. Vester, L., Thyssen, J.P., Menné, T., Johansen, J.D. 2012. Consequences of occupational food-related hand dermatoses with a focus on protein contact dermatitis. *Contact Dermatitis* 67:328–33.

20. Scalone, L., Cortesi, P.A., Mantovani, L.G., Belisari, A., Ayala, F., Fortina, A.B., Bonamonte, D., Borroni, G., Cannavò, S.P., Guarneri, F., Cristaudo, A., De Pità, O., Gallo, R., Girolomoni, G., Gola, M., Lisi, P., Pigatto, P.D., Satta, R., and Giannetti, A. 2015. Clinical epidemiology of hand eczema in patients accessing dermatological reference centres: Results from Italy. *Br J Dermatol* 172:187–95.

21. Kersh, A.E., Helms, S., De La Feld, S. 2018. Glove-related allergic contact dermatitis. *Dermatitis* 29:13–21.

22. Bauer, A., Geier, J., Elsner, P. 2002. Type IV allergy in the food processing industry: Sensitization profiles in bakers, cooks and butchers. *Contact Dermatitis* 46:228–35.

23. Nettis, E., Assennato, G., Ferrannini, A., Tursi, A. 2002. Type I allergy to natural rubber latex and type IV allergy to rubber chemicals in health care workers with glove-related skin symptoms. *Clin Exp Allergy* 32:441–7.

24. Hamnerius, N., Svedman, C., Bergendorff, O., Björk, J., Bruze, M., Engfeldt, M., and Pontén, A. 2018. Hand eczema and occupational contact allergies in healthcare workers with a focus on rubber additives. *Contact Dermatitis* 79:149–56.

25. Buttazzo, S., Prodi, A., Fortina, A.B., Corradin, M.T., and Larese Filon, F. 2016. Sensitization to rubber accelerators in Northeastern Italy: The Triveneto Patch Test Database. *Dermatitis* 27:222–6.

26. Shaffrali, F.C., Gawkrodger, D.J. 1999. Allergic contact dermatitis from natural rubber latex without immediate hypersensitivity. *Contact Dermatitis* 40:325–6.

27. Leuzzi, M., Vincenzi, C., Sechi, A., Tomasini, C., Giuri, D., Piraccini, B.M., and La Placa, M. 2019. Delayed hypersensitivity to natural rubber latex: Does it exist or not? *Contact Dermatitis* 81:404–5.

28. Pesonen, M., Jolanki, R., Larese, F.F., Wilkinson, M., Kręcisz, B., Kieć-Świerczyńska, M., Bauer, A., Mahler, V., John, S.M., Schnuch, A., and Uter, W. 2015. Patch test results of the European baseline series among patients with occupational contact dermatitis across Europe - analyses of the European Surveillance System on Contact Allergy network, 2002–2010. *Contact Dermatitis* 72:154–63.

29. Carøe, T.K., Ebbehøj, N., Agner, T. 2014. A survey of exposures related to recognized occupational contact dermatitis in Denmark in 2010. *Contact Dermatitis* 70:56–62.

30. Siegel, P.D., Fowler, J.F., Storrs, F.J., Sasseville, D., Pratt, M., Bledsoe, T.A., Law, B.F., Beezhold, D., Zug, K., and Fowler, L.M. 2010. Allergen content of patient problem and nonproblem gloves: Relationship to allergen-specific patch-test findings. *Dermat Contact, Atopic, Occup Drug* 21:77–83.

31. Warburton, K.L., Bauer, A., Chowdhury, M.M.U., Cooper, S., Kręcisz, B., Chomiczewska-Skóra, D., Kieć-Świerczyńska, M., Filon, F.L., Mahler, V., Sánchez-Pérez, J., Schnuch, A., Uter, W., and Wilkinson, M. 2015. ESSCA results with the baseline series, 2009–2012: Rubber allergens. *Contact Dermatitis* 73:305–12.

32. Miri, S., Pourpak, Z., Zarinara, A., Heidarzade, M., Kazemnejad, A., Kardar, G., Firooz, A., and Moin, A. 2007. Prevalence of type I allergy to natural rubber latex and type IV allergy to latex and rubber additives in operating room staff with glove-related symptoms. *Allergy Asthma Proc* 28:557–63.

33. Geier, J., Lessmann, H., Mahler, V., Pohrt, U., Uter, W., and Schnuch, A. 2012. Occupational contact allergy caused by rubber gloves - Nothing has changed. *Contact Dermatitis* 67:149–56.

34. Cao, L.Y., Taylor, J.S., Sood, A., Murray, D., and Siegel, P.D. 2010. Allergic contact dermatitis to synthetic rubber gloves: Changing trends in patch test reactions to accelerators. *Arch Dermatol* 146:1001–7.

35. Goodier, M.C., Ronkainen, S.D., Hylwa, S.A. 2018. Rubber accelerators in medical examination and surgical gloves. *Dermatitis* 29:66–76.

36. Aalto-Korte, K., Koskela, K., Pesonen, M. 2020. 12-year data on dermatologic cases in the Finnish Register of Occupational Diseases I: Distribution of different diagnoses and main causes of allergic contact dermatitis. *Contact Dermatitis* 82:337–42.

37. Sukakul, T., Chaweekulrat, P., Limphoka, P., Boonchai, W. 2019. Changing trends of contact allergens in Thailand: A 12-year retrospective study. *Contact Dermatitis* 81:124–9.

38. Scheman, A., Hylwa-Deufel, S., Jacob, S.E., Katta, R., Nedorost, S., Warshaw, E., Eifrid, K., Geiser, A.J., McGaughey, L., Scheman, N., Kimyon, R., Rundle, C., and Shaver, R. 2019. Alternatives for allergens in the 2018 American Contact Dermatitis Society Core Series: Report by the American Contact Alternatives Group. *Dermatitis* 30:87–105.

39. Warburton, K.L., Uter, W., Geier, J., Spiewak, R., Mahler, V., Crépy, M.N., Schuttelaar, M.L., Bauer, A., and Wilkinson, M. 2017. Patch testing with rubber series in Europe: A critical review and recommendation. *Contact Dermatitis* 76:195–203.

40. Bains, S.N., Nash, P., Fonacier, L. 2019. Irritant contact dermatitis. *Clin Rev Allergy Immunol* 56:99–109.

41. Slodownik, D., Lee, A., Nixon, R. 2008. Irritant contact dermatitis: A review. *Australas J Dermatol* 49:1–11.

42. Ramsing, D.W., Agner, T. 1996. Effect of glove occlusion on human skin (II). Long-term experimental exposure. *Contact Dermatitis* 34:258–62.

43. Wetzky, U., Bock, M., Wulfhorst, B., John, S.M. 2009. Short- and long-term effects of single and repetitive glove occlusion on the epidermal barrier. *Arch Dermatol Res* 301:595–602.

44. Jiang, A., Maibach, H. 2018. Contact urticaria and protein contact dermatitis—A frequently hidden diagnosis. *Curr Treat Options Allergy* 5:302–9.

45. Caballero, M.L., Quirce, S. 2015. Identification and practical management of latex allergy in occupational settings. *Expert Rev Clin Immunol* 11:977–92.

46. Higuero, N.C., Igea, J.M., de la Hoz, B. 2012. Latex allergy: Position paper. *J Investig Allergol Clin Immunol* 22:313–30.

47. Giménez-Arnau, A.M. 2014. Contact urticaria syndrome: How it is clinically manifested and how to diagnose it. In *Contact Urticaria*. Gimenez-Arnau, A.M., and Maibach, H.I., eds, 1st ed. Boca Raton, FL: CRC Press, 21–8.

48. Hadjiliadis, D., Banks, D.E., Tarlo, S.M. 1996. The relationship between latex skin prick test responses and clinical allergic responses. *J Allergy Clin Immunol* 97:1202–6.

49. Blanco, C., Carrillo, T., Ortega, N., Alvarez, M., Dominguez, C., and Castillo, R. 1998. Comparison of skin-prick test and specific serum IgE determination for the diagnosis of latex allergy. *Clin Exp Allergy* 28:971–6.

50. Garnier, L., Selman, L., Rouzaire, P., Bouvier, M., Roberts, O., Bérard, F., Bienvenu, J., and Bienvenu, F. 2012. Molecular allergens in the diagnosis of latex allergy. *Eur Ann Allergy Clin Immunol* 44:73–9.

51. Vandenplas, O., Froidure, A., Meurer, U., Rihs, H.P., Rifflart, C., Soetaert, S., Jamart, J., Pilette, C., and Raulf, M. 2016. The role of allergen components for the diagnosis of latex-induced occupational asthma. *Allergy Eur J Allergy Clin Immunol* 71:840–9.

52. Ünsel, M., Mete, N., Ardeniz, Ö., Göksel, S., Ersoy, R., Sin, A., Gulbahar, O., and Kokuludag, A. 2009. The importance of nasal provocation test in the diagnosis of natural rubber latex allergy. *Allergy Eur J Allergy Clin Immunol* 64:862–7.

53. Vandenplas, O., Suojalehto, H., Cullinan, P. 2017. Diagnosing occupational asthma. *Clin Exp Allergy* 47:6–18.

54. Uter, W., Warburton, K., Weisshaar, E., Simon, D., Ballmer-Weber, B., Mahler, V., Fuchs, T., Geier, J., and Wilkinson, M. 2016. Patch test results with rubber series in the European Surveillance System on Contact Allergies (ESSCA), 2013/14. *Contact Dermatitis* 75:345–52.

55. Hamann, C.P., Rodgers, P.A., Sullivan, K.M. 2004. Management of natural rubber glove sensitivity. In *Protective Gloves for Occupational Use*. Boman, A., Estlander, T., Wahlberg, J.E., Maibach, H.I., eds, 2nd ed. Boca Raton, FL: CRC Press, 155–87.

56. Allmers, H., Schmengler, J., Skudlik, C. 2002. Primary prevention of natural rubber latex allergy in the German health care system through education and intervention. *J Allergy Clin Immunol* 110:318–23.

57. Trapé, M., Schenck, P., Warren, A. 2000. Latex gloves use and symptoms in health care workers 1 year after implementation of a policy restricting the use of powdered gloves. *Am J Infect Control* 28:352–8.

58. Paul, M.A., Fleischer, A.B., Scherertz, E.F. 1995. Patients' benefit from contact dermatitis evaluation: Results of a follow-up study. *Am J Contact Dermat* 6:63–6.

59. Edman, B. 1988. The usefulness of detailed information to patients with contact allergy. *Contact Dermatitis* 19:43–7.

60. Truscott, W. 2002. Glove powder reduction and alternative approaches. *Methods* 27:69–76.

61. Hunt, L.W., Kelkar, P., Reed, C.E., Yunginger, J.W. 2002. Management of occupational allergy to natural rubber latex in a medical center: The importance of quantitative latex allergen measurement and objective follow-up. *J Allergy Clin Immunol* 110 Supplement:S96–106.

62. Allmers, H., Brehler, R., Chen, Z., Raulf-Heimsoth, M., Fels, H., and Baur, X. 1998. Reduction of latex aeroallergens and latex-specific IgE antibodies in sensitized workers after removal of powdered natural rubber latex gloves in a hospital. *J Allergy Clin Immunol* 102:841–6.

63. Baur, X., Chen, Z., Allmers, H. 1998. Can a threshold limit value for natural rubber latex airborne allergens be defined? *J Allergy Clin Immunol* 101:24–7.

64. Mitakakis, T.Z., Tovey, E.R., Yates, D.H., Toelle, B.G., Johnson, A., Sutherland, M.F., O'Hehir, R.E., and Marks, G.B. 2002. Particulate masks and non-powdered gloves reduce latex allergen inhaled by healthcare workers. *Clin Exp Allergy* 32:1166–9.

65. FDA. 2021. Recommendations for labeling medical products to inform users that the product or product container is not made with natural rubber latex. FDA. https://www.fda.gov/regulatory-information/search-fda-guidance-documents/recommendations-labeling-medical-products-inform-users-product-or-product-container-not-made-natural [accessed on 6 March 2021].

66. Federal Register. 2021. Recommendations for Labeling Medical Products To Inform Users That the Product or Product Container Is Not Made With Natural Rubber Latex; Guidance for Industry and Food and Drug Administration Staff; Availability. https://www.federalregister.gov/documents/2014/12/02/2014-28265/recommendations-for-labeling-medical-products-to-inform-users-that-the-product-or-product-container [accessed on 6 March 2021].

67. Vandenplas, O., Raulf, M. 2017. Occupational latex allergy: The current state of affairs. *Curr Allergy Asthma Rep* 17:14. DOI: 10.1007/s11882-017-0682-5.

68. Wrangsjö, K., Boman, A., Lidén, C., Meding, B. 2012. Primary prevention of latex allergy in healthcare - Spectrum of strategies including the European glove standardization. *Contact Dermatitis* 66:165–71.

69. Tarlo, S.M. 2001. Natural rubber latex allergy and asthma. *Curr Opin Pulm Med* 7:27–31.

70. Allmers, H., Schmengler, J., John, S.M. 2004. Decreasing incidence of occupational contact urticaria caused by natural rubber latex allergy in German health care workers. *J Allergy Clin Immunol* 114:347–51.

71. Liss, G.M., Tarlo, S.M. 2001. Natural rubber latex-related occupational asthma: Association with interventions and glove changes over time. *Am J Ind Med* 40:347–53.

72. Tarlo, S.M., Easty, A., Eubanks, K., Parsons, C.R., Min, F., Juvet, S., and Liss, G.M. 2001. Outcomes of a natural rubber latex control program in an Ontario teaching hospital. *J Allergy Clin Immunol* 108:628–33.

73. Nienhaus, A., Kromark, K., Raulf-Heimsoth, M., van Kampen, V., and Merget, R. 2008. Outcome of occupational latex allergy - Work ability and quality of life. *PLoS One* 3:1–5.

74. Vandenplas, O., Jamart, J., Delwiche, J.-P., Evrard, G., and Larbanois, A. 2002. Occupational asthma caused by natural rubber latex: Outcome according to cessation or reduction of exposure. *J Allergy Clin Immunol* 109:125–30.

75. Turjanmaa, K., Kanto, M., Kautiainen, H., Reunala, T., and Palosuo, T. 2002. Long-term outcome of 160 adult patients with natural rubber latex allergy. *J Allergy Clin Immunol* 110 Supplement:S70–4.

17 Allergic Responses to Powdered Natural Rubber Latex Gloves in Healthcare Workers

A.M. Giménez-Arnau and A. Salman

CONTENTS

17.1 INTRODUCTION

Natural rubber latex (NRL) is a polymer of isoprene primarily procured from the *Hevea brasiliensis* tree. Considering its advantages including easy processing, flexibility, good mechanical properties, and ozone resistance, it is still being used in manufacturing medical gloves and medical devices.[1]

Allergic reactions to natural rubber latex significantly increased following the recommendations on the regular use of latex gloves during the HIV epidemic in the 1980s. In addition to increased exposure, altered manufacturing quality due to mass

DOI: 10.1201/9781003126874-20

production might have caused an increase in the allergenic potential of NRL gloves and attributed to the NRL sensitization.[2]

In this chapter, the clinical characteristics, diagnosis, and management of the NRL-induced allergic reactions in healthcare workers (HCWs) will be addressed.

17.2   NATURAL RUBBER LATEX GLOVES: AN OVERVIEW

Fifteen latex allergens with IgE-binding properties have been identified to date in natural rubber. These allergens show different distributions over the gloves and may have different clinical significance. The primary allergens also differ among different risk groups. A study has shown that Hev b 2, 5, 6.01, and 13 were the primary allergens among HCWs.[3] Another study found that Hev b 6.02 was the main allergen in HCWs occupationally sensitized to NRL.[4] These differences might be related to the differences in sensitization routes and allergen distribution on medical gloves. Accordingly, a study has shown that concentrations of Hev b 1 and Hev b 3 were significantly higher on external surfaces, while internal surfaces had higher levels of Hev b 5 and Hev b 6.02, which are frequent sensitizers in HCWs.[5] Identified natural rubber allergens are given in detail in Table 17.1.

17.3   NRL ALLERGY AND RISK FACTORS
IN HEALTHCARE WORKERS

The identification of risk factors for NRL allergy might allow to pre-define the high-risk groups and implement effective prevention strategies. Also, educational programs on NRL allergy targeting high-risk groups might be of benefit. The educational programs are needed even for HCWs, which are among the highest risk occupations (i.e. rubber industry workers, housekeepers, food handlers) for NRL allergy. Accordingly, a study investigating the level of knowledge among HCWs about NRL allergy has demonstrated that only 1% of the study population correctly matched the appropriate gloves to a specific procedure and every three of four participants failed to recognize the characteristics of type I allergy to NRL.[6]

The prevalence and incidence of NRL allergy were higher in HCWs compared to the general population. Although an earlier systematic review did not show an increased risk of latex sensitization in HCWs compared to other occupations,[7] another systematic review has demonstrated that the frequency of latex allergy (4.32% vs 1.37%), positive skin prick test (SPT) to latex (6.9%–7.8% vs 2.1%–3.7%), and the mean percentage of NRL-specific serum IgE were higher in HCWs when compared to the general population. The same review concluded that HCWs exposed to latex had an increased risk of hand dermatitis, asthma/wheezing, and rhinoconjunctivitis in comparison to the general population.[8] Accordingly with the latter review, a study of 1171 patients comparing NRL sensitization between healthcare and non-healthcare workers showed that NRL sensitization (positive prick test and specific IgE levels) was more frequent in HCWs (16.7% vs 2.3%). NRL-induced contact urticaria was also much more common among the HCWs (71.4% vs 28.6%).[9] In addition to HCWs, a study has shown that dental hygiene students are at higher risk for NRL

TABLE 17.1

Allergens in Natural Rubber Latex and Their Clinical Significance (allergen.org)

Allergen	Biochemical Name	Molecular Weight (kDa)	Clinical Implications
Hev b 1	Rubber elongation factor	14	Major allergen in spina bifida
Hev b 2	beta-1,3-Glucanase; glucan endo-1,3-beta-glucosidase, basic vacuolar isoform	35, 36.5 and 38	
Hev b 3	Small rubber particle protein (SRPP)	24	Major allergen in spina bifida
Hev b 4	Lecithinase homolog; GDSL lipase/esterase family member	53–55	Minor allergen in HCWs
Hev b 5	Acidic protein, unknown function	16	HCWs and patients with spina bifida. Homology with kiwi acid protein
Hev b 6	Hevein precursor Hev b 6.01	20	Main allergen in HCWs. Homology with chitinases from banana, avocado, and chestnut causing latex-fruit syndrome
	Hevein Hev b 6.02	4.7	
	Win-like protein Hev b 6.03	14	
Hev b 7	Patatin-like protein	42	
Hev b 8	Profilin	15	
Hev b 9	Enolase	51	
Hev b 10	Superoxide dismutase (Mn)	26	
Hev b 11	Class I chitinase	30	
Hev b 12	Non-specific lipid transfer protein type 1 (nsLTP1)	9	
Hev b 13	Esterase	42	Major allergen in HCWs
Hev b 14	Hevamine	30	
Hev b 15	Serine protease inhibitor	7.5	

exposure and sensitization.[10] In a school of dentistry, the rate of positive skin prick test response increased with the student year, and the symptoms of asthma, rhino-conjunctivitis, and contact urticaria were more common in students with a positive skin test.[11]

Additional risk factors have been identified for NRL allergy in HCWs. In a survey from Sri Lanka, the duration of the service and the use of gloves for more than an hour per day increased the risk of sensitization in HCWs.[12] From 2000-2009, 2,053

TABLE 17.2

The Risk Groups for NRL Allergy

Patients with spina bifida, cerebral palsy

Patients who underwent multiple surgeries esp. during childhood

Patients who underwent multiple mucosal procedures

Individuals with food allergy (kiwi, avocado, banana etc.)

Individuals with atopy

Healthcare workers

   Physicians

   Nurses

   Medical students

   Janitors at hospitals

   Personnel at ambulances

Workers in the latex-related industry (glove factory, toy factory)

HCWs in Italy presented respiratory symptoms and urticaria that were positively correlated with latex sensitization, common allergic respiratory symptoms, and familial atopy.[13] In Taiwan, high levels of total serum IgE and self-report of symptoms associated with atopy were more frequent in HCWs with NRL allergy.[14] In a study of HCWs presenting with glove-related symptoms, female sex was associated with the presence of type I allergy to latex.[15] Nevertheless, a small study consisting of dentists and dental assistants has failed to show an association between filaggrin mutations and type I hypersensitivity to latex.[16]

Several other risk factors for NRL allergy in both the general population and healthcare workers (HCWs) are summarized in Table 17.2.[17]

Despite a trend of decrease in the incidence of NRL allergy among HCWs and the general population following the regulations in glove use and implementation of prevention strategies, it is still a problem in already sensitized individuals that can cause absenteeism and morbidities, thus an increase in healthcare costs.

17.4 CLINICAL MANIFESTATIONS OF NRL ALLERGY IN HEALTHCARE WORKERS

Two types of allergic reactions may occur due to natural rubber latex gloves. The clinical picture and the severity of the symptoms depend on the route of exposure, i.e. direct contact with skin, mucous membranes (nose, throat, lung airway) exposed to inhalational aerosolized glove powder, the amount of allergens, and host factors.[17]

Type I hypersensitivity reaction, or immediate type reaction, develops in the presence of latex-specific IgE and may present with contact urticaria, generalized urticaria, wheezing, and anaphylaxis. The onset of symptoms is within 30 minutes following exposure to latex. Also, due to the cross-reaction of latex allergens with food allergens (e.g. banana, kiwi, avocado, chestnut), the latex-fruit syndrome may occur.

Contact urticaria is the most common presentation of type I NRL allergy. It may occur as an isolated reaction or precede a systemic reaction. In the case of mucosal involvement, angioedema may develop. As the contact urticaria becomes chronic, type IV hypersensitivity to latex may lead to the development of protein contact dermatitis which presents with eczematous lesions. Exposure to NRL through inhalation may result in the development of allergic rhinitis and/or asthma. Powdered gloves are the primary source of exposure in this case as latex proteins may attach to the cornstarch used in powdered gloves.[18]

Type IV hypersensitivity, or delayed-type reaction, occurs in individuals who are sensitized to either latex proteins themselves or more frequently additive substances (e.g. thiurams, carbamates) added during the glove manufacturing processes. This type of reaction presents with allergic contact dermatitis. Because type IV hypersensitivity to latex proteins is very rare, contact allergy to rubber additives such as carbamates and thiurams should also be considered in the case of NRL glove-related allergic contact dermatitis. In a study of 190 gloves, carbamates were, by far, the most frequent accelerator (90.5%) followed by thiurams (5.8%).[19] In a study analyzing skin prick tests and patch test results in operating room staff presenting with glove-related symptoms, 30.5% of the HCWs had type I latex allergy, whereas 16.7% and 14.6% of them had type IV allergy to latex and rubber additives (most common additive tetramethyl thiuram monosulfide), respectively.[15] Contact allergy to rubber gloves is most commonly associated with sensitization to accelerators. Thiurams and dithiocarbamates are the most frequent allergens. In a study of 3448 patients, of which one-third were HCWs, 13% were sensitized to thiurams followed by dithiocarbamates, mercaptobenzothiazole, and thioureas.[20]

On the other hand, irritant contact dermatitis, which may be confused with allergic contact dermatitis, may also develop due to the mechanical and frictional effects associated with the use of NRL gloves rather than an immunologic reaction. The characteristics of NRL-induced reactions have been summarized in Table 17.3.

TABLE 17.3
Characteristics of Natural Rubber Latex-Associated Reactions

	Allergic Reactions		Irritant Reaction
Pathophysiology	Type I IgE-mediated hypersensitivity	Type IV hypersensitivity	Non-allergic, mechanical friction
Clinical findings	Contact urticaria, rhinoconjunctivitis, asthma, anaphylaxis	Allergic contact dermatitis: erythematous scaly patches extending proximally from hands	Irritant contact dermatitis: dryness, fissures, cracks, erythema
Causative component	Latex allergens	Chemical accelerators, thiurams, rarely latex	Glove powder, soaps, water

17.5 DIAGNOSTIC TESTS FOR NRL ALLERGY

The history of exacerbation of allergic symptoms (itchy wheals, watery eyes, runny nose, dry cough, shortness of breath) during workdays and improvement during holidays is suggestive of an occupational allergy. The medical history of a patient presenting with suspected NRL allergy should focus on the following aspects:[21,22]

- History of other allergies
- Personal history of atopy
- Previous latex exposure
- Possible source of exposure
- Possible cross-reaction with fruits
- Presence of risk factors

In addition to a thorough medical history and workplace visits, various in vivo and in vitro tests have been used to confirm NRL allergy.

In a study from 2005, the most common test to diagnose NRL allergy was latex-specific IgE measurement in serum among British dermatologists and allergologists. The glove use tests were used by almost half of the physicians. It was interesting that approximately every one of five specialists avoided performing prick testing and glove challenges because of the risk of anaphylaxis which underlies the need for guidance for the diagnosis of NRL allergy.[23]

17.5.1 Serum-Specific IgE Levels

In vitro radioallergosorbent test (RAST) is used to detect the presence of specific IgE antibodies against latex allergens. *Hevea brasiliensis* latex serum is used for in vivo and in vitro diagnosis of NRL allergy. However, a study investigated the allergen concentration in the serum and reported that the concentration of Hev b 6 is up to a thousand times higher than the other seven allergens measured (Hev b 1, 2, 3, 4, 5, 7, and 13). Thus, the tests using the latex serum might not be able to detect the patients sensitized to allergens other than Hev b 6 and cause false-negative test results.[24] The false-negative results were seen in 2%–10% of tests. Thus, the clinical relevance of the test results should be interpreted carefully with a detailed patient history.[21,25]

The most relevant allergens for specific IgE measurement are Hev b 6.01 and Hev b 5. Hev b 6.01 had the highest correlation with in vivo tests, while Hev b 5 is of particular benefit in case of discordance between clinical history and skin tests.[26]

17.5.2 Skin Prick Testing

The in vivo diagnosis of type I NRL allergy is made using skin prick testing in which the allergen is introduced into the skin through a prick made by prick lancets. Although the sensitivity may vary depending on the commercial extract, the SPT has a high specificity (92%) and is usually used in conjunction with RAST. Screening for NRL allergy with SPT in patients with a history of intolerance NRL is recommended.[9] The degree of the SPT response is related to the clinical severity of the symptoms.[27]

17.5.3 Patch Testing

Delayed-type hypersensitivity to NRL gloves may also occur. The gold standard in the diagnosis of type IV hypersensitivity is patch testing. In addition to standard series (i.e. European Baseline Series, North American Baseline Series) and rubber additive series, patch testing with patients' own glove materials is highly recommended in patients with glove-related symptoms.[28] The glove can be cut off into 2 × 2 cm pieces, and both the internal and external surfaces of the gloves should be tested as the allergens on these surfaces may differ. The glove pieces can be applied to the upper back using adhesive tapes, and the first reading is done at 48 hours. The rubber compounds in the European Baseline Series are detailed in Table 17.4. In a study of 148 patients with suspected rubber-related ACD, 2% had a positive patch test reaction to NRL. An important point in patch testing with NRL is that an early reading at 20–30 minutes is essential to detect patients with immediate hypersensitivity.[29]

17.5.4 Glove Use Test

In the glove use test, a finger portion of a latex glove is cut off and placed on the finger of the patient for 15–30 minutes. A non-NRL glove may be used as a negative control, and the test may be repeated with the whole glove in case of a negative result and high clinical suspicion.[21]

In a study, the glove use test had a sensitivity of 81% and specificity of 90%.[30] An important pitfall with the glove use test is that some of the NRL gloves may contain cow's milk casein and positive reactions to casein might be interpreted as NRL allergy.[31]

17.5.5 Nasal Challenge Test

Nasal challenge tests (NCTs) have also been used to confirm the diagnosis of NRL allergy. In a study, the sensitivity, specificity, positive predictive value, and negative predictive value of NCT were 96%, 100%, 100%, and 98%, respectively.[30] Caution

TABLE 17.4
Rubber compounds included in the European Baseline Series

Thiuram mix (dithiocarbamates)	Accelerator
Mercapto mix	Accelerator
2-Mercaptobenzothiazole	Accelerator
N-isopropyl-N-phenyl-p-phenylenediamine (IPPD)	Antioxidant

is advised during the challenge tests, particularly in patients with a previous history of anaphylaxis or asthma.

17.5.6   DIAGNOSIS OF NRL-INDUCED OCCUPATIONAL ASTHMA

Immunological tests, serial assessments of work-related changes in peak expiratory flow (PEF) rate with pulmonary function tests, serial assessments of work-related changes in sputum eosinophils, specific inhalation challenges in the laboratory, and workplace inhalation challenges can be used in the diagnosis of occupational asthma.[32]

Although the gold standard is specific inhalation challenges, the test is expensive, is often time consuming, and may induce severe asthma episodes.

A diagnostic algorithm for the diagnosis of occupational asthma has been proposed. In HCWs with work-related asthma symptoms, the first step is the assessment of non-specific bronchial hyperresponsiveness and the immunological sensitization (via skin prick tests or measurement of specific IgE). In patients with negative or weakly positive test results, serial measurements of PEF, sputum eosinophils at/off work, and specific inhalation challenges may be performed to confirm the diagnosis.[32]

17.6   TREATMENT OF NRL ALLERGY

Despite the lack of commercially available latex extracts for subcutaneous or sublingual therapy, there is a low-to-moderate level of evidence on the effectiveness of immunotherapy in occupational NRL allergy.[33] In a randomized double-blinded study of subcutaneous immunotherapy (SCIT) in 20 HCWs, the therapy led to lower rhinitis, conjunctivitis, and cutaneous scores at 12 months; however, the asthma scores did not differ significantly.[34] Sublingual immunotherapy failed to show any benefit in a small study of the general population with latex allergy.[35]

Omalizumab, an anti-IgE monoclonal antibody, was also used successfully in the treatment of occupational NRL allergy in HCWs. In a randomized, placebo-controlled study of 18 HCWs with NRL-related rhinitis, conjunctivitis, and/or asthma, treatment with omalizumab led to a significant decrease in mean conjunctival challenge scores compared to placebo. At the end of the study overall ocular response rate was 93.6% and the glove use test was negative in 11 of 15 patients.[36]

Topical barrier gel containing zinc provided a decrease in skin irritation in patients with known type IV hypersensitivity to latex gloves.[37]

17.7   PREVENTION

The replacement of HCWs due to NRL allergy-related clinical symptoms can cause cost up to billions of dollars to the medical industry.[38] Thus, the prevention strategies should aim to decrease the absenteeism of individuals with type I or type IV hypersensitivity to NRL. In addition to general regulations, continuing education of the staff, proper labeling of the gloves, limiting unnecessary exposure, the use of protective clothes, reducing airborne exposure via better ventilation, and the use of low-allergen, non-powdered glove alternatives are the main approaches in prevention.[17,39]

17.7.1 LABELING

The measurement of the four NRL allergens (Hev b 1, 3, 5, and 6) in medical gloves was used to classify gloves as low and moderate-to-high allergenic. The threshold value of 0.15 mcg/g had a sensitivity and specificity of 93% and 90%, respectively. This approach can help choose appropriate gloves for HCWs.[40]

In a study, the rates of sensitization to rubber gloves did not decline between 2002 and 2010. The authors suggested that the allergen declaration on the gloves and gloves with reduced accelerator concentrations are needed.[20]

17.7.2 PRIMARY PREVENTION

Primary prevention of latex allergy by switching from powdered gloves to powder-free alternatives for all HCWs is suggested.[41] Previous studies have shown a significant decrease in the development of new cases of NRL allergy following the use of non-powdered gloves over powdered gloves.[42,43] Another study from Germany examined the NRL-related contact urticaria incidence among HCWs and found that despite an increasing frequency until 1998, the incidence has decreased since then with the wider availability of powder-free NRL gloves.[44] A similar benefit of primary prevention was also demonstrated in a study from Canada.[45] Switching to low-powdered, low-protein examination gloves led to a significant decline in the incidence of NRL allergy in a hospital.[46]

The following recommendations have been made for the primary prevention of NRL allergy:[47]

- Restriction of the use of NRL gloves only to specific scenarios (i.e. procedures requiring high tactile sensitivity, e.g. medical interventions).
- The use of non-NRL gloves should be implemented in non-sterile medical procedures.
- Sterile powdered NRL gloves should be replaced with non-powder, low-allergen NRL or non-NRL gloves.
- The unnecessary use of NRL gloves should be limited.

17.7.3 SECONDARY PREVENTION

The use of non-powdered latex gloves for all staff and non-latex gloves for HCWs sensitized to NRL helped to a significant decrease in the incidence of glove-related symptoms.[13] Similarly, in a study of 196 HCWs with reported NRL allergy, the symptom intensity decreased significantly following the implementation of powder-free gloves. In addition to symptom reduction, the work ability index scores increased significantly. However, almost every six out of ten patients reported that they continued to experience NRL-related symptoms during the last six months.[48] Another study from Denmark supported these earlier findings with a decrease in NRL sensitization and clinical NRL allergy rates from 2002 to 2013.[49] In a study of HCWs with occupational asthma due to NRL, a significant number of staff could continue to work in the same workplace by limiting the latex exposure at work.[50] Even normally powdered but low-allergenic gloves have been reported to be a sufficient strategy in a previous study.[51] A follow-up study of 1040 HCWs in Italy has demonstrated that symptoms significantly improved and disappeared in most patients. The authors concluded that basic measures including avoiding unnecessary exposure, the use of non-powdered latex gloves by all HCWs, and the use of non-latex gloves by HCWs sensitized to latex are very helpful in halting the progression of symptoms and new sensitizations.[39]

17.8 CONCLUSION

Although the initial epidemic of NRL allergy in HCWs is currently controlled to some point with legislation and measures, the maintenance of improvement is critical with vigilant follow-up of the measures and continuing education of the healthcare workers.

REFERENCES

1. Rahimi, A., and Mashak, A. 2013. Review on rubbers in medicine: Natural, silicone and polyurethane rubbers. *Plast Rubber Compos* 42:223–30.
2. Shah, D., and Chowdhury, M.M.U. 2011. Rubber allergy. *Clin Dermatol* 29:278–86.
3. Raulf-Heimsoth, M., Rihs, H.P., Rozynek, P., Cremer, R., Gaspar, A., Pires, G., Yeang, H.Y., Arif, S.A., Hamilton, R.G., Sander, I., Lundberg, M., and Brüning, T. 2007. Quantitative analysis of immunoglobulin E reactivity profiles in patients allergic or sensitized to natural rubber latex (*Hevea brasiliensis*). *Clin Exp Allergy* 37:1657–67.
4. Yagami, A., Suzuki, K., Saito, H., and Matsunaga, K. 2009. Hev b 6.02 is the most important allergen in health care workers sensitized occupationally by natural rubber latex gloves. *Allergol Int* 58:347–55.
5. Peixinho, C., Tavares-Ratado, P., Tomás, M.R., Taborda-Barata, L., and Tomaz, C.T. 2008. Latex allergy: New insights to explain different sensitization profiles in different risk groups. *Br J Dermatol* 159:132–6.
6. Al-Niaimi, F., Chiang, Y.Z., Chiang, Y.N., and Williams, J. 2013. Latex allergy: Assessment of knowledge, appropriate use of gloves and prevention practice among hospital healthcare workers. *Clin Exp Dermatol* 38:77–80.
7. Garabrant, D.H.,and Schweitzer, S. 2002. Epidemiology of latex sensitization and allergies in health care workers. *J Allergy Clin Immunol* 110 Supplement:S82–95.
8. Bousquet, J., Flahault, A., Vandenplas, O., Ameille, J., Duron, J.J., Pecquet, C., Chevrie, K., and Annesi-Maesano, I. 2006. Natural rubber latex allergy among health care workers: A systematic review of the evidence. *J Allergy Clin Immunol* 118:447–54.
9. Valks, R., Conde-Salazar, and L., Cuevas, M. 2004. Allergic contact urticaria from natural rubber latex in healthcare and non-healthcare workers. *Contact Dermatitis* 50:222–4.
10. Gautrin, D., Ghezzo, H., Infante-Rivard, C., and Malo, J.L. 2000. Incidence and determinants of IgE-mediated sensitization in apprentices. A prospective study. *Am J Respir Crit Care Med* 162:1222–8.

11. Tarlo, S.M., Sussman, G.L., and Holness, D.L. 1997. Latex sensitivity in dental students and staff: A cross-sectional study. *J Allergy Clin Immunol* 99:396–401.

12. Amarasekera, M., Rathnamalala, N., Samaraweera, S., and Jinadasa, M. 2010. Prevalence of latex allergy among healthcare workers. *Int J Occup Med Environ Health* 23:391–6.

13. Larese, F.F., Bochdanovits, L., Capuzzo, C., Cerchi, R., and Rui, F. 2014. Ten years incidence of natural rubber latex sensitization and symptoms in a prospective cohort of health care workers using non-powdered latex gloves 2000–2009. *Int Arch Occup Environ Health* 87:463–9.

14. Wan, K.S., and Lue, H.C. 2007. Latex allergy in health care workers in Taiwan: Prevalence, clinical features. *Int Arch Occup Environ Health* 80:455–7.

15. Miri, S., Pourpak, Z., Zarinara, A., Heidarzade, M., Kazemnejad, A., Kardar, G., Firooz, A., and Moin, A. 2007. Prevalence of type I allergy to natural rubber latex and type IV allergy to latex and rubber additives in operating room staff with glove-related symptoms. *Allergy Asthma Proc* 28:557–63.

16. Carlsen, B.C., Meldgaard, M., Hamann, D., Hamann, Q., Hamann, C., Thyssen, J.P., Meyer, D.M., Gruninger, S.E., and Hamann, C. 2011. Latex allergy and filaggrin null mutations. *J Dent* 39:128–32.

17. Ranta, P.M., and Ownby, D.R. 2004. A review of natural-rubber latex allergy in health care workers. *Clin Infect Dis* 38:252–6.

18. Poulos, L.M., O'Meara, T.J., Hamilton, R.G., and Tovey, E.R. 2002. Inhaled latex allergen (Hev b 1). *J Allergy Clin Immunol* 109:701–6.

19. Goodier, M.C., Ronkainen, S.D., and Hylwa, S.A. 2018. Rubber accelerators in medical examination and surgical gloves. *Dermatitis* 29:66–76.

20. Geier, J., Lessmann, H., Mahler, V., Pohrt, U., Uter, W., and Schnuch, A. 2012. Occupational contact allergy caused by rubber gloves - Nothing has changed. *Contact Dermatitis* 67:149–56.

21. Higuero, N.C., Igea, J.M., and de la Hoz, B. 2012. Latex allergy: Position paper. *J Investig Allergol Clin Immunol* 22:313–30.

22. Caballero, M.L., and Quirce, S. 2015. Identification and practical management of latex allergy in occupational settings. *Expert Rev Clin Immunol* 11:977–92.

23. Lowe, J.G., Green, C.M., and Nasser, S.M. 2005. Investigative methods for natural rubber latex allergy in the UK. *Contact Dermatitis* 52:11–3.

24. Yeang, H.Y., Hamilton, R.G., Bernstein, D.I., Arif, S.A., Chow, K.S., Loke, Y.H., Raulf-Heimsoth, M., Wagner, S., Breiteneder, H., and Biagini, R.E. 2006. Allergen concentration in natural rubber latex. *Clin Exp Allergy* 36:1078–86.

25. Blanco, C., Carrillo, T., Ortega, N., Alvarez, M., Dominguez, C., and Castillo, R. 1998. Comparison of skin-prick test and specific serum IgE determination for the diagnosis of latex allergy. *Clin Exp Allergy* 28:971–6.

26. Garnier, L., Selman, L., Rouzaire, P., Bouvier, M., Roberts, O., Bérard, F., Bienvenu, J., and Bienvenu, F. 2012. Molecular allergens in the diagnosis of latex allergy. *Eur Ann Allergy Clin Immunol* 44:73–9.

27. Hadjiliadis, D., Banks, D.E., and Tarlo, S.M. 1996. The relationship between latex skin prick test responses and clinical allergic responses. *J Allergy Clin Immunol* 97:1202–6.

28. Crepy, M.N. 2016. Rubber: New allergens and preventive measures. *Eur J Dermatology* 26:523–30.

29. Bendewald, M.J., Farmer, S.A., and Davis, M.D.P. 2010. Patch testing with natural rubber latex: The Mayo Clinic experience. *Dermatitis* 21:311–6.

30. Ünsel, M., Mete, N., Ardeniz, Ö., Göksel, S., Ersoy, R., Sin, A., Gulbahar, O., and Kokuludag, A. 2009. The importance of nasal provocation test in the diagnosis of natural rubber latex allergy. *Allergy Eur J Allergy Clin Immunol* 64:862–7.

31. Ylitalo, L., Mäkinen-Kiljunen, S., Turjanmaa, K., Palosuo, T., and Reunala, T. 1999. Cow's milk casein, a hidden allergen in natural rubber latex gloves. *J Allergy Clin Immunol* 104:177–80.
32. Vandenplas, O., Suojalehto, H., and Cullinan, P. 2017. Diagnosing occupational asthma. *Clin Exp Allergy* 47:6–18.
33. Smith, A.M., and Sastre, J. 2020. The role of immunotherapy and biologic treatments in occupational allergic disease. *J Allergy Clin Immunol Pract* 8:3322–30.
34. Leynadier, F., Herman, D., Vervloet, D., and Andre, C. 2000. Specific immunotherapy with a standardized latex extract versus placebo in allergic healthcare workers. *J Allergy Clin Immunol* 106:585–90.
35. Gastaminza, G., Algorta, J., Uriel, O., Audicana, M.T., Fernandez, E., Sanz, M.L., and Muñoz, D. 2011. Randomized, double-blind, placebo-controled clinical trial of sublingual immunotherapy in natural rubber latex allergic patients. *Trials* 12:1–10.
36. Leynadier, F., Doudou, O., Gaouar, H., Le Gros, V., Bourdeix, I., Guyomarch-Cocco, L., and Trunet, P. 2004. Effect of omalizumab in health care workers with occupational latex allergy. *J Allergy Clin Immunol* 113:360–1.
37. Hamann, C.P., and Rodgers, P.A. 2005. A topical cream containing a zinc gel (Allergy Guard) as a prophylactic against latex glove-related contact dermatitis. *Dermatitis* 16:152–3; author reply 153–4.
38. Kelly, K.J., and Sussman, G. 2017. Latex allergy: Where are we now and how did we get there? *J Allergy Clin Immunol Pract* 5:1212–6.
39. Filon, F.L., and Radman, G. 2006. Latex allergy: A follow up study of 1040 healthcare workers. *Occup Environ Med* 63:121–5.
40. Palosuo, T., Reinikka-Railo, H., Kautiainen, H., Alenius, H., Kalkkinen, N., Kulomaa, M., Reunala, T., and Turjanmaa, K. 2007. Latex allergy: The sum quantity of four major allergens shows the allergenic potential of medical gloves. *Allergy Eur J Allergy Clin Immunol* 62:781–6.
41. Wrangsjö, K., Boman, A., Lidén, C., and Meding, B. 2012. Primary prevention of latex allergy in healthcare - Spectrum of strategies including the European glove standardization. *Contact Dermatitis* 66:165–71.
42. Tarlo, S.M. 2001. Natural rubber latex allergy and asthma. *Curr Opin Pulm Med* 7:27–31.
43. Hunt, L.W., Kelkar, P., Reed, C.E., and Yunginger, J.W. 2002. Management of occupational allergy to natural rubber latex in a medical center: The importance of quantitative latex allergen measurement and objective follow-up. *J Allergy Clin Immunol* 110 Supplement:S96–106.
44. Allmers, H., Schmengler, J., and John, S.M. 2004. Decreasing incidence of occupational contact urticaria caused by natural rubber latex allergy in German health care workers. *J Allergy Clin Immunol* 114:347–51.
45. Liss, G.M., and Tarlo, S.M. 2001. Natural rubber latex-related occupational asthma: Association with interventions and glove changes over time. *Am J Ind Med* 40:347–53.
46. Tarlo, S.M., Easty, A., Eubanks, K., Parsons, C.R., Min, F., Juvet, S., and Liss, G.M. 2001. Outcomes of a natural rubber latex control program in an Ontario teaching hospital. *J Allergy Clin Immunol* 108:628–33.
47. Vandenplas, O., and Raulf, M. 2017. Occupational latex allergy: The current state of affairs. *Curr Allergy Asthma Rep* 17:14. DOI:10.1007/s11882-017-0682-5.
48. Nienhaus, A., Kromark, K., Raulf-Heimsoth, M., van Kampen, V., and Merget, R. 2008. Outcome of occupational latex allergy - Work ability and quality of life. *PLoS One* 3:1–5.

49. Blaabjerg, M.S.B., Andersen, K.E., Bindslev-Jensen, C.,and Mortz, C.G. 2015. Decrease in the rate of sensitization and clinical allergy to natural rubber latex. *Contact Dermatitis* 73:21–8.
50. Vandenplas, O., Jamart, J., Delwiche, J.-P., Evrard, G., and Larbanois, A. 2002. Occupational asthma caused by natural rubber latex: Outcome according to cessation or reduction of exposure. *J Allergy Clin Immunol* 109:125–30.
51. Turjanmaa, K., Kanto, M., Kautiainen, H., Reunala, T., and Palosuo, T. 2002. Long-term outcome of 160 adult patients with natural rubber latex allergy. *J Allergy Clin Immunol* 110 Supplement:S70–4.

18 Other Reactions from Gloves

T. Bullock, A. Sood, and J.S. Taylor

CONTENTS

18.1 INTRODUCTION, GLOVE COMPOSITION, AND COVID-19

Classic allergic reactions to gloves occur as allergic contact dermatitis to the major rubber accelerators and antioxidants and as immunologic contact urticaria (ICU) to natural rubber latex. Among the easiest adverse reactions to document,[1] they are a particular problem for people whose occupations demand that they wear gloves. Though ICU reactions to natural rubber latex proteins were common in the 1980s and 1990s, they are now rare and affect less than 1% of the general population in the USA.[2-5] Aside from these classic allergic reactions, less commonly reported glove reactions also occur. This chapter discusses these other reactions, both irritant and allergic, as well as other mechanisms. Glove reactions are classified in Table 18.1.

Critical to assessing patients with putative glove reactions is knowledge of glove composition, much of which is now proprietary. A 2009 article reviewed materials potentially present in latex, nitrile, Neoprene, and polyvinyl chloride (PVC) gloves, whether or not they had been reported as glove allergens, and suggested specific chemicals for both patch and prick testing.[10] A 2019 EU study identified the presence of sulfites in multiple natural rubber latex and synthetic rubber gloves and postulated their potential role in inducing or eliciting glove reactions.[12] A 2020 multidisciplinary engineering publication[11] from East Asia proposes using (1) antimicrobial agents, e.g., brilliant green and cyclohexadiene for surgical glove coatings, (2) metal ions (chromium, aluminum, and iron) as crosslinkers in gloves, and (3) bioadditives from food waste and plants in nitrile glove manufacture which would enhance biodegradation.[11] Mislabeling of glove components is possible, and chemical analysis of glove extracts may be needed in some cases to identify occult causes.[38]

DOI: 10.1201/9781003126874-21

TABLE 18.1
Classification of Glove Reactions

Irritation from occlusion, friction, and maceration; worse with dermographism[6,7]

    Pseudomonas folliculitis[8]

    See Table 18.3 for other examples of glove irritation

Allergy to glove material

    Contact dermatitis

        Classic from major glove components

        Other potential allergens: NRL itself, sulfites, and multiple other potential additives

    Contact urticaria,[1]angioedema, and anaphylaxis

        Classic from NRL proteins

        Other: cornstarch; accelerators; phthalates, nitrile, PVC, polyethylene, and gloves contaminated with NRL; Physical urticaria (pressure urticaria);[9] multiple other potential additives[10–12]

Aggravation of pre-existing dermatoses by gloves, e.g., atopic eczema, psoriasis, chronic urticaria, dermographism, etc.

Penetration of chemicals through gloves—epoxy, acrylics, permanent wave chemicals, etc.

Other:

    Chemical leukoderma[13–24, 94–98]

    Endotoxin reaction[25, 100–111]

    Ethylene oxide and other sterilization reactions[26–37, 112–134]

Key: NRL natural rubber latex; PVC polyvinylchloride.

Sources: Adapted from Chew, A.L. and H.I. Maibach, Irritant Dermatitis, 2006: Springer; Estlander, T. and Jolanki, R., *Dermatol. Clin.,* 6, 105, 1988; and McSweeney SM and White IR. Contact urticaria to non-latex synthetic glove material: A case report. Contact Dermatitis, 2020;83:417–418.

COVID-19 has had a major impact on healthcare workers (HCWs) with shortages of all types of personal protective equipment, including gloves, and concerns over HCWs' well-being and safety from infectious exposures through re-use of personal protective equipment, especially masks. There has been an increase in double gloving, and data show that one-step removal of gloves and gowns and sanitizing gloves before doffing with quaternary ammonium or bleach, but not with alcohol-based hand sanitizers, may decrease contamination.[39–41]

18.2 IRRITANT REACTIONS

Irritant contact dermatitis is probably the most frequent adverse glove reaction, especially among those with occupational exposure to latex gloves. This non-immunological cutaneous response manifests as dry, crusted lesions on glove-exposed areas.[42] The nationwide voluntary reporting program for adverse events associated with medical devices maintained by the U.S. Food and Drug Administration (U.S. FDA) received 2396 reports from 1985 to 1999, describing either local or systemic reactions associated with the use of medical gloves.[43] Irritation as a symptom was reported by 15% of individuals, and 3% were reported with a diagnosis of irritant dermatitis. Heese et al.[44] found that of 432 latex glove intolerant reactions, irritation occurred in 40%, type I latex allergy in 33.1%, type IV allergic contact dermatitis in 20.4%, and both type I and type IV reactions in 6.5%.

Two studies based on questionnaires among hospital and dental personnel showed that 37% and 29%, respectively, complained of irritation from gloves.[45,46] In the latter study, Burke et al.[46] noted a strong association between patterns of glove use and incidence of skin irritation, with routine glove users developing skin irritation more often than the occasional users. Additionally, female respondents were more likely to have experienced skin irritation than male respondents. Another study, which examined the effect of glove occlusion on normal skin, showed a significantly negative effect on skin barrier function as measured by transepidermal water loss, concluding that gloves may be a substantial factor in the pathogenesis of cumulative irritant contact dermatitis.[47]

Heese et al.[48] suggest that irritation from gloves occurs especially in atopic individuals and that the reactions may be mechanically provoked by glove powder. The FDA banned the use of powdered gloves in medical and surgical practice in 2016 due to wound infections, surgical complications, and latex allergy promoted by cornstarch powder.[49] Powdered gloves continue to be used outside of the hospital setting due to their cost effectiveness and ease of fit. Cornstarch is the most common glove powder used today and has replaced club moss (*Lycopodium*) powder and talc.[50,51] Lactose has also occasionally been used, and on some gloves, silicone has been used.[52] In addition, glove powders have been employed in latex glove dipping to facilitate glove removal from porcelain molds. According to Dr D. Hogan (personal communication, May 1991), Tolbert and Brown's[50] study of glove powder showed that because the powder is applied before gloves are fully cured, particles become embedded in the soft rubber. Thus, once powdered, a glove can never be made powder-free. Brehler et al.[53] studied the effect of glove powder on skin irritation and concluded that skin roughness increased after using certain powdered gloves. A large variation in the pH of the gloves tested was also found, with a higher pH noted on powdered gloves. They proposed that the variation of glove chemicals and powder, and glove pH, might be responsible for skin irritation from gloves, as the dissociation constant of chemicals is associated with their irritant capability.[54] In another study for irritant reactions to glove powder, Held et al.[55] found that glove powder caused significantly lower skin hydration levels, with the result that this drying effect could be the first sign of irritant contact dermatitis.

Gloves can produce occlusion and maceration, especially following prolonged use, which are major factors in glove irritation.[48,56,57] Compounding these factors may be the practice of double gloving for infectious cases, friction from gloves rubbing against skin, and frequent hand washing with surgical scrubs and brushes. Cutaneous exposure to soaps, detergents, and other cleaning agents is also a major factor in the high prevalence of irritant dermatitis in occupations such as hospital cleaning.[48] Rietschel[58] has emphasized that in certain industrial situations gloves may serve as wicks, absorbing chemicals and then aggravating or producing dermatitis. Rarely is bacterial endotoxin released by gamma-irradiated gloves and ethylene oxide-sterilized gloves an irritant factor[48] (see separate discussion of these two entities). Penetration of chemicals through gloves and aggravation of existing skin disease are other contributing causes.[59] Mathias[60] believes that gloves should not be worn over inflamed skin unless worn for short periods and topical corticosteroids are first applied. Irritation may also be caused by increased glove use and overuse in unnecessary tasks. One study found glove use was appropriate at rates of only 59% on hospital wards vs. 90% in the laboratory. Only 52% of nurses washed their hands upon doffing their gloves.[61] Variations in the thickness and tightness of examination, surgical, utility, and industrial gloves may be factors in producing irritation. Tight ambidextrous gloves can cause pain, particularly in the thumb area, if worn for long periods of time.[62]

The type of glove material may also be important (Table 18.2). Cut-resistant work gloves are typically produced with yarn that contains an inner core made from materials such as fiberglass, steel, or basalt. This inner core is then enclosed by an outer shell made of cut-resistant materials such as high-performance polyethylene (HPPE) composite yarn or Kevlar (para-aramid fibers), and a filler made of polyester, spandex, or nylon. Over time, the fibers of the inner core can become fragmented and irritate the skin of workers who are prone to developing irritant contact dermatitis. Recently, manufacturers have begun producing cut-resistant gloves specifically for individuals who are prone to contact dermatitis. These gloves are produced with yarn that lacks the inner core and are claimed to not cause skin irritation. These gloves continue to be cut resistant due to the infusion of strength-enhancing microparticles.[63]

Some of the published literature on irritation is relevant to glove reactions. Lammintausta and Maibach[42] classify irritation from all causes into eight clinical types: (1) acute irritant dermatitis (primary irritation), (2) irritant reactions, (3) delayed acute irritant dermatitis, (4) cumulative irritant contact dermatitis, (5) traumatic irritant dermatitis, (6) pustular and acneiform dermatitis, (7) non-erythematous

---

TABLE 18.2
Glove Materials

Rubber polymers (cause of most glove reactions)—Natural rubber latex; synthetic rubbers: synthetic polyisoprene, butyl, nitrile, Neoprene, polyurethane, and Viton®

Plastic polymers—Polyvinyl chloride, polyethylene, polyvinyl alcohol

Multilayered laminate—Ethylene vinyl alcohol co-polymer is laminated with polyethylene on both sides (Silver Shield 4H™-gloves), polyethylene-nylon-polyethylene laminate

Leather—Chrome or vegetable tanned

Textiles—Natural or synthetic; woven from fabrics, knit or terry cloth; may be coated with rubber or plastic

Special material—Wire cloth

Source: Adapted from Estlander, T. et al., Protective gloves, in *Hand Eczema,* Menné, T. and Maibach, H.I., Eds., CRC Press, Boca Raton, FL, 2000, chap 18.

TABLE 18.3

Types and Examples of Irritation and Associated Glove Dermatitis

Type of Irritation	Examples of Direct Chemical, Physical, or Mechanical Causes	Examples of Possible Associated Skin Reactions to Gloves
Acute irritant dermatitis	Strong acid or alkali burn	Excess ETO in gloves
Irritant reactions	Wet work, perm chemicals, detergents, soaps	Chemicals penetrating gloves
Delayed acute irritant reaction	ETO and HF burns; hexanediol, and butanediol diacrylates[64]	Excess ETO in gloves; HF penetrating gloves
Chronic (cumulative) irritant contact dermatitis	Wet work	Sweating and maceration from gloves; chemical gloves
Traumatic irritant dermatitis	Burn; laceration	Possible aggravation by gloves
Pustular and acneiform dermatitis	Tar, oil, grease, metals	Acne mechanica from glove or gauntlet friction
Non-erythematous irritation	Cosmetics; textiles	Possible glove occlusion as a direct cause
Subjective irritation	Lactic acid	Possible enhancement by gloves
Friction dermatitis[65]	Low-grade friction, e.g., paperwork	Gloves stiffened by tar or dirtied with abrasive materials

Note: ETO = ethylene oxide; HF = hydrofluoric acid.

Source: Modified from Lammintausta, K. and Maibach, H.I., in *Occupational Skin Diseases,* Adams, R.M., Ed., W.B. Saunders, Philadelphia, 1990, chap. 1; and Chew, A.L. and H.I. Maibach, Irritant Dermatitis, 2006.

irritation, and (8) subjective irritation. Table 18.3 lists the types and causes of irritation as well as examples of possible glove-associated dermatitis.

Clinical features that may suggest a specific direct chemical, physical, or mechanical cause of irritant dermatitis include (1) ulceration, (2) folliculitis and acne, (3) miliaria, (4) pigmentary changes, (5) alopecia, (6) urticaria, and (7) granulomas.[42] Of these, gloves may directly cause or have been reported to cause ulceration from severe ethylene oxide (ETO) burns (see Section 18.6 on ETO); folliculitis, miliaria, or both from friction or occlusion; hypopigmentation from glove antioxidants, usually an immunologic reaction (see Section 18.4 on chemical leukoderma); ICU from natural rubber latex proteins; and possibly nonimmunologic contact urticaria from glove powder.[1,48,59] In other cases gloves may indirectly aggravate ulceration caused by chemicals or directly prevent ulceration, pigmentary changes, urticaria, and granulomas by acting as a barrier between chemicals and the skin.

Noncutaneous granulomas from talc have been reported in wound scars and intra-abdominal adhesions. Talc has been replaced by starch, but granulomas from starch also have been reported in the peritoneum, pleura, pericardium, synovium, cranium, and eye.[51] Starch-free (powder-free) gloves are now available from many glove suppliers.

The diagnosis of irritant dermatitis is generally based on the exclusion of allergic contact dermatitis and ICU. Rietschel's[66] criteria for irritant dermatitis include (1) a rapid onset of symptoms (minutes to hours), (2) discomfort, especially in the early stages (especially stinging and burning), and less so (3) onset of dermatitis within two weeks of exposure, and (4) the identification of other persons similarly affected.[67]

In Maibach's view (personal communication, February 1993), irritant reactions specific to gloves are suggested by three observations. First, patch testing with pieces of some gloves results in macular erythema at 48 h that largely resolves at 96 h. A similar patch test response occurs in 21-day cumulative assay studies. Also, some patients with neither allergic contact dermatitis nor ICU can tolerate a latex glove only with a liner. Silk, nylon, and cotton liners are available. Silk (Sensi Touch®) liners are claimed by the manufacturer to preserve tactile sensation while absorbing sweat and reducing friction.[67]

The moist, cotton-lined interior of rubber gloves may also be an ideal location for the growth of *Pseudomonas aeruginosa*, which is a gram-negative bacillus that thrives in warm, damp environments and can cause infection by entering through disruptions in the skin barrier. Though *Pseudomonas* is known for causing infections after the use of whirlpools, hot tubs, and saunas, rubber gloves were reported to be the source of infection in a woman who has been diagnosed with *Pseudomonas* folliculitis of the hands.[8] Though *Pseudomonas* infection is typically benign and self-limited in the immunocompetent, it is an important public health concern due to infections in the immunocompromized. To prevent rubber gloves from being a source of infection, rubber gloves should be cleaned and dried after each use.

The use of protective gloves is necessary when direct contact with hazardous substances cannot be prevented. Though gloves can offer protection for the skin, they can also cause irritant reactions. Proper use of protective gloves can decrease the occurrence of these reactions. Gloves should be selected according to the tasks being performed and the materials being handled and should only be impermeable if necessary for protection against the hazardous agent. Disposable gloves should not be reused, and reusable gloves should only be reused if they are clean. If gloves are to be reused, cotton inner gloves are recommended. When doffing gloves, the user should be careful to avoid making contact between the skin and the soiled outer surface of the gloves.[68]

Glove irritation needs continued study with *in vitro*, *in vivo*, and predictive cumulative irritation studies. All glove components and materials should be investigated.

18.3   CONTACT AND OTHER URTICARIA

CU due to natural rubber latex (NRL), especially NRL gloves was a major global occupational health issue in the 1980s and 1990s, reaching a peak of 17% of HCW and 70% of spina bifida patients affected. Although today less than 1% of the population is affected,[2-5] NRL allergy is still an important consideration in HCW with hand dermatitis, asthma, and urticaria, and it is important for patients with spina bifida to avoid all NRL from birth. The latter is critical for neurosurgeons, urologists, and orthopedists who care for these patients. The Finnish occupational health register listed NRL allergy as the third most common cause of contact urticaria from 2005 to 2016 but is decreasing in frequency.[4] There is still no FDA-cleared latex skin test reagent in the USA, and the use of a highly specific immunologic test (ImmunoCAP, immuno solid-phase allergen chip [ISAC], or cellular antigen stimulation test [CAST]) may produce false-negative results.[3] NRL allergy should still be considered in those with a positive history and negative immunologic test. CU to NRL is most frequently the result of IgE-mediated immediate-type allergy to one of 26 *Hevea brasiliensis* allergens identified by the WHO/International Union of Immunological Societies.

CU to other components of gloves is uncommon but should be considered in patients with symptoms of CU due to synthetic rubber gloves, as well as in patients without latex allergy but who still develop CU to latex gloves.[69] CU due to non-latex gloves may also be caused by contamination with latex allergens during the manufacturing process.[70] Immediate-type reactions due to glove powder itself have been reported, although infrequently. Absorbable dusting powder consists of mainly cornstarch, which initially contains a small part of corn (maize) protein, which is the main suspect. The glove manufacturing process is supposed to remove this soluble maize protein almost completely; however, electrophoretic analysis of glove powders has detected the presence of proteins.[48,71] This suggests that besides causing irritant dermatitis and acting as a vehicle for other allergens, cornstarch powder may act as a type I allergen itself.

Van der Meeren[71] was the first to report a 29-year-old male nurse with severe CU from cornstarch glove powder. Prick tests on the powdered glove were strongly positive, although IgE antibodies to corn could not be detected. In another report of anaphylaxis due to cornstarch, the authors were unable to demonstrate a positive RAST to corn.[72] Fisher[73] reported a case with CU to a surgical powdered glove in which patch testing with a piece of the powdered glove produced an immediate urticarial reaction, whereas patch tests to washed glove gave negative results; a RAST for corn was not performed. Seggev et al.[74] reported two nurses with anaphylaxis due to powdered gloves who also developed respiratory symptoms. One of the nurses also developed symptoms when several coworkers donned powdered gloves, possibly in response to exposure to airborne cornstarch powder. This individual developed anaphylaxis following a prick test to cornstarch powder, while the second had a positive skin test. IgE antibodies to natural corn or cornstarch powder were not present in either patient. Both could wear nonpowdered latex gloves and ate corn without incident. The authors hypothesized that the altered, polymerized cornstarch caused *in vivo* mast cell activation and mediator release by some unknown mechanism. Crippa et al.[75] evaluated eight hospital personnel for suspected type I allergic symptoms from cornstarch powder; two had respiratory symptoms in addition to urticaria. The serum IgE test for corn was positive in three individuals, three others had positive IgE antibodies to both corn and latex, and two were negative to both. In the two patients with negative IgE antibodies, prick tests were positive: one for corn and the other for both corn and latex. All the patients had symptoms only in the workplace, and none had food allergies to corn.

Allergens in various rubber products can also cause CU. For example, CU to the carbamate accelerator in rubber has been reported.[76–78] Belsito reported three patients with CU to carbamates, mercaptobenzothiazole (MBT), and black rubber mix.[77] Two of these patients had a combined CU and delayed hypersensitivity to carbamates and MBT. CU was confirmed with scratch/chamber and open scratch tests. RAST testing for these rubber chemicals was not available, so it could not be confirmed if these reactions were IgE mediated. In another study of 31 patients with hand dermatitis, urticarial test reactions were reported to tetramethyl thiuram disulfide, mercapto mix, and p-phenylenediamine (PPD) mix.[79] CU to MBT in nitrile gloves in a latex-allergic patient has been reported.[80] However, type I allergy to rubber chemicals is quite rare; Brehler and Sedlmayr[81] prick-tested 75 patients allergic to natural rubber latex (NRL) with rubber chemicals and found no relevant positive tests. They concluded that prick tests with rubber chemicals are unnecessary in the routine diagnosis of latex-allergic patients. Contamination of non-latex gloves with latex allergens during the manufacturing process can also cause CU. Five workers in a hospital presented with immediate reactions (contact urticaria and/or rhinoconjunctivitis) with the use of three lots of Dermagrip® nitrile gloves. All five had previously been diagnosed with IgE-mediated hypersensitivity to latex and had tolerated nitrile gloves in the past from other lots from the same and other manufacturer(s). IgE immunoblotting showed that latex allergens were detected in the three lots of contaminated gloves, while no latex allergens were detected in nitrile gloves from other manufacturers.[70] In a more recent case contact urticaria was reported to an unknown component of a blue nitrile glove in a physician who developed urticaria on her hands and other touch points (e.g., face) shortly after donning nitrile gloves. A closed patch for 20 min on her forearm was strongly positive for urticaria. Coworkers were not affected, and she substituted Neoprene gloves without reaction.[82]

Sugiura et al.[83] reported CU to di(2-ethylhexyl)phthalate in the dotted PVC grip of cotton gloves. They subsequently reported CU to polyethylene gloves in another patient.[84] This patient had positive scratch test reactions to octadecanoic acid methyl ester, 2,6-di-tert-butylphenol, di(2-ethylhexyl)phthalate, cis-13-docosenoic acid amide, and octadecyl 3-(3,5-di-tert-butyl-4-hydroxy-phenyl) propionate; these chemicals are used as antioxidants and lubricants in polyethylene. Both patients were brothers who had chronic urticaria, which worsened when they wore gloves at work. Cow's milk casein is used as a stabilizer in glove manufacturing and can cause CU syndrome in individuals with cow's milk allergy.[85] CU was also reported to be caused by polyvinylchloride (PVC) gloves in a patient who developed three episodes of pruritus of the hands and wrists, each within minutes of donning the gloves. Her symptoms of localized pruritus progressed to generalized pruritus, edema of the lips and tongue, and dyspnea. This patient showed early patch test reactions to pieces of the PVC glove, but no other early or delayed patch test reaction to any of the additives usually found in PVC gloves.[86]

According to Heese et al.[48] nonimmunologic contact urticaria (NICU) from gloves has not been reported, but sorbic acid, a known NICU agent, is sometimes added to glove powder and should be considered in evaluating patients with glove-induced CU.

Pressure urticaria and cholinergic urticaria associated with glove use should be diagnosed by the patient's history and cutaneous examination.[48] Armstrong et al.[6] reported a case of glove-related urticaria of the hands in a hospital worker who did not have type I allergy to latex or type IV hypersensitivity to rubber chemicals. The patient developed a dermographic urticarial response whenever she scratched her hands while wearing the gloves; dermographism could also be elicited at other skin sites. A diagnosis of glove irritation leading to a secondary dermographic response was made. Thomson et al.[7] reported three healthcare workers with a history of itching and inflammation of hands related to latex glove use; localized dermographism could be demonstrated in all patients. Patch and prick testing to latex was negative. The dermographism was thought to be precipitated by pressure or shearing forces produced by the recurrent application and removal of tight-fitting surgical gloves.

Pressure urticaria, a form of physical urticaria, is either localized at the stimulus site (contact type) or associated with distant reactions, such as hypotension, tachycardia, tickle, or pruritus of the nose or fingertips (reflex type).[9] Atopy is frequently absent, and lesions do not occur at night. Pressure urticaria arises after a single stimulus, and the skin reaction is not a typical wheal but rather a reddened, deeper, sometimes painful swelling of the angioedema type. Urticarial dermographism may be associated with pressure urticaria. Pressure urticaria and urticarial dermographism can be classified as immediate (3–30 minutes) or delayed (2–6 h) types.[9,87]

Cholinergic (sweat or exertion) urticaria follows an increase in body temperature. Tiny, confluent, pruritic wheals on patchy erythema develop; lesions usually occur on the upper body after physical exertion or sweating and urticarial dermographism may be present.[9]

Distinguishing irritant reactions in NICU may be difficult. Lahti[88] points out that strong irritants, such as hydrochloric acid, formaldehyde, and phenol, can cause immediate whealing followed by erythema, and either scaling or crusting, which lasts 20 h or longer. Nicotinic acid esters produce only CU; sodium lauryl sulfate is a pure irritant while phenol and dimethyl sulfoxide have both features. Diagnostic tests for NICU and ICU include the rub, use, open application, patch, and chamber tests, usually performed in that order. Prick, RAST, and passive transfer tests are negative in NICU.

In 1984, Anderson and Maibach[89] described multiple-application, delayed-onset CU to formalin as possibly related to certain textile reactions. The reaction appeared on normal skin after repeated open applications but only after a single application on diseased skin. Although they described this reaction as possibly a non-clinically relevant epiphenomenon, it could be relevant to unexplained glove reactions.

In 2015 Hawkey and Ghaffar reported 17 patients with glove-related hand urticaria as an increasing problem among healthcare workers, 11 of whom had concurrent dermatitis; 10 had CU from NRL gloves, 12 CU from nitrile gloves, and 5 to both types; and three had underlying idiopathic urticaria.[90] They proposed a testing algorithm including a 20-minute closed patch test on the forearm with a 5 × 5 cm glove piece to avoid possible false positives with the one finger and subsequent whole hand glove challenges. Idiopathic urticaria and dermographism are confounding factors. The authors also emphasize the importance of a correct diagnosis noting that some patients may have both immediate urticarial and delayed eczematous reactions.

ICD and atopic eczema along with other entities described in this chapter are important to consider as differential and concomitant diagnoses.[90,91] These include psoriasis[92] and other reasons for developing hand eczema associated with glove use, especially in a group of hairdressers: (1) Inappropriate glove use with increased exposure to allergens from internal contamination, e.g., turning disposable gloves inside out and reusing them; and washing disposable gloves and dusting them with talcum powder before turning them inside out; (2) incorrect doffing of gloves with chemical contamination of the hands; and (3) wearing incorrectly sized gloves—too big or small or too short with contamination of the forearms.[93]

18.4   CHEMICAL LEUKODERMA

The first cases of chemical leukoderma occurred in tannery workers wearing heavy rubber gloves and were reported in 1939 and 1940 by Schwartz, Oliver, and Warren of the US Public Health Service.[13,14] These reports are classics in the annals of occupational dermatology. Depigmentation of the skin was caused by the rubber antioxidant "Agerite Alba," also known as monobenzylether of hydroquinone (MBEH). In one tannery 25 (52%) of 48 workers who wore heavy acid-cured rubber gloves with MBEH present at 0.5% were affected. The workers wore rubber gloves for many months before the leukoderma developed. According to the 1940 report, "itching and in some case mild dermatitis" preceded the appearance of the depigmentation without "great discomfort." However, in a 1947 review, Schwartz[15] stated, "There was [sic] no inflammatory symptoms at any time." This discrepancy may be explained by 1940 report[14] that no signs of acute or chronic dermatitis were present in the areas of leukoderma at the time of examination. In some workers, the leukoderma occurred on the hands and halfway up the forearms with a uniform sharp cutoff line corresponding to areas covered by the gloves. In others, there was a patchy, guttate, confetti-like pigment loss. The face and trunk were also involved in some workers, probably from direct contact with the gloves. Hair in the leukodermic areas remained pigmented. The depigmentation was most marked in African-Americans, less intense in Hispanics, and noticeable in Caucasians only in the summer.

Patch testing with various chemicals in the gloves confirmed MBEH as the cause.[14] Eight different patch tests with unspecified concentrations of the glove ingredients were occluded for seven days on ten workers. When one of the MBEH patch test sites (site 3) was read at 14 days on each of the ten workers, all showed a positive eczematous reaction and six of the ten showed leukoderma. After six months, three more workers had developed leukoderma at the patch test sites. There was no direct "correlation between intensity of skin reaction to the MBEH patch tests and the subsequent development of leukoderma"[14] Other MBEH patch tests occluded for 72 h caused leukoderma to develop three to five months after the patches were removed. Hydroquinone was present as an impurity at less than 1% and was not a factor in the leukoderma.

Several months after workers stopped using the gloves, partial repigmentation occurred. Repigmentation was perifollicular, spreading peripherally; was more rapid in some than in others; and was "practically completed in all the cases three years later. The general health of the workers was not affected."[14] Further investigation by the US Public Health Service showed that a considerable percentage of workers wearing the same make of gloves in the tanneries and other industries were also affected. According to Ortonne, Mosher, and Fitzpatrick, in 1939 McNally[16] reported depigmentation in 34 employees in a tannery. Leukoderma also occurred at remote sites and was attributed to accidental direct contact with the gloves. In 1959, Botvinick[17] reported dermatitis and secondary leukoderma from a fabric-lined household glove. MBEH was identified in one of the gloves, and dermatitis and leukoderma were reproduced by patch testing.

In 1985, one of us (JST) evaluated a patient with chemical leukoderma on the hands associated with wearing a glove manufactured in Germany but distributed in the USA. The company stated that MBEH was not present in the glove, and the cause of the leukoderma remains unknown. In 1992, Bajaj et al.[18] identified a patient with depigmentation at the site of a hearing aid. High-pressure liquid chromatography revealed that the hearing aid contained MBEH.

Leukoderma caused by MBEH has been reported from a number of other rubber devices including tape, diaphragms, condoms, finger cots, clothing, aprons, dolls, and shoes.[19,20] It has also been identified in synthetic Neoprene® rubber.[21] The US rubber industry has not used MBEH as an antioxidant for many years.[1]

Some chemicals related to MBEH that also produce pigment loss include hydroquinone,[19] monomethylether of hydroquinone (p-methoxyphenol or p-hydroxyanisole), and monoethyl-ether of hydroquinone (p-ethoxyphenol). Hydroquinone rarely produces complete depigmentation, does not produce pigment loss at distant sites as does MBEH, and is a weaker allergen than MBEH.

Several other depigmenting chemicals have now been identified, including alkylphenol p-tertiary butylphenol (PTBP), pyrethroid insecticides, hexamethylenetetramine, mercurial, arsenics, and sulfhydryls. When present in excess in Neoprene rubber glue containing p-tertiary butylphenol formaldehyde resins, PTBP has been associated with depigmentation in industrial workers and consumers when present in wristwatch adhesive and plastic shoes.[1,19] To our knowledge, PTBP has not been found in gloves.

Pyrethroid insecticides (cypermethrin and beta-cyfluthrin) from an insect sprayer were reported to have caused chemical leukoderma on the head, trunk, and extremities of a patient who worked for 15 years spraying insecticides.[94] Hexamethylenetetramine, a chemical found in adhesives and sealants, was reported to cause chemical leukoderma in a factory worker who mixed adhesives, chemicals, and other raw materials together to produce automobile materials.[95] In China, two cases of chemical leukoderma due to dimethyl sulfate, a chemical used in the production of pharmaceuticals, perfumes, and pesticides, were recently described.[96]

No other reported cases of chemical leukoderma from gloves were found after a literature search for the past 45 years. Occupational vitiligo was reported after the appearance of allergic contact dermatitis in a firefighter. He initially had vitiligo and thiuram allergy and developed disseminated dermatitis and depigmentation after wearing firefighting gear.[21] In another report, occupational depigmentation from dinoterbe (2-t-butyl 4,6-dinitrophenol structurally related to PTBP and present in the herbicide Herbogil®) began as depigmentation on the hands and improved when the worker started wearing gloves.[22]

Chemical leukoderma may be difficult to differentiate from idiopathic vitiligo.[23] While chemical leukoderma is limited to the part of the body exposed to the chemical agent, idiopathic vitiligo most commonly causes lesions that are symmetrically distributed on the dorsal hands and forearms and around the mouth and eyes. Idiopathic vitiligo usually occurs in the second decade of life, and patients often have a family history of similar lesions.[97] The "mode of spread may be helpful for diagnosis—a history of gradual coalescence of small discrete macules, rather than the development of large macules with perifollicular sparing suggests chemical leukoderma."[20] Scalp hair is rarely involved, and eye color does not change. The period for exposure ranges from two weeks to approximately six months.[23] Depigmentation is not always preceded by inflammation of the affected skin but is frequently associated with allergic contact dermatitis to the same chemical responsible for the pigment loss, although the latter is not a prerequisite.[16] The absence of preceding inflammation may be explained by the resistance of some idiopathic vitiligo patients to developing a contact allergy in depigmented skin sites.[24] Wood's light examination of the skin in a dark room may identify areas of leukoderma not obvious on routine visual inspection of the skin.

Diagnosis of chemical leukoderma is more easily made when a number of cases are clustered in a factory, and there is a history of worker exposure to a known depigmenting agent; when pigment loss follows contact dermatitis; or when the person affected is an adult without childhood or family history of vitiligo.[23] Patch tests with putative depigmenting agents may result in leukoderma at the sites of positive or negative tests for up to six weeks or more after application. Satellite depigmentation may occur, and patch testing should be done cautiously (we prefer to patch test on the buttocks) with unknown chemicals. Application of the putative chemicals to black guinea pigs[23] and identification of unknown depigmenting agents by HPLC[18] are alternative test methods.

Table 18.4 lists a number of reported causes of chemical leukoderma.

18.5 ENDOTOXINS

Endotoxin is an inflammatory agent made by gram-negative bacteria that can irritate the skin and induce respiratory problems, fever, and shock. It is an adjuvant for both delayed hypersensitivity and IgE production and has been known to magnify antigen-specific mediator release. Endotoxin reactions are "an ever-present danger in the preparation of biological agents for intravenous and intramuscular use."[25] The problems associated with endotoxin reactions are usually systemic and characterized by fever, chills, and hypotension. Local reactions may also occur. Generalized and localized Schwartzman reactions "are older terms used in reference to these reactions." Endotoxins may have an immunomodulatory effect on the development

TABLE 18.4
Selected Reported Causes of Chemical Leukoderma

Phenol/catechol derivatives
  Monobenzylether of hydroquinone (MBH)
  Monomethylether of hydroquinone (MMH, p-methoxyphenol, or p-hydroxyanisole)
  Monoethyl-ether of hydroquinone (MEH, p-ethoxyphenol)
  Hydroquinone
  p-tert-Butylcatechol (PTBC)
  p-tert-Butylphenol (PTBP)
  p-tert-Amylphenol (PTAP)
Sulfhydryls
  Cysteamine
  Sulfanolic acid
  Cystamine dihydrochloride
Others
  Mercurials
  Arsenic
  Ammoniated mercury
  Dimethyl sulfate[96]
  Cinnamic aldehyde
  Tretinoin
  Azo dyes
  Benzoyl peroxide
  Red alta
  Rhododendrol[98]
  Fluorouracil
  Chloroquine
  Imatinib mesylate
  Fluphenazine
  Paraphenylenediamine (PPD)
  Azelaic acid
  Corticosteroids
  Brilliant lake red R
  Soymilk and derived protein Thiotepa (inhibits PAR-2)
  Methylphenidate[99]
  Pyrethroid insecticides (cypermethrin and beta-cyfluthrin) [94]
  Hexamethylenetetramine[95]

Source: Adapted from Harris JE. Chemical-Induced Vitiligo. Dermatol Clin. 2017;35(2):151–161. doi:10.1016/j.det.2016.11.006

of latex allergy.[100,101] The pathogenesis of fever in endotoxin reactions "is due to the release of endogenous pyrogens from activated granulocytes rather than a direct response to bacterial endotoxin. The exogenous stimuli can be bacteremia, viremia, or endotoxemia."[102] NRL gloves can be contaminated with endotoxin.[103,104] Glove powder may both support the growth of microbes and act as a vehicle for endotoxin.[105]

Williams et al.[106] reported that nonsterile examination gloves had an average of 135 times more endotoxin than sterile surgical gloves, with powdered gloves containing higher amounts of endotoxin. Endotoxin was found mostly on the inside of the gloves, suggesting that contamination occurred at the time of manufacture. They hypothesize that endotoxin may be responsible for some of the irritation associated with latex glove use, considering their proinflammatory properties. In addition, it may also be responsible for the enhancement of the immediate and delayed hypersensitivity reactions to proteins and chemicals found in gloves. Interestingly, paradoxical increases in endotoxin levels have been reported with steam sterilization (autoclaving)[107] and gamma irradiation.[25]

Shmunes and Darby[25] reported the only known case of contact dermatitis apparently due to endotoxin present in irradiated latex gloves worn by a hospital phlebotomist. The patient developed "vivid erythema along the sides and back of the finger shafts with vesiculation and relative sparing of the palms."[25] The source of the irritation, which occurred clinically and on usage tests 12–24 h after wearing gloves (Micro Touch® by Arbrook, Inc.) for 10–20 minutes, was linked to bacterial endotoxin in sterile latex gloves. The reaction repeatedly recurred within the same timeframe. On one occasion after handling a rubber tourniquet enclosed in a sterile intravenous catheter packed for several minutes, isolated patches and linear streaks developed under the patient's chin, neck, cheek, and eyelid. A rubbing test using a tourniquet from a freshly opened catheter pack produced a positive response. Patch tests done with the standard screening tray were negative. The gloves, however, were not patch tested. There was no immediate itching within the first hours suggestive of CU. The lag time of at least 12 h between testing and the development of the erythema and vesicles made delayed CU seem unlikely. RAST or prick testing was not performed. Glove samples from the same lot were analyzed, and all were found to contain endotoxin levels higher than permitted. Sterilization of the gloves by gamma irradiation was reported to increase endotoxin levels when the bacterial count was elevated. Water-soluble endotoxin was absorbed onto powder inside the gloves, and sweating under the gloves may have enhanced entry into the skin. No systemic symptoms, which may occur in cases of endotoxin reactions from contaminated biological agents intended for intramuscular or intravenous use, were reported. Shmunes and Darby[25] postulate that dyshidrosis from cutting fluids could also be based on bacterial endotoxins.

Recently, a group in Japan evaluated four types of single-use sterile surgical gloves and found that three of the four gloves showed endotoxin contamination. Contaminated gloves were also found to have increased cytokine production in comparison to uncontaminated gloves.[108] In addition to finding increased endotoxin levels on unused gloves, another study found that the gloves had a high variability of endotoxin contamination across brands and between various lots ranging between <1.5 and 5810 endotoxin units.[109] Though there is a minimum allowable endotoxin level on medical devices, a permissible endotoxin concentration for gloves has not been established.[110,111] Establishing a minimum allowable endotoxin concentration for gloves may prevent future glove-related reactions to endotoxin.

18.6   ETHYLENE OXIDE AND OTHER STERILIZATION METHODS

Ethylene oxide (ETO) was first used as a sterilizing agent for medical supplies in 1962. It has now become the most widely used gaseous sterilization agent in the world.[112,113] The ability of ETO to sterilize depends on its alkylating properties and irreversible bactericidal effect on cell metabolism. Over the years it has been used to sterilize several reusable medical supplies susceptible to heat, such as those made of plastic and rubber, in which ETO is soluble and retained in large amounts after sterilization. Chemical ETO treatment is very useful for sterilizing gloves in forensic science due to its ability to destroy contaminating DNA from saliva, blood, and skin cells. Treatment with chemical ETO was shown to be superior to gamma irradiation and electron beam treatment in reducing the amount of PCR-amplifiable DNA.[114] Hazards associated with inadequate aeration of ETO-sterilized devices and equipment include cutaneous burns (e.g., from rubber gloves), tracheal inflammation (e.g., endotracheal tubes), hemolysis (e.g., from plastic tubing), and anaphylaxis (e.g., plastic and rubber tubing used for hemodialysis).[26,115,116] Adequate aeration of the devices is therefore imperative to ensure that all ETO residues are eliminated.[26–28,117]

There have been reports of ETO irritation and burns from industrial[29] and medical gloves.[30] Royce and Moore[29] report ETO irritation in microbiology workers. A hermetically sealed glove box, devised for performing aseptic operations in a microbiology laboratory, was sterilized with ETO vapor. When the box's long rubber gloves were used without adequate aeration, all the operators developed dermatitis. The problem was solved by extending the whole of the glove and gauntlet outside of the box and allowing the rubber to "air off" for 1.5 h before work started.[29] Rendell-Baker et al.[31] cited instances of burns on surgeons' hands from ETO residues in gloves. In another case, he cited hand irritation from ethylene chlorohydrin and ethylene glycol residues in ETO-sterilized gloves.[32] Other studies have shown these two compounds to be much less irritating than ETO.[26] In 1988, Fisher[30] reported ETO burns on the hands of a hospital worker wearing heavy-duty rubber gloves.

ETO burns continue to be reported, although not from gloves. A 1998 report from Mexico and a 2000 report from Turkey described burns from silicone mammary implants and a blood pressure cuff, respectively.[33,34] In both reports the devices were sterilized with ETO but probably inadequately aerated. In 2010, around 20 employees of a department of surgery in Germany developed eczematous skin reactions at the contact areas of wrist bands from surgical gowns that had undergone ETO sterilization.[118] Furthermore, burns due to ETO sterilization have been reported with anesthesia masks, hospital linens, endotracheal tubes, and other medical devices. Commercially sterilized nitrofurazone gauze dressings have also been cited as a cause of first- and second-degree burns. In addition, a number of industrial workers exposed to ETO have suffered burns, irritant contact dermatitis, and allergic contact dermatitis.[26]

The amount of residual ETO after sterilization is greater on rubber products, such as rubber gloves, as compared to metallic objects.[35] Accordingly, when ETO is used, adequate aeration is imperative and probably best handled by mechanical aeration. Special handling of PVC plastic, rubber, and previously gamma-irradiated equipment is indicated. Most equipment now combines the ETO sterilization with aeration cycles.[119]

Not only is ETO a potent irritant, but it also can cause delayed hypersensitivity (allergic contact dermatitis) and immediate hypersensitivity (anaphylaxis).[26,27,29] In 1986, one of us (JST) evaluated an operating room nurse with allergic contact dermatitis of the hands that occurred only after she wore ETO-sterilized gloves. Her patch test reactions to the standard tray, rubber chemicals, a steam-sterilized glove provided by the same manufacturer, and gamma-irradiated gloves were all negative. Her only positive patch test reactions were to pieces of ETO-sterilized gloves, results of which were confirmed several months later after re-testing pieces from the same ETO-sterilized glove. Other batches of the same ETO-sterilized gloves and other brands of ETO-sterilized gloves produced the same clinical and patch test reactions. Her only alternative was to wear gamma-irradiated gloves. Highly reactive ETO can combine with several other chemicals, such as rubber accelerators and iodine. The reaction in this nurse may have been caused by ETO itself or by an ETO rubber-chemical reaction product.[1] Downey showed that the mercaptobenzothiazole vulcanization accelerators in rubber react rapidly with ETO to produce (hydroxyethyl-mercapto)-thiazole, despite the fact that residual ETO concentration in the rubber tubing has been reported to dissipate after 5 h of aeration. Thus, small amounts of free ETO may remain in the rubber matrix and can be a contributing factor in allergic contact dermatitis.[37]

Patch testing for thresholds of ETO irritation and allergy has been carried out with ETO-impregnated materials such as gauze, rubber, PVC, and petrolatum.[28] Fisher[28] reviewed these studies, one of which revealed an irritation threshold of 1000 ppm ETO in thick PVC or petrolatum and atypical mild delayed allergy at 100 ppm in PVC.[37]

Though ETO sterilization is widely used for medical devices, active pharmaceuticals, pharmaceutical packaging and containers, and drug/device containers, most sterile medical gloves are now commercially processed by gamma irradiation. However, gloves may undergo ethylene oxide sterilization if they are prepackaged in kits, such as many catheterization kits,[116,120,121] and male circumcision surgical kits,[122,123] due to being packaged with components that are less suitable for other methods of sterilization. In addition, gloves sterilized with ethylene oxide may be used in forensic science.[114]

Sterilization with hydrogen peroxide vapor (V-PRO), a cold sterilization process, is an alternative to ETO sterilization that has gained popularity. This process uses hydrogen peroxide vapor to penetrate the target and sterilize exposed surfaces. Hydrogen peroxide sterilization has cycle times that typically last less than an hour and is very safe; these sterilization systems are self-contained and only produce water and oxygen as byproducts.[124,125] Vaporized peracetic acid sterilization is another cold sterilization process that uses reactive molecules found in the vapor phase between acetic acid and peracetic acid to denature proteins, disrupt cell wall permeability, and oxidize sulfhydryl and disulfide bonds. This type of sterilization is typically used for medical devices and ideal for stainless steel and many polymers. Residues of vaporized peracetic acid sterilization include acetic acid, peracetic acid, water, and oxygen, which have low concerns for toxicity.[113,125] Though no skin reactions have been reported due to residual peracetic acid or acetic acid from vaporized peracetic acid sterilization or residual hydrogen peroxide from hydrogen peroxide vapor sterilization, these corrosive chemicals have the potential to cause skin irritation or type I hypersensitivity reactions[126] if remaining after sterilization. These reactions could occur due to penetration of the chemicals through the gloves with direct contact of materials sterilized or through sterilization of gloves themselves. Ozone sterilization, which is safe and cost effective and does not leave a residue like ETO, may replace hospital use of ETO in the future but remains less commonly used.[127]

Ortho-phthalaldehyde (OPA) is a disinfectant for heat-sensitive medical equipment that has recently been introduced to the hospital setting and is gaining popularity. It is often used as an alternative to glutaraldehyde sterilization due to its superior anti-mycobactericidal activity. Though OPA is more effective than glutaraldehyde at disinfecting, it appears to be more irritating, even when compared in lower concentrations of OPA.[128] Ortho-phthalaldehyde is an aromatic dialdehyde that has a barely perceptible odor and might be a dermal and respiratory sensitizer. Many allergic reactions including anaphylaxis, urticaria, angioedema, and severe pruritus have been reported.[129] Many protective gloves are permeable to OPA, and individuals working with OPA-sterilized equipment should take proper precautions. Nitrile gloves appear to be much more resistant to OPA than vinyl gloves.[130]

The COVID-19 pandemic has brought a new focus on the sterilization of medical equipment with ozone, ethylene oxide, air ionization, hydrogen peroxide vapor, and UV rays.[131,132] Hydrogen peroxide vapor is being used to sterilize used N95 masks and face shields at many hospitals.[133] Recently, ETO treatment of used and expired N95 respirators showed unchanged fitted filtration efficiencies, suggesting that used or expired N95 respirators treated with ETO can be acceptable alternatives when new N95 respirators are unavailable.[134] Skin reactions should be further investigated as changes in sterilization methods and techniques occur due to COVID-19.[60]

REFERENCES

1. Taylor, J.S. 1986. Rubber, in *Contact Dermatitis*, L. Febiger, Ed. Philadelphia, PA: Fisher AA, Chapter 36.
2. Kelly, K.J., and Sussman, G. 2017. Latex allergy: Where are we now and how did we get there? *J Allergy Clin Immunol Pract* 5(5):1212–6. DOI: 10.1016/j.jaip.2017.05.029.
3. Raulf, M. 2020. Current state of occupational latex allergy. *Curr Opin Allergy Clin Immunol* 20(2):112–6. DOI: 10.1097/ACI.0000000000000611.
4. Pesonen, M., Koskela, K., and Aalto-Korte, K. 2020. Contact urticaria and protein contact dermatitis in the Finnish Register of Occupational Diseases in a period of 12 years. *Contact Dermatitis* 83(1):1–7. DOI: 10.1111/cod.13547.
5. Liberatore, K., and Kelly, K.J. 2018. Latex allergy risks live on. *J Allergy Clin Immunol Pract* 6(6):1877–8. DOI: 10.1016/j.jaip.2018.08.007.
6. Armstrong, D.K.B., Smith, H.R., and Rycroft, R.J.G. 1999. Glove-related hand urticaria in the absence of type I latex allergy. *Contact Dermatitis* 41:42.
7. Thomson, K.F., and Wilkinson, S.M. 1999. Localized dermographism: A differential diagnosis of latex glove allergy. *Contact Dermatitis* 41:103.

8. Mazza, J., Borkin, M., Buchholz, R., and Deleo, V. 2013. Pseudomonas folliculitis contracted from rubber gloves: A public health concern. *J Am Acad Dermatol* 69(2):e93–4.
9. Braun-Falco, O., Plewig, G., Wolff, H.H., and Winkelmann, R.K. 1991. Urticaria, angioedema and anaphylaxis, in *Dermatology, Second Edition*. Berlin, Germany: Springer-Verlag, chap. 11.
10. Rose, R.F., Lyons, P., Horne, H., and Wilkinson, S.M. 2009. A review of the materials and allergens in protective gloves. *Contact Dermatitis* 61(3):129–37. DOI: 10.1111/j.1600-0536.2009.01580.x.
11. Yew, G.Y., Tham, T.C., Show, P.L., Ho, Y.C., Ong, S.K., Law, C.L., Song, C., and Chang, J.S. 2020. Unlocking the secret of bio-additive components in rubber compounding in processing quality nitrile glove. *Appl Biochem Biotechnol* 191(1):1–28. DOI: 10.1007/s12010-019-03207-7.
12. Dendooven, E., Darrigade, A.S., Foubert, K., Pieters, L., Lambert, J., Goossens, A., and Aerts, O. 2020. The presence of sulfites in 'natural rubber latex' and 'synthetic' rubber gloves: An experimental pilot study. *Br J Dermatol* 182(4):1054–5. DOI: 10.1111/bjd.18608.
13. Oliver, E.A. 1993. Chemical hypomelanosis, in *Vitiligo and Other Hypomelanoses of Hair and Skin*, Ortonne, J.-R, Mosher, D.B., and Fitzpatrick, T.B., Eds. New York: Plenum Press, chap. 5.
14. Schwartz, L., Oliver, E.A., and Warren, L.H. 1940. Occupational leukoderma. *Public Health Service Rep* 55:1111.
15. Schwartz, L. 1947. Occupational pigmentary changes in the skin. *Arch Dermatol Syph* 56:592.
16. McNally. 1993. Chemical hypomelanosis, in *Vitiligo and Other Hypomelanoses of Hair and Skin*, Ortonne, J.-P, Mosher, D.B., and Fitzpatrick, T.B., Eds. New York: Plenum Press, chap. 5.
17. Botvinick, I. 1951. Dermatitis and secondary leukoderma due to fabric-lined rubber gloves. *Arch Dermatol Syph* 53:334.
18. Bajaj, A.K., Gupta, S.C., and Chatterjee, A.K. 1992. Hearing aid depigmentation. *Contact Dermatitis* 27:126.
19. Fisher, A.A. 1976. Vitiligo due to contactants. *Cutis* 17:431.
20. Ortonne, J.-P, Mosher, D.B., and Fitzpatrick, T.B. 1993. Chemical hypomelanosis, in *Vitiligo and Other Hypomelanoses of Hair and Skin*. New York: Plenum Press, chap. 5.
21. Riordan, A.T., and Nahass, G.T. 1996. Occupational vitiligo following allergic contact dermatitis. *Contact Dermatitis* 34:371.
22. Sabourad, S., Testud, E., Rogerie, M.J., Decotes, J., and Evreux, J.C. 1997. Occupational depigmentation from dinoterbe. *Contact Dermatitis* 36:227.
23. Gellin, G.A., and Maibach, H.I. 1985. Chemically induced depigmentation, in *Models in Dermatology*, Maibach, H., and Low, N., Eds. Basel: Karger, pp. 282–286.
24. Uehara, M., Miyauchi, H., and Tanaka, S. 1984. Diminished contact sensitivity response in vitiliginous skin. *Arch Dermatol* 120:195.
25. Shmunes, E., and Darby, T. 1984. Contact dermatitis due to endotoxin in irradiated latex gloves. *Contact Dermatitis* 10:240.
26. Taylor, J.S. 1977. Dermatologic hazards from ethylene oxide. *Cutis* 19:189.
27. Glaser, Z.R. 1977. *Use of Ethylene Oxide as a Sterilant in Medical Facilities*. DHEW (NIOSH) Publ. 77–200. Cincinnati, OH: NIOSH, CDC.
28. Fisher, A.A. 1984. Ethylene oxide dermatitis. *Cutis* 34:20.
29. Royce, A., and Moore, W.K.S. 1955. Occupational dermatitis caused by ethylene oxide. *Br J Ind Med* 12:169.
30. Fisher, A.A. 1988. Burns of the hands due to ethylene oxide used to sterilize gloves. *Cutis* 42:267.

31. Rendell-Baker, L., Roberts, R.B., and Watson, B.M. 1969. Problems in sterilization of medical equipment. *Hosp Bur Res News* 16:1.
32. Smith, E.A. 1969. As cited by Rendell-Baker, L. in Problems in sterilization of medical equipment. *Hosp Bur Res News* 16:1.
33. Cardenas-Camerana, L. 1998. Ethylene oxide burns from improperly sterilized mammary implants. *Ann Plast Surg* 41:361.
34. Karacalar, A., and Karacalar, S.A. 2000. Chemical burns due to blood pressure cuff sterilized with ethyl oxide. *Burns* 26:760.
35. Arimoto, H., Wakui, H., Sakagami, M., Magara, K., Yohkoh, N., and Kami, T. 1989. [Studies on the method of sterilization with ethylene oxide gas. Residual EO gas on sterilized objects]. *Shigaku* 77:1349.
36. Downey, P.M. 1977. As referenced in Glasser, Z.R., *Use of Ethylene Oxide as a Sterilant in Medical Facilities*. DHEW (NIOSH) Publ. 77–200. Cincinnati, OH: NIOSH, CDC.
37. Shupack, J.L., Anderson, S.R., and Romano, S.J. 1981. Human skin reactions to ethylene oxide. *J Lab Clin Med* 98:723.
38. Higgins, C., and Nixon, R. 2016. Facial allergic contact dermatitis without hand involvement caused by disposable latex gloves. *Contact Dermatitis* 74(4):251–3. DOI: 10.1111/cod.12502.
39. Tabah, A., Ramanan, M., Laupland, K.B., Buetti, N., Cortegiani, A., Mellinghoff, J., Conway Morris, A., Camporota, L., Zappella, N., Elhadi, M., Povoa, P., Amrein, K., Vidal, G., Derde, L., Bassetti, M., Francois, G., Ssi Yan Kai, N., and De Waele, J.J. 2020. Personal protective equipment and intensive care unit healthcare worker safety in the COVID-19 era (PPE-SAFE): An international survey. *J Crit Care* 59:70–5. DOI: 10.1016/j.jcrc.2020.06.005. Erratum in: J Crit Care. 2020.
40. Kim, H., Hegde, S., LaFiura, C., Raghavan, M., Sun, N., Cheng, S., Rebholz, C.M., and Seidelmann, S.B. 2021. Access to personal protective equipment in exposed healthcare workers and COVID-19 illness, severity, symptoms and duration: A population-based case-control study in six countries. *BMJ Global Health* 6:e004611.
41. Hegde, S. 2020. Which type of personal protective equipment (PPE) and which method of donning or doffing PPE carries the least risk of infection for healthcare workers? *Evid Based Dent* 21(2):74–6. DOI: 10.1038/s41432-020-0097-3.
42. Lammintausta, K., and Maibach, H.I. 1990. Contact dermatitis due to irritation, in *Occupational Skin Diseases*, 2nd ed., Adams, R.M., Ed. Philadelphia, PA: W.B. Saunders, chap. 1.
43. Dillard, S.F., Hefflin, B., Kaczmarek, R.G., Petsonk, E.L., and Gross, T.P. 2002. Health effects associated with medical glove use. *AORN J* 76(1):88–96.
44. Heese, A., Peters, K.P., and Koch, H.U. 1997. Type I allergies to latex and the aeroallergenic problem. *Eur J Surg Suppl* 579:19–22.
45. Wrangsjö, K., Osterman, K., and Van Hage-Hamsten, M. 1994. Glove-related skin symptoms among operating theatre and dental care unit personnel (I). Interview investigation. *Contact Dermatitis* 30(2):102–7.
46. Burke, F.J.T., Wilson, N.H.F., and Cheung, S.W. 1995. Factors associated with skin irritation of the hands experienced by general dental practitioners. *Contact Dermatitis* 32(1):35–8.
47. Ramsing, D.W., and Agner, T. 1996. Effect of glove occlusion on human skin (II). Long-term experimental exposure. *Contact Dermatitis* 34(4):258–62.
48. Heese, A., van Hintzenstern, J., Peters, K.P., Koch, H.U., and Hornstein, O.P. 1991. Allergic and irritant reactions to rubber gloves in medical health services. Spectrum, diagnostic approach, and therapy. *J Am Acad Dermatol* 25(5 Pt 1):831–9.
49. Baid, R., and Agarwal, R. 2017. Powdered gloves: Time to bid adieu. *J Postgrad Med* 63(3):206. DOI: 10.4103/jpgm.JPGM_80_17.

50. Tolbert, T.W., and Brown, J.L. 1980. Surface powders on surgical gloves. *Arch Surg* 115(6):729–32.

51. Beck, W.C. 1992. Issues related to surgical gloves. *Biomed Instr Technol* 26:225.

52. Korniewsicz, D., and Martin, C. 2001. Is it time to stop using powder as a donning agent for gloves? *Infection Control Today*, February 2001.

53. Brehler, R., Voss, W., and Müller, S. 1998. Glove powder affects skin roughness, one parameter of skin irritation. *Contact Dermatitis* 39(5):227–30.

54. Nangia, A., Andersen, P.H., Berner, B., and Maibach, H.I. 1996. High dissociation constants (pKa) of basic permeants are associated with in vivo skin irritation in man. *Contact Dermatitis* 34(4):237–42.

55. Held, E., and Agner, T. 2002. Irritant reaction to glove powder. *Contact Dermatitis* 46(Suppl. 4):50.

56. Agrup, G. 1969. Hand eczema. *Acta Dermatol Venereol* 49(Suppl. 61):1.

57. Fay, M.F., and Sullivan, R.W. 1992. Changing requirements for glove selection and hand protection. *Biomed Instrum Technol* 26(3):227–32.

58. Rietschel, R.L. 1988. Irritant contact dermatitis lecture, in *Symp. Occupational Skin Disease*, American Academy of Dermatology, December 1988.

59. Estlander, T., and Jolanki, R. 1988. How to protect the hands. *Dermatol Clin* 6(1):105–14.

60. Mathias, C.G.T. 1993. Treatment of occupational contact dermatitis, in *Syllabus, Occupational Skin Disease Sem.*, American College of Occupational and Environmental Medicine, April 1993.

61. DeGroot-Kosolcharoen, J. 1991. Pandemonium over gloves: Use and abuse. *Am J Infect Control* 19(5):225–7. DOI: 10.1016/s0196-6553(05)80252-4.

62. Christensen, G.J. 2001. Operating gloves. The good and the bad. *J Am Dent Assoc* 132:1145.

63. Sutherland, M.B. 2019. Innovations in cut-resistant work gloves solve common problems. *Industrial Safety and Hygiene News: Cutting-Edge Answers*, 7 February 2019.

64. Chew, A.L., and Maibach, H.I. 2006. *Irritant Dermatitis*. London: Springer.

65. Hodgson, G.A. 1966. Industrial dermatitis. *Postgrad Med J* 42(492):643–51.

66. Rietschel, R.L. 1988. Patch testing and occupational hand dermatitis. *Dermatol Clin* 6:43.

67. Maso, M.J., and Goldberg, D.J. 1990. Contact dermatoses from disposable glove use: A review. *J Am Acad Dermatol* 23:733.

68. Aalto-Korte, K., Alanko, K., Henriks-Eckerman, M.-L., Estlander, T., and Jolanki, R. 2003. Allergic contact dermatitis from bisphenol A in PVC gloves. *Contact Dermatitis* 49(4):202–5.

69. Field, E.A., and King, C.M. 1990. Skin problems associated with routine wearing of protective gloves in dental practice. *Br Dent J* 168:281.

70. Gonzalo-Garijo, M.A., Caballero, M.L., Gil-Micharet, M.S., Moneo, I., Pérez-Calderón, R., and García-Borruel, L. 2012. Hypersensitivity reactions due to nitrile gloves. *J Allergy Clin Immunol* 129(2):562–4. DOI: 10.1016/j.jaci.2011.09.016.

71. van der Meeren, H.L.M., and van Erp, P.E.J. 1986. Life-threatening contact urticaria from glove powder. *Contact Dermatitis* 14:190.

72. Assalve, D., Cicioni, C., Pemo, P., and Lisi, P. 1988. Contact urticaria and anaphylactoid reaction from cornstarch glove powder. *Contact Dermatitis* 19:61.

73. Fisher, A.A. 1986. Contact urticaria due to cornstarch surgical glove powder. *Cutis* 38:307.

74. Seggev, J.S., Yunginger, J.W., and Braun, S.R. 1990. Anaphylaxis due to cornstarch surgical glove powder. *Ann Allergy* 65:152.

75. Crippa, M., and Pasolini, G. 1997. Allergic reactions due to glove-lubricant powder in health care workers. *Int Arch Occup Environ Health* 70:399.

76. Wrangsjo, K., Mellstrom, G., and Axelsson, G. 1986. Discomfort from rubber gloves indicating contact urticaria. *Contact Dermatitis* 15:79.

77. Belsito, D.V. 1990. Contact Urticaria caused by rubber. *Dermatol Clin* 8:61.

78. Helander, I., and Makels, A. 1983. Contact urticaria to zinc diethyldithiocarbamate (ZDC). *Contact Dermatitis* 9:327.

79. Fuchs, T., and Wahl, R. 1992. Immediate reactions to rubber products *Allergy Proc* 13:61.

80. Brehler, R. 1996. Contact urticaria caused by latex-free nitrile gloves. *Contact Dermatitis* 34:296.

81. Brehler, R., and Sedlmayr, S. 1997. Contact urticaria due to rubber chemicals? *Contact Dermatitis* 37:125.

82. McSweeney, S.M., White, I.R., McFadden, J.P., and Tziotzios, C. 2020. Contact urticaria to non-latex synthetic glove material: A case report. *Contact Dermatitis* 83:417–8. DOI: 10.1111/cod.13627.

83. Sugiura, K., Sugiura, M., Hayakawa, R., and Sasaki, K. 2000. Di (2-ethyl-hexyl) phthalate (DOP) in the dotted polyvinyl-chloride grip of cotton gloves as a cause of contact urticaria syndrome. *Contact Dermatitis* 43:237.

84. Sugiura, K., Sugiura, M., Shiraki, R., Hayakawa, R., Shamoto, M., Sasaki, K., and Itoh, A. 2002. Contact urticaria due to polyethylene gloves. *Contact Dermatitis* 46:262.

85. Ylitalo, L., Makinen-Kiljunen, S., Turjanmaa, K., Palosuo, T., and Reunala, T. 1999. Cow's milk casein, a hidden allergen in NRL gloves. *J Allergy Clin Immunol* 104:177.

86. Sasseville, D., and Thériault, M. 2012. Occupational contact urticaria caused by polyvinylchloride gloves. *Contact Dermatitis* 66(1):49–50.

87. Kanani, A., Betschel, S.D., and Warrington, R. 2018. Urticaria and angioedema. *Allergy Asthma Clin Immunol* 14 (Suppl 2):59.

88. Lahti, A., and Maibach, H.I. 1989. Immediate contact reactions. *Immunol Allergy Clin North Am* 9:463.

89. Anderson, K.E., and Maibach, H.I. 1984. Multiple application delayed onset contact urticaria. *Contact Dermatitis* 10:227.

90. Hawkey, S., and Abdul Ghaffar, S. 2016. Glove-related hand urticaria: An increasing occupational problem among healthcare workers. *Br J Dermatol* 174(5):1137–40. DOI: 10.1111/bjd.14318.

91. Taylor, J.S., and Praditsuwan, P. 1996. Latex allergy. Review of 44 cases including outcome and frequent association with allergic hand eczema. *Arch Dermatol* 132(3):265–71. DOI: 10.1001/archderm.132.3.265.

92. Silva, L., Miroux-Catarino, A., Pimentel, B.V., Amaro, C., and Viana, I. 2020. An overlooked allergic contact dermatitis to rubber. *Contact Dermatitis* 83(3):226–7. DOI: 10.1111/cod.13556.

93. Havmose, M., Thyssen, J.P., Zachariae, C., and Johansen, J.D. 2020. Use of protective gloves by hairdressers: A review of efficacy and potential adverse effects. *Contact Dermatitis* 83(2):75–82. DOI: 10.1111/cod.13561.

94. O'Reilly, K.E., Patel, U., Chu, J., Patel, R., and Machler, B.C. 2011. Chemical leukoderma. *Dermatol Online J* 17(10):29.

95. Jung, J.Y., Yeom, K.B., and Eun, H.C. 2010. Chemical leukoderma improved by low-dose steroid pulse therapy. *Ann Dermatol* 22(2):241–4.

96. Gozali, M.V., Zhang, J-N., Yi, F., Zhou, B-R., and Luo, D. 2016. Chemical leukoderma induced by dimethyl sulfate. *Anais brasileiros de dermatologia* 91(5 suppl 1):26–8.

97. Attarchi, M.S., Mohammadi, S., and Asghari, E. 2009. Evaluation of skin diseases and disorders in photographers. *Indian J Occup Environ Med* 13(2):88–91.

98. Ito, S., and Wakamatsu, K. 2018. Biochemical mechanism of rhododendrol-induced leukoderma. *Int J Mol Sci* 19(2):552.

99. Cheng, C., La Grenade, L., Diak, I.L., Brinker, A., and Levin, R.L. 2017. Chemical leukoderma associated with methylphenidate transdermal system: Data from the US Food and Drug Administration Adverse Event Reporting System. *J Pediatr* 180:241–6.

100. Howell, M.D., Tomazic, V.J., Leakakos, T., Truscott, W., and Meade, B.J. 2004. Immunomodulatory effect of endotoxin on the development of latex allergy. *J Allergy Clin Immunol* 113(5):916–24.

101. Slater, J.E., Paupore, E.J., Elwell, M.R., and Truscott, W. 1998. Lipopolysaccharide augments IgG and IgE responses of mice to the latex allergen Hev b 5. *J Allergy Clin Immunol* 102(6 Pt 1):977–83.

102. Barth, E., Talbott, N., Gable, R., Richter, S., and Reponen, T. 2002. Evaluation of bioaerosol exposures during conditioning of biofilter organic media beds. *Appl Occup Environ Hyg* 17(1):10–4.

103. Haishima, Y., Murai, T., Nakagawa, Y., Hirata, M., Yagami, T., and Nakamura, A. 2001. Chemical and biological evaluation of endotoxin contamination on natural rubber latex products. *J Biomed Mater Res* 55(3):424–32.

104. Peiró, S.A., Kulander, L., and Eriksson, O. 1990. Quantitative determination of endotoxins on surgical gloves. *J Hosp Infect* 16(2):167–72.

105. Abraham, E.K., and Ramesh, P. 2002. Natural rubber latex products: Concerns in health care. *J Macromolecular Sci Part C* 42(2):185–234.

106. Williams, P.B., and Hasley, J.F. 1997. Endotoxin as a factor in adverse reactions to latex gloves. *Ann Allergy Asthma Immunol* 79:303.

107. Alfa, M.J. 2012. The 'Pandora's box' dilemma: Reprocessing of implantable screws and plates in orthopedic tray sets. *Biomed Instrum Technol* Suppl:55–9.

108. Takahashi, G., Kan, S., Hoshikawa, K., Sato, K., Fujita, Y., Inada, K., and Inoue, Y. 2020. Endotoxin contamination of single-use sterile surgical gloves. *Future Microbiol* 15:1425–1430.

109. Thorne, P.S., Metwali, N., Avol, E., and McConnell, R.S. 2005. Surface sampling for endotoxin assessment using electrostatic wiping cloths. *Ann Occup Hyg* 49(5):401–6.

110. Althomali, T.A. 2016. Viscoelastic substance in prefilled syringe as an etiology of toxic anterior segment syndrome. *Cutan Ocul Toxicol* 35(3):237–41.

111. Nomura, Y., Fukui, C., Morishita, Y., and Haishima, Y. 2017. A biological study establishing the endotoxin limit for in vitro proliferation of human mesenchymal stem cells. *Regen Ther* 7:45–51. DOI: 10.1016/j.reth.2017.08.004.

112. International Irradiation Association. 2017. *White Paper - A Comparison of Gamma, E-Beam, X-Ray and Ethylene Oxide Technologies for the Industrial Sterilization of Medical Devices and Healthcare Products.*

113. McEvoy, B., and Rowan, N.J. 2019. Terminal sterilization of medical devices using vaporized hydrogen peroxide: A review of current methods and emerging opportunities. *J Appl Microbiol* 127(5):1403–20.

114. Neureuther, K., Rohmann, E., Hilken, M., Sonntag, M.L., Herdt, S., Koennecke, T., Jacobs, R., Adamski, M., Reisbacher, S., Alfs, K., Strain, P., and Bastisch, I. 2014. Reduction of PCR-amplifiable DNA by ethylene oxide treatment of forensic consumables. *Forensic Sci Int Genet* 12:185–91.

115. Akhavan, B.J., Osborn, U.A., and Mathew, R. 2019. Anaphylactic reaction to ethylene oxide in a hemodialysis patient. In *SAGE Open Med Case Rep* 7:2050313X19838744. DOI: 10.1177/2050313X19838744.

116. Bache, S., Petersen, J.T., and Garvey, L.H. 2011. Anaphylaxis to ethylene oxide - A rare and overlooked phenomenon? *Acta Anaesthesiol Scand* 55(10):1279–82.

117. Ayliffe, G. 2000. Decontamination of minimally invasive surgical endoscopes and accessories. *J Hosp Infect* 45(4):263–77.

118. Breuer, K., Worm, M., Skudlik, C., and John, S.M. 2017. Ethylene oxide as an occupational contact allergen - An underestimated problem? *Allergol Select* 1(1):9–13.
119. Mendes, G.C., Brandão, T.R., and Silva, C.L. 2007. Ethylene oxide sterilization of medical devices: A review. *Am J Infect Control* 35(9):574–81.
120. McCook, A. 2020. COVID-19 further complicates existing sterilization problems. *Clinical News*, July 8, 2020.
121. Mohapatra, S. 2017. Sterilization and disinfection, in *Essentials of Neuroanesthesia*, Prabhakar, H., Ed. Cambridge, MA: Academic Press (Elsevier), chap. 59.
122. SCMS. 2011. *SCMS Male Circumcision Core List: Male Circumcision Kit Options 1, 2 & 3: Supply Chain Management System (SCMS)*. Available at: https://www.malecircumcision.org/sites/default/files/document_library/GD3.%20SCMS%20E-catalog%20including%20all%20MC%20Kit%20Options.pdf.
123. USAID. 2020. *GHSC-PSM Voluntary Medical Male Circumcision (VMMC) Reference Guide. USAID Global Health Supply Chain Program Procurement and Supply Management*. Available at: https://www.ghsupplychain.org/sites/default/files/2018-03/2018_03_02_VMMC_Reference_Guide_1.pdf.
124. Boiano, J.M., and Steege, A.L. 2015. Ethylene oxide and hydrogen peroxide gas plasma sterilization: Precautionary practices in U.S. hospitals. *Zentralsterilisation (Wiesb)* 23(4):262–8.
125. U.S. FDA. 2019. *Executive Summary*. In Prepared for the November 6–7, 2019 meeting of the General Hospital and Personal Use Devices Panel of the Medical Devices Advisory Committee. Washington, DC: U.S. Food and Drug Administration.
126. Walters, G.I., Burge, P.S., Moore, V.C., Thomas, M.O., and Robertson, A.S. 2019. Occupational asthma caused by peracetic acid-hydrogen peroxide mixture. *Occup Med (Lond)* 69(4):294–7.
127. Sousa, C.S., Torres, L.M., Azevedo, M.P., de Camargo, T.C., Graziano, K.U., Lacerda, R.A., and Turrini, R.N. 2011. [Sterilization with ozone in health care: An integrative literature review]. *Rev Esc Enferm USP* 45(5):1243–9.
128. Anderson, S.E., Umbright, C., Sellamuthu, R., Fluharty, K., Kashon, M., Franko, J., Jackson, L.G., Johnson, V.J., and Joseph, P. 2010. Irritancy and allergic responses induced by topical application of ortho-phthalaldehyde. *Toxicol Sci* 115(2):435–43.
129. Pala, G., and Moscato, G. 2013. Allergy to ortho-phthalaldehyde in the healthcare setting: Advice for clinicians. *Expert Rev Clin Immunol* 9(3):227–34.
130. Marena, C., Lodola, L., Marone Bianco, A., Maestri, L., Alessio, A., Negri, S., and Zambianchi, L. 2003. [Monitoring air dispersed concentrations of aldehydes during the use of ortho-phthalaldehyde and glutaraldehyde for high disinfection of endoscopes]. *G Ital Med Lav Ergon* 25(2):131–6.
131. Sarada, B.V., Vijay, R., Johnson, R., Narasinga Rao, T., and Padmanabham, G. 2020. Fight against COVID-19: ARCI's technologies for disinfection. *Transactions Indian Nat Acad Eng* 5:349–354.
132. Cumbo, E., Gallina, G., Messina, P., and Scardina, G.A. 2020. Alternative methods of sterilization in dental practices against COVID-19. *Int J Environ Res Public Health* 17(16):5736.
133. DeFabio, C. 2020. Personal communication. October 30, 2020. Cleveland Clinic.
134. Sickbert-Bennett, E.E., Samet, J.M., Clapp, P.W., Chen, H., Berntsen, J., Zeman, K.L., Tong, H., Weber, D.J., and Bennett, W.D. 2020. Filtration efficiency of hospital face mask alternatives available for use during the COVID-19 pandemic. *JAMA Intern Med* 180(12):1607–1612. DOI: 10.1001/jamainternmed.2020.4221.

19 Occlusion vs. Contact Dermatitis*

T. Tran and H. I. Maibach

CONTENTS

19.1 INTRODUCTION

Occlusion enhances skin hydration and increases absorption of most applied substances, which may increase irritant and allergic contact dermatitis.[1–4] In addition, occlusion may compromise skin barrier function by impairing passive transepidermal water loss at the application site and therefore aggravate the irritant effect of applied compounds.[2,4–7]

Transdermal drug delivery systems (TDDS) are typically occlusive patches placed on the skin surface for 1–7 days while delivering drugs into the systemic circulation[5] and have been extensively investigated because of potential advantages over traditional oral or other administration routes.[7–13] However, local reactions (i.e., irritation and/or sensitization) have become obstacles in the design and application of TDDS in clinical situations.[7–13] This chapter summarizes the effects of occlusion on contact dermatitis.

19.2 SKIN AND EFFECTS OF OCCLUSION

Skin envelops the body surface as a flexible shield, acting as a two-way barrier, minimizing water loss, electrolytes, and other body constituents and decreasing the entry of noxious substances from the external environment. The stratum corneum is a principal barrier and normally contains 10%–20% water.[14] Skin barrier function may be perturbed by physical, chemical, therapeutic, and pathological factors; even changes in environmental humidity may also induce pathophysiologic

---

* Adapted from Zhai, H. and Maibach, H.I. 2001. Skin occlusion and irritant and allergic contact dermatitis: an overview. *Contact Dermatitis* 44(4):201–206.

DOI: 10.1201/9781003126874-22

alterations.[15] Increasing stratum corneum hydration can progressively reduce its barrier efficiency.[1–5,16,17]

Occlusion is created by covering the skin with tape, gloves, impermeable dressings, or transdermal devices.[5] In addition, certain topical vehicles such as those containing fats and oils (petrolatum, paraffin, etc.) may be occlusive.[6,18] Moisturizers and emollients may functionally be occlusive. Most studies demonstrated an effective duration of moisture of minutes to hours. Lodén[19] has provided extensive documentation of this area.

Occlusion can completely block passive transepidermal water loss.[5] This leads to an increase in stratum corneum hydration, thereby swelling the corneocytes and promoting the uptake of water into intercellular lipid domains.[2,4,20] Occlusion alters many factors that may influence percutaneous absorption: (1) increasing the water content of stratum corneum from a normal range of 10%–20% up to 50% and thus altering the partitioning between the surface chemical and skin;[2,4] (2) swelling the corneocytes and altering the intercellular lipid phase organization;[2,4,20] (3) increasing the skin surface temperature from a normal range of 32°C to 37°C;[2,4] (4) increasing blood flow;[2,4] (5) preventing accidental wiping or evaporation (volatile compound) of an applied compound, in essence of maintaining a higher applied dose;[21] and (6) serving as a reservoir of the drug for penetration as a result of hydration.[21] Initially, a drug enters the stratum corneum under occlusion conditions. After dressing removal and stratum corneum dehydration, the movement of the drug slows and the stratum corneum becomes a reservoir.[21] However, occlusion does not enhance penetration of all chemicals.[1–4] Skin hydration increased penetration of lipid-soluble, nonpolar molecules but had less effect on polar molecules.[13] In humans, occlusion enhanced the absorption of more lipophilic steroids but did not enhance the absorption of water-soluble materials.[1] The effect of occlusion on absorption may also be influenced by physicochemical properties (such as volatility, partition coefficient, and aqueous solubility), anatomic site, and vehicle.[1,4,22,23]

In addition, the effects of occlusion are complex and may produce profound changes. Occlusion can alter epidermal lipids, DNA synthesis, epidermal turnover, microbial flora, pH, epidermal morphology, sweat glands, Langerhans cell stresses, wound healing, etc.[5,6,15,24–28]

19.3 LOCAL REACTIONS OF OCCLUSION

Bucks et al.[2,4] observed that about one-third of normal, healthy, male volunteers experienced plastic chamber occlusion-induced irritation following contact with TDDS when contact periods were greater than 24 h. However, no irritation was observed on the same volunteers when a nonocclusive patch system was used following identical contact periods with the same penetrant.

Hurkmans et al.[29] documented irritation produced by transdermal therapeutic systems (TTS) during long-term (5 days) application in humans. Different types of TTS were applied to the back of male volunteers for 120 h, and sweat accumulation and bacterial growth were studied. Hydrogel discs of systems had less skin irritation, but intense bacterial growth was observed when compared to other systems. They concluded that water accumulation is a major cause of skin irritation under TDDS during long-term application and that bacteria and/or yeasts play only a minor role; in addition, the incorporation of hydrogels in the TDDS may reduce skin irritation by absorbing water.

Nieboer et al.[30] investigated the effects of occlusion with TTS on Langerhans cell and skin irritation. In their study, 25 healthy volunteers were divided into 5 groups of 5 volunteers and occluded with a placebo TTS and a silver-patch test for five different periods (6 h, 1, 2, 4, and 7 days). Irritation was judged on morphology, histopathologic and immunofluorescence findings, and changes in the Langerhans cell systems. Occlusion with their systems provoked only slight or no skin irritation.

Van der Valk and Maibach[31] utilized a post-application occlusion human model to assess if occlusion increases the irritant response of the skin to repeated short-term sodium lauryl sulfate (SLS) exposure in ten healthy subjects. In an open application procedure, the volar side of the forearm was treated by repeated application of SLS. One test site on either arm was exposed for 5 consecutive days, and one adjacent skin site was exposed on alternate days. After the open exposure, the skin was either left open or occluded with plastic wrap. Skin irritancy was measured by visual grading and transepidermal water loss (TEWL). The occluded skin sites had a significant increase in the visual grading system and TEWL values (every day and alternate-day schedule) when compared to unoccluded sites. They indicated that post-exposure occlusive treatment markedly enhanced irritant response.

Bircher et al.[32] evaluated the adverse skin reactions to nicotine in a TTS in 14 volunteers with a history of former adverse skin reactions to this device. Individual components of TDDS were tested for immediate- and delayed-type reactions. In the study, nine subjects developed mild irritant erythematous reactions due to occlusion (reacted to both of the adhesive and matrix layers), and five individuals had positive allergic patch test reactions to nicotine base. The optimal test agent and concentration for eliciting the adverse skin reaction was an aqueous solution of 10% nicotine base. They suggested that nicotine should be added to the expanding list of TDDS that may elicit contact dermatitis.

Emtestam and Ollmar[33] measured the electrical impedance index in human skin after occlusion in five anatomical regions and areas of mild irritant contact dermatitis. The volunteers were divided into three groups. In the occlusion group with 11 subjects, the test sites were occluded on the back for 24 h using empty aluminum chambers and chambers with water, physiological saline, a paper disc, or 0.002% of SLS. In the normal skin group of ten subjects, electrical impedance was measured at five body sites for 5 consecutive days. In the long-term study group of three subjects, daily measurements for 1 month were performed on normal skin and skin following the application of 2% SLS. The irritation index based on electrical skin impedance gave little day-to-day variation at the same test site, in comparison to the variations between different test sites on the same subject and the interindividual variations observed. Occlusion did not affect readings taken 24 h or later after removal, but it increased variance for readings taken 1 h after removal.

Matsumura et al.[25] investigated the effect of occlusion on the skin in humans. The flexor sides of both upper arms were covered with column-shaped polyethylene foam closed chambers. The chambers' tops were sealed by plastic films with various levels of water vapor permeability to control moisture in each chamber. After 24 h application, morphological changes on the surface of occluded skin were observed using the nitrocellulose-replica method. The number of deepened skin furrows on the skin surface was increased by lower water vapor permeability of the film, as well as increasing temperature and humidity on the test day. This result suggested that simple occlusion with water vapor permeability below 30 g/m²h can induce morphological alternations on the skin surface and implied that prolonged exposure by simple occlusion may act as a primary irritant.

Kligman[5] studied hydration dermatitis in humans; 1 week of an impermeable plastic film did not injure the skin; 2 weeks were moderately harmful to some but not all subjects; and 3 weeks regularly induced hydration dermatitis. Hydration dermatitis was independent of race, sex, and age. They examined the potential role of microorganisms in developing hydration dermatitis by using antibiotic solutions immediately following occlusion with plastic wrapping. Results showed the microorganisms had no impact. In addition, they noticed that some hydrogels did not appreciably hydrate or macerate the surface by visual inspection when left in place for 1 week. But some TDDS may, indeed, provoke dermatitis when applied twice weekly to the same site. From a histologic study, they demonstrated marked cytotoxicity to Langerhans cells, melanocytes, and keratinocytes.

Graves et al.[34] assessed the detrimental effect of occlusive glove patches in humans. Four test sites were assigned on both forearms of each subject. On day 1: two sites were occluded with glove patch for 4 and 8 h, respectively; the third site was left unoccluded as a control. On day 2: the fourth site was covered with a transparent dressing (without a glove patch) for 8 h as an active control. The effects on the skin barrier were evaluated by percomeal permeability, TEWL, skin surface roughness, and skin surface compliance. Results show that percomeal permeability, TEWL, and compliance parameter were significantly increased after occlusion for 4 and 8 h, and skin surface roughness was significantly reduced in terms of roughness parameters Ra and Rz by 4 and 8 h occlusion. They concluded that the glove patches caused a temporary impairment in barrier function and suggested the repeated occlusion by gloves may have a cumulative effect.

Wilhelm[35] investigated the effects of surfactants on stratum corneum (SC) hydration in nine human subjects: a series of sodium alkyl sulfates were applied to the volar forearm using occlusive plastic chambers for 24 h. SC hydration was evaluated by measurements of electrical capacitance (CAP) at 30 min after removal of the patches and thereafter at daily intervals for 7 days. All alkyl sulfates, except for SLS, resulted in a temporary decrease of SC hydration 1 h after patch removal. On day 2, SC hydration levels of surfactant-treated skin were not significantly different from controls. Thereafter, the second decrease in CAP value was observed with the lowest hydration on day 7.

Wood et al.[28] observed impacts of occlusion on epidermal cytokine with essential fatty acid-deficient and normal mouse and noted that occlusion lowers cytokine mRNA levels in essential fatty acid-deficient and normal mouse epidermis, but not after acute barrier disruption.

Welzel et al.[36,37] evaluated the effect of occlusive treatments on the repair of the human skin permeability barrier under controlled experimental conditions. Barrier perturbation was induced either by application of SLS or by repeated tape stripping. This was followed by treatment with occlusive and semipermeable dressings, partly after pretreatment with petrolatum. Repair of water barrier function was evaluated by daily measurements of TEWL for 1 week. SLS irritation and tape stripping led to a sixfold increase in TEWL as a sign of severe water barrier perturbation, followed by a stepwise decrease over the following days. Occlusion did not significantly delay barrier repair as measured by TEWL.

Ramsing and Agner[38] evaluated the effect of glove occlusion on normal and compromised human skin by non-invasive methods in two studies (A and B). Each subject wore an occlusive glove on the one hand, while the other hand served as control. Hypoallergenic non-latex gloves were used. In study A, 20 volunteers wore a glove on normal skin 6 h/day for 3 days; in study B, 20 wore a glove on SLS-compromised skin 6 h/day for 3 days. Skin barrier function was evaluated by measurement of TEWL, skin hydration by electrical capacitance, and inflammation by erythema index. Glove occlusion on normal skin for short-term exposure (6 h/day for 3 days) did not significantly change the water barrier function but caused a significantly negative effect on SLS-compromised skin for the same period.

They also evaluated the effect of long-term glove occlusion on normal skin (6 h/day for 14 days) in two studies (A and B).[39] The effect of a cotton glove worn under the occlusive glove was also determined. In study A, 19 volunteers wore an occlusive glove on normal skin 6 h/day for 14 days on one hand only, while the other hand served as control. In study B, 18 volunteers wore occlusive gloves on both hands, on normal skin. A cotton glove was worn under the occlusive glove on one hand only, while the other hand utilized the glove only (no inner cotton glove). This long-term glove occlusion on normal skin (6 h/day for 14 days) caused a significant negative effect on skin barrier function, as measured by TEWL, which was prevented by the cotton glove. They concluded that occlusion may be an additional factor in the pathogenesis of cumulative irritant contact dermatitis. The use of an inner cotton glove provided protection against the effects of occlusion.

Fluhr et al.[40] evaluated the barrier damage by prolonged occlusion in humans. Five sites were assigned on the volar forearm: four were occluded by a plastic chamber and one served as a control on day 0. Occlusion was then removed at site 1 after 24 h, site 2 after 48 h, site 3 after 72 h, and site 4 after 96 h. At 2 h after occlusion removal, TEWL and skin hydration were measured and a sorption-desorption test was performed. TEWL increased, reaching a plateau on day 2. Hydration and water-holding capacity did not show significant changes. They concluded that occlusion-induced barrier damage without skin dryness.

Angelova-Fischer et al.[41] studied the cumulative effects of n-propanol concentrations in healthy individuals and those with atopic dermatitis (AD). The study consisted of healthy adults and AD adults who were exposed to n-propanol concentrations ranging from 30% to 75%. Measurements of erythema, TEWL, capacitance, and natural moisturizing factor (NMF) levels were measured at baseline and after 96 h. The results showed that even at the lowest concentrations, n-propanol still had a significant barrier-damaging effect.

With respect to NMF levels, exposure to all concentrations of n-propanol significantly reduced NMF levels. Prior exposure to low-grade trauma (occlusion/water exposure) before n-propanol reduced the skin irritation threshold in both healthy and AD groups. Finally, there were significant differences in the severity of barrier function impairment after exposure to the same concentration of n-propanol between the two groups.

Antonov et al.[42] investigated the effect of glove occlusion with and without an antibacterial hand cleanser. In addition, the effects of a pre-exposure cream (petrolatum) and a post-exposure cream (Eucerin® hand cream) on irritant dermatitis were studied. A modified repeated short-term occlusive irritation test was performed on 20 healthy volunteers with the application of irritants over 4 days, with pre-exposure cream, post-exposure cream, and overnight occlusion. SLS served as the positive control. Changes in TEWL were used to document irritant damage to the epidermal barrier. When combined, the antibacterial cleanser followed by glove occlusion had a significant increase in TEWL, similar to that seen with SLS than either on their own. The use of a pre-exposure and a post-exposure cream significantly alleviated the cumulative irritation when both creams were used.

Bock et al.[43] evaluated the impact of semipermeable gloves on barrier recovery after standardized irritation with SLS. Twenty-five healthy volunteers were exposed to 1% SLS for 24 h on 4 test areas on normal skin on the upper back. Each test area was covered with semipermeable membranes (Goretex, Sympatex) and an occlusive membrane (Meditrate Vinyl), and one test area was left uncovered as control, respectively. Barrier repair on each test area was measured by TEWL and erythema. Results showed that areas covered with semipermeable membrane had enhanced barrier recovery and reduced inflammatory response compared to occluded areas and control. TEWL in areas covered with semipermeable membranes were significantly lower than in occluded areas and uncovered areas. This indicates that a semipermeable membrane can aid with barrier recovery rates by providing optimal water vapor gradient during the healing process.

Buraczewska et al.[44] investigated the long-term effects of using a semipermeable membrane on normal skin and the occlusive properties of urea cream and lipid-rich cream. TEWL and skin susceptibility to SLS irritation were measured to evaluate skin barrier function after treatment with a semipermeable membrane, a urea cream, a lipid-rich cream, or no treatment (control). Results suggest that long-term use (23 h/day for 3 weeks) of a semipermeable membrane improved skin barrier function. No significant changes were found for using a semipermeable membrane for 8 h a day. In addition, no obvious differences in occlusion were found between urea creams and lipid-rich creams.

Fartasch et al.[45] studied the differences between water exposure and occlusion on the skin barrier. In this study, the term "wet work" refers to both occlusion and water exposure. Seventy-three participants were randomized into four groups (A, B, C, and D). Group A had 2 h of daily exposure to water and occlusion for 7 consecutive days. Group B had 3 h of daily exposure to water and occlusion for 7 consecutive days. Group C had 4 h of daily exposure to water and occlusion for 7 consecutive days. Group D had 6 h of occlusion versus 3 h of occlusion followed by 3 h of water exposure. Two application areas were marked on each volar forearm. Water exposure was in the form of a wet cotton patch, while occlusion was in the form of polyvinyl glove material. One arm had no treatment, and the other had water exposure and occlusion. After 1 week of exposure, participants were subjected to SLS irritation on each test site. Visual inspection (clinical score), TEWL, skin hydration, and erythema were used to evaluate skin barrier conditions after wet work.

Results suggested that skin reacted in a time-dependent manner in both forms of wet work. Water exposure for more than 3 h daily had a significant increase in TEWL as compared to the control area. SLS irritation in water-exposed test sites had higher TEWL and clinical scores than in occluded test sites. Both water-exposed sites and occluded sites had higher TEWL and clinical scores than control sites. They concluded that previous occlusion and water exposure were capable of bringing about higher susceptibility to SLS irritation. Occlusion also had a different biological effect than water exposure. In addition, short occlusion times were less harmful to the skin barrier than water exposure for the same duration.

Fluhr et al.[46] studied the effects of sequential application of mechanical irritation combined with 0.5% SLS and occlusion on skin barrier impairment. Twenty healthy volunteers were exposed to mechanical irritation and occlusion with water or mechanical irritation with 0.5% SLS solution for 4 consecutive days in a combined tandem repeated irritation test (TRIT). The application areas were the volar forearms. Permeability barrier function was measured, while irritation was evaluated with a colorimeter and a visual score.

Results suggested that barrier disruption was rated as follows with most barrier disruption to least barrier disruption: occlusion with SLS and mechanical irritation > occlusion with SLS > occlusion with water and mechanical irritation > mechanical irritation and occlusion with water > occlusion with a glove and mechanical irritation > mechanical irritation > occlusion with water. Barrier disruption resulting from occlusion or mechanical irritation was worsened by tandem application. Other factors that affected barrier disruption were the choice of irritant under occlusion, time of occlusion, and order of tandem application. The study concluded that the use of physical irritants and detergents should be minimized as they significantly increase irritation risk, as shown in the TRIT model.

Jungbauer et al.[47] investigated the effectiveness of two measures recommended for reducing exposure to skin irritants for nurses: (1) using hand alcohol instead of soap and water when the hands are not visibly dirty and (2) using gloves in wet activities. There were two models in the study: regular and prevention. The regular exposure model emulated the mean daily wet work nurses usually do. The prevention model was the implementation of the two recommended measures. Thirty-nine healthy volunteers were recruited and randomly sorted into either regular or prevention models. Participants were asked to expose their hands 5 days a week for 3 weeks to their allocated models with gloves only used on the one hand in each model. Wet work cleaning activity in nursing was simulated with Glorix wet cleaning towels. Sterillium hand alcohol was used for hand disinfection. Hand washing was done with water and a commercially available cationic pH-neutral soap.

Results indicated an increase in TEWL after a 3-week exposure to the regular model and a decrease in TEWL after a 3-week exposure to the prevention model.

In addition, skin irritation from occlusion appeared to be more prominent in the regular model compared to the prevention model. Although there was more glove occlusion in the prevention model, there was no additional irritant effect, possibly due to the absence of soap exposure. In conclusion, hand alcohol is preferable as a disinfectant in nursing work, and gloves should be used in wet activities.

Jungersted et al.[48] investigated the impact of occlusion on healthy and irritated skin barriers. Two independent studies were done: study A examined response of occlusion on normal skin, and study B the response of occlusion on skin with a damaged barrier. Nineteen healthy volunteers were enrolled in study A. The volar forearm on each volunteer was divided into three areas and randomized on each participant for different occlusion regimens. Area 1 was occluded for 8 h a day for 7 consecutive days. Area 2 was occluded for 72 consecutive hours. Area 3 was not occluded and served as a control. TEWL, erythema, and capacitance were measured 4 h after occlusion removal. After that, an SLS patch was placed on each area for 24 h. A cyanoacrylate stratum corneum sample adjacent to the SLS patches was taken for lipid analysis. TEWL, erythema, and capacitance were measured 1 h after SLS patch removal.

Nineteen healthy volunteers were recruited for study B. The volar forearm on each volunteer was divided into four areas. SLS patches were applied on areas 1 and 2 for 24 h. On day 2, the SLS patches were removed, and after 1 h, area 1 was occluded for 72 h and area 2 was left as control. Areas 3 and 4 were untouched for 1 day and were tape stripped on day 2. After that, area 3 was occluded for 72 h, and area 4 was left as control. On day 5, TEWL, erythema, and capacitance were measured 4 h after the occlusion was removed.

Study A results showed no statistical differences for any of the measurements between the occlusion regimens and control. Study B results showed that occlusion of the skin resulted in significantly higher levels of TEWL after SLS irritation than in areas not occluded. However, occluded skin had lower levels of TEWL after tape stripping. There were no differences in erythema of electrical capacitance.

Mirza et al.[49] studied the effect of glove wearing on skin pH, compared the effect of study gloves with standard gloves on skin pH, and determined if study gloves reduced skin irritation. Study gloves were non-powdered natural rubber latex gloves that were designed to keep skin at pH 5.5. Twenty healthy subjects participated and were randomized into two groups: group 1 and group 2. Group 1 wore the study glove on the right hand and the control glove on the left hand for 8 h a day, 5 days per week over a 4-week duration. Group 2 wore the study glove on the left hand and the control glove on the right hand 8 h a day, 5 days per week over a 4-week duration. Subjects were instructed to wash their hands with a gentle wash every 45 min to 2 h and wear new gloves after each hand wash. TEWL, skin pH, physician skin assessment, and subject skin assessment were measured prior to glove use at week 2, week 4, and 2 days before the end of the study.

Glove wearing led to a significant increase in pH in both study and control groups at all times compared to baseline levels. However, the skin surface pH of the study hand was significantly lower than the control hand and had less irritation. Scaling and dryness were reported on both hands in week 4, but the study hand had significantly less dryness than the control hand. In conclusion, pH 5.5 gloves kept lower skin pH levels and may reduce irritation in long-term glove wearers.

Tiedemann et al.[50] reviewed the literature on the effects of glove occlusion on skin barrier function and found that data on the negative effect of occlusion is limited and only extensive and long-term occlusion will cause barrier impairment. Studies investigating the combined effects of occlusion and exposure to detergents show that occlusion significantly increases skin barrier damage caused by detergents in a dose-dependent manner.

Weistenhofer et al.[51] studied the effects of wearing occlusive gloves throughout the entire workday without exposure to hazardous substances on skin condition and skin barrier function. Three hundred and twenty-three employees of a semiconductor production company in Germany were assessed: 177 cleanroom employees wore occlusive gloves during the whole shift (exposed group) and 146 were administration employees (control). TEWL and stratum corneum hydration of both hands were measured. In addition, the skin condition of both hands was studied using the quantitative score hand eczema score for occupational screenings (HEROS).

The results showed no significant difference in skin condition between the two groups. TEWL and skin hydration were significantly higher for the exposed group, but TEWL values were similar to control if gloves were taken off at least 30 min before measurements. Therefore, the effect of occlusion on skin barrier function seems temporary which possibly indicates that prolonged glove use on clean hands without exposure to hazardous substances was not negative.

Wetzky et al.[52] analyzed the occlusive effects of short-term and long-term glove wear on skin barrier function. In addition, two different glove materials were compared for their effect on the skin barrier. Twenty healthy participants were recruited: ten participants wore PVC gloves on the right hand and natural rubber latex (NRL) gloves on the left hand, and ten participants wore PVC gloves on their left hands and NRL gloves on their right hands. TEWL, capacitance, skin surface color, and skin pH were measured. Short-term occlusion was defined as wearing gloves once for 4 h. To measure the short-term effects of glove occlusion, measurements were taken before occlusion, 30 min after occlusion, and 3 h after occlusion. Long-term glove occlusion was defined as wearing gloves for 4 h a day, 7 days a week. Measurements were taken 1 day after the 1-week occlusion.

Capacitance increased significantly for both types of gloves 30 min after 4 h of occlusion compared to baseline. The NRL glove site capacitance significantly decreased 3 h after single occlusion compared to 30 min after occlusion. There were no significant capacitance differences between long-term and short-term glove wear. TEWL increased significantly 30 min after single occlusion compared to baseline in both test sites. TEWL went down to baseline 3 h after removal of gloves. There were no differences in TEWL between long-term occlusion and baseline. For skin color, there was a significant difference between 30 min after occlusion and baseline in the NRL glove but not the PVC glove. No significant difference was seen 3 h after glove removal. Regarding pH, skin pH decreased significantly after short-term glove wear. This is contrasted with previous studies, which showed an increase in skin pH after glove wear, possibly indicating that different glove materials affect skin pH differently.

Brief data of local reactions of occlusion are in Table 19.1.

TABLE 19.1
Brief Data of Local Reactions of Occlusion

Occlusion	Local Reactions and References
TDDS for greater than 24 h	One-third of volunteers experienced plastic chamber occlusion-induced irritation.[2,4]
TTS for 5 days	Hydrogel discs of systems had less skin irritation when compared to other systems.[29]
TTS and a silver-patch test for five time periods: 6 h, 1, 2, 4, and 7 days	Occlusion with their systems provokes only slight or no skin irritation.[30]
Post-application occlusion on SLS-induced compromised skin	Post-exposure occlusive treatment markedly enhanced irritant response.[31]
Nicotine TTS and its device	Nine of 14 subjects developed mild irritant erythematous reactions due to occlusion (reacted to both of the adhesive and matrix layers).[32]
Aluminum chambers and chambers with water, physiological saline, a paper disc, or 0.002% of SLS for 24 h	Occlusion did not affect readings of electrical skin impedance taken 24 h or later after removal but increased variance for readings taken 1 h after removal.[33]
Polyethylene foam closed chambers for 24 h	Number of deepened skin furrows on skin surface was increased by lower water vapor permeability of the film, as well as increasing temperature and humidity on test day.[25]
Impermeable plastic films for 1, 2, and 3 weeks and various TDDS	One week of an impermeable plastic film did not injure skin; 2 weeks were moderately harmful to some, but not all, subjects; 3 weeks regularly induced hydration dermatitis; some hydrogels did not appreciably hydrate or macerate the surface by visual inspection when left in place for 1 week; but some TDDS may indeed provoke a dermatitis when applied twice weekly to the same site.[5]
Glove patch for 4 and 8 h, and empty dressing; hexyl nicotinate (HN) as an indicator	Percomeal permeability, TEWL, and compliance parameters were significantly increased after 4 and 8 h occlusion, and skin surface roughness was significantly reduced in terms of roughness parameters Ra and Rz by 4 and 8 h occlusion.[34]
Plastic chambers with sodium alkyl sulfates for 24 h	All alkyl sulfates except for SLS resulted in a temporary decrease of SC hydration 1 h after patch removal; at day 2, SC hydration levels of surfactant-treated skin were not significantly different from controls; thereafter, a second decrease in capacitance value was observed with the lowest hydration at day 7.[35]
Occlusion on essential fatty acid-deficient and normal mouse for 8, 24, and 48 h	Occlusion lowers cytokine mRNA levels in essential fatty acid-deficient and normal mouse epidermis, but not after acute barrier disruption.[28]
Different occlusive and semipermeable dressings for 23 and 46 h on irritation and tape stripping skins	Occlusion did not significantly delay barrier repair.[36-37]

(Continued)

TABLE 19.1 (CONTINUED)
Brief Data of Local Reactions of Occlusion

Occlusion	Local Reactions and References
Short-term (6 h/day for 3 days) gloves on normal skin and gloves on SLS-compromised skin	Glove occlusion on normal skin for short-term exposure did not significantly change water barrier function but caused a significantly negative effect on SLS-compromised skin for same period.[38]
Long-term (6 h/day for 14 days) gloves on normal skin and a cotton glove worn under the occlusive glove	This long-term using glove occlusion on normal skin caused a significant negative effect on skin barrier function, as measured by TEWL and prevented by cotton glove.[39]
Plastic chambers at 24, 48, 72, and 96 h	A significantly progressive increase under occlusion and reaching a plateau on day 2; hydration and water-holding capacity did not show significant changes.[40]
Occlusion with and without antibacterial hand cleanser	Antibacterial hand cleanser followed by glove occlusion had a significant TEWL increase.[42]
Impact of semipermeable gloves on barrier recovery and TEWL compared to occluded areas	Areas covered with semipermeable membranes showed enhanced barrier recovery than occluded areas. TEWL in areas covered with semipermeable membranes had significantly lower than occluded areas.[43]
Long-term use of semipermeable membrane	Long-term use (23 h/day for 3 weeks) of semipermeable membrane improved skin barrier function.[44]
SLS irritation in water-exposed sites vs. SLS irritation in occluded sites	SLS irritation in water-exposed sites had higher TEWL and clinical scores than occluded test sites.[45]
Effects of sequential application of irritation combined with SLS and occlusion on skin barrier	Barrier disrupted rated from most disruption to least disruption: occlusion with SLS and mechanical irritation > occlusion with SLS > occlusion with water and mechanical irritation > mechanical irritation and occlusion with water > occlusion with a glove and mechanical irritation > mechanical irritation > occlusion with water.[46]
Effect of hand alcohol and gloves in wet activities on TEWL.	Decrease in TEWL when hand alcohol was used in place of soap when hands were not visibly dirty and when gloves were used in wet activities.[47]
Impact of occlusion on healthy vs. irritated skin	Occlusion in irritated skin resulted in significantly higher levels of TEWL.[48]
Effect of pH 5.5 gloves on skin irritation	pH 5.5 gloves kept lower skin pH levels and may reduce irritation.[49]
Effects of glove occlusion on skin barrier.	Data on the negative effect of occlusion is limited. Only long-term and extensive occlusion will cause barrier impairment.[50]
Effect of wearing occlusive gloves on skin condition if gloves are worn throughout entire work day	TEWL and skin hydration were significantly higher for those who wore occlusive gloves for the entire work day. However, TEWL dropped after gloves were removed for at least 30 min.[51]

(Continued)

TABLE 19.1 (CONTINUED)
Brief Data of Local Reactions of Occlusion

Occlusion	Local Reactions and References
Occlusive effect of short-term (wearing once for 4 h) and long-term (wearing gloves for 4 h a day, 7 days a week) glove wear	TEWL was seen 30 min after 4 h occlusion as compared to baseline. Three hours later, there was a full recovery to baseline. A significant long-term effect after daily occlusion of 4 h for 1 week could not be shown.[52]

19.4 CONCLUSIONS

Most studies presented here are related to occlusive effects on normal skin. Data on compromised skin are unfortunately limited.[28,31,36–38] As noted above, occlusion alone may produce cytological skin damage, which has been termed *hydration dermatitis* by Kligman.[5] With the application of chemicals/drugs under occlusion conditions, it can increase the penetration of chemicals and antigens into the skin and therefore also increases dermatitis.[5,6] These side effects should be considered whenever applying occlusion manner in clinical situations. The application of optimal hydrocolloid patches that absorb water in both liquid and vapor form can decrease the irritant reaction.[26,53,54] Topical corticoids are another alternative, but their role in the suppression of TDDS-induced dermatitis needs to be better defined, especially for patients who require continued treatment with the long-term application of such devices.[7] The hope is that more efficacious and realistic approaches to abrogating contact dermatitis will be developed. Taken together, the experimental data presented here documents how far we have progressed in understanding the effects of occlusion on the skin in recent decades. Fortunately, the overwhelming majority of individuals now extensively utilizing occlusive gloves tolerate them well. That does not mean that future improvements will not be possible. Those few intolerant to occlusive gloves are dealt with in Chapter 22.

We conclude with the most important findings:

1. Occlusion decreases skin barrier function.
2. Occlusion increases skin irritants and allergic contact dermatitis, in particular on compromised skin.
3. An optimal design like hydrogel and semipermeable membranes can reduce such dermatitis.
4. Occlusion does not significantly delay barrier repair in humans and may hasten the healing time.[6,55–61]

REFERENCES

1. Bucks, D.A., McMaster, J.R., Maibach, H.I., and Guy, R.H. 1988. Bioavailability of topically administered steroids: A "mass balance" technique. *J Invest Dermatol* 91:29.

2. Bucks, D., Guy, R., and Maibach, H.I. 1991. Effects of occlusion. In *In vitro Percutaneous Absorption: Principles, Fundamentals, and Applications*. Bronaugh, R.L., and Maibach, H.I., Eds. Boca Raton, FL: CRC Press, 85.

3. Treffel, P., Muret, P., Muret-D'Aniello, P., Coumes-Marquet, S., and Agache, P. 1992. Effect of occlusion on *in vitro* percutaneous absorption of two compounds with different physicochemical properties. *Skin Pharmacol* 5:108.

4. Bucks, D., and Maibach, H.I. 1999. Occlusion does not uniformly enhance penetration *in vivo*. In *Percutaneous Absorption: Drug-Cosmetics-Mechanisms-Methodology*, 3rd ed. Bronaugh, R.L., and Maibach, H.I., Eds. New York: Marcel Dekker, 81.

5. Kligman, A.M. 1996. Hydration injury to human skin. In *The Irritant Contact Dermatitis Syndrome*. Van der Valk, P.G.M., and Maibach, H.I., Eds. Boca Raton, FL: CRC Press, 187.

6. Berardesca, E., and Maibach, H.I. 1988. Skin occlusion: Treatment or drug-like device? *Skin Pharmacol* 1:207.

7. Hogan, D.J., and Maibach, H.I. 1991. Transdermal drug delivery systems: Adverse reaction — dermatologic overview. In *Exogenous Dermatoses: Environmental Dermatitis*. Menne, T., and Maibach, H.I., Eds. Boca Raton, FL: CRC Press, 227.

8. Bodde, H.E., Verhoeven, J., and van Driel, L.M.J. 1989. The skin compliance of transdermal drug delivery systems. *Crit Rev Ther Drug Carrier Syst* 6:87.

9. Cleary, G.W. 1993. Transdermal delivery systems: A medical rationale. In *Topical Drug Bioavailability, Bioequivalence, and Penetration*. Shah, V.P., and Maibach, H.I., Eds. New York: Plenum Press, 17.

10. Cleary, G.W. 1993. Transdermal drug delivery. In *Skin Permeation, Fundamentals and Application*. Zatz, J.L., Ed. Wheaton, IL: Allured Publishing, 207.

11. Sobel, S. 1993. Clinical considerations of transdermal drugs. In *Topical Drug Bioavailability, Bioequivalence, and Penetration*. Shah, V.P., and Maibach, H.I., Eds. New York: Plenum Press, 431.

12. Ghosh, T.K., and Pfister, W.R. 1997. Transdermal and topical delivery systems: An overview and future trends. In *Transdermal and Topical Drug Delivery Systems*. Ghosh, T.K., Pfister, W.R., and Yum, S.I., Eds. Buffalo Grove, IL: Interpharm Press, 1.

13. Kydonieus, A.F., Wille, J.J., and Murphy, G.F. 2000. Fundamental concepts in transdermal delivery of drug. In *Biochemical Modulation of Skin Reactions, Transdermals, Topicals, Cosmetics*. Kydonieus, A.F., and Wille, J.J., Eds. Boca Raton, FL: CRC Press, 1.

14. Baker, H. 1972. The skin as a barrier. In *Textbook of Dermatology*, 2nd ed. Rook, A., Wilkinson, D.S., and Ebling, F.J.G., Eds. Oxford: Blackwell Scientific, 249.

15. Denda, M., Sato, J., Tsuchiya, T., Elias, P.M., and Feingold, K.R. 1998. Low humidity stimulates epidermal DNA synthesis and amplifies the hyperproliferative response to barrier disruption: Implication for seasonal exacerbations of inflammatory dermatoses. *J Invest Dermatol* 111:873.

16. Tsai, T.-F., and Maibach, H.I. 1999. How irritant is water? An overview. *Contact Dermatitis* 41:311.

17. Warner, R.R., Boissy, Y.L., Lilly, N.A., Spears, M.J., McKillop, K., Marshall, J.L., and Stone, K.J. 1999. Water disrupts stratum corneum lipid lamellae: Damage is similar to surfactants. *J Invest Dermatol* 113:960.

18. Orth, D.S., and Appa, Y. 2000. Glycerine: A natural ingredient for moisturizing skin. In *Dry Skin and Moisturizers. Chemistry and Function*. Lodén, M., and Maibach, H.I., Eds. Boca Raton, FL: CRC Press, 213.

19. Lodén, M. 2000. Moisturizers. In *Cosmeceuticals. Drugs vs. Cosmetics*. Eisner, P., and Maibach, H.I., Eds. New York: Marcel Dekker, 73.

20. Haftek, M., Teillon, M.H., and Schmitt, D. 1998. Stratum corneum, corneodesmosomes and *ex vivo* percutaneous penetration. *Microsc Res Tech* 43:242.

21. Wester, R.C., and Maibach, H.I. 1983. Cutaneous pharmacokinetics: 10 steps to percutaneous absorption. *Drug Metab Rev* 14:169.
22. Hotchkiss, S.A., Miller, J.M., and Caldwell, J. 1992. Percutaneous absorption of benzyl acetate through rat skin *in vitro*. 2. Effect of vehicle and occlusion. *Food Chem Toxicol* 30:145.
23. Qiao, G.L., Chang, S.K., and Riviere, J.E. 1993. Effects of anatomical site and occlusion on the percutaneous absorption and residue pattern of 2,6-[ring-^{14}C] parathion *in vivo* in pigs. *Toxicol Appl Pharmacol* 122:131.
24. Leow, Y.H., and Maibach, H.I. 1997. Effect of occlusion on skin. *J Dermatol Treat* 8:139.
25. Matsumura, H., Oka, K., Umekage, K., Akita, H., Kawai, J., Kitazawa, Y., Suda, S., Tsubota, K., Ninomiya, Y., Hirai, H., Miyata, K., Morikubo, K., Nakagawa, M., Okada, T., and Kawai, K. 1995. Effect of occlusion on human skin. *Contact Dermatitis* 33:231.
26. Faergemann, J., Aly, R., Wilson, D.R., and Maibach, H.I. 1983. Skin occlusion: Effect on *pityrosporum orbiculare*, skin P CO_2, pH, transepidermal water loss, and water content. *Arch Dermatol Res* 275:383.
27. Kömvües, L.G., Hanley, K., Jiang, Y., Katagiri, C., Elias, P.M., Williams, M.L., and Feingold, K.R. 1999. Induction of selected lipid metabolic enzymes and differentiation-linked structural proteins by air exposure in fetal rat skin explants. *J Invest Dermatol* 112:303.
28. Wood, L.C., Elias, P.M., Sequeira-Martin, S.M., Grunfeld, C., and Feingold, K.R. 1994. Occlusion lowers cytokine mRNA levels in essential fatty acid-deficient and normal mouse epidermis, but not after acute barrier disruption. *J Invest Dermatol* 103:834.
29. Hurkmans, J.F., Bodde, H.E., van Driel, L.M., van Doorne, H., and Junginger, H.E. 1985. Skin irritation caused by transdermal drug delivery systems during long-term (5 days) application. *Br J Dermatol* 112:461.
30. Nieboer, C., Bruynzeel, D.P., and Boorsma, D.M. 1987. The effect of occlusion of the skin with transdermal therapeutic system on Langerhans cells and the induction of skin irritation. *Arch Dermatol* 123:1499.
31. van der Valk, P.G.M., and Maibach, H.I. 1989. Post-application occlusion substantially increases the irritant response of the skin to repeated short-term sodium lauryl sulfate (SLS) exposure. *Contact Dermatitis* 21:335.
32. Bircher, A.J., Howald, H., and Rufli, T. 1991. Adverse skin reactions to nicotine in a transdermal therapeutic system. *Contact Dermatitis* 25:230.
33. Emtestam, L., and Ollmar, S. 1993. Electrical impedance index in human skin: Measurements after occlusion, in 5 anatomical regions and in mild irritant contact dermatitis. *Contact Dermatitis* 28:104.
34. Graves, C.J., Edwards, C., and Marks, R. 1995. The occlusive effects of protective gloves on the barrier properties of the stratum corneum. In *Irritant Dermatitis. New Clinical and Experimental Aspects. Current Problems in Dermatology.* Eisner, P., and Maibach, H.I., Eds. Basel: Karger, 23, 87.
35. Wilhelm, K.P. 1995. Effects of surfactants on skin hydration. In *Exogenous Dermatology. Current Problems in Dermatology.* Surber, C., Eisner, P., and Bircher, A.J., Eds. Basel: Karger, 22, 72.
36. Welzel, J., Wilhelm, K.P., and Wolff, H.H. 1995. Occlusion does not influence the repair of the permeability barrier in human skin. In *Irritant Dermatitis. New Clinical and Experimental Aspects. Current Problems in Dermatology.* Eisner, P., and Maibach, H.I., Eds. Basel: Karger, 23, 180.
37. Welzel, J., Wilhelm, K.R., and Wolff, H.H. 1996. Skin permeability barrier and occlusion: No delay of repair in irritated human skin. *Contact Dermatitis* 35:163.

38. Ramsing, D.W., and Agner, T. 1996. Effect of glove occlusion on human skin. (I). Short-term experimental exposure. *Contact Dermatitis* 34:1.

39. Ramsing, D.W., and Agner, T. 1996. Effect of glove occlusion on human skin (II). Long-term experimental exposure. *Contact Dermatitis* 34:258.

40. Fluhr, J.W., Lazzerini, S., Distante, F., Gloor, M., and Berardesca, E. 1999. Effects of prolonged occlusion on stratum corneum barrier function and water holding capacity. *Skin Pharmacol Appl Skin Physiol* 12:193.

41. Angelova-Fischer, I., Soltanipoor, M., Stilla, T., Fischer, T.W., Kezic, S., and Jakasa, I. 2020. Barrier damaging effects of n-propanol in occlusion-modified tandem repeated irritation test: Modulation by exposure factors and atopic skin disease. *Contact Dermatitis* 82:1–9.

42. Antonov, D., Kleesz, P., Elsner, P., and Schliemann, S. 2013. Impact of glove occlusion on cumulative skin irritation with or without hand cleanser–comparison in an experimental repeated irritation model. *Contact Dermatitis* 68:293–299.

43. Bock, M., Damer, K., Wulfhorst, B., and John, S.M. 2009. Semipermeable glove membranes–effects on skin barrier repair following SLS irritation. *Contact Dermatitis* 61:276–280.

44. Buraczewska, I., Broström, U., and Lodén, M. 2007. Artificial reduction in transepidermal water loss improves skin barrier function. *Br J Dermatol* 157:82–86.

45. Fartasch, M., Taeger, D., Broding, H.C., Schöneweis, S., Gellert, B., Pohrt, U., and Brüning, T. 2012. Evidence of increased skin irritation after wet work: Impact of water exposure and occlusion. *Contact Dermatitis* 67:217–228.

46. Fluhr, J.W., Akengin, A., Bornkessel, A., Fuchs, S., Praessler, J., Norgauer, J., Grieshaber, R., Kleesz, P., and Elsner, P. 2005. Additive impairment of the barrier function by mechanical irritation, occlusion and sodium lauryl sulphate in vivo. *Br J Dermatol* 153:125–131.

47. Jungbauer, F.H.W., Harst, J.J.V.D., Groothoff, J.W., and Coenraads, P.J. 2004. Skin protection in nursing work: Promoting the use of gloves and hand alcohol. *Contact Dermatitis* 51:135–140.

48. Jungersted, J.M., Høgh, J.K., Hellgren, L.I., Jemec, G.B.E., and Agner, T. 2010. Skin barrier response to occlusion of healthy and irritated skin: Differences in trans-epidermal water loss, erythema and stratum corneum lipids. *Contact Dermatitis* 63:313–319.

49. Mirza, R., Maani, N., Liu, C., Kim, J., and Rehmus, W. 2006. A randomized, controlled, double-blind study of the effect of wearing coated pH 5.5 latex gloves compared with standard powder-free latex gloves on skin pH, transepidermal water loss and skin irritation. *Contact Dermatitis* 55:20–25.

50. Tiedemann, D., Clausen, M.L., John, S.M., Angelova-Fischer, I., Kezic, S., and Agner, T. 2016. Effect of glove occlusion on the skin barrier. *Contact Dermatitis* 74:2–10.

51. Weistenhöfer, W., Wacker, M., Bernet, F., Uter, W., and Drexler, H. 2015. Occlusive gloves and skin conditions: Is there a problem? Results of a cross-sectional study in a semiconductor company. *Br J Dermatol* 172:1058–1065.

52. Wetzky, U., Bock, M., Wulfhorst, B., and John, S.M. 2009. Short- and long-term effects of single and repetitive glove occlusion on the epidermal barrier. *Arch Dermatol Res* 301:595–602.

53. Fairbrother, J.E., Hollingsbee, D.A., and White, R.J. 1992. Hydrocolloid dermatological patches — corticosteroid combinations. In *Topical Corticosteroids*. Maibach, H.I., and Surber, C., Eds. Basel: Karger, 503.

54. Hollingsbee, D.A., White, R.J., and Edwardson, P.A.D. 1995. Use of occluding hydrocolloid patches. In *Percutaneous Penetration Enhancers*. Smith, E.W., and Maibach, H.I., Eds. Boca Raton, FL: CRC Press, 35.

55. Eaglstein, W.H., Mertz, P.M., and Falanga, V. 1991. Wound dressings: Current and future. *Prog Clin Biol Res* 365:257.

56. Winter, G.D. 1962. Formation of the scab and the rate of epithelization of superficial wounds in the skin of the young domestic pig. *Nature* 193:293.

57. Hinman, C.D., and Maibach, H.I. 1963. Effect of air exposure and occlusion on experimental human skin wounds. *Nature* 200:377.

58. Alvarez, O.M., Mertz, P.M., and Eaglstein, W.H. 1983. The effect of occlusive dressings on collagen synthesis and re-epithelization in superficial wounds. *J Surg Res* 35:142.

59. Fisher, L.B., and Maibach, H.I. 1972. Effect of occlusive and semipermeable dressings on the mitotic activity of normal and wounded human epidermis. *Br J Dermatol* 86:593.

60. Pinski, J.B. 1987. Human dermabrasion as a wound healing model. In *Models in Dermatology*. Maibach, H.I., and Lowe, N., Eds. Basel: Karger, 196.

61. Silverman, R.A., Lender, J., and Elmets, C.A. 1989. Effects of occlusive and semiocclusive dressings on the return of barrier function to transepidermal water loss in standardized human wounds. *J Am Acad Dermatol* 20:755.

Section IV

Protection against Chemical and Microbial Agents

20 Gloves and Dermal Exposure to Chemicals

K.S. Galea and J.W. Cherrie

CONTENTS

20.1 INTRODUCTION

There is an enormous range of chemical protective gloves available. These differ in design, method of fabrication, and materials used to protect against chemical attacks. Gloves and other protective clothing are designed either to protect the environment from the person, such as in semiconductor manufacture, or to guard the body against environmental insult. The health protection goals for gloves may focus on two purposes: to prevent localized damage to the skin from irritant, corrosive, or other harm or to limit the systemic uptake of chemicals through the skin. In this chapter, we focus specifically on the latter use, although many of the concepts that we discuss can also be applied to the protection of the hands from acute hazards.

Many glove users wrongly believe that gloves provide complete protection from all chemicals; however, there is a wealth of laboratory data that demonstrates that chemicals may permeate through gloves. In these circumstances, if the challenge

DOI: 10.1201/9781003126874-24

chemical remains present, after a period of time there will be a steady mass flux of the chemical through the glove material.[1] When this occurs, the wearer will generally not be aware of contamination of the inside of the glove because the flux will be insufficient to produce any sensation on the skin surface. However, it may still be high enough to make a significant contribution to the systemic uptake of the chemical into the body.

There is also much anecdotal information and published literature that suggests that glove users do not always wear their gloves and that removing and replacing gloves may potentially contaminate the inside of the gloves leading to additional exposure for the wearer.[2,3] This is not surprising, as occupational hygienists have, in terms of the hierarchy of control, asserted that all forms of personal protection should be considered the last resort in controlling hazardous agents, primarily because their effectiveness is highly dependent on the wearer.[4] Contaminant may also bypass the glove barrier and flow between the glove and the skin; for example, a liquid splash to the forearm may run down the arm and inside the glove. This is particularly true when short wrist-length gloves are employed instead of gauntlets for hand immersion activities. Finally, gloves may become damaged, and this can result in chemicals flowing through the breach onto the skin.

The integrity of gloves may be particularly important when they are reused. Work by El-Ayouby and co-workers[5] showed that repeated use of nitrile and butyl gloves and decontamination using alcohol compromised the chemical resistance of the gloves to solvents after only one or two use/decontamination cycles. When conditions are likely to involve stretching the glove materials (e.g., through repeated clenching of the hands), this may stress the glove material, resulting in tears and a potential influx of the chemical agents into the skin.[6] Contact with objects may lead to accidental puncture holes.

We can therefore distinguish three causes of skin contamination while wearing gloves:

1. Factors related to the glove material or glove design, for example, permeation and penetration through the glove.
2. Selection factors where there is an interaction between the glove design and the exposure scenario, e.g., direct deposition onto the skin because an area potentially exposed was not covered by the glove.
3. Human factors related to use, e.g., contamination of the skin because of the unnecessary removal of gloves during work.

Despite a good understanding of the possible mechanisms by which people may become exposed to chemicals while wearing gloves, it is uncertain how important each of these is in reality or how effective gloves are overall in protecting the hands during work activities. The effectiveness of other personal protective equipment (PPE), particularly respiratory protection, has been investigated in detail. In this case, the effectiveness of respiratory protective equipment (RPE) is assessed by measuring the ratio of the contaminant concentration inside the respirator face piece and the corresponding concentration outside the respirator. This ratio is known as the protection factor (PF), and if the study is undertaken in a real work environment, we may measure the workplace protection factor. There have been numerous respirator workplace protection factor studies published in the peer-review literature, some of which are summarized in a review by Janssen et al.[7]

Information from studies on the effectiveness of RPE may be used to determine appropriate risk management strategies, and this has led to the development of the use of the term *assigned protection factor* (APF). The APF is the minimum level of protection that is expected to be achieved by a trained wearer using a properly fitted, correctly functioning respirator.[8] For example, if the estimated inhalation exposure level in a workplace is 10 mg/m^3, then wearing a respirator with an APF of ten would, with a high degree of certainty, reduce the inhaled concentration to 1 mg/m^3, one-tenth the original value. If this value is less than the occupational exposure limit (OEL) value, then it may be concluded that the risks from inhaling the chemical are sufficiently well controlled by respiratory protection. This approach has been a powerful tool in selecting RPE, and so one must ask: Why do we not have a comparable approach for dermal exposure and gloves?

Various national regulatory authorities assign a skin notation for a variety of substances. According to Banaee and Que Hee,[1] the major guidance in the USA is based on a system of American Conference of Governmental Industrial Hygienists (ACGIH) notations, to denote systemic and sensitizing effects, with the National Institute for Occupational Safety and Health (NIOSH) also publishing guidelines that incorporate skin irritation and absorption. Viegas et al.[9] present a list of all the EU Occupational Safety and Health legislation that mentions skin as a possible exposure route to chemicals in the workplace or uses the skin notation for specific chemicals. In this last case, the commonest description in the legal text is "a skin notation assigned to the OEL value indicates the possibility of significant uptake through the skin." In the Directive 2004/37/EC, the text is different, but the meaning is similar "substantial contribution to the total body burden via dermal exposure possible." Some authors have also proposed the introduction of dermal OELs as a quantitative measure of maximum acceptable exposure during a work shift.[10,11] Several regulations already demand OELs for dermal exposure, e.g., dermal acceptable operator exposure levels (AOELs) for pesticides and biocides in the EU,[12] and local and systemic derived no-effect levels under the Registration, Evaluation, Authorization, and Restriction of Chemicals (REACH) regulations.[13] While limits are in place and recognized by some agencies, the measurement of dermal exposure is far less well developed than the corresponding techniques used for inhalation exposure. There is little standardization of methodology and no real agreement about the most appropriate exposure metric to assess risk. The main reason for this is the lack of an agreed theoretical picture of how people become exposed to chemicals on their skin and then subsequently how the chemicals are taken up into the body.

In this chapter, the methods available to measure dermal exposure are discussed, and a summary of the literature that helps clarify the effectiveness of gloves is presented. We also present a conceptual model of the processes involved in dermal exposure and discuss what an appropriate exposure metric might be for risk evaluation. In particular, we focus on how this model illuminates the approach that should be used to evaluate the effectiveness of gloves in the workplace. Finally, we discuss how the assessment of the effectiveness of gloves may be improved in the future.

20.2 A CONCEPTUAL MODEL OF DERMAL EXPOSURE

Schneider and a group of other European researchers devised a conceptual model of dermal exposure.[14] This describes the processes and "compartments" involved, from the source of the hazardous chemical in the workplace through to permeation of the chemical through the outer skin layers, i.e., uptake. This section briefly describes their model and uses it to provide some insight into the protection provided by gloves.

The uptake of the chemical into the body is mediated by diffusion across the stratum corneum. For this to occur the chemical must be within the "skin contamination layer," a liquid layer in contact with the stratum corneum. Diffusion will cause an uptake flux of the chemical if there is a difference in concentration between the skin contamination layer and the peripheral blood flow or extracellular fluids. At a steady state, the flux is described by Fick's law of diffusion:

$$J = k_p dC \qquad (20.1)$$

where J is the flux of contaminant, for example, mg/cm²/h, k_p is the permeability constant, and dC is the concentration difference (mg/cm³).

For systemic effects, the mass of contaminant taken into the body will play an important role in determining the consequent risk and so we believe that the most appropriate measure of exposure is the product of the concentration in the skin contamination layer (C_{sk}), the area exposed (A_{sk}), and the duration of exposure (t_{sk}), so E_{sk} the dermal exposure is

$$E_{sk} = C_{sk} A_{sk} t_{sk} \qquad (20.2)$$

With this approach, the mass uptake through the skin (U_{sk}) may be estimated as:

$$U_{sk} = k_p E_{sk} \qquad (20.3)$$

This analysis assumes that the concentration is constant over the exposed area throughout the exposure period and that the concentration in the skin contamination layer may be approximated as the concentration difference, i.e., C_{sk} is approximately equal to dC.

Note that we also assume that the flux is the same across the whole skin area exposed, although there are large differences in flux rate between different anatomical locations.[15] This simplifying assumption is made because we are primarily interested in "external" exposure rather than internal body burden. We believe differences in actual uptake because of the location of exposure on the body should be accounted for in a risk assessment as part of the evaluation of the dose received by the individual. However, it is less important in assessing the effectiveness of gloves.

These equations are also only valid if there is an unlimited supply of the contaminant available for uptake. If this is not the case, then the mass of the contaminant chemical in the skin contaminant layer minus any losses from evaporation or cleaning (M_{sk}) would be equal to the uptake. Mathematically, if $k_pE_{sk} > M_{sk}$, then $U_{sk}=M_{sk}$; otherwise, $U_{sk}=k_pE_{sk}$. From this, we can see that the uptake is the most relevant exposure metric for the assessment of risk and hence glove effectiveness.

The model that Schneider and his co-workers devised is shown in Figure 20.1. It comprises compartments, such as the skin contamination layer, and transfer processes that allow contaminant mass to move from one compartment to another. The skin contamination layer is toward the bottom of the figure, with the uptake shown

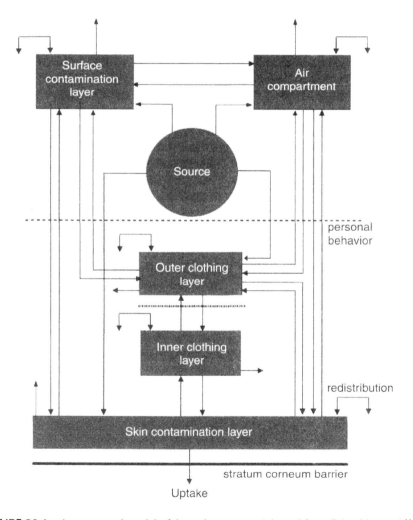

FIGURE 20.1 A conceptual model of dermal exposure. Adapted from Schneider et al.[14]

schematically as an arrow toward the stratum corneum. It should be noted that the model focuses on the processes at a conceptual level to help analyze how people may become exposed, and it is not intended to provide a basis for the prediction of exposure.

The uppermost compartments in the model figure relate to the indoor environment where exposure takes place: the room air and the internal surfaces. There are two compartments for clothing, which include gloves, and in the remainder of this chapter we refer specifically to gloves in relation to clothing. The upper of these two compartments represents the outer surface of the gloves, and the lower compartment the inner surface of the gloves. The flow between the two compartments is regulated by a permeation barrier, i.e., the glove material, and then onto the skin contamination layer. However, it is clear that this is not the only way that contamination can enter the skin contamination layer from the outside because there are transfer processes shown between the outside of the gloves and the skin or directly onto the skin from the source or other compartments. A full description of each of the compartments and transfer processes is given in Schneider et al.[14]

20.3 MONITORING EXPOSURE TO ASSESS THE PROTECTION AFFORDED BY GLOVES

20.3.1 AVAILABLE METHODS FOR MONITORING DERMAL EXPOSURE

The methods currently available to monitor dermal exposure can be divided into three categories, these being: interception, removal, and in situ methods. The WHO's International Programme on Chemical Safety (IPCS) document on dermal exposure[15] and the ISO technical report[16] are two key references that provide a more detailed description of these methods; however, the main points are summarized in the following sections. We particularly focus on the use of these techniques to measure hand and forearm contamination to chemicals; however, many can be applied to assess whole-body exposure.

In addition to these three categories, we should highlight the recent advancements in the use of silicon wristbands as passive sampling devices to evaluate personal chemical exposure. These were first introduced by O'Connell and colleagues,[17] in 2014, and these simple-to-use, inexpensive, and unobtrusive methods have been used to detect chemical exposure too, for example, flame retardants, pesticides, and polycyclic aromatic hydrocarbons (PAHs).[18,19] They are used to detect chemicals in the wearers' external environment and thus can incorporate both the inhalation and dermal exposure routes simultaneously, although not in isolation.[18,20] A major limitation of these devices is the lack of quantitative assessment of concentration.

20.3.1.1 Interception Methods

Interception (also known as surrogate skin) methods generally comprise absorbent or retentive patches or garments (whole suits and gloves) that are attached to the skin or clothing. When worn, they intercept and retain the chemicals that would otherwise have come into contact with the clothing or skin. Following exposure, these dosimeters are removed, and the amount of chemical retained by them is determined by an appropriate analytical method, with the mass recovered being a surrogate of the dermal exposure mass.

Patches are often made from absorptive material (e.g., cotton gauze, rayon/cotton cloth), backed with impervious material such as aluminum foil or polyethylene to avoid losses of the collected contaminant to the skin (i.e., absorption into the body) or clothing as well as provide greater integrity and robustness to the sampler. The sizes of the patches also vary, although for sampling on the hands/forearm the largest size used has an area of about 100 cm^2 and the smallest about 9 cm^2 in area[21]. "Generic" protocols that prescribe sizes, numbers, location, and method of attachment of patches are available,[22–24] with some chemical-specific patch methods also being published.[16]

Patch samples are generally located at strategic points on the body. If, for example, a person receives a single splash to the forearm, then it will probably not be sampled, although occasionally some high measurements will be recorded by chance. It is, therefore, possible that patch samples may under- or overestimate whole-body exposure from irregular random processes. While close-fitting whole suit samplers can address this limitation (as the surface areas of the sampler may be more approximate to the equivalent body area), the use of larger whole suits worn over clothing may lead to oversampling due to the increased surface area (as well as the potential discomfort and restriction of movement).

Patches are difficult to locate on the hands, and so cotton sampling gloves are often worn as an alternative. These also have the advantage of sampling the whole hand area rather than a specific area. Where sampling gloves are worn, they are normally worn inside any protective gloves, which makes it difficult to derive any measure of protection from studies that have been undertaken to measure dermal exposure using these methods. In addition, these may impede the manual dexterity of the wearer.

Interception methods do have their limitations. Firstly, different collection materials may have different absorption, retention, and repellence characteristics, and it is important to understand and quantify these before applying them in a dermal exposure assessment study. In addition, their absorbent capacity may be much greater than that the skin contamination layer could contain. Therefore, interception methods tend to measure the total mass of a chemical that has come into contact with the sampling medium rather than the mass of contaminant that might reside on the skin. Dividing the mass on the sampling medium by the duration allows an estimate to be made of the average flux onto the skin, i.e., the mass of chemical per unit time, but gives no indication of the likely mass that will "runoff" or evaporate from the skin before absorption takes place.[21] It is also recommended that when a sampler becomes saturated that it should be replaced with a fresh one although there is no available guidance to help determine whether or not a sampler is saturated.

All of the absorbent interception techniques are limited to low-volatility liquid chemicals or solids; volatile chemicals rapidly evaporate from this type of sampler. Some researchers have used activated charcoal cloth (ACC) pads or patches to assess dermal exposure to more volatile agents, mainly benzene and toluene;[25,26] Creta et al.[27] reported a study where ACC was found to be a suitable sampling material for quantitatively assessing dermal exposure to 181 volatile organic compounds in terms of sensitivity and desorption efficiency. Cherrie and Robertson proposed a novel patch sampler for volatile agents. [28] Their design relies on a semipermeable membrane to regulate the adsorption of chemicals by an activated charcoal layer. The semipermeable membrane should ideally mimic the barrier properties of the stratum corneum, and this sampler will then directly measure the uptake through the skin.

20.3.1.2 Removal Methods

Removal methods rely on recovering the chemicals directly from the skin contamination layer, normally using some variation of washing or wiping the skin.[15,16] The mass that has evaporated or fallen or been absorbed by the skin during the exposure process is not sampled using these methods.

Wiping may either be carried out using dry materials or with some absorbent solid material moistened with water, alcohol, or some proprietary solvent mixture. The absorbent material can be filter papers, cotton balls, surgical cotton pads, or proprietary moist wipes. If a sample is to be obtained from the hands, then subjects may be asked to thoroughly wipe the whole of both hands or each hand individually may be swabbed by the investigator. Alternatively, a template (e.g., circular, square, or rectangular) may be used to enable a swab sample to be collected from a defined area of skin, e.g., on the dorsal or palmar regions of the hand. There are no standardized protocols that specify the amount of pressure to be applied when wiping, the pattern of wiping, or indeed the number of consecutive wipes to be collected from the same area, which is a limitation of the wipe sampling method.[29] However, in a recent pan-European hexavalent chromates biomonitoring study, a standardized hand wipe protocol was adopted, specifying the wiping pattern, the number of wipes to be collected, and the sampling strategy.[30]

Brouwer et al.[31] described the sampling efficiencies for pesticide residues reported by various investigators. These ranged from approximately 40% up to more than 100%, although the majority of results were less than about 60%. Other studies have shown higher and more consistent sampling efficiency for metal particles, where typically more than 95% of the contamination can be consistently removed with three sequential wipes using proprietary moist wipes.[32] Galea et al.[33] reported mean sampling efficiencies (at both ambient and elevated environmental conditions) of 102, 96%, and 91% for wipes collected 10–15 min, 2 h, and 4 h after pigs' trotters were spiked with known quantities of crude oil. Sampling efficiencies of over 90% were also reported for diesel, engine, and bike oil spiked directly on pigs' trotters.[34] Wipe sampling efficiencies using various procedures and for several compounds including metals, pyrene, and pesticides from the published literature are summarized in the WHO IPCS document on dermal exposure, and readers are encouraged to review this reference should they require further information.[15] The WHO IPCS document notes that the wiping pattern (e.g., S/Z movement, left to right or circular) is also considered to be important in terms of the sampling efficiency, but a comparison of the sampling efficiencies related to these approaches could not be identified in the literature.

Colorimetric wipe indicators are commercially available for substances such as isocyanates, amines, phenol, and acids/base.[35] After contact the color change of the wipe provides a qualitative indicator of exposure which can be a quick, easy technique for assessing skin contamination. These techniques have also been used to provide a semi-quantitative assessment of exposure and will be used in a planned pan-European study of workers exposed to di-isocyanates, again with a standardized wipe and collection protocol being adopted.[36,37,38]

Washing or rinsing techniques are invariably applied to hands. Typically for rinsing, a hand is placed into a plastic bag containing water or some other solvent, and this is then sealed around the wrist. The hand is then vigorously shaken for a defined period or a fixed number of "shakes." During hand washing, the subject is asked to wash using a "normal" technique, with washing and rinsing repeated several times. All of the rinse liquid is collected for later analysis. The ISO document summarizes the materials and procedures associated with hand washing and rinsing techniques.[16]

Sampling efficiency for washing various pesticide residues was again reported by Brouwer and colleagues.[39] Here the mean sampling efficiency typically ranged from about 50% to 96%, although most of the results were greater than 70%. The within-test standard deviation of the sampling efficiencies was generally less than that for wiping (mostly less than 10%).

Where removal techniques are used to sample, it is normally recommended that there should be an assessment of the actual sampling efficiency achieved, and as sampling efficiency may not be constant across all sample loading levels (mass and mass per unit area), it is important that the efficiency assessment is undertaken in conditions that are representative of the workplace. The WHO IPCS document also highlights that the recovery efficiency from the sampling medium being used in the assessment should also be determined. [15]

Wipe and washing/rinsing removal techniques remove what is present on the skin at the time of collection and so do not sample that which has been absorbed by the body or lost from the skin surface by, for example, evaporation or removal. Measurements should therefore generally be made before breaks when persons might be expected to wash to avoid losses from this activity.[16] Care must also be taken to ensure that the barrier function of the skin is not disrupted during sampling (e.g., minimizing the number of wipes, washes per day). The major limitation of hand wash methods is that they can really only be applied to a single body location (i.e., hands, wrists, and parts of the forearms), whereas wipe samples can be applied to other body regions such as the forehead, peri-oral region, and chest. One specific limitation of standardized wipe sampling is the person-dependent variability of applied pressure for wiping. Despite their limitations, removal techniques have been widely used, perhaps because of their simplicity and low cost. They can also be used to take samples from work surfaces, and work tools.[29]

Tape stripping is a well-established method in dermatology used for sampling the stratum corneum and is a technique that can be used to assess dermal exposure. Adhesive tapes are applied to the skin surface and peeled off, removing the most exterior skin layer along with substances deposited in this layer. As tape stripping reaches deeper skin areas, the amount of substance removed may also be taken to represent the amount absorbed into the skin. A number of adhesive tapes, each with different properties, are available. The WHO IPCS document on dermal exposure summarizes several studies which described the sampling efficiencies of tape-stripping methods.[15] These studies included a range of substances (e.g., methylene bisphenyl isocyanate, naphthalene in jet fuel, pyrene, etc.), tape types, and exposure durations. While comparison of the studies is difficult, it was noted that the properties of the adhesive tape itself may influence sampling and recovery efficiency and that recovery can be improved with a higher number of strips. Properties of the skin itself, substances being sampled, and the amount on the skin contaminant layer compartment, can also impact recovery efficiency. Limitations of the tape-stripping method are summarized in the ISO technical report.[16] They are related to sampling area and body locations covered by hair and the number of samples per day that may be reasonably collected. Another limitation of tape stripping is when sampling chemicals that have high transport rates from the skin contaminant layer. Also, the amount of stratum corneum which is removed in the first few tape strips can be influenced by how dirty or wet the skin is. The application of this sampling method may also be limited by the analytical limit of detection; however, pooled analysis of repeated tape stripping may overcome this problem. Finally, this method is subject to within- and between-operator operator variation, which may influence sampling parameters such as pressure and time tape is applied for and removal speed.

20.3.1.3   In Situ Methods

Dermal exposure can also be quantified by measuring the quantity of the agent or by adding a tracer (e.g., fluorescent material or visible dye) to the substance directly on the clothing or skin. The sampling principle is "in situ detection of a surrogate tracer present at the skin or clothing surface" [16]. Three approaches are cited as falling within this dermal exposure category, these being video imaging, Fourier transform infrared spectroscopy with attenuated total reflectance (ATR-FTIR), and detection via light sensor or probe. The use of qualitative and quantitative visualization techniques has also been reviewed by Cherrie et al.[40]

These methods can be based on the ultraviolet (UV) fluorescence of the hazardous substance itself, e.g., for PAHs. If the agent itself cannot be detected directly on the skin, a fluorescent or colored dye or an infrared absorbing chemical may be added before the individual starts working normally with the product. As the tracers are being used as surrogates for the substance of interest, their ratio to the substance must be known and should be constant during the exposure process. It is also important that the tracer does not significantly alter the physical properties of the product.[15] Cohen Hubal et al.[41] highlight that it may not always be possible to identify a tracer with the same deposition and retention characteristics as the substance of interest.

Typical fluorescent materials used include Uvitex OB, Tinopal, and Calcofluor.[40] For a qualitative evaluation, it may be sufficient to illuminate the person's body with long-wavelength UV light (i.e., wavelength 320–400 nm) in an area of subdued general lighting. For example, if the purpose of an investigation is to show whether contamination may enter a glove, then it may be sufficient for the worker to work normally with the hazardous substance containing the tracer, wearing their gloves, and then afterward inspect the hands under UV light, with any contamination shown clearly as fluorescence. Most of the fluorescent agents bind effectively to the skin, and so the estimate is essentially equivalent to the cumulative amount of tracer landing in the skin contamination layer.

Quantitative visualization uses the same basic approach although the systems for assessing the extent and intensity of fluorescence are much more sophisticated. The two main variants of this technique are known as Video Imaging Techniques for Assessing Dermal Exposure, developed initially by Fenske et al.,[42] and the Fluorescent Interactive Video Exposure System, developed by Roff.[43] In these systems the quantitative assessment is achieved by acquiring the image with a video camera and transferring it to a digital computer where the intensity of individual picture elements (pixels) is assessed using a previously derived relationship between the pixel intensity and the mass of tracer. From this information, the mass of a contaminant chemical in the skin contamination layer can be estimated. However, since each pixel represents an area of contaminated skin, the number of pixels that are detected to be "exposed" indicates the area of exposed skin.

Small areas of the skin (typically up to 5 cm^2) can be quantified by fluorescence using a small probe and a light fiber. The use of this technique has been fairly limited to, for example, the measurement of PAHs on the skin. An optic fiber is used to transport the light (typically UV-A, although UV-B has been used [with caution] in some devices) from the source to the surface and back to the detector, measuring the fluorescence emitted by the skin in response to being irradiated. The use of an "SMF 2" light probe was reported to be labor intensive, and not user friendly, with the probe needing to be applied to flat surfaces to obtain the correct readings.[44]

ATR-FTIR spectroscopy may be used for skin surface analysis of optically dense non-volatile infrared-active compounds. This technique can be used for identification purposes and is typically limited to smaller areas of the body. When infrared light is internally reflected off the crystal surface from beneath the instrument, an evanescent wave is produced extending out of the crystal surface and penetrating the skin in direct contact with it. The infrared absorption of this evanescent wave by the surface can be measured and qualitatively and quantitatively analyzed, representing the amount of the agent or tracer material present in the skin contaminant layer at the time of sampling.[16] Any agents with a suitable infrared spectrum would be suitable for detection by this method; however, the method is limited to small, selected areas, usually less than 2 cm^2 in area.[44]

Quantitative visualization techniques cannot be used in some circumstances where it is impracticable to add fluorescent tracers to the source. They are also labor intensive, and the hardware and software are relatively expensive. Many additional technical aspects need to be resolved, either by technical equipment, software, or study design, e.g., anthropometric adjustment, natural and variable fluorescence of the skin, removability of the tracer, etc.[15] However, this is the only technique that allows both the area exposed and the mass contamination that has been deposited in the skin contamination layer to be estimated. In addition, this dermal exposure assessment technique can be an incredibly powerful tool for training purposes, as workers can clearly see where they are experiencing exposure and understand better how this exposure is occurring and how it can be controlled.

20.3.1.4　Comparison of Dermal Exposure Monitoring Techniques

A number of studies have compared various dermal exposure assessment techniques. This section does not aim to provide a comprehensive overview of these but rather highlights some selected recent publications.

In 2019, the results of the large-scale SysDEA "Systematic Analysis of Dermal Exposure to Hazardous Chemical Agents at the Workplace" project were published.[44,45] This aimed to generate knowledge to improve/standardize dermal exposure measurement methods and compare several methods. In this study, different methods (body sampling using coveralls and patches, hand sampling utilizing 100% cotton gloves and washing, and head sampling using headbands and wiping) and the fluorescence method were compared during several tasks using both liquid formulations and powders. Just focusing on the hand exposure results, significantly higher exposure values were measured with the cotton glove method for rolling and manually handling objects with liquids. For spraying and pouring activities, higher values were measured with the cotton glove method compared to the hand washing method, although these were not statistically significant. The glove method resulted in significantly higher exposure values for handling contaminated objects, but not for dumping powders. In short, exposure values found on the cotton gloves were on average higher than the exposure values found in the hand wash solution, although the difference varied depending on the exposure situation. Estimates of body exposure using the fluorescence method resulted in much lower exposure values compared to the methods based on chemical analysis for both liquids and powders.

Tape-stripping, rinsing, and wiping of the hands were not included in the SysDEA study, although these are also commonly used methods to measure dermal exposure of the hands. Lundgren et al.[46] compared vacuum sampling with patches and tape stripping. Comparing tape stripping (two strips) with vacuuming, a small underestimation (an average of 9% lower values) was observed, whereas an overestimation (up to 21%) was observed with the patch method. Gorman Ng et al.[47] compared wipes, rinses, and gloves in side-by-side experiments. Wipe and rinse methods generally yielded similar results for the test substance, i.e., Epsom salts and zinc oxide (geometric mean [GM] ratios of wipe-to-rinse measurements of 0.6 and 1.4, respectively), but they did not for calcium acetate (GM wipe-to-rinse ratio of 4.6). For glycerol solutions, measurements from the glove samplers were consistently higher than wipe samples. At lower levels of exposure, the relative difference between these two methods was greater than at higher levels. Galea et al.[34] also carried out a direct comparison of a wipe and cotton glove sampling method using pigs' trotters as a surrogate for human skin. The trotters (placed into a cotton glove in instances when the cotton glove sampler was being assessed) were placed onto a clean metal surface, where known quantities of drilling fluid or crude oil had been loaded, with a weight of 5 kg being applied for 5 seconds. Significantly higher removal of both fluids from the metal surface was observed with the glove samples compared with the wipe samples (on average 2.5 times higher), with the authors concluding that glove samplers may overestimate the amount of fluid transferred to the skin.

Gorman Ng et al.[47] highlighted that further research would be necessary to enable conversion of exposure measurements from one metric to another. Franken et al.[44] explored whether it was possible to derive conversion factors based on the results of the different methods they assessed. The factor differences in exposure between the patch method and the whole-body method were found to vary greatly, with the differences being dependent on the type of liquid being used. Considering also that extrapolation of the patch method to a reference surface led the authors to conclude that there is too much uncertainty to reliably establish a generally applicable conversion factor. They also considered it inappropriate to derive a conversion factor based on the glove and hand wash results as they viewed the uncertainty around the factor would be too high. Marquat et al.[48] had also previously concluded that derivation of a general conversion factor between interception (gloves and patches) and removal (wipes, hand washes, and tape strips) sampling methods was unlikely to be feasible following an analysis of dermal exposure data as a part of the validation study of the ECETOC Targeted Risk Assessment (TRA) exposure model (this model will be discussed later in this chapter).

Franken et al.[44] concluded that no "golden standard" with regard to a preferred measurement method for dermal exposure could be identified from the methods investigated although some considerations are put forward. With respect to exposure to the hands, they considered that removal methods like a hand wash are a more appropriate way to determine exposure, while an interception method like gloves generally results in higher exposure values, which are assumed to resemble a worst-case exposure estimate. When measuring dermal exposure for, e.g., REACH dossiers, where a conservative/worst-case exposure assessment is preferred, it was considered that the glove method might be the more appropriate option.

It's recommended that before embarking on a dermal exposure assessment campaign that persons carefully consider their reasons for doing so and devise a suitable sampling strategy for this, taking into account the benefits and limitations of the respective techniques.[16,49] For example, if the purpose is to assess the effectiveness of protective gloves in the workplace, then consideration should be given to the evaporation rate of the hazardous substances from the skin and their uptake rate through the skin. Consideration should be given as to whether the wearing of interception samplers under (or over) protective gloves is possible or if these could compromise manual dexterity. Frequency and timing of sample collection from the hands require careful planning, given that gloves are frequently removed throughout the work shift for comfortable/refreshment breaks.

20.3.2 Role of Biological Monitoring in Assessing Dermal Exposure

Biological monitoring is the measurement of the body's burden of chemical compounds, elements, or their metabolites, in biological fluids (usually blood or urine, although other biological media have been used including breath, saliva, hair, nails, etc.).[50] A summary of the respective advantages and limitations of various biological matrices used in biomonitoring studies to assess environmental exposures to humans is provided in the WHO document on biomonitoring.[51] Such measurements may reflect the amount of substance stored in the body from previous exposure, sometimes from exposure that has occurred many weeks or months prior (e.g., persistent organic pollutants, lead, and cadmium).[51] When considering dermal exposure, it reflects both exposure and subsequent absorption of the agent into the systemic circulation, rather than potential exposure.[15] However as biological monitoring generally evaluates some form of integrated exposure by inhalation, dermal contact, and any other possible routes into the body, the amount of exposure by the dermal route may not be distinguishable from that by the inhalation or ingestion route.

The use of biological monitoring to reflect dermal exposure has been proposed as one approach for assessing the potential risks when chemicals may come into contact with the skin.[52] Boogaard[53] discusses various methods for dermal risk assessment, focusing on the advantages and disadvantages of dermal exposure and absorption models versus biomonitoring, and concludes that biomonitoring should be considered the method of choice to assess (dermal) exposure. The ISO[16] document states that for risk assessment purposes, where removal, evaporation, and resuspension rates for agents are high, irrespective of whether the uptake rates are high or low, biomonitoring is suggested. However, if dermal exposure is to be estimated based on biomonitoring, extensive additional studies (i.e., on absorption, metabolism, and physiologically based pharmacokinetics) are needed.[15,29] Given that biological monitoring measures are mediated by internal physiological and biochemical processes, as well as external exposure, they also reflect inter-individual variations that can also complicate interpretation. Kielhorn et al.[54] in the WHO IPCS document on dermal absorption highlight that unless a worker is breathing clean air, it may not be possible to separate dermal exposure from inhalation exposure, and thus observation of the worker and work practices is important for defining the routes of exposure. Recent large-scale biomonitoring studies have included the comprehensive collection of inhalation, dermal samples, and contextual data in their sampling strategy to allow for a more robust interpretation of the collected biomonitoring data,[30] thus allowing sources of exposure to be identified.

Biological monitoring has been used to evaluate the efficiency of PPE. For example, Chang et al.[55] evaluated the protective effect of gloves from occupational exposure to 2-methoxyethanol using the biomarkers of 2-methoxyacetic acid levels in the urine and plasma. The authors reported that rubber gloves provided a significant reduction in 2-ME uptake, whereas cotton gloves provided little protection with fluctuating effectiveness, based on estimates of protective effectiveness indices. Chang et al.[56] also successfully evaluated the effectiveness of chemical protective suits and gloves worn by spray painters by using biomarkers. Some have suggested that the measurement of "internal" exposure is superior to "external" exposure measurement to assess glove and PPE protection because it is more closely linked to the dose of the chemical in the body and any consequent adverse health effects.[57] However, there is often no strong statistical link between measures of internal and external exposure, and this leaves us with a dilemma regarding how best to reduce exposure to control unacceptable risks because it is mostly in relation to external exposure that we can effectively intervene.

20.3.3 What Can These Methods Measure?

It is possible to make measurements that reflect dermal exposure, both inside the body and on external body parts. However, none of the outlined approaches provides a method that is clearly superior to the others; each method has its limitations, and all methods measure different things. Table 20.1 summarizes the pros and cons of each of the approaches. Here we focus on four key parameters that may help quantify exposure: the mass of the hazardous substance in the skin contamination layer (M_{sk}), the area of skin exposed (A_{sk}), the concentration of the contaminant chemical in the skin contamination layer (C_{sk}), and, lastly, the duration of exposure (t_{sk}).

Although interception techniques can provide a measure of the chemical contaminant mass flux onto the skin, they do not provide any real indication of the mass in the skin contamination layer. This is because the collection efficiency of the absorbent materials used for these purposes is in no way comparable to that of the skin. Imagine pouring 10 ml of water onto a cotton gauze pad and then doing the same thing onto the back of your hand. In the former case, almost all of the liquid will be retained and, in the latter, almost none of it will remain on the hand. Removal and in situ methods (washing, wiping, and fluorescent methods) can provide an estimate of the amount of substance that has been retained in the skin contamination layer, although they each provide a slightly different measure. For example, the material that can be wiped from the skin at the end of a workday is the mass of contaminant that has landed on the skin, minus that was taken up into the body and the material lost to the work environment. Using a fluorescent tracer in the same circumstance would provide a measure of the mass of the contaminant that landed on the skin and remained there long enough for the tracer to bind to the skin protein. Normally, fluorescent tracers are neither taken up into the body nor lost in any significant quantity to the environment.

As we mentioned earlier, only tape strip methods can provide an estimate of the exposure loading or the concentration present in the skin contaminant layer covering the skin area at the time of sampling (concentration of the substance in the skin contamination layer $[C_{sk}]$), which is an important parameter to our evaluation of how much of a chemical may be taken up into the body.

20.3.4 Modeling Dermal Exposure and Uptake

Several model tools are available to estimate skin exposure to chemical agents for workers, particularly stimulated by regulations in Europe for the REACH regulations.[58] The accuracy of these models is poor, and they are mostly used as screening tools in a regulatory risk assessment, i.e., they are expected to overestimate true exposure to provide an appropriate margin of safety in use. Two of the most widely used tools are the ECETOC TRA, which provides a way to estimate consumer, environmental and occupational inhalation and dermal exposures, and Stoffenmanager, which can be used to estimate inhalation and dermal exposure to hazardous substances in workplaces.

The TRA was developed by the European chemical industry specifically for REACH, and it is freely available to download as an Excel workbook

TABLE 20.1

Methods for Measuring Dermal Exposure

Method Type	Description	Advantages	Disadvantages	M_{sk}	A_{sk}	t_{sk}	C_{sk}
					Measurement of Key Parameters		
Interception technique—patches	Small square cotton or other cloth patches attached to the body	Standard method for pesticides	Only low-volatility substances, only a small proportion of body sampled	✗	✗	✓	✗
Interception technique—suit sampling and gloves	Workers wear lightweight cotton overalls with hood	Whole-body sample	Only low-volatility substances, practical difficulties in sampling and analysis	✗	✗	✓	✗
Removal method—washing or wiping	Defined areas of skin washed with a solvent or wiped with a moist cloth	Low cost, easy to use	Only for low-volatility substances that do not quickly penetrate through the skin	✓	✗	✓	✗
Removal method—tape stripping	Removal of an agent from the skin using adhesive tape	Offers the potential to recover or measure agents in the stratum corneum	Sampling area/body locations covered by the hair; sampling chemicals from the skin that have high transport rates from the skin contaminant layer	✓	✗	✓	✓
In situ—fluorescence	Fluorescent compound added to source and then the intensity of fluorescence on the worker's body	Accurate assessment of area exposed to whole-body sample	Requires specialist equipment, must add a fluorescent agent to source	✓	✓	✓	✗
Biological monitoring	Measurement of the concentration of the substance or its metabolites in body fluids or tissues	Assessment of uptake into the body	Remote from the impact of control measures such as wearing gloves	?	?	?	?

M_{sk} mass of the hazardous substance in the skin contamination layer, A_{sk} area of skin exposed, t_{sk} duration of exposure, and C_{sk} concentration of the substance in the skin contamination layer. ✗ means "no", ✓ means "yes", ? means unknown.

(www.ecetoc.org/tools/targeted-risk-assessment-tra/). The basic concept of the TRA is that it combines the degree of exposure, based on physical-chemical properties such as molecular weight, vapor pressure, water solubility, octanol-water partition coefficient, exposure scenario data, and the hazard of a chemical to provide a way to demonstrate safe use. The worker protection section included provisions for the use of respiratory and dermal protection, including its efficiency. The output is provided as the estimated intake (mg per kg-body weight per day) and a risk characterization ratio, i.e., the ratio of the estimated exposure to a reference value.

Marquart and colleagues carried out a study to try to validate the TRA (version 3.1) using published dermal exposure data and unpublished sources.[48] They identified 106 cases where contextual data were available to derive a model estimate, and for each of these, the 75th percentile of the measurements was calculated. The model explained just 37% of the variance in the measurement data, although in about 80% of cases the model estimate was higher than the 75th percentile of the measurement. In particular, the authors showed that the impact of wearing protective gloves was underestimated in the model compared with the data, a reduction of five to ten times was assumed in the model, whereas the data showed exposures were 34 times lower when wearing gloves. Franken et al.[59] reported an experimental study with human volunteers designed to further validate the TRA with scenarios representing "use in a closed batch process," "mixing or blending in a partly open batch process," "rolling," "immersion," and "stirring." The TRA overestimated dermal hand exposure for all scenarios investigated between about 50 and 15,000 times, depending on the scenario; the most conservative estimates were for liquid in a partially enclosed process.

Stoffenmanager was originally developed as a simple tool to help small companies manage chemical exposure in specific workplaces using a risk (control) banding approach. The basic version of the software tool is available free online (www.stoffenmanager.nl). The tool is designed to use categorical estimates of exposure (in categories from 1 for "negligible" to 6 for "extreme") and hazard (in categories from A for "low" to E for "extreme") to provide the final outcome as one of three risk categories, from "low" to "high." There is no explicit account taken of wearing protective gloves, although the user can choose whether to exclude covered parts of the body, e.g., the hands. This tool has not been validated for dermal exposure assessment.

There are also mathematical models to estimate the dermal uptake of chemicals through the skin for simple exposure scenarios. For example, the American Industrial Hygiene Association's (AIHA) IH-SkinPerm© is an Excel tool that can be freely downloaded (www.aiha.org/public-resources/consumer-resources/topics -of-interest/ih-apps-tools). This tool works for pure substances based on information on how the chemical deposits on the skin, e.g., instantaneous deposition, the mass deposited, the area exposed, and the duration of exposure. The tool takes account of the evaporative loss of the chemical from the skin.

All of these tools have their limitations, and they clearly have poorer accuracy than measurements. However, particularly when using the exposure and uptake tools in combination they can provide a useful basis for risk management. Using this type of approach, Cherrie demonstrated for a rubber processing task involving toluene that the estimated dermal uptake was likely to be a small fraction of the maximum allowable inhalation uptake.[60]

20.4 STUDIES THAT HAVE ATTEMPTED TO ASSESS THE WORKPLACE EFFECTIVENESS OF GLOVES

Standardized laboratory tests for chemical protective gloves are available that provide estimates of breakthrough time and steady-state permeation flux. Permeation data is generated from permeation "standards" of the American Society for Testing and Materials International (ASTM International), the European Committee for Standardization (EN), and the International Organization for Standardization (ISO). It is evident that the actual, real-life performance of protective gloves can vary considerably, and protective efficacy in the workplace may be significantly different from those derived in standardized laboratory tests. However, there is no consensus view on how the actual workplace effectiveness of protective gloves against chemical challenges should be assessed.

Data may be reported as percent effectiveness, which represents the reduction in measured exposure achieved by wearing the gloves, or as a protection factor that represents the ratio of measured exposure outside a glove to that inside, or alternatively as the ratio of the exposure when not wearing gloves and when gloves are worn. It is straightforward to convert between these two measures of efficacy because the protection factor is just one divided by one minus the effectiveness expressed as a fraction; for example, 99% effectiveness corresponds to a protection factor of 100 and 90% effectiveness to a protection factor of 10.

Several regulatory authorities use a set of default values for assessing the effectiveness of the exposure reduction provided by protective gloves, as summarized in Table 20.2. As Oltmanns et al.[61] highlight, the Human Exposure Expert Group (HEEG) Opinion 9 assumes "that the worker has a good occupational hygiene approach in his/her behavior and uses, where appropriate, gloves with long sleeves to prevent exposure via the openings around the wrists. It is also assumed that gloves are taken off carefully, without touching the outside of the contaminated gloves with bare hands" (EC, 2010).[62] Oltmanns et al.[61] also highlight that ECETOC TRA assumes that "specific activity training" (95% effectiveness for gloves) can only be considered in the industrial setting, but not for professional workers and that "specific activity training" must include procedures for glove removal and disposal. Oltmanns et al.[61] state that while the scope of default effectiveness values for protective gloves in the areas of chemicals (REACH) and biocides (BPR) shows some differences, the scientific basis of these default values and their justification is limited.

With this background, Oltmanns et al.[61] provided a comprehensive literature review that aimed to quantify the effectiveness of PPE, including protective gloves, against dermal exposure. The review was limited to publications since 2000 and cross-referenced other known and relevant reviews or project reports.[64–66] For those requiring a more in-depth understanding of the literature, it is recommended that the final study report is consulted; however, key aspects of the review are summarized in the following sections.

TABLE 20.2

Default Effectiveness Values for Protective Gloves

Effectiveness (%)	Description	Context
90	Operators, liquids 10% penetration factor	EFSA guidance, cited by
95	Operators, solids 5% penetration factor	Garrigou [63]
90	Workers, solids 10% penetration factor	
80	Chemically resistant gloves conforming to EN374 REACH	REACH (ECHA, 2012),[1] ECETOC TRA
90	Chemically resistant gloves conforming to EN374 with basic employee training	(ECETOC, 2012)
95	Chemically resistant gloves conforming to EN374 with specific activity training; industrial users only	
90	For challenges by a liquid	BPR, HEEG Opinion 9[62]
95	When new gloves for each work shift are used	
95	For challenges by a solid	

[1] Application of an efficiency of 98% for gloves is possible under certain conditions but requires specific justification.

Modified and adapted from Table 1.1 in Oltmanns et al.,[61] page 9.

Oltmanns et al.[61] review identified 410 datasets, of which 35% (142) related to dosimetry studies (those measuring exposure outside the body, using the interception, removal, or in situ techniques) focused on protective gloves. Where efficiency values were reported in the corresponding references, they were used as reported; however, if this was not possible or not considered reasonable, they were calculated from raw data by the study team. Limiting the database entries to those studies providing minimum information on the protective gloves investigated (e.g., about glove length and material) resulted in 120 database entries being considered, and average efficiency factors of 88.1% were observed, ranging from 12% to 100%. Fransman and colleagues reported efficiency factors of 100% for gloves used during hospital activities involving exposure to cyclophosphamide although it was also reported that both values (outside and inside the gloves) were below the limit of detection.[67,68] These data entries were not considered in subsequent analyses by Oltmanns and colleagues. The lowest efficiency factor corresponded to information published by Shih et al.[69] where exposure to 2-ethoxyethyl acetate in a silk-screening shop had been assessed using a tape-stripping method in a cross-sectional study. For those database entries without minimum glove information being available (corresponding to 18 entries), an average exposure reduction of 64% was observed, ranging from 4.4% from exposure to pesticides during harvesting activities to 99.4% during biocide wood impregnation activities.[70,71] It was considered that the low exposure reduction value reported by Baldi et al.[70] may be due to the lack of hand exposure values, as the publication only included overall exposure in qualitative units. One negative efficiency was identified using data published by Cattani et al.[72] when leather rigger gloves were worn during pesticide application activities involving chlorpyrifos.

It was observed that the database entries were biased toward studies involving pesticides and nitrile glove materials, with only a small or limited number of entries for other categories which leads to uncertainty in reaching firm conclusions for other scenarios. In order to reduce at least some of the issues of variability, a further refinement of the analyses was carried out whereby gloves for which minimum information was available were categorized as either "textile" (cloth, cotton, waterproofed cotton, nylon), disposable gloves, or protective gloves (nitrile, neoprene, rubber, PVC). Oltmanns et al.[61] further analyzed the exposure reduction data for the database entries, with respect to various factors such as prior use, glove length, duration, user behavior, and so forth. A summary of some of the key points identified in their report is listed below; however, the authors repeatedly highlight that "no final conclusions" can be made. For further information and supporting references, readers are again invited to review the report:

- Use status of protective gloves—a mixture of new and used gloves (neoprene/rubber) showed smaller efficiencies than new (nitrile, rubber, or undefined material) gloves; 76 vs. 90% efficiency.
- Glove length—short gloves were found to provide a much lower efficiency than longer gloves (89% less contamination), suggesting that significant exposure reductions may be possible using long instead of short gloves for at least some exposure scenarios.
- Glove material – neoprene, nitrile, and rubber gloves were reported to show efficiencies of 96%, 90%, and 87%, respectively. No clear tendency for highest efficacy could be identified as all the identified studies were based (at least partly) on pesticide activities, and there was limited other information on other factors, for example, substance-specific differences or behavior or training influences.
- Disposable gloves—only a comparison of different materials was possible. The highest efficiency was observed for latex/nitrile/vinyl (97%) and latex gloves (94%).
- Textile gloves—the highest efficiency has been found for "cloth" (94%), followed by nylon (89%). New gloves seemed to show higher efficiencies (91%–93%) than used gloves (84%), resulting in a 44%–54% reduction of exposure when changing from used to new gloves. The high efficiency of textile gloves seems at odds when considering the glove materials' high penetration potential.
- User behavior and training—the effect of user behavior and training measures could not be evaluated in detail because of a lack of information. There was a suggestion of a large influence (messy vs. tidy worker leads to 51% reduction), but no firm conclusion could be made.

Oltmanns et al.[61] also separately considered biomonitoring studies in their literature review. Despite the large amount of biomonitoring research found in their searches, only six studies were identified that could be used to derive a dermal protection efficacy, based on the following equation (note the authors refer to this as a protection factor but it is actually protection efficacy, PE):

$$PE(\%) = \frac{(\text{post exposure value with gloves - pre exposure value with gloves})}{(\text{post exposure value without gloves - pre exposure value without gloves})} \times 100$$

(20.4)

The reasons for this were that many studies were not designed to test the effectiveness of dermal protection (i.e., they do not assess the use of the substance with and without dermal protection); several were focused on evaluating current exposure then, and it was not possible to derive a protection factor due to a lack of baseline data (or indeed how a reasonable baseline could be defined). Finally, the lack of availability of a pre-shift value, providing background exposure to the substance (or its metabolites) being investigated. The resulting protection factors from the six biomonitoring studies are listed in Table 20.3; due to the limitations of the studies, these protection factors should be used with caution, with Section 6.2 in Oltmanns et al.[61] providing further discussion on the uncertainty of these values.

Due to the lack of available studies, criteria for biomonitoring studies to be suitable for deriving dermal protection factors were proposed by Oltmanns et al.[61] This criterion included the following elements: compliance with good epidemiological and biomonitoring study requirements; sufficient data; consideration of background exposure; detailed information about the evaluated PPE and tasks; correct application/use of PPE; reliable pre-shift values; individual evaluation of protection factor, not group means; and other exposure routes should be excluded (e.g., inhalation) or controlled.

Oltmanns et al.'s[61] review was very comprehensive; however, when they tried to compare the data extracted from the literature with the default protective glove efficiencies of the HEEG opinion or ECETOC TRA (Table 20.2), the exposure reductions were sometimes higher or lower. The authors note that such a comparison involves significant uncertainty, for example, due to literature data potentially reflecting inappropriate PPE being used and the level of training in the use of PPE is rarely documented. It was also raised that the influence of the challenge of exposure, personal behavior/level of training, and substances enhancing passage through PPE (not skin)/carrier substances has not been evaluated in their review, all of these being areas for future research.

20.5 IMPACT OF GLOVES ON UPTAKE THROUGH THE SKIN

In occupational situations, the route of exposure may have important consequences for dermal uptake. If someone is handling a liquid chemical without any gloves, then a splash of the liquid onto the skin or immersion of the hand in the chemical will completely overwhelm and compromise the skin contamination layer. If the material is undiluted, then uptake will proceed rapidly as there will be a large concentration difference between the skin contamination layer and the peripheral blood supply, as

TABLE 20.3

Glove Effectiveness Derived From Biomonitoring Studies

Citation	Effectiveness (%)	Setting
Scheepers et al.[73]	74	Uptake of polycyclic aromatic hydrocarbons (PAH) in nurses applying ointments containing coal tar to patients in a dermatology clinic in The Netherlands. Also investigated the effectiveness of skin protection methods.
Chang et al.[56]	49 (53.6) (methyl hippuric acid) 69 (72.4) (mandelic acid)	Male spray painters at a ship coating factory in Taiwan. Painters used an airless spray gun to apply ethyl benzene- and xylene-containing paints. Week 1—workers wore no protective clothing. Week 2—provided with protective suits and gloves. During both weeks, all workers wore respirators during spray painting.
Chang et al.[55]	74.7 (metabolites in urine) 68.9 (metabolites in plasma)	Evaluated the protective effectiveness of gloves from exposure to 2-methoxyethanol (2-ME) and examined the association of 2-methoxyacetic acid (MAA) in urine and plasma collected simultaneously from low 2-ME and high 2-ME exposure workers in a semiconductor copper laminate circuit board manufacturing plant in Taiwan.
Wang et al.[74]	49	Protective effectiveness of various PPE against N,N-dimethylformamide (DMF) in a synthetic leather factory in Taiwan.
Lander and Hinke[75]	7.69	Relationship between plasma cholinesterase and uptake of anti-cholinesterase agents (organophosphate insecticides) in greenhouse workers in Denmark.
Aprea et al.[76]	87.8 (rubber gloves) 85.3 (waterproofed cotton gloves) 98.4 (cotton gloves) 90.3 (cotton gloves, no control of inhalation exposure)	Population of workers exposed to chlorpyrifos-methyl and azinphos-methyl during work (thinning immature peaches) in a previously sprayed peach orchard presumably in Italy.

Modified and adapted from Table 6.3 in Oltmanns et al.,[61] page 143.

indicated by Equations 20.2 and 20.3. Conversely, if the contaminant material is in a dilute form, there will be relatively slow uptake.

However, if the person is wearing a glove, the situation will be different. Assuming the chemical only comes into contact with the outer glove surface, there will be no flux into the inner glove contamination layer until the chemical breaks through the glove material. Thereafter, there will, in an ideal situation with a large external reservoir of a contaminant, be a steady flux of the chemical into the inner surface compartment. The chemical must first partition into the glove and then diffuse toward the inner glove surface. Then the chemical must partition into the skin contamination layer. Sweat will accumulate while wearing gloves, and there is no possibility of this sweaty layer being washed away by the diffusive flux. Therefore, the maximum concentration that can be achieved in the sweat will be the saturated water concentration for that chemical. Diffusion through the stratum corneum is then dependent on this concentration, which if the worker is handling the chemical in a concentrated form is likely to be much less than is present on the outer surface of the glove. Therefore, the flux through the glove will ultimately be limited by the flux through the skin from a saturated water concentration; in some situations, the glove permeation rate may be the determinant of the flux through the skin, but only if this is less than the flux from the saturated water solution.

We explore the consequences of this model in a hypothetical work scenario. In an aircraft factory, nitrile rubber gloves are used to protect the hands of a worker who cleans special components with toluene. The work is done inside a fume cupboard to control inhalation exposure. The worker takes approximately 60 min to complete the task, and throughout this time the palms of her gloves are covered with toluene. At the end of this work, the gloves are removed and placed in a waste container.

The dermal uptake that might occur if no gloves were worn can be estimated from the work of Kĕzić et al.[77] who exposed volunteers to a range of solvents over a 27 cm^2 area on the forearm for 3 min. They carefully controlled the experimental conditions so that it was not possible to inhale toluene during the test and then measured the toluene vapor in expired air for about an hour after exposure. The dermal toluene flux was calculated from comparative data for the exhaled toluene concentrations resulting from inhalation exposure, with the assumption that regardless of the route of exposure for the same toluene mass uptake the concentration in expired air would be the same. The permeation rate of toluene averaged over the exposure period was approximately 1.2 mg/cm^2/h. The results from such a short exposure period are perhaps not representative of steady-state diffusion conditions that would occur in a longer exposure scenario, and the palm will be less permeable to toluene than the forearm. Nevertheless, these data provide some basis to estimate the risk from uncontrolled work. Assuming that if gloves are not worn, 500 cm^2 of the hands* are exposed for 60 min, then the uptake might be 600 mg, which is quite a substantial contribution to this worker's risk. For example, someone inhaling toluene vapor throughout this task at the level permitted in the United Kingdom (191 mg/m^3)[78] and a breathing rate of 0.025 m^3/min would inhale 286 mg.

The glove manufacturer has provided data that suggest the breakthrough time for these nitrile gloves is 45 min and the steady-state flux is 8.3 mg/cm^2/h.[†] If we assume there is no uptake until breakthrough and then the flux through the glove and skin corresponds to the steady-state value quoted by the manufacturer, then the uptake would be 1040 mg. This is greater than we might even expect without protection and so seems an implausible basis on which to assess risk. It is possible for the

---

* A surface area of 445 cm^2 per female hand (total 890 cm^2 for both hands) (US EPA, 2011), therefore assuming around 50% of hands exposed.

† Note that these tests are primarily undertaken to assess the breakthrough time and not to provide data that would be used as we have done here to estimate uptake.

flux through the glove to be so high when tested in the laboratory, but when the skin provides better resistance than the glove one must ask whether the permeation data from these tests are relevant to real-use situations.

Boeniger and Klingner[79] report the results of *in vivo* laboratory experiments carried out to investigate the protection afforded by gloves. They found that even for highly permeable glove membranes, where the permeation rate reported by the manufacturer exceeded the skin absorption rate, a reduction in uptake was seen when the membrane was covering the skin. For example, a glove had a permeation rate in an *in vitro* test system of 18 mg/cm^2/h, whereas the measured permeation rate through miniature pigskin was only about 0.3 mg/cm^2/h. The authors speculate that the aqueous layer under the glove may reduce the concentration gradient between the stratum corneum and the subcutaneous tissues because of the necessity for the toluene to dissolve in the sweat.

It may therefore be more appropriate and a more reliable basis to assess uptake if we assume that the highest toluene concentration that could be in the skin contamination layer is the saturated water concentration (which for toluene is 515 mg/l). The uptake can then be estimated using the software program AIHA IHSkinPerm©, which has been developed as a general-purpose tool to estimate uptake in this type of situation (see Section 20.3.4). The predicted uptake flux is 0.03 mg/cm^2/h and the uptake, again for the last 15 min of the task, would be 8 mg, although this does not properly account for the occlusion of the skin and assumes the gloves are removed immediately after the exposure.

We believe that the protection factor provided by gloves should be assessed by comparing the estimated mass uptake of the chemical through the skin when no protection is worn ($U_{sk,hands}$) with the uptake while the gloves are worn ($U_{sk,gloves}$). By analogy with what is done for respirators, we can calculate the protection factor for the gloves (PF_{gloves}) as the ratio of these two uptake values. In this way, the protection factor properly indicates the reduction in risk that might be expected from wearing gloves.

$$PF_{gloves} = U_{sk,hands} / U_{sk,gloves} \qquad (20.4)$$

For the toluene scenario outlined above, the estimated protection factor is 75. However, it might be expected that if the task took longer than 60 min then the protection factor would be lower than this value (and if it were shorter the protection factor would be higher). Overall, the PF_{gloves} will tend toward the ratio of the flux through the skin without gloves and the flux through the skin when the gloves are worn; in this case, this would be 40.

The above analysis assumes that the only way in which the skin inside the glove may become contaminated is by diffusion through the glove. However, it is also possible for chemicals to be introduced inside the glove through the gap between the wrist and the glove cuff. In the hypothetical cleaning task with toluene, if we assume that on average every 15 min a splash of liquid of 0.1 ml (approximately 87 mg of toluene) lands inside the gloves and spreads to cover 5 cm^2, then we can estimate the uptake by this route as 1.5 mg over 15 min. The estimate is based on the uptake rate

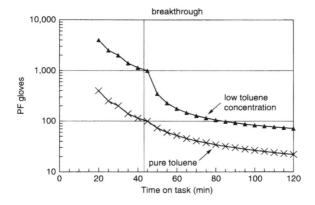

FIGURE 20.2 The hypothetical protection factor for nitrile gloves against toluene in a cleaning task.

for pure toluene, i.e., 1.2 mg/cm²/h. This, of course, assumes that the uptake is the same as we have assumed when the hand is not occluded by the glove and that the toluene does not all evaporate, both of which seem to be reasonable assumptions. Note that most of the toluene from splashes will remain inside the glove after a splash and will eventually be lost to the air by evaporation, either while the glove is worn or more likely after it is removed.

Using this type of analysis, Cherrie et al.[80] showed that the protection factor, assuming there is splashing of pure toluene inside the glove along with permeation through the glove material, results in a protection factor that decreases over time (Figure 20.2). The graph shows the modeled change in protection factor for task duration between about 20 min and 2 h for a low and high concentration of toluene in the product, with the protection factor about 10–100 times greater for the low concentration material. It is clear from this graph that in this scenario the glove breakthrough time has little relevance to the degree of protection provided and the protection factor decreases steadily as the task continues. This type of pattern is probably always going to arise when there is a significant reduction in the efficacy of gloves because of contamination bypassing the glove barrier. The dependence of the glove protection factor on the duration of the task is very different from what is assumed in the case of respirators, where it is assumed that the protection factor is constant and independent of the concentration of contaminant challenging the device.

Figure 20.3 compares the hypothetical protection for the original nitrile glove and an alternative Viton glove with the same assumptions about exposure as assumed by Cherrie et al.[80] The manufacturer's data suggested that the Viton gloves had a breakthrough time of 240 min and so it was assumed the task could last up to 8 h to illustrate the relative difference in the performance of the two glove types. Before the breakthrough of the nitrile gloves, both types of gloves give identical protection; thereafter, the protection factor of the nitrile gloves decreased rapidly, and there is

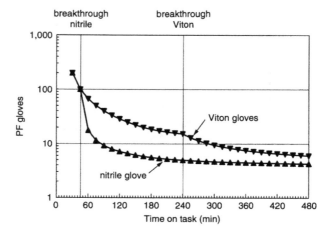

FIGURE 20.3   The hypothetical protection factor for nitrile and Viton gloves against toluene in a cleaning task.

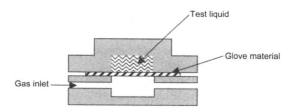

FIGURE 20.4   Schematic diagram of the apparatus used to evaluate permeation through a glove material.

about a four to five times greater protection factor from the Viton gloves. The performance of the nitrile and Viton gloves comes closer to each other after the toluene breakthrough with the Viton gloves.

20.6   IMPLICATIONS FOR TESTING THE EFFECTIVENESS OF GLOVES

These theoretical arguments suggest some important implications for laboratory and field-testing of glove efficacy. Laboratory measurements are generally made using a permeation cell where the glove material is securely held, with the test liquid in contact with the outer glove surface and a gas flow passing the inner surface (Figure 20.4 shows a schematic diagram of this apparatus).

Standard methods are described by the ASTM,[81] CEN,[82] ISO,[16] and others. It has been argued that these tests are designed to provide "worst-case" information on breakthrough time as a screening test for glove suitability. However, as we have

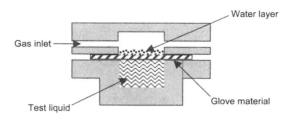

FIGURE 20.5   Schematic of a modified test cell to evaluate biologically relevant permeation.

seen these systems essentially have an infinite capacity to maintain steady-state permeation and may therefore provide an erroneous impression of the real-life chemical flux through gloves. In the example described earlier in this chapter, we saw that using this type of test the glove permeation rate might in fact be greater than that which would be expected through the unprotected skin. An alternative proposal for a perhaps more realistic test cell is shown in Figure 20.5. In this system, the glove is arranged so that there is a thin layer of water covering the inner surface. We believe this type of approach could provide an alternative, perhaps more realistic measure of glove performance than the existing standard approaches. However, this is dependent on the theoretical model we have outlined being realistic, and it is clear that further work is needed to investigate the potential of this type of test.

There are other aspects of the standardized test systems that probably do not properly reflect real work situations. Klingner and Boeniger[83] highlight five areas where the current laboratory tests may be inadequate to characterize workplace performance:

1. Permeation of mixtures through gloves may be different from pure compounds.
2. The permeation test is generally carried out at less than skin temperature, and permeation may increase with temperature.
3. Pressure, stretching, and abrasion of gloves in real-life situations may degrade performance.
4. Gloves may be reused, and this may affect the acceptable use time.
5. Manufacturing tolerances may mean different batches of gloves from the same manufacturer may show considerable variation in permeation characteristics.

In a number of cases, researchers have tried to assess the permeation of chemicals through gloves in the workplace using adsorbent or absorbent pads located inside gloves. This type of design may again overestimate the permeation through the glove because the pad will generally provide a more extensive reservoir for permeating chemicals than the skin contamination layer could offer, which is exactly what we saw with the hypothetical example involving toluene described in the previous section. Ideally, we need a sampler that more accurately reflects the way that chemicals are taken up through the skin, i.e., a "biologically relevant" sampler.

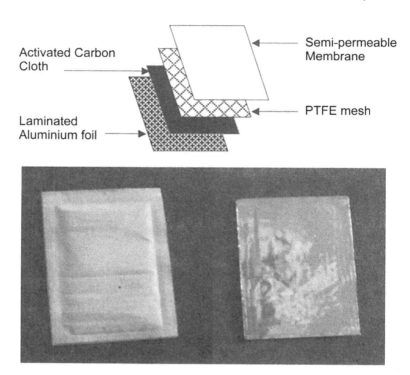

FIGURE 20.6 Exploded diagram of the prototype IOM dermal sampler plus photographs of an assembled sampler.

Lindsay and colleagues at the Institute of Occupational Medicine (IOM) describe some preliminary studies to design such a sampler for exposure to toluene.[84] This prototype IOM dermal patch sampler is based on a simple "sandwich" design: impervious backing, activated charcoal adsorbent, and then a semipermeable membrane with permeation characteristics similar to human skin (Figure 20.6). We believe this design is likely to be suitable for occupational exposures, whereas we suggested the volume of contaminant liquid contacting the skin is sufficient to predominate in the skin contamination layer. However, if we wished to sample under gloves, we would ideally need to have a water coating over the surface of the sampler, and this could perhaps be achievable by using some form of gel. Unfortunately, such samplers are not yet available.

How then should we attempt to evaluate the protection afforded by chemical protective gloves? We have used the toluene cleaning scenario described earlier to explore two possible suggestions for a practical assessment technique:

1. Using adsorbent materials over and under the glove, similar to that used by Creely and Cherrie[85]
2. Using a fluorescent tracer to assess the area of the glove and the area of the hand contaminated

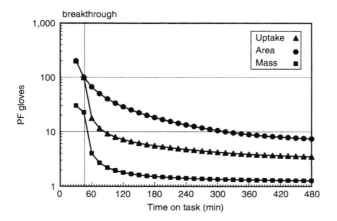

FIGURE 20.7   The hypothetical protection factor for nitrile gloves based on uptake, mass, and area data.

In each case, the protection factor was calculated as the ratio of the outside exposure metric (mass or area) to the inside glove metric. Both alternative approaches were compared with the glove protection factor calculated from the uptake estimates (Figure 20.7).

To estimate the mass of chemicals that might be inside the glove, we used the mass of toluene that was notionally splashed inside the glove and assumed that the adsorbent sampling glove was sufficient to retain it all. To that, we added the estimated mass flux through the glove assuming that it was not limited by the necessity to dissolve in water, i.e., we used the flux rate quoted by the manufacturer on the assumption that the adsorbent in the inner sampling glove would sustain the higher permeation rate. For the external exposure, we have assumed that a 1-μm layer of toluene would come into contact with the exposed outer glove surface every 5 min. It is difficult to judge exactly how much toluene would be in contact with the hand, and so this choice is rather arbitrary.

For the area exposed under the glove, we have used the same assumptions involved in the calculation of uptake, although we did not take into account permeation on the assumption that the fluorescent tracer would not pass through the glove. The outside exposed area was again based on the assumption used in the calculation of uptake. All calculations were made for the nitrile gloves assuming pure toluene was used.

Interestingly, all three measures show similar changes in the estimated protection factor as the task duration increases, although each graph is systematically displaced from the others. The protection factors differ by approximately an order of magnitude. However, there is no guarantee that, for example, the assessment of the area will always produce the highest estimated protection factor or that the assessment of the mass will always be the lowest. If, for example, the task had been carried out with a material containing a lower concentration of toluene, then the protection factor estimated from uptake would have been much higher, although the protection factor estimated from the area would probably have been comparable to that shown in the figure.

However, it might be possible to use measurements of contaminant mass and surface area exposed to estimate uptake, provided there was additional information about the concentration of the contaminant in the bulk liquid or where an estimate of the uptake flux was available for the substance.

Perhaps the best approach would be to use biological monitoring to evaluate the protection factor of gloves. As previously discussed in Section 20.4, Oltmanns et al.[61] identified criteria for biomonitoring studies to be suitable for deriving dermal protection factors which should be considered. This would necessarily need to be carried out in a semi-experimental study to ensure that the measurements reflected the protection afforded by the gloves and not other influences, e.g., background levels of the material in the body from prior/background exposure. Workers would need to wear a high level of respiratory protection to ensure that there was no contribution to exposure from inhalation of the contaminant substance. In addition, it would be necessary to ensure that it was ethically acceptable to have the work carried out without wearing protective gloves because the protection factor would be obtained from the level measured without wearing gloves to that while wearing gloves. If we adopted an intervention study design, then it would not be necessary to take into account inter-individual variation in metabolism.

20.7   DISCUSSION

In this chapter, we have outlined current theoretical concepts about dermal exposure and the practical methods that are available to measure exposure. The conceptual model developed by Schneider and colleagues[14] points toward a logical definition of the workplace protection factor for gloves based on the ratio of uptake through the unprotected skin to the corresponding uptake through the hands when protective gloves are worn. Unfortunately, there are currently no standardized methods to measure uptake and so there are real difficulties in assessing workplace glove protection.

Assessment of workplace protection using the mass of a chemical on the skin and glove surface or other measures of external exposure may be undertaken. However, our analysis suggests that these tests may give estimates of exposure that are systematically biased and that this bias may be either positive or negative. In addition, the calculations we have done also incorporate several assumptions that may or may not be justified, although we believe they are a reasonable basis for comparing the possible measurement strategies. However, further work is needed to ensure that the conclusions we have arrived at are truly robust.

The concept of protection factors for gloves appears to be quite different from what is often assumed for other PPE, particularly respirators used to protect from inhalation exposure. For gloves, the protection factor will not be constant either with the duration of exposure or with the concentration of the challenge chemical, both of which are fundamental assumptions for respiratory protection. This means that the protection factor is less an intrinsic property of the glove and more a reflection of the exposure scenario and the glove. It is therefore not likely to provide such a simple basis for glove selection as we are used to for respirator selection.

In addition, the concept of breakthrough time may also be a less reliable indicator of glove performance in the workplace than has been previously assumed. In our hypothetical calculations, there was often little change in the trend of decreasing protection factor with time, before and after breakthrough. This is because the concept of breakthrough is strongly premised on the assumption that the only route for contaminant onto the hand of someone wearing protective gloves is permeation through the protective layer. However, this is patently not the case and there may be quite significant quantities of the chemical that bypass the glove protective layer.

A central element of the calculations we have made is the assumption that if the hand is exposed to a bulk chemical, then this will swamp the skin contamination layer (containing sweat), and uptake through the skin will be dictated by the concentration of the chemical in the bulk liquid. However, if the chemical permeates through the glove, we have assumed that the flux is insufficient to overwhelm the skin contamination layer and the chemical must therefore dissolve into the sweat before permeating through the skin. For toluene, this meant that the estimated permeation through the glove was lower than the data provided by the glove manufacturer because of the lower flux from a saturated toluene water solution. This may not always be the case and, for some chemicals, it is possible that the flux from a saturated solution in sweat might be equal to or greater than the glove permeation rate and so the glove would become the rate-limiting factor for uptake.

The overall conclusion of this analysis is that measurement of a workplace protection factor is practicable, and we believe this type of study should be undertaken more widely. The best approaches that are currently available are to use the available measures of external exposure to estimate uptake with and without the protective gloves. Alternatively, a carefully controlled biological monitoring intervention study could be used to provide similar data. However, it is most important that these studies are carried out according to a standard protocol.

ACKNOWLEDGMENTS

This chapter is an update and revision of Chapter 17, published in Protective Gloves for Occupational Use, 2nd Edition (CRC Press), and we would like to thank Prof. Sean Semple and Prof. Derk H. Brouwer for their earlier contributions.

The contents, including any opinions and/or conclusions expressed in this chapter are those of the authors alone and do not necessarily reflect the opinions or policy of the organization in which they are employed.

REFERENCES

1. Banaee, S., and Hee, S.S.Q. 2019. Glove permeation of chemicals: The state of the art of current practice, Part 1: Basics and the permeation standards. *J Occup Environ Hyg* 16 (12):827–839.

2. Rawson, B.V., Cocker, J., Evans, P., and Akrill, P.M. 2005. Internal contamination of gloves: Routes and consequences. *Ann Occup Hyg* 49 (6):535–541.

3. Roff, M. 2007. *Use of chemical protective gloves to control dermal exposures in the UV lithographic printing sub-sector.* Report RR525. Sudbury: United Kingdom Health and Safety Executive (HSE).

4. NIOSH. 2021. *Hierarchy of controls.* Available at: https://www.cdc.gov/niosh/topics/hierarchy/default.html (accessed 21st Feb 2021).

5. El-Ayouby, N.S., Gao, P., Wassell, J.T., and Hall, R.C. 2002. Effect of cycles of contamination and decontamination on chemical glove performance. Paper read at *Int Conf Occup Environ Exp Skin Chem: Sci Pol*, Crystal City, VA.

6. Phalen, R., and Que Hee, S.S. 2008. A moving robotic hand system for whole-glove permeation and penetration: Captan and nitrile gloves. *J Occup Environ Hyg* 5 (4):258–270.

7. Janssen, L., Zhuang, Z., and Shaffer, R. 2014. Criteria for the collection of useful respirator performance data in the workplace. *J Occup Environ Hyg* 11 (4):218–226.

8. HSE. 2013. *Respiratory protective equipment at work: A practical guide.* Sudbury: United Kingdom Health and Safety Executive (HSE) Books.

9. Viegas, S., Zare Jeddi, M., Hopf, N.B., Bessems, J., Palmen, N., Galea, K.S., Jones, K., Kujath, P., Duca, R.C., Verhagen, H., Santonen, T., and Pasanen-Kase, R. 2020. Biomonitoring as an underused exposure assessment tool in occupational safety and health context - Challenges and way forward. *Int J Environ Res Public Health* 17 (16):5884.

10. McDougal, J.N., and Boeniger, M.F. 2002. Methods for assessing risks of dermal exposure in the workplace. *Crit Rev Toxicol* 32 (4):291–327.

11. Bos, P.M., Brouwer, D.H., Stevenson, H., Boogaard, P.J., de Kort, W.L., and van Hemmen, J.J. 1998. Proposal for the assessment of quantitative dermal exposure limits in occupational environments: Part 1. Development of a concept to derive a quantitative dermal occupational exposure limit. *Occup Environ Med* 55 (12):795–804.

12. Sanco, DG. 2006. *Draft guidance for the setting and application of acceptable operator exposure levels (AOELs): Working document.* Brussels: DG Sanco.

13. ECHA. 2012. *Guidance on information requirements and chemical safety assessment. Chapter R.8: Characterisation of dose [concentration]-response for human health.* Version 2.1. Helsinki: European Chemicals Agency (ECHA).

14. Schneider, T., Vermeulen, R., Brouwer, D.H., Cherrie, J.W., Kromhout, H., and Fogh, C.L. 1999. Conceptual model for assessment of dermal exposure. *Occup Environ Med* 56 (11):765–773.

15. Mangelsdorf, I., Dobrev, I., Cherrie, J.W., Schroder, K., and Costa Pinheiro, N. 2014. *Dermal exposure.* Geneva: International Programme on Chemical Safety (IPCS).

16. ISO. 2013. *ISO 6529:2013 Protective clothing — Protection against chemicals — Determination of resistance of protective clothing materials to permeation by liquids and gases.* Geneva: International Organization for Standardization (ISO).

17. O'Connell, S.G., Kincl, L.D., and Anderson, K.A. 2014. Silicone wristbands as personal passive samplers. *Environ Sci Technol* 48 (6):3327–3335.

18. Wang, S., Romanak, K.A., Stubbings, W.A., Arrandale, V.H., Hendryx, M., Diamond, M.L., Salamova, A., and Venier, M. 2019. Silicone wristbands integrate dermal and inhalation exposures to semi-volatile organic compounds (SVOCs). *Environ Int* 132:105104.

19. Anderson, K.A., Points 3rd, G.L., Donald, C.E., Dixon, H.M., Scott, R.P., Wilson, G., Tidwell, L.G., Hoffman, P.D., Herbstman, J.B., and O'Connell, S.G. 2017. Preparation and performance features of wristband samplers and considerations for chemical exposure assessment. *J Expo Sci Environ Epidemiol* 27 (6):551–559.

20. Dixon, H.M., Armstrong, G., Barton, M., Bergmann, A.J., Bondy, M., Halbleib, M.L., Hamilton, W., Haynes, E., Herbstman, J., Hoffman, P., Jepson, P., Kile, M.L., Kincl, L., Laurienti, P.J., North, P., Paulik, L.B., Petrosino, J., Points, G.L. 3rd, Poutasse. C.M., Rohlman, D., Scott, R.P., Smith, B., Tidwell, L.G., Walker, C., Waters, K.M., and Anderson, K.A. 2019. Discovery of common chemical exposures across three continents using silicone wristbands. *R Soc Open Sci* 6 (2):181836.
21. Soutar, A., Semple, S., Aitken, R.J., and Robertson, A. 2000. Use of patches and whole body sampling for the assessment of dermal exposure. *Ann Occup Hyg* 44 (7):511–518.
22. WHO. 1982. *Field surveys of exposure to pesticides, standard protocol.* Geneva: World Health Organization (WHO).
23. EPA. 2011. *Exposure factors handbook.* EPA/600/R-09/052F. Washington, DC: U.S. Environmental Protection Agency (EPA).
24. OECD. 1997. Guidance document for the conduct of occupational exposure to pesticides during agricultural application, in *OECD environmental and safety publications series on testing and assessment,* No. 9 OECD/GD (97) 148. Paris: Organisation for Economic Co-operation and Development (OECD).
25. van Wendel de Joode, B., Tielemans, E., Vermeulen, R., Wegh, H., and Kromhout, H. 2005. Dermal exposure assessment to benzene and toluene using charcoal cloth pads. *J Expo Sci Environ Epidemiol* 15 (1):47–50.
26. Vermeulen, R., Lan, Q., Li, G., Rappaport, S.M., Kim, S., van Wendel de Joode, B., Shen, M., Bohong, X., Smith, M.T., Zhang, L., Yin, S., and Rothman, N. 2006. Assessment of dermal exposure to benzene and toluene in shoe manufacturing by activated carbon cloth patches. *J Environ Monitor* 8 (11):1143–1148.
27. Creta, M., Poels, K., Thoelen, L., Vranckx, K., Collaerts, P., Jansen, F., Vangeel, M., Godderis, L., Duca, R.C., and Vanoirbeek, J.A.J. 2017. A method to quantitatively assess dermal exposure to volatile organic compounds. *Ann Work Expo Health* 61 (8):975–985.
28. Cherrie, J., and Robertson, A. 1995. Biologically relevant assessment of dermal exposure. *Ann Occup Hyg* 39 (3):387–392.
29. Behroozy, A. 2013. On dermal exposure assessment. *Int J Occup Environ Med* 4 (3):113–127.
30. Santonen, T., Alimonti, A., Bocca, B., Duca, R.C., Galea, K.S., Godderis, L., Göen, T., Gomes, B., Hanser, O., Iavicoli, I., Janasik, B., Jones, K., Kiilunen, M., Koch, H.M., Leese, E., Leso, V., Louro, H., Ndaw, S., Porras, S.P., Robert, A., Ruggieri, F., Scheepers, P.T.J., Silva, M.J., Viegas, S., Wasowicz, W., Castano, A., and Sepai, O. 2019. Setting up a collaborative European human biological monitoring study on occupational exposure to hexavalent chromium. *Environ Res* 177:108583.
31. Brouwer, D.H., Boeniger, M.F., and van Hemmen, J. 2000. Hand wash and manual skin wipes. *Ann Occup Hyg* 44 (7):501–510.
32. Hughson, G.W., and Cherrie, J.W. 2001. *Validation of the EASE model in relation to dermal zinc exposures.* Edinburgh: Institute of Occupational Medicine (IOM).
33. Galea, K.S., Mueller, W., Arfaj, A.M., Llamas, J.L., Buick, J., Todd, D., and McGonagle, C. 2018. Laboratory validation and field assessment of petroleum laboratory technicians' dermal exposure to crude oil using a wipe sampling method. *Ann Work Expo Health* 62 (6):733–741.
34. Galea, K.S., Davis, A., Todd, D., MacCalman, L., McGonagle, C., and Cherrie, J.W. 2014. Dermal exposure from transfer of lubricants and fuels by consumers. *J Expo Sci Environ Epidemiol* 24 (6):665–672.
35. SKC. 2021. *Colorimetric SWYPEs.* Available at: https://www.skcltd.com/products2/surface-skin-sampling/colorimetric-swypes.html#skin-swypes (accessed March 20, 2021).

36. Ceballos, D.M., Yost, M.G., Whittaker, S.G., Camp, J., and Dills, R. 2009. Objective color scale for the SWYPE surface sampling technique using computerized image analysis tools. *J Occup Environ Med* 6 (10):604–611.

37. Liu, Y., Bello, D., Sparer, J.A., Stowe, M.H., Gore, R.J., Woskie, S.R., Cullen, M.R., and Redlich, C.A. 2007. Skin exposure to aliphatic polyisocyanates in the auto body repair and refinishing industry: A qualitative assessment. *Ann Occup Hyg* 51 (5):429–439.

38. Jones, K. 2021. *A22 diisocyanates. SOP-6 collection of hand wipe samples.* Available at: https://www.hbm4eu.eu/online-library/ (accessed March 20, 2021).

39. Brouwer, D.H., de Vreede, J.A.F., Meuling, W.J.A., and van Hemmen, J.J. 2000. *Determination of the efficiency for pesticide exposure reduction with protective clothing: A field study using biological monitoring.* Baton Rouge, FL: CRC Press.

40. Cherrie, J., Brouwer, D.H., Roff, M., Vermeulen, R., and Kromhout, H. 2000. Use of qualitative and quantitative fluorescence techniques to assess dermal exposure. *Ann Occup Hyg* 44 (7):519–522.

41. Cohen Hubal, E.A., Suggs, J.C., Nishioka, M.G., and Ivancic, W.A. 2005. Characterizing residue transfer efficiencies using a fluorescent imaging technique. *J Expo Anal Environ Epidemiol* 15 (3):261–270.

42. Fenske, R.A., Wong, S.M., Leffingwell, J.T., and Spear, R.C. 1986. A video imaging technique for assessing dermal exposure. II. Fluorescent tracer testing. *Am Ind Hyg Assoc J* 47 (12):771–775.

43. Roff, M.W. 1994. A novel lighting system for the measurement of dermal exposure using a fluorescent dye and an image processor. *Ann Occup Hyg* 38 (6):903–919.

44. Franken, R., Spaan, S., Kasiotis, K., Tsakirakis, A., Chartzala, I., Nikolopoulou, D., Anastasiadou, P., Snippe, A., Schoen, E., Baan, J., Engel, R., Turkenburg, J., Machera, K., and Gerritsen-Ebben, R. 2019. *SysDEA: Systematic analysis of dermal exposure to hazardous chemical agents at the workplace.* Dortmund: Bundesanstalt für Arbeitsschutz und Arbeitsmedizin (BAuA).

45. Kasiotis, K.M., Spaan, S., Tsakirakis, A.N., Franken, R., Chartzala, I., Anastasiadou, P., Machera, K., Rother, D., Roitzsch, M., Poppek, U., Lucadei, G., Baumgärtel, A., Schlüter, U., and Gerritsen-Ebben, R.M. 2019. Comparison of measurement methods for dermal exposure to hazardous chemicals at the workplace: The SysDEA Project. *Ann Work Expo Health* 64 (1):55–70.

46. Lundgren, L., Skare, L., and Liden, C. 2006. Measuring dust on skin with a small vacuuming sampler--A comparison with other sampling techniques. *Ann Occup Hyg* 50 (1):95–103.

47. Ng, M.G., de Poot, S., Schmid, K., Cowie, H., Semple, S., and van Tongeren, M. 2014. A preliminary comparison of three dermal exposure sampling methods: Rinses, wipes and cotton gloves. *Environ Sci: Process Impacts* 16 (1):141–147.

48. Marquart, H., Franken, R., Goede, H., Fransman, W., and Schinkel, J. 2017. Validation of the dermal exposure model in ECETOC TRA. *Ann Work Expo Health* 61 (7):854–871.

49. CEN. 2006. *Workplace exposure - Strategy for the evaluation of dermal exposure (NPR-CEN-TR-15278).* London: British Standards Institution (BSI).

50. Jones, K. 2020. Human biomonitoring in occupational health for exposure assessment. *Portuguese J Public Health* 38 (1):2–5.

51. WHO. 2015. *Human biomonitoring. Facts and figures.* Copenhagen: World Health Organization (WHO).

52. Garrod, A.N.I., Phillips, A.M., and Pemberton, J.A. 2001. Potential exposure of hands inside protective gloves - A summary of data from non-agricultural pesticide surveys. *Ann Occup Hyg* 45 (1):55–60.

53. Boogaard, P.J. 2008. Biomonitoring as a tool in the human health risk characterization of dermal exposure. *Hum Exp Toxicol* 27 (4):297–305.

54. Kielhorn, J., Melching-Kollmub, S., and Mangelsdorf, I. 2006. *Dermal Absorption. Environmental Health Criteria 235*. Geneva: World Health Organization (WHO).
55. Chang, H.-Y., Lin, C.-C., Shih, T.-S., Chan, H., Chou, J.S., and Huang, Y.S. 2004. Evaluation of the protective effectiveness of gloves from occupational exposure to 2-methoxyethanol using the biomarkers of 2-methoxyacetic acid levels in the urine and plasma. *Occup Environ Med* 61 (8):697–702.
56. Chang, F.K., Chen, M.L., Cheng, S.F., Shih, T-S., and Mao, I.F. 2007. Field protection effectiveness of chemical protective suits and gloves evaluated by biomonitoring. *Occup Environ Med* 64 (11):759–762.
57. Lauwerys, R.R., and Hoet, P. 2001. *Industrial chemical exposure. Guidelines for biological monitoring*, Third Edition. Boca Raton, FL: CRC Press.
58. ECHA. 2016. *Guidance on information requirements and chemical safety assessment. Chapter R.14: Occupational exposure estimation. Version: 3*. Helsinki: European Chemicals Agency (ECHA).
59. Franken, R., Kasiotis, K.M., Tsakirakis, A.N., Chartzala, I., Anastasiadou, P., Machera, K., Fransman, W., Gerritsen-Ebben, R.M., and Spaan, S. 2020. Experimental assessment of inhalation and dermal exposure to chemicals during industrial or professional activities in relation to the performance of ECETOC TRA. *Ann Work Expo Health* 64 (9):944–958.
60. Cherrie, J.W. 2018. How to quantitatively assess dermal exposure to volatile organic compounds. *Ann Work Expo Health* 62 (2):253–254.
61. Oltmanns, J., Kaiser, E., Heine, K., Schneider, K., Hesse, S., and Hahn, St. 2016. *Effectiveness of personal protective equipment against dermal exposure – A comparative survey*. Dortmund: BAuA.
62. EC. 2010. *HEEG opinion. Default protection factors for protective clothing and gloves*. Inspra: Joint Research Centre, Institute for Health and Consumer Protection, Chemical Assessment and Testing.
63. Garrigou, A., Laurent, C., Berthet, A., Colosio, C., Jas, N., Daubas-Letourneux, V., Jackson Filho, J.-M., Jouzel, J.-N., Samuel, O., Baldi, I., Lebailly, P., Galey, L., Goutille, F., and Judon, N. 2020. Critical review of the role of PPE in the prevention of risks related to agricultural pesticide use. *Safety Sci* 123:104527.
64. Gerritsen-Ebben, R., Brouwer, D.H., and van Hemmen, J.J. 2007. *Effective Personal Protective Equipment (PPE). Default setting of PPE for registration purposes of agrochemical and biocidal pesticides*. Zeist: [Netherlands Organisation for Applied Scientific Research] (TNO).
65. Spaan, S., Valenzuela, N.M., Glass, R., and Gerritsen, R. 2014. *BROWSE. Bystanders, Residents, Operators and Workers Exposure models for plant protection products*. York: U.K. Food and Environment Research Agency (FERA).
66. Tsakirakis, A., Kasiotis, K.M., Arapaki, N., Charistou, A., Tsatsakis, A., Glass, C.R., and Machera, K. 2011. Determination of operator exposure levels to insecticide during bait applications in olive trees: Study of coverall performance and duration of application. *Int J Hyg Environ Health* 214 (1):71–78.
67. Fransman, W., Vermeulen, R., and Kromhout, H. 2004. Occupational dermal exposure to cyclophosphamide in Dutch hospitals: A pilot study. *Ann Occup Hyg* 48 (3):237–244.
68. Fransman, W., Vermeulen, R., and Kromhout, H. 2005. Dermal exposure to cyclophosphamide in hospitals during preparation, nursing and cleaning activities. *Int Arch Occup Environ Health* 78 (5):403–412.
69. Shih, T.-S., Kuo, Y.-C., Liang, R.-H., Liou, S.H., Chang, H.Y., and Chou, T.C. 2009. Assessment of airborne and dermal exposure to 2-ethoxyethyl acetate in an occupational environment. *Am J Ind Med* 52 (8):654–661.

70. Baldi, I., Lebailly, P., Rondeau, V., Bouchart, V., Blanc-Lapierre, A., Bouvier, G., Canal-Raffin, M., and Garrigou, A. 2012. Levels and determinants of pesticide exposure in operators involved in treatment of vineyards: Results of the PESTEXPO Study. *J Expo Sci Environ Epidemiol* 22 (6):593–600.

71. Garrod, A.N.I., Guiver, R., and Rimmer, D.A. 2000. Potential exposure of amateurs (consumers) through painting wood preservative and antifoulant preparations. *Ann Occup Hyg* 44 (6):421–426.

72. Cattani, M., Cena, K., Edwards, J., and Pisaniello, D. 2001. Potential dermal and inhalation exposure to chlorpyrifos in Australian pesticide workers. *Ann Occup Hyg* 45 (4):299–308.

73. Scheepers, P.T., van Houtum, J., Anzion, R.B., Champmartin, C., Hertsenberg, S., Bos, R.P., and van der Valk, P. 2009. The occupational exposure of dermatology nurses to polycyclic aromatic hydrocarbons – Evaluating the effectiveness of better skin protection. *Scand J Work Environ Health* 35 (3):212–221.

74. Wang, S.M., Shih, T-S., Huang, Y-S., Chueh, M.R., Chou, J.S., and Chang, H.Y. 2006. Evaluation of the effectiveness of personal protective equipment against occupational exposure to N,N-dimethylformamide. *J Haz Mater* 138 (3):518–525.

75. Lander, F., and Hinke, K. 1992. Indoor application of anti-cholinesterase agents and the influence of personal protection on uptake. *Arch Environ Contam Toxicol* 22 (2):163–166.

76. Aprea, C., Sciarra, G., Sartorelli, P., Desideri, E., Amati, R., and Sartorelli, E. 1994. Biological monitoring of exposure to organophosphorus insecticides by assay of urinary alkylphosphates: Influence of protective measures during manual operations with treated plants. *Int Arch Occup Environ Health* 66 (5):333–338.

77. Kezic, S., Monster, A.C., van de Gevel, I.A., Krüse, J., Opdam, J.J., and Verberk, M.M. 2001. Dermal absorption of neat liquid solvents on brief exposures in volunteers. *AIHAJ* 62 (1):12–18.

78. HSE. 2020. *EH40/2005 workplace exposure limits. Containing the list of workplace exposure limits for use with the Control of Substances Hazardous to Health Regulations 2002 (as amended)*. Norwich: United Kingdom Health and Safety Executive (HSE) Books.

79. Boeniger, M.F., and Klingner, T.D. 2002. In-use testing and interpretation of chemical-resistant glove performance. *Appl Occup Environ Hyg* 17 (5):368–378.

80. Cherrie, J., Semple, S., and Brouwer, D. 2004. Gloves and dermal exposure to chemicals: Proposals for evaluating workplace effectiveness. *Ann Occup Hyg* 48 (7):607–615.

81. ASTM International. 2020. *ASTM F739-20, standard test method for permeation of liquids and gases through protective clothing materials under conditions of continuous contact*. West Conshohocken, PA: ASTM International.

82. CEN. 2018. *EN 16523-1:2015+A1: 2018. Determination of material resistance to permeation by chemicals. Permeation by potentially hazardous liquid chemicals under conditions of continuous contact*. London: British Standards Institution (BSI).

83. Klingner, T.D., and Boeniger, M.F. 2002. A critique of assumptions about selecting chemical-resistant gloves: A case for workplace evaluation of glove efficacy. *Appl Occup Environ Hyg* 17 (5):360–367.

84. Lindsay, F.E., Semple, S., Robertson, A., and Cherrie, J. 2006. Development of a biologically relevant dermal sampler. *Ann Occup Hyg* 50 (1):85–94.

85. Creely, K.S., and Cherrie, J. 2001. A novel method of assessing the effectiveness of protective gloves - Results from a pilot study. *Ann Occup Hyg* 45 (2):137–143.

21 Percutaneous Absorption of Chemicals from Fabric (Textile)*

J. L. Bormann, A. S. F. Acipayam, and H. I. Maibach

CONTENTS

21.1 INTRODUCTION

Percutaneous penetration of chemicals from fabric can occur when contaminated clothing comes in contact or proximity with human skin. Such situations can range from sleeping in night clothes mercerized by a protective chemical to the battlefields where chemically treated military uniforms are utilized to defend against insect vector diseases. Occupational exposure to pesticides in the agricultural industry extends itself to high exposure risk, leading to chronic illness, or in more severe cases, acute toxicity and death. Here we review the literature and summarize what is known about the percutaneous penetration of chemicals from fabric in quantifiable terms. We also summarize dermal protection from pesticides and other chemicals, or lack thereof, offered by the many types of fabric worn for occupational use. It is imperative to consider the percutaneous penetration of pesticides and other toxins from textiles due to the local and systemic toxicities that may occur.

---

* Reprinted with permission from *Journal of Applied Toxicology.*

DOI: 10.1201/9781003126874-25

21.2　METHODS

We searched PubMed, Embase, Web of Science, and Google Scholar with extensive bibliographical review from January 1980 to May 2020, with the search words: "textile", "fabric", "percutaneous penetration," "percutaneous absorption," "protection," "pesticides," "dermal absorption," "dermal penetration," "skin absorption," and "clothing." We included *in vitro* and *in vivo* studies (rabbit and human). The cutaneous barrier penetration results along with description/use of chemicals and description of fabric used in each study are summarized in tables.

21.3　RESULTS

We found 22 publications pertaining to the percutaneous penetration of chemicals from fabrics. Tables 21.1 and 21.2 capsule this limited experimented data. Table 21.1 includes *in vitro* data, and Table 21.2 includes *in vivo* data.

21.3.1　PERCUTANEOUS PENETRATION: IN VITRO STUDIES

21.3.1.1　Liquids

Military personnel may be exposed to chemicals as a means of attack through chemical warfare. Chemicals in the organophosphate family, such as Agent VX, are widely studied. Agent VX is a chemical warfare agent with lethal properties when dermally absorbed. Due to the lethality of Agent VX, parathion, a common pesticide with similar chemical properties as VX, was used to estimate percutaneous penetration of the more lethal Agent VX when transferred from clothing.[1] Standard army issue coat, hot weather woodland camouflage, combat pattern, 50% nylon and 50% cotton (American Apparel, Inc.) was utilized as the uniform material. Arms, head, and neck were unprotected by the military uniform. Parathion absorption was measured at 1, 8, and 96 hours after contact with the contaminated fabric, or, in the case of naked skin, after chemical contamination with no uniform barrier.

A 1-hour time frame simulated exposure and quick removal of the exposed clothing or decontamination. An 8-hour time frame simulated the average workday, and the 96-hour window reproduced the conditions experienced by military personnel in the field where a change of clothing may not be available for an extended time. Military uniform, both dry and wet, offered significantly more protection against parathion than naked skin alone ($p = 0.000$). The mean percentages of parathion absorbed after 96 hours by a military worker with no uniform, a wetted uniform, and a dry uniform, were 1.8%, 0.7%, and 0.3%, respectively. Their study showed significant differences in chemical percutaneous penetration of dry clothing and moist clothing at 1, 8, and 96 hours after exposure ($p = 0.007$). The calculated VX systemic dose from their in vitro study showed total dermal absorption of 9.9, 79.0, and 947.8 mg at 1, 8, and 96 hours, respectively, in military workers wearing a moist uniform. In a military worker wearing a dry uniform, 6.4, 51.2, and 614.2 mg were absorbed at 1, 8, and 96 hours, respectively (Table 21.1).

TABLE 21.1

Summary of *In Vitro* Studies

Reference	Fabric Description	Chemical(s)	Cutaneous System	Findings
			Liquids	
Wester et al. (2000)[1]	Standard army issue coat, 50% cotton, and 50% nylon	Parathion (pesticide)	Human skin	Parathion absorption was significantly less through uniformed skin when compared to naked skin. A dry uniform offered significantly more protection than a moist uniform.
Wester et al. (1996)[2]	100% cotton sheet	Glyphosate (herbicide), malathion (insecticide)	Human skin	Allowing fabric contaminated with a chemical to dry before skin contact decreased the amount of percutaneous penetration. Adding water to the dried contaminated cloth to simulate perspiration increased percutaneous absorption. Pesticides exhibit unique chemical properties and their percutaneous absorption from fabric can vary.
Obendorf et al. (2003)[3]	Bleached and bleached/ mercerized: print fabric (102–107 g/m^2) and denim (274 g/m^2)	Methyl parathion (pesticide)	Model membrane	There was significantly less pesticide absorption through starched fabrics compared to non-starched fabrics. Thicker fabric may increase absorption and decrease percutaneous penetration of the pesticide.
Welch and Obendorf (1997)[4]	Unfinished 100% cotton denim, 274 g/m^2	Methyl parathion (pesticide)	Human skin	Denim fabric decreased pesticide transport through human skin.
Moore et al. (2014)[5]	Cotton shirt material	Chlorpyrifos, dichlorvos (pesticides)	Human skin	Removing contaminated clothing after exposure can limit dermal absorption. Everyday clothing can protect against dermal absorption of pesticides in a variety of applicator formulations.
Iadaresta et al. (2018)[6]	Textile fabric	Benzothiazole (many industrial uses)	Strat-M® artificial membranes	Greater than 60% of the benzothiazole penetrated through the artificial membrane in 24 hours.

(Continued)

TABLE 21.1 (CONTINUED)
Summary of *In Vitro* Studies

Reference	Fabric Description	Chemical(s)	Cutaneous System	Findings
		Gaseous Chemicals		
Wester et al. (1997)[7]	100% polyester material	Ethylene oxide (fumigant)	Human skin	Ethylene oxide was rapidly absorbed through the skin from contaminated fabric. Occlusion of the fabric by latex gloves resulted in increased percutaneous penetration.
Gaskin et al. (2013a)[8]	100% cotton (denim)	Ammonia gas (HAZMAT)	Human skin	Denim material covering the cutaneous barrier resulted in negligible systemic absorption of ammonia gas at a concentration of 2000 ppm.
Gaskin et al. (2013b)[9]	100% cotton (denim)	Hydrogen cyanide, chlorine gases (HAZMAT)	Human skin	Hydrogen cyanide gas negligibly penetrated the cutaneous barrier with and without denim covering. Chlorine gas penetration significantly increased with denim fabric over the skin.
Gaskin et al. (2019)[10]	100% cotton (denim)	Nitric oxide, nitrogen dioxide, sulfur dioxide gases (HAZMAT)	Human skin	The study showed no significant absorption of nitric oxide or nitrogen dioxide with or without denim covering. There was slightly increased absorption of sulfur dioxide in the presence of denim covering.
Gaskin et al. (2017)[11]	100% polyester and 100% cotton (denim)	Methyl bromide, sulfuryl fluoride, and chloropicrin (pesticides)	Human skin	Clothing was protective against percutaneous penetration of methyl bromide. Percutaneous penetration of sulfuryl fluoride and chloropicrin was minimally affected by the addition of cloth covering the skin.
Heath et al. (2017)[12]	Denim fabric	Ethylene oxide gas (sterilant, fumigant)	Human skin	There were no significant differences in percutaneous penetration of ethylene oxide with or without denim covering the cutaneous barrier.

Chemical characteristics and various fabric properties influenced percutaneous absorption.

TABLE 21.2
Summary of *In Vivo* Studies

Reference	Fabric Description	Chemical	Subject	Findings
			Liquids	
Blum et al. (1978)[13]	Children's sleepwear	Tris(2,3-dibromopropyl) phosphate (tris-BP) (flame retardant)	Human	Sleepwear treated with tris-BP caused significantly elevated urinary excretion levels of 2,3-dibromopropanol.
Ulsamer et al. (1978)[14]	Polyester cloth (3 oz/sq yd)	Radiolabeled tris(2,3-dibromopropyl) phosphate (tris-BP) (flame retardant)	Rabbit	Sweat- and urine-soaked cloth resulted in greater percutaneous penetration of chemicals than from dry cloth over 96 hours.
Snodgrass (1992)[15]	100% cotton military uniform (Type III) and 50% nylon/50% cotton military uniform (NYCO)	Permethrin (insecticide)	Rabbit	The study showed percutaneous absorption of permethrin from 100% cotton or 50/50 cotton and nylon fabric over a 7-day study. Environment and fabric type were not significant variables.
Rossbach et al. (2010)[16]	Battle dress uniforms	Permethrin (insecticide)	Human	Significantly higher levels of permethrin metabolites were found in the urine of soldiers wearing permethrin-impregnated uniforms.
Rossbach et al. (2016)[17]	Forestry worker pants (two separate distributors)	Permethrin (insecticide)	Human	Workers wearing permethrin-impregnated pants resulted in higher amounts of permethrin urinary metabolites compared to workers wearing non-impregnated pants.
Rossbach et al. (2014)[18]	Commercially available permethrin-impregnated forestry work clothing	Permethrin (insecticide)	Human	Increased physical workload, temperature, and humidity resulted in higher levels of urinary permethrin metabolites.
Meinke et al. (2009)[19]	Polyester/cotton fabric (65/35)	Dianix® Leuchtgelb 10G (textile dye)	Human	Sweat greatly increased chemical migration from the fabric into the skin.

(Continued)

TABLE 21.2 (CONTINUED)
Summary of *In Vivo* Studies

Reference	Fabric Description	Chemical	Subject	Findings
		Gaseous Chemicals		
Morrison et al. (2016)[20]	Cotton clothing articles	Airborne phthalates (semi-volatile organic compounds)	Human	Exposed cotton clothing led to increased dermal uptake of phthalates, while clean clothing protected against uptake.
Morrison et al. (2017)[21]	100% cotton long sleeve shirts	Airborne benzophenone-3 (UV light filter)	Human	Wearing clothing with previous exposure to airborne benzophenone-3 resulted in increased urinary levels of benzophenone-3.
Bekö et al. (2017)[22]	Cotton clothing articles, unexposed or exposed to nicotine	Nicotine (drug)	Human	Wearing clean clothing resulted in four times less absorption of airborne nicotine than when wearing nicotine-exposed clothing.

Various pesticides, organic compounds, and HAZMAT simulation exposures were studied in regard to their percutaneous penetration through clothing.

In another in vitro study utilizing human skin, percutaneous absorption of the herbicides glyphosate (water-soluble) and malathion (water-insoluble) from solution were compared to their percutaneous absorption from contaminated 100% cotton fabric.[2] The fabric was in contact with human skin on day 0, day 1, or day 2 after contamination occurred. By day 2, the contaminated cotton fabric had dried, and water was added to simulate wet conditions such as perspiration on a hot day.

Percutaneous absorption was measured for the wetted fabric. 1.4% of the 1% glyphosate solution control was absorbed across the skin, while 0.7%, 0.1%, 0.1%, and 0.4% of the glyphosate were absorbed across the skin from cotton fabric on day 0, day 1, day 2, and day 2 with the addition of water, respectively. 8.8% of the 1% malathion solution control was absorbed across the skin, while 3.9%, 0.6%, 0.6%, and 7.3% of the malathion was absorbed across the skin from cotton fabric on day 0, day 1, day 2, and day 2 with the addition of water, respectively. These results suggest that chemical drying decreased the absorption but wetting the dried chemical increased its absorption. This study reinforces the increased protection offered by some fabrics against chemicals involved in occupational exposures and the importance of removing contaminated clothing as soon as feasible after contamination (Table 21.1).

Franz diffusion cell technique was utilized to study the percutaneous penetration of the pesticide from contaminated textiles.[4] Using the pesticide, methyl parathion, and an unfinished 100% cotton denim, they observed a statistical difference in pesticide transferred through human skin between pesticide exposure without fabric compared to the same system with protection from denim fabric. While 0.08 mg of methyl parathion was transferred through the skin with no fabric barrier, only 0.01 mg was transferred when utilizing denim fabric during the primary exposure and 0.02 mg utilizing fabric under secondary exposure conditions (Table 21.1).

Obendorf et al.[3] utilized a synthetic membrane system to determine the absorption of the pesticide methyl parathion from dry cotton fabric. Cotton fabric in print cloth, simulating the thickness of shirt material, showed 2.1% absorption of the pesticide 8 hours after fabric contamination. Bleached print cloth, mercerized print cloth, and carboxymethylated print cloth revealed 1.4%, 2.4%, and 2.6% absorption after 8 hours, respectively. Absorption by bleached, mercerized, and carboxymethylated cloth was significantly decreased with the addition of starch to the fabric; absorption after 8 hours was 0.8%, 0.6%, and 1.9%, respectively. In the second part of their study, they used a denim fabric, thicker than the print fabric to simulate absorption through pant material. They compared pesticide penetration through human skin from the denim fabric to pesticide penetration through human skin with no fabric barrier. At 50 hours post-exposure, ~4% of the pesticide had transported through human skin with no fabric, while only ~1% of the pesticide was transported through human skin protected by denim fabric. Their results suggest that thickness and weave of fabric can significantly affect pesticide's percutaneous penetration. They also suggest that starching aids in absorbing the pesticide, which reduces pesticide exposure and subsequent penetration (Table 21.1).

Moore et al.[5] measured percutaneous penetration of chemicals from clothing using chlorpyrifos and dichlorvos to contaminate fabric. Dichlorvos is a moderately lipophilic liquid, while chlorpyrifos is a lipophilic solid. Pesticides were applied in two different vehicles: isopropanol (IPA) and propylene glycol (PG). Fabrics contaminated with chlorpyrifos in both IPA and PG solutions showed significantly reduced cutaneous penetration compared to contaminated unclothed human skin. There was no statistical significance in chlorpyrifos's cutaneous penetration between the 4- and 24-hour periods between fabric removal and skin decontamination in the IPA solution, while there was a statistical difference in the PG vehicle between those two time points. Percentages of absorbed chlorpyrifos in IPA with clothing decontamination at 4 hours, clothing decontamination at 24 hours, and unclothed decontamination at 4 hours were 2.3%, 1.0%, and 1.0%, respectively. There was, however, a statistical difference in percutaneous penetration of chlorpyrifos in the PG solution when decontamination occurred at 4 hours instead of 24 hours. Percentages of absorbed chlorpyrifos in PG with clothing decontamination at 4 hours, clothing decontamination at 24 hours, and unclothed decontamination at 4 hours were 2.2%, 0.6%, and 1.1%, respectively. Percentages of absorbed dichlorvos in IPA solution were 1.3%, 2.6%, and 10.1% for decontamination at 30 minutes, decontamination at 24 hours, and unclothed decontamination at 30 minutes, respectively. Percentages of absorbed dichlorvos in PG solution were 1.2%, 2.0%, and 6.4% for decontamination at 30 minutes, decontamination at 24 hours, and unclothed decontamination at 30 minutes, respectively. This study reveals that a significant reduction of pesticide cutaneous absorption can occur with the swift removal of contaminated clothing. Different chemicals absorb into the skin at different rates, and it is imperative to remove the contaminated clothing as soon as possible (Table 21.1).

Keeble et al.[23] utilized an *in vitro* test system to determine the percutaneous absorption of azinphos-methyl, paraoxon, and malathion from glove fabrics. Absorption was quantified as the amount of acetylcholinesterase inhibition that occurred within the *in vitro* test system. Out of the fabrics tested, 100% cotton in 13-cut and 7-cut displayed the lowest rates of acetylcholinesterase inhibition through the *in vitro* system, therefore providing the best protection against the organophosphate pesticides.[23] A later study by Keeble et al.[24] used *in vitro* test systems to study the effect of laundering on permeation properties of the fabric and subsequent percutaneous penetration.[24] They found that fabric contaminated with azinphos-methyl in petroleum distillates provided protection regardless of fabric laundering status, whereas fabric contaminated with paraoxon in ethanolic solution displayed decreased protection against percutaneous absorption when the fabric had been laundered (Table 21.1).

Iadaresta et al.[6] studied penetration of benzothiazole with a Strat-M® artificial membrane system utilizing a flow-through diffusion cell method. Fifty microliters of benzothiazole solution (0.228 mg/mL in H_2O:EtOH, 50:50 v:v) was applied to 0.5 cm^2 t-shirt material over the membrane. After 24 hours, 56.9% ± 3.2% of the chemical applied to the textile was recovered, with 26.9% ± 1.9% having penetrated through the artificial membrane into the receiving chamber. The textile contained 13.3% ± 4.6% of the recovered chemical, and the artificial membrane contained 16.7% ± 2.4% of the chemical recovered (Table 21.1).

21.3.1.2 Gaseous Chemicals

Gaskin et al.[8] simulated a hazardous material (HAZMAT) incident scenario with ammonia gas at 2000 ppm to determine percutaneous penetration through a human abdominal skin/Franz diffusion cell system with denim fabric as protection. They found negligible absorption; however, the fabric acted as a reservoir with potential for secondary exposure. Systemic absorption was also negligible with the addition of a post-exposure ventilation period, but there was a significant reduction in the amount of ammonia contained within the denim fabric compared to no post-exposure ventilation period (Table 21.1). In an additional study by Gaskin et al.,[9] similar protocols were followed utilizing chlorine and hydrogen cyanide gases. A significant increase in chlorine gas penetration at 500 ppm occurred in the presence of denim fabric. Elevated levels of hydrogen cyanide gas (800 ppm) resulted in marginal percutaneous penetration; however, the presence of denim covering slightly increased penetration compared to no denim covering (Table 21.1).

Gaskin et al.[10] performed a similar study with nitrogen and sulfur gases. Nitrogen dioxide, nitric oxide, and sulfur dioxide gases were exposed to denim covering a human abdominal skin/Franz diffusion cell system. Nitrogen dioxide and nitric oxide were minimally absorbed with or without the presence of denim. Only sulfur dioxide absorption slightly increased in the presence of fabric; there were similar findings in the setting of a post-exposure ventilation period (Table 21.1). An additional study by Gaskin et al.[11] found clothing to protect skin from percutaneous penetration of methyl bromide, while textiles minimally affected penetration of chloropicrin and sulfuryl fluoride (Table 21.1).

Heath et al.[12] simulated a HAZMAT incident with ethylene oxide gas exposure. Negligible dermal penetration occurred at 800 ppm, and increased penetration occurred at concentrations of 3000 ppm. Denim present on the skin resulted in increased percutaneous penetration, but values were insignificant. There was, however, a more than five times increase in chemical residue in fabric and human skin at the 3000 ppm concentration, potentially acting as a reservoir for further future penetration (Table 21.1).

Wester et al.[7] created an *in vitro* model to determine hazardous gas percutaneous penetration from contaminated fabric. A 100% polyester material was contaminated with ethylene oxide, an alkylating agent. The contaminated fabric was placed in contact with human skin in the *in vitro* system. A portion of the fabric was left exposed to normal air conditions, while another portion was occluded with double-layer latex glove material. Results revealed expeditious absorption through skin in under 4 hours. 1.3% of the ethylene oxide was percutaneously absorbed under non-occluded conditions, while 46.0% of the ethylene oxide was absorbed under occluded conditions (Table 21.1)

21.3.2 Percutaneous Penetration: In Vivo Studies

21.3.2.1 Liquids

A pioneering study regarding percutaneous penetration from fabrics performed by Blum et al.[13] investigated the flame retardant, tris(2,3-dibromopropyl)phosphate (tris-BP), used on children's sleepwear from 1973 until its banning in 1977. Morning urine collection from a 7-year-old female with a history of wearing well-worn tris-BP-treated sleepwear was performed for 12 days. On the first two mornings, the level of 2,3-dibromopropanol in the urine was 0.4 ng/ml. On the second through the sixth night, the subject wore new pajamas treated with tris-BP and dibromopropanol levels in the female's urine increased significantly; measurements showed 11, 29, 21, and 18 ng/ml on nights 2, 3, 5, and 6, respectively. Urine collection was lost from night 4.

Five months after banning the sale of tris-BP-treated sleepwear, Blum et al.[13] tested the urine of ten children and one adult. No urinary excretion of 2,3-dibromopropanol was detected in one child or adult; both reported no past use of tris-BP-treated sleepwear. Seven of the children who reported wearing washed tris-BP-treated sleepwear had levels of about 0.5 ng/ml in their urine, while an additional child's urine revealed 5 ng/ml of 2,3-dibromopropanol. The last child stopped wearing tris-BP-treated sleepwear around 6 months prior to the study, and his urine demonstrated only trace amounts of 2,3-dibromopropanol (Table 21.2).

Ulsamer et al.[14] also studied the percutaneous absorption of tris-BP from radio-labeled polyester cloth. A gauze patch was used to secure the cloth in place on white rabbits over a 96-hour study period. When controlling for exhaled radio-label in the form of CO_2, dry cloth led to 4.31% absorption, sweat-treated cloth resulted in 4.79% absorption, and human urine-soaked cloth caused the greatest amount of absorption: 15.84%. The increased absorption may have resulted from a dermatitis-like reaction that developed on cloth-covered areas of the urine-soaked cloth group. Absorption was measured from the dose remaining in the body, urine, and feces (Table 21.2).

Although organophosphates can be used as chemical warfare agents against military personnel, similar agents may be used to the military's benefit in uniforms as protection against insect vector diseases. A widely used clothing insect repellant is permethrin. Snodgrass[15] used permethrin-treated military uniform fabric and measured the absorption of the pesticide from fabric through rabbit skin. One hundred percent cotton or a 50/50 blend of cotton and nylon military uniform fabric swatch contaminated with permethrin was attached to the hairless back of a rabbit for 7 days. The percentage absorbed was measured by the amount of radiolabeled permethrin excreted in both urine and feces. The 100% cotton fabric contamination led to 0.9% percutaneous absorption under a temperate environment (no sweat), while a subtropical environment (sweat present) increased absorption to 3.2%. The 50/50 blend of cotton and nylon fabric contamination led to 1.7% percutaneous absorption in the temperate environment and 2.0% absorption in the subtropical environment. Authors suggest the absorption percentages may be higher in their study compared to those found when wearing a military uniform because uniforms are more loosely fitting than the apparatus applied to the rabbits in their study. The exposure dose to humans from wearing permethrin-treated (0.125 mg/cm^2) military clothing is predicted to be 6×10^{-4} mg/kg/d. They did not find the environment or type of fabric to be statistically significant variables (Table 21.2).

Rossbach et al.[16] studied percutaneous absorption of permethrin from military uniforms in a study comprised of 187 participants who wore a permethrin-impregnated or non-impregnated uniform for 40–72 hours per week for 4 weeks. Urine was collected and analyzed for permethrin metabolites at set time points throughout the study, which revealed significantly higher metabolite levels in the soldiers wearing permethrin-impregnated clothing compared to the collection at initiation of the study. Of note, permethrin metabolites were still present 4 weeks after the study concluded (Table 21.2).

Rossbach et al.[17] showed similar findings of increased permethrin uptake from permethrin-impregnated work pants in forestry workers, with the highest levels of permethrin urinary metabolites found 1 week into the 16-week study period. It was suggested that washing the pants throughout the study may have resulted in decreased permethrin concentrated within the pants, resulting in decreased percutaneous penetration. Interestingly, there were significant differences in permethrin percutaneous penetration between two different brands of pants used in the study, although chemical concentrations were advertised as similar (Table 21.2). Rossbach et al.[18] measured urinary metabolites of permethrin from commercial work outfits under different environmental and work conditions, finding that increased physical workload, temperature, and humidity resulted in higher levels of urinary permethrin metabolites (Table 21.2).

Meinke et al.[19] approached measurement of chemical migration into and through the cutaneous barrier differently, using tape stripping and tape extraction. Twelve volunteers wore a piece of cloth treated with textile dye on their lower backs for 12 hours; six of the participants performed no sports activity during the study, while the other half of the cohort performed 30 minutes of physical activity while wearing the textile-dyed clothing. The level of activity more significantly affected dye migration than did the time elapsed from first contact with the dyed material (Table 21.2). In vitro studies performed by Meinke et al.[19] correlated with the in vivo results described here.

21.3.2.2 Gaseous Chemicals

Several volatile organic compounds are encountered in the workplace, and percutaneous absorption of such compounds can occur.[25] Morrison et al.[20] studied dermal absorption of airborne phthalates under conditions of bare skin, clean cotton clothing, and cotton clothing exposed to phthalates for at least 1 week. Individuals wearing cotton clothing exposed to phthalates (diethylphthalate and di-n-butylphthalate) for at least 1 week exhibited increased excretion of chemical metabolites in their urine, while clean cotton clothing was protective against dermal absorption. Compared to bare skin, exposed clothing led to 6.5 and 3.3 times higher absorption of diethylphthalate and di-n-butylphthalate, respectively. Clean clothing resulted in 5.6 and 3.2 times lower dermal uptake of diethylphthalate and di-n-butylphthalate, respectively, compared to bare skin (Table 21.2). A similar study by Morrison et al.[21] found significantly higher levels of benzophenone-3 in the urine of individuals wearing clothing with previous exposure to airborne benzophenone-3 compared to that of urine samples from the same individuals before contact with the contaminated clothing (Table 21.2).

Bekö et al.[22] determined dermal uptake of nicotine from air under conditions of bare skin, cotton clothing, and exposed cotton clothing by urinary measurements of nicotine and its metabolites. Two bare-skinned individuals wearing only shorts were exposed to nicotine for 3 hours (estimated nicotine air concentration 420 μg/m³); urinary excretion of nicotine and its metabolites was measured for 60 hours after removal from the airborne nicotine chamber. A third individual wearing clean cotton clothing entered and left the chamber at the same time points as the two bare-skinned individuals, and urinary excretion was measured for 24 hours. At 24 hours after exiting the chamber, that individual reentered the chamber wearing clean clothing except for a nicotine-exposed shirt (5-day exposure at estimated >200 μg/m³) for an additional 3 hours. Urinary excretion of nicotine and its metabolites was measured for 60 hours after his exit from the chamber. Both exposed and unexposed clothing resulted in decreased dermal uptake of nicotine compared to bare skin; however, clean clothing resulted in four times less absorption than exposed clothing (Table 21.2).

21.4 DISCUSSION

Percutaneous penetration of pesticides from clothing in the occupational worker is a nearly inevitable process unless full personal protective equipment is worn. Depending on the chemical being used, exposure can result in chronic illness or acute toxicity. Such exposure over decades of work may be related to the increased incidence of cancer and other health conditions. Oftentimes, environmental conditions, such as heat and humidity, limit the practicability of full personal protective equipment use. Continuous innovation and modification of everyday clothing materials to create protective gear that is user friendly while still preventing the penetration of chemicals is imperative.

It is necessary to consider the variable properties of protective fabrics when choosing appropriate clothing for occupational workers. Fabrics that decrease the penetration of a pesticide ultimately result in less pesticide reaching the skin and, therefore, decreased opportunity for dermal penetration. Tyvek, a 100% olefin spun-bonded nonwoven, exhibited the lowest transmission level, followed by 100% cotton and cotton/polyester blend fabrics, whereas woven fabrics made of 100% synthetic fibers exhibited high levels of pesticide transmission.[26] Tyvek provided more protection than cotton with azinphos-methyl exposure.[27] In a study by Lillie et al.,[28] chlordane, diazinon, carbaryl, and prometon penetrated 100% polyester more than 100% cotton. In addition to the type of fabric, the motion of the worker in contaminated clothing while performing occupational duties could transfer up to 12% of the pesticide to human skin through friction.[29]

Oftentimes the comfort of occupational clothing is inversely related to the protection it provides. A full personal protective equipment outfit revealed penetration factor values of 0.0%–2.1%, while average work clothing of a cotton shirt, pants, and tennis shoes or rubber boots yielded penetration factor values of 0.0%–24.0%.[30] Certain body regions are more likely to be contaminated with pesticides than others.[31] Certain pesticide application methods also yield increased deposition of pesticide contamination compared to an alternate method.[32] More data is needed to determine which common textiles afford the best protection, as occupational workers will most likely choose comfort and convenience over the increased efficacy of the personal protective equipment available today.

To understand percutaneous penetration from contaminated fabric, more in vitro and in vivo studies must be performed. The limited data summarized here show that the type of fabric influences the pesticide's transfer from fabric to human skin or a model membrane. Certain properties such as weave, thickness, starch, carboxymethylation, and mercerization can influence the fabric's ability to either allow permeation of the pesticide or absorb the pesticide to prevent the transfer to the skin surface.[3] Other environmental conditions such as heat, humidity, and worker perspiration can also affect the transfer of the pesticide from clothing to skin.[1]

The absorption and permeability of fabric can be influenced by how the pesticide distributes within the fabric itself. In a study by Solbrig et al.,[33] both cotton and polyester fabrics revealed malathion distributed on the surface of the fibers; however, only the cotton fabric had malathion distributed within the fibers themselves. Information about the distributive properties of the pesticide could aid in creating more defensive clothing. Distributive information has the potential to determine which fabrics retain their protective qualities after multiple washings or uses. The hydrophilic or hydrophobic properties of each pesticide should also be considered.

Limited studies described percutaneous penetration from contaminated fabric utilizing an *in vivo* system. Of interest, one of the included studies utilized rabbits (Table 21.2).[15] Rabbits display increased permeability of their skin compared to humans, rats, and pigs.[34] Further, Sidon et al.[35] investigated the permeability of permethrin through monkey and rat skin. Although *in vivo* studies in humans are not readily available due to the illness and toxicity that may ensue, future *in vivo* studies utilizing a myriad of pesticides and fabric conditions could lead to a better understanding of the mechanisms involved in percutaneous penetration from fabrics. Law et al.[36] provided detail as to the factors involved in cutaneous penetration; a further investigation must be directed toward understanding the interplay between those factors and fabric permeability.

REFERENCES

1. Wester, R.M., Tanojo, H., Maibach, H.I., and Wester, R.C. 2000. Predicted chemical warfare agent VX toxicity to uniformed soldier using parathion in vitro human skin exposure and absorption. *Toxicol Appl Pharmacol* 168:149–152. DOI: 10.1006/taap.2000.9028.
2. Wester, R.C., Quan, D., and Maibach, H.I. 1996. In vitro percutaneous absorption of model compounds glyphosate and malathion from cotton fabric into and through human skin. *Food Chem Toxicol* 34:731–735. DOI: 10.1016/0278-6915(96)00030-0.
3. Obendorf, S.K., Csiszár, E., Maneefuangfoo, D., and Borsa, J. 2003. Kinetic transport of pesticide from contaminated fabric through a model skin. *Arch Environ Contam Toxicol* 45:283–288. DOI: 10.1007/s00244-003-0211-5.
4. Welch, O., and Obendorf, S.K. 1997. Limiting dermal exposure of workers to pesticides from contaminated clothing. In *Performance of Protective Clothing*, 6th volume. Still, J., and Schwope, A., Eds. West Conshohocken, PA: American Society for Testing and Materials. DOI: 10.1520/STP19900S.

5. Moore, C.A., Wilkinson, S.C., Blain, P.G., Dunn, M., Aust, G.A., and Williams, F.M. 2014. Use of a human skin in vitro model to investigate the influence of 'every-day' clothing and skin surface decontamination on the percutaneous penetration of organophosphates. *Toxicol Letters* 229:257–264. DOI: 10.1016/j.toxlet.2014.06.007.

6. Iadaresta, F., Manniello, M.D., Östman, C., Crescenzi, C., Holmbäck, J., and Russo, P. 2018. Chemicals from textiles to skin: An in vitro permeation study of benzothiazole. *Environ Sci Pollution Res* 25:24629–24638. DOI: 10.1007/s11356-018-2448-6.

7. Wester, R.C., Hartway, T., Serranzana, S., and Maibach, H.I. 1997. Human skin in vitro percutaneous absorption of gaseous ethylene oxide from fabric. *Food Chem Toxicol* 35:513–515. DOI: 10.1016/s0278-6915(97)00016-1.

8. Gaskin, S., Pisaniello, D., Edwards, J.W., Bromwich, D., Reed, S., Logan, M., and Baxter, C. 2013. Application of skin contamination studies of ammonia gas for management of hazardous material incidents. *J Haz Mater* 252–253:338–346. DOI: 10.1016/j.jhazmat.2013.02.048.

9. Gaskin, S., Pisaniello, D., Edwards, J.W., Bromwich, D., Reed, S., Logan, M., and Baxter, C. 2013. Chlorine and hydrogen cyanide gas interactions with human skin: In vitro studies to inform skin permeation and decontamination in HAZMAT incidents. *J Haz Mater* 262:759–763. DOI: 10.1016/j.jhazmat.2013.09.040.

10. Gaskin, S., Heath, L., Pisaniello, D., Logan, M., and Baxter, C. 2019. Skin permeation of oxides of nitrogen and sulfur from short-term exposure scenarios relevant to hazardous material incidents. *Sci Total Environ* 665:937–943. DOI: 10.1016/j.scitotenv.2019.02.205.

11. Gaskin, S., Heath, L., Pisaniello, D., Edwards, J.W., Logan, M., and Baxter, C. 2017. Dermal absorption of fumigant gases during HAZMAT incident exposure scenarios-methyl bromide, sulfuryl fluoride, and chloropicrin. *Toxicol Indust Health* 33:547–554. DOI: 10.1177/0748233716689651.

12. Heath, L., Gaskin, S., Pisaniello, D., Crea, J., Logan, M., and Baxter, C. 2017. Skin absorption of ethylene oxide gas following exposures relevant to HAZMAT incidents. *Ann Work Exposures Health* 61:589–595. DOI: 10.1093/annweh/wxx030.

13. Blum, A., Gold, M.D., Ames, B.N., Jones, F.R., Hett, E.A., Dougherty, R.C., Horning, E.C., Dzidic, I., Carroll, D.I., Stillwell, R.N., and Thenot, J.P. 1978. Children absorb tris-BP flame retardant from sleepwear: Urine contains the mutagenic metabolite, 2,3-dibromopropanol. *Science* 201:1020–1023. DOI: 10.1126/science.684422.

14. Ulsamer, A.G., Porter, W.K., and Osterberg, R.E. 1978. Percutaneous absorption of radiolabeled TRIS from flame-retarded fabric. *J Environ Pathol Toxicol* 1:543–549.

15. Snodgrass, H.L. 1992. Permethrin transfer from treated cloth to the skin surface: Potential for exposure in humans. *J Toxicol Environ Health* 35:91–105. DOI: 10.1080/15287399209531598.

16. Rossbach, B., Appel, K.E., Mross, K.G., and Letzel, S. 2010. Uptake of permethrin from impregnated clothing. *Toxicol Lett* 192:50–55. DOI: 10.1016/j.toxlet.2009.06.863.

17. Rossbach, B., Kegel, P., Süß, H., and Letzel, S. 2016. Biomonitoring and evaluation of permethrin uptake in forestry workers using permethrin-treated tick-proof pants. *J Exposure Sci Environ Epidemiol* 26:95–103. DOI: 10.1038/jes.2015.34.

18. Rossbach, B., Niemietz, A., Kegel, P., and Letzel, S. 2014. Uptake and elimination of permethrin related to the use of permethrin treated clothing for forestry workers. *Toxicol Lett* 231:147–153. DOI: 10.1016/j.toxlet.2014.10.017

19. Meinke, M., Abdollahnia, M., Gähr, F., Platzek, T., Wolfram, S., and Lademann, J. 2009. Migration and penetration of a fluorescent textile dye into the skin - in vivo versus in vitro methods. *Exper Dermatol* 18:789–792. DOI: 10.1111/j.1600-0625.2009.00885.x.

20. Morrison, G.C., Weschler, C.J., Bekö, G., Koch, H.M., Salthammer, T., Schripp, T., Toftum, J., and Clausen, G. 2016. Role of clothing in both accelerating and impeding

dermal absorption of airborne SVOCs. *J Exposure Sci Environ Epidemiol* 26:113–118. DOI: 10.1038/jes.2015.42.

21. Morrison, G.C., Bekö, G., Weshcler, C., Schripp, T., Salthammer, T., Hill, J., Andersson, A-M., Toftum, J., Clausen, G., and Frederiksen, H. 2017. Dermal uptake of benzophenone-3 from clothing. *Environmental Science and Technology* 51:11371–11379. DOI: 10.1021/acs.est.7b02623.

22. Bekö, G., Morrison, G., Weschler, C.J., Koch, H.M., Pälmke, C., Salthammer, T., Schripp, T., Toftum, J., and Clausen, G. 2017. Measurements of dermal uptake of nicotine directly from air and clothing. *Indoor Air* 27:427–433. DOI: 10.1111/ina.12327.

23. Keeble, V.B., Corell, L., and Ehrich, M. 1993. Evaluation of knit glove fabrics as barriers to dermal absorption of organophosphorus insecticides using an in vitro test system. *Toxicology* 81:195–203. DOI: 10.1016/0300-483x(93)90012-h.

24. Keeble, V.B., Corell, L., and Ehrich, M. 1996. Effect of laundering on ability of glove fabrics to decrease the penetration of organophosphate insecticides through in vitro epidermal systems. *J Appl Toxicol* 16:401–406. DOI: 10.1002/(SICI)1099-1263(199609)16:5<401::AID-JAT364>3.0.CO;2-F.

25. Rehal, B., and Maibach, H. 2011. Percutaneous absorption of vapors in human skin. *Cutaneous Ocular Toxicol* 30:87–91. DOI: 10.3109/15569527.2010.534522.

26. Raheel, M. 1991. Pesticide transmission in fabrics: Effect of particulate soil. *Bull Environ Contam Toxicol* 46:845–851. DOI: 10.1007/bf01689728.

27. Orlando, J., Branson, D., Ayres, G., and Leavitt, R. 1981. The penetration of formulated guthion spray through selected fabrics. *J Environ Sci Health, Part B* 16:617–628. DOI: 10.1080/03601238109372283.

28. Lillie, T.H., Livingston, J.M., and Hamilton, M.A. 1981. Recommendations for selecting and decontaminating pesticide applicator clothing. *Bull Environ Contam Toxicol* 27:716–723. DOI: 10.1007/bf01611087.

29. Yang, Y., and Li, S. 1993. Frictional transition of pesticides from protective clothing. *Arch Environ Contam Toxicol* 25:279–284. DOI: 10.1007/bf00212142.

30. Protano, C., Guidotti, M., and Vitali, M. 2009. Performance of different work clothing types for reducing skin exposure to pesticides during open field treatment. *Bull Environ Contam Toxicol* 83:115–119. DOI: 10.1007/s00128-009-9753-1.

31. Guy, R.H., and Maibach, H.I. 1985. Calculations of body exposure from percutaneous absorption data. In *Percutaneous Absorption*, 4th ed. Bronaugh, R., and Maibach, H.I., Eds., 461–466. New York: CRC Press. DOI: 10.3109/9780203904015-22.

32. Chan, H.P., Honbo, Z., Wester, R.C., and Maibach, H.I. 2010. Agricultural chemical percutaneous absorption and decontamination. In *Hayes' Handbook of Pesticide Toxicology*. Krieger, R.I., Ed., 683–700. New York: Marcel Dekker. DOI: 10.1016/B978-0-12-374367-1.00027-6.

33. Solbrig, C.M., and Obendorf, S.K. 1985. Distribution of residual pesticide within textile structures as determined by electron microscopy. *Textile Res J* 55:540–546. DOI: 10.1177/004051758505500904.

34. Bartek, M.J., LaBudde, J.A., and Maibach, H.I. 1972. Skin permeability in vivo: Comparsion in rat, rabbit, pig and man. *J Investigative Dermatol* 58:114–123. DOI: 10.1111/1523-1747.ep12538909.

35. Sidon, E.W., Moody, R.P., and Franklin, C.A. 1988. Percutaneous absorption of cis- and trans-permethrin in rhesus monkeys and rats: Anatomic site and interspecies variation. *J Toxicol Environ Health* 23:207–216. DOI: 10.1080/15287398809531107.

36. Law, R.M., Ngo, M.A., and Maibach, H.I. 2020. Twenty clinically pertinent factors/observations for percutaneous absorption in humans. *Am J Clin Dermatol* 21:85–95. DOI: 10.1007/s40257-019-00480-4.

22 Practical Considerations When Selecting and Using Gloves for Chemical Protection

C.L. Packham and H.E. Taylor

CONTENTS

DOI: 10.1201/9781003126874-26

22.1 INTRODUCTION

Millions of gloves are worn every day around the world in an attempt to protect workers from chemical hazards. Unfortunately, in all too many cases, the protection that employers and employees believe the gloves provide is not achieved. This is simply because neither have adequate knowledge of the factors that affect glove performance when used with chemicals. Assumptions are made about glove performance that do not conform to the reality. Gloves are not simple membranes that, provided they do not disintegrate, protect the worker. The way gloves perform in contact with chemicals is complex and affected by a wide range of factors.

22.2 SHOULD WE BE PROVIDING GLOVES
FOR CHEMICAL PROTECTION?

It is a basic principle in the management of workplace dermal exposure that we should control the process, not the person. In other words, we need to take appropriate steps to ensure that the process is intrinsically safe and independent of the worker's actions. In fact, in many countries, this is a legal requirement.

There are several good reasons why we should adopt this policy. In the first place, when controlling the process, we are not relying upon one or more individuals to perform in a predetermined manner. The process determines the level of safety that we are achieving. Human nature is such that even the most conscientious worker will not always perform in the way anticipated. Furthermore, when controlling the process, we can take steps to ensure that this is fail-to-safe. In other words, should the splash guard not be in place, then the machine will not start. If relying upon local exhaust ventilation, if this is not achieving the required airflow, then either the process is shut down or, at least, a warning is sounded. We have yet to develop a process that ensures that people are fail-to-safe!

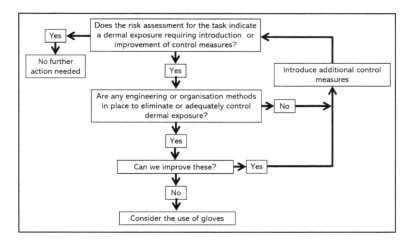

FIGURE 22.1   Factors to consider when deciding if gloves should be provided. Printed with permission of the authors and EnviroDerm Services (UK), Ltd.

As a final consideration, we also need to consider the cost. Although a single pair of gloves may not appear expensive, regular use of gloves can result in significant costs to the employer. This is particularly the case where the nature of the chemical requires a more expensive glove to be used and changed frequently.

So before deciding to provide gloves for chemical protection, we need to consider a number of factors and reach appropriate decisions, as shown in Figure 22.1.

Only when we have concluded that we have no alternative course of action open to us but to resort to gloves to achieve that final protection should we start to consider which type of glove we should be providing and how it should be used. The only exception to this would be an emergency situation not predicted by our risk assessment, where there is no time to consider alternative strategies and where gloves may be used for a relatively short period until other measures can be implemented.

22.3   WHAT FACTORS THAT AFFECT GLOVE PERFORMANCE DO WE NEED TO CONSIDER

Firstly, it is essential to work on the basis that each task has its own particular characteristics and hazards. The risk assessment must be based on the real hazard that exists when chemicals are used for that task. This can be very different from the data provided by a safety data sheet, and in many cases, there may not be a safety data sheet as this is not seen as necessary as is the case with water. Skin exposure to water is one of the most common causes of occupational irritant contact dermatitis.

We purchase chemicals to use to achieve some outcome. In the process, they will almost inevitably undergo some form of change. Table 22.1 explains many of these.

TABLE 22.1

Factors That Can Affect Glove Performance

Factor	Examples
Contamination	Cleaning chemicals or solvents used for degreasing will have possibly unknown substances added
Mixing/diluting	If we mix two or more chemicals, this may change the effect should contact occur
Reaction	A reaction between two or more chemicals to produce a different substance, e.g. bleach and acid-based toilet cleaner can produce chlorine
Processing	Can change the properties of the chemicals, e.g. vulcanizing rubber
Heating	Can affect the properties of the chemical and cause the release of chemicals that may be harmful, e.g. solder flux
Metabolization	Within the skin, e.g. methanol can metabolize into formaldehyde
Other changes	That occur over time, e.g. biocides that are formaldehyde releasers
Physical changes	Such as the leaching of metals into metalworking fluid, grinding dust, etc.

It is beyond the scope of this chapter to describe in detail how these may affect the hazard and the consequences of any skin exposure. Indeed, there are no simple means of doing this.

For the time being, there is no EU-wide system in place to assess the combination effects and risks of chemicals.
From "Chemicals in our life," ECHA (European Chemicals Agency)[1]

In many situations, it is not too difficult to identify the hazardous properties that will arise from the use of the chemical. In others, it may require specialist knowledge or support from someone such as an industrial chemist.

22.4 WHY SOME GLOVES CAN FAIL TO PROTECT

No glove will provide more than momentary protection against all chemicals. Indeed, for some chemicals, no glove would be suitable as protection. In many cases, the only glove that would provide the protection needed possesses properties that render it unusable for the task.

The main reasons for gloves failing to provide adequate protection fall into four main categories:

1. Misuse
2. Physical damage
3. Degradation
4. Permeation

22.4.1 MISUSE

22.4.1.1 Using the Wrong Glove

Given that the knowledge about gloves appears often to be inadequate among those who need to decide which glove to use for a particular task, it is not surprising that all too often the gloves being used are not the ones that are really needed. In addition, experience suggests that those who are responsible for supplying the gloves, such as a general distributor of industrial health and safety equipment, do not have the knowledge needed to ensure that their customer receives the correct advice. Furthermore, as will be shown later in this chapter, the technical information provided to meet regulatory requirements can be misleading.

22.4.1.2 Not Donning or Removing the Glove Correctly

It is essential when donning gloves to ensure that only clean hands are placed in clean gloves. This is generally less of an issue when single-use gloves are being used. Provided that the hands are clean (or for biological protection decontaminated) there should be no problem. Where gloves are being reused, the possibility that the interior of the gloves has become contaminated with the very chemicals against which the glove had been providing protection is something that should be considered. One of the most common causes of this is when gloves are worn that are either too short or where the nature of the task can result in the chemical entering the glove through the cuff.

The significance of this is that due to the effect on the skin of the occlusion the effect of any internal contamination can be enhanced.

Wearing internally contaminated gloves led to higher systemic absorption than was gained from the equivalent skin contamination when not wearing gloves.
(Rawson, Cocker, et al.)[2]

A very common problem, particularly where relatively tight-fitting single-use gloves are worn, is when on removing the gloves the wearer's hands come into contact with the contaminated outer surface of the gloves. The result is to largely negate the protection that the gloves may have been providing. In one study with hairdressers, it was found that following shampooing, even with the use of disposable gloves, every single person had contaminated their hands with the shampoo. Even after training on the proper use of gloves, the result was that 55% still had contaminated hands.[3] Given that the skin barrier of the hands will have been reduced due to the occlusion, this could increase the damage that could result.

22.4.1.3 Using Gloves beyond the Time for Which They Can Provide Protection

All chemical protective gloves have a limited life. This will depend on several factors, as described later in this chapter. Unfortunately, as will become apparent, deciding in any one situation what the duration during which protection will be provided is, in many cases, anything but simple. Manufacturers' published performance data is not a reliable guide.

Particularly with the single-use gloves so often encountered, this life can be very short. Moreover, experience shows that with many suppliers of this type of glove the information provided on the packaging is either inadequate or simply missing.

Furthermore, as will become apparent, the point in time at which the glove ceases to protect will, in many cases, not be easily identifiable. As will be explained, the gloves can fail without there being any visible or sensory indication that this has happened.

Perhaps an extreme example, but indicative of the potential consequences, is the case of Professor Karen Wetterhahn.[4] Working in a laboratory with dimethyl mercury she inadvertently spilled "several drops" on her gloved hand. As she was wearing a glove made from the recommended material (latex), there appeared to be no effect on the glove, and she couldn't feel anything passing through the glove, she completed the task. Without her realizing it, the chemical was able to migrate through the glove at a molecular level and be absorbed into her skin. Six months later she noticed symptoms of a rapid decline in health. Despite aggressive treatment, she became unresponsive and died from the resulting brain damage 10 months after the initial exposure.

22.4.1.4   Improper Storage of Gloves When Temporarily Not in Use

When gloves are used on more than one occasion, then it is essential to ensure that they are stored in such a manner that they are not damaged during the period when they are not being used. Ideally, the gloves would be washed and dried prior to removal. Not only will this reduce the potential for skin contamination on removal, but it should prevent any chemical left on the glove from continuing to degrade or pass through (permeate) the glove material while not being worn.

Ideally when stored, this should be so that air can circulate inside the glove to encourage any moisture left on the inside of the glove to evaporate.

22.4.1.5   Incorrect Disposal

Gloves that have become contaminated with a hazardous chemical must be considered as contaminated waste and disposed of accordingly. We need also to consider the glove material itself and the requirements that this imposes on our disposal method. For example, gloves manufactured from Viton™ rubber should not be incinerated, unless appropriate steps have been taken to ensure that the hydrofluoric acid that will result from the incineration is safely dealt with. The same is true for gloves manufactured from polyvinylchloride (PVC or "vinyl"). Incineration of PVC results in the creation of several toxic chemicals, in particular dioxins.

22.4.2   Physical Damage

When the task for which the gloves are provided is for a situation where physical hazards are also present, then consideration should be given to protecting both the hands and the glove by wearing a separate glove outside the chemical glove that is designed to provide the relevant protection. All too often a physical protective glove with an outer coating is provided. Very quickly, upon use, the chemical protective coating can become compromised. When both chemical and physical protection is required, a chemical protective glove needs to be provided inside of the physical protection.

22.4.3 DEGRADATION

Degradation is when the chemical in contact with the glove causes damage to the glove material itself. Note that no glove material can withstand all chemicals. Usually, degradation is detectable by the user as it involves a change in the properties of the glove materials themselves.

With regard to degradation, in the EU there is now a standard, EN374-4:2019—Normative Puncture Degradation Resistance test. Degradation is where the chemical when in contact with the glove material adversely changes the material's physical properties. Not only does this eventually destroy the glove, but it can also have the effect of reducing permeation breakthrough time. Unfortunately, as can be the case with laboratory-based tests imitating real-life situations, the new standard for degradation—EN374-4:2019—has limitations with some chemicals, which means it is not a reliable indicator of what will happen in real use. The test involves exposing a sample of the glove to the chemical and then measuring the force required for a needle to penetrate. The lesser the force, the greater the assumed degradation.

However, with some forms of degradation, the effect is initially to harden the material, the glove goes brittle and eventually splits. The hardening effect will increase the force needed for the needle to penetrate, thus perhaps creating the impression that the effect of the chemical on the glove material is in fact improving its properties! Currently, the degradation test is optional.

22.4.4 PERMEATION

Permeation is the passage of the chemical through the glove at a molecular level. Apart from any simultaneous degradation, there will be no visible change to the glove. As the chemical eventually desorbs from the glove's interior surface, there is no sensory effect to alert the wearer that the glove is no longer protecting them. Thus, it is essential when deciding whether a particular glove is suitable for use with the chemical for which protection is required to know how long it will take for the chemical to arrive in the interior of the glove, usually referred to as the permeation breakthrough time (BTT). It was a lack of knowledge of the short permeation breakthrough time that led to the hazardous exposure and ultimate death of Karen Wetterhahn.

In most industrial countries, manufacturers or suppliers of chemical protective gloves are required to provide permeation breakthrough times for the chemicals against which they are claimed to provide protection. Unfortunately, this data is of very limited help when attempting to establish for how long the glove will protect when used for a particular task.

As will be seen, determining the real BTT is far from simple, yet it is essential to understand the complexities of permeation if we are to ensure that gloves are not worn for longer than they can provide protection.

The permeation of chemicals through gloves is explained in more detail in other chapters. The concern of this chapter is to consider how permeation affects our choice of glove for a particular task and how it affects the glove use protocol.

Firstly, what do the data provided by the manufacturer tell us about the suitability of the particular glove used for the task for which we are attempting to ensure adequate protection? The simple answer is that they will certainly indicate where the glove is unsuitable. Even where it appears that the glove will provide protection, albeit, during a limited time of use, a variety of factors will affect what is achieved in practice. These include the integrity of the glove as a membrane, temperature, extent of exposure, stretching and flexing, and, in particular, the nature of the chemical hazard.

Standards, such as ISO EN 374 and ASTM F 739, lay down how such permeation breakthroughs should be determined. What is important for the selection of the appropriate glove and decision as to how it can be used for the task in question is an understanding of how the conditions under which the gloves will be used will affect the permeation breakthrough time.

Several factors, discussed in the next sections, can affect chemical permeation through gloves.

22.4.4.1 Chemical Coverage, Flexing, and Stretching of the Glove

The standardized tests involve total coverage of the membrane being tested. In reality, this will often not be the case. Recent research developing new methods for glove permeation testing has shown that permeation through the glove material is significantly affected by the coverage of the chemical on the glove.[5] This is backed up by in-use testing, as described later in this chapter, and shows how the extent of the exposure affects the actual permeation that is likely to be experienced depending on the nature of the exposure. These studies along with others have also shown or alluded to the impact that flexing and stretching have on the permeation of chemicals through gloves.

22.4.4.2 Impact of Temperature on Glove Permeation

Both the two standardized tests mentioned stipulate that the test be carried out at room temperature, specified as 23 ± 1 °C. In reality, it is unlikely that the glove will be at this temperature during the time it is worn. A very simple test of temperature change when a glove is donned is shown in Table 22.2.

The effect on permeation time that the increase in temperature can cause is considerable. One manufacturer published performance data according to EN374-1 at two different temperatures. Table 22.3 shows how variable the actual breakthrough time was for the same glove when tested with a variety of chemicals. Note how there is no consistency in the changes. In other words, there can be no formula that indicates a percentage reduction in BTT for each given increase in temperature. This is due to the impact of the temperature increase being linked to the nature of the chemical, e.g. the temperature at which the chemical evaporates.

Other studies such as that carried out on behalf of the association of German statutory insurance providers (Hauptverband der gewerblichen Berufsgenossenschaften)

TABLE 22.2
Changes in Temperature of the Glove and Hands before, during, and after Use

Conditions	Temperature (°C)
Ambient temperature	23.0
Hand temperature at the start	30.1
Glove temperature at the start	22.8
Elapsed time 2 min—glove temperature	30.3
Elapsed time 5 min—glove temperature	30.4
Hand temperature on glove removal	30.6

TABLE 22.3
Effect of Temperature on Breakthrough Time (BTT) in Minutes

Chemical	BTT at 23 °C (min)	BTT at 35 °C (min)	Percentage of Original BTT with Increased Temperature
n-Butanol	>480	240	Half (50%)
Diethylamine	60	6	Significantly reduced (10%)
Dipentene	>480	36	Significantly reduced (7.5%)
Isobutanol	>240	>240	No change (100%)
Methyl ethyl ketone	>1440	>240	Significantly reduced (17%)

in 1999 tested gloves for permeation not only at different temperatures but also when stretched and showed significant changes in the actual time achieved.

22.4.4.3 Effects of Mixtures on Glove Permeation

There is also the question of the actual chemical. Most of the permeation data provided by manufacturers are for the glove performance against a single chemical. The reality is that in many cases we will be dealing with mixtures. How gloves perform against mixtures of chemicals is uncertain. Table 22.4 shows the permeation breakthrough time for a specific glove when tested against two chemicals individually and also when mixed at a ratio of 1:1. Keep in mind that in a large number of situations the mixture may vary during the task, both in the nature and concentration of the chemicals and the potential effect of the combination. It should also be mentioned that not all mixtures will have the same impact on the breakthrough time.

22.4.4.4 At What Point Do We Consider Permeation to Be Significant?

As shown in Figure 22.2, the current test procedures consider the permeation breakthrough to be the time at which a certain permeation rate has been measured. These range from 1 $\mu g/min\cdot cm^2$ (EN 374) to 0.1 $\mu g/min\cdot cm^2$ (ASTM F 739). However,

TABLE 22.4

Changes in Breakthrough Time (BTT) for a Glove for a Mixture of Two Chemicals

Chemical/Mixture	BTT at 35 °C
Methyl ethyl ketone (MEK)	>240 min
Toluene	>240 min
MEK + Toluene (1:1)	9 min

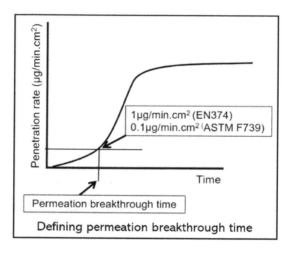

FIGURE 22.2 Permeation curve showing the determination of the breakthrough time based on a permeation rate of 1 µg/min·cm^2 (EN 374) to 0.1 µg/min·cm^2 (ASTM F 739). Printed with permission of the authors and EnviroDerm Services (UK), Ltd.

factors such as the nature of the chemical, its potency as a skin sensitizer, and the condition of the skin barrier can potentially lower the level at which a reaction will occur. Prudence suggests that it is the time that the chemical is first detected that is used as the key to deciding when the glove should be considered to have failed to prevent exposure. Obviously, this will be less than the time shown in the manufacturer's published performance data, nor can one assume a figure based on calculating a given percentage of the published data.

22.4.4.5 Establishing the SMUT (Safe Maximum Use Time)

As should by now be apparent, there is no simple method for determining the permeation breakthrough time. Many different factors can affect how long a particular glove will protect. It should be clear that the manufacturer's published data does not indicate what will be achieved in practice. Table 22.5 outlines various factors that may be present during the task in question and could affect glove performance.

TABLE 22.5
Factors That Can Either Increase or Decrease Breakthrough Time (BTT)

Factors That Can *Decrease* the BTT	Factors That Can *Increase* the BTT
Degradation of glove	Volatility of chemical
High temperature during use	Intermittent chemical contact
Mechanical damage to the glove	Incomplete chemical contact
Chemical mixtures	Low temperature during use
Abrasion of glove	Mixture strength of chemical (e.g. lower)
Flexing of the glove (in use)	Frequent glove washing
Aging of the glove	
Poor glove maintenance	

Questions such as how each of the factors shown in the table affects permeation breakthrough time, possibly interact with each other, possibly in a synergistic manner, or by inhibiting the effect of a different factor, have yet to be determined.

22.5   THE EFFECT OF OCCLUSIVE GLOVES ON THE SKIN

While the selection and use of gloves to protect against chemical hazards is important, we should not lose sight of the fact that all occlusive gloves, regardless of material, will cause some damage to the skin. This is because inside the occlusive glove the skin will become hyperhydrated. It is often assumed that it is sweating inside the glove that is the cause of this condition. While sweat may play an important role, it will not be the only cause; indeed, hyperhydration can occur in situations where the hands inside the glove are unlikely to sweat at all.

Sweating occurs due to one of several stimuli. It is a primary way in which our body can lose excess heat. Sweating is the passage of what is largely water from sweat glands in the skin through ducts to emerge through pores onto the surface of the skin. One of the main causative factors is the need to maintain a largely constant body temperature. The evaporation of sweat can remove large amounts of heat from the skin. However, this is not the only way in which we lose water through the skin. Sweating is an on/off function that occurs as a result of specific conditions, e.g. increase in body temperature or emotions; however, our skin is continuously losing water across its surface. This is generally referred to as transepidermal water loss, generally shortened to TEWL. Skin in normal condition can result in the loss of up to around 700 ml of water every 24 hours. Normally this loss of water is not visible or detectable without the use of special measurement instruments. However, inside an occlusive glove, the TEWL cannot evaporate so is reabsorbed into the stratum corneum. Underneath an occlusive glove sweat also cannot evaporate and will also be absorbed into the skin. This changes the way in which certain cells respond, with a resultant negative effect on the formation of what are called natural moisturizing factors. The result is that the cells (corneocytes) in the stratum corneum are unable to bind the water needed for them to maintain the barrier performance of the skin. The loss of barrier performance has implications both on the ability of the skin to prevent ingress of chemicals and also on its ability to inhibit colonization by transient micro-organisms.

22.6   A STRUCTURED APPROACH TO SELECTION AND USE OF GLOVES

A risk assessment for chemical exposure must relate to the conditions under which a task is carried out, the risks arising from actual or potential exposure, and the consequent damage to health. It is no different when we consider the selection and use protocol for the glove, or gloves, to be used during the task. This must reflect the actual residual exposure for which they are being provided. In other words, the concept that one glove will provide the same level of protection for several different tasks or across a whole complex workplace is rarely one that will stand up to critical examination.

So we need a structured system that is matched to the conditions that exist during the specific task for which the gloves will be worn. The gloves selected and how they are used should be able to provide adequate protection for the wearer. Note, however, that our knowledge of the many factors that may exist in any given workplace or during a particular task is far from complete. As a result, we should always attempt, so far as possible, to limit the use of gloves to where there is no satisfactory alternative. We should also keep in mind that all protective gloves have potential to fail and we must take into account in our risk assessment the consequences of such failure. Figure 22.3 provides an example of a common procedure for the selection and use of gloves for protection against chemical hazards.

The following is only a brief explanation of each of the steps in this process. Each organization, or site, will have its own structure, and the system based on this outline will almost certainly need to be adapted to the particular circumstances and conditions that prevail there.

22.6.1   SELECT TASK

As has already been stated, the concept of a "one glove fits all" presents a significant risk of failure for at least one of the tasks for which the gloves are being worn. While a glove may perform to a certain extent against a particular chemical, the performance will almost certainly vary according to the nature of the task for which it is being worn. As an example of this when conducting a study on permeation breakthrough times under actual conditions of use, a nitrile glove being used as protection against xylene, with a manufacturer's permeation breakthrough time given by the manufacturer of 37 minutes, showed in one task no breakthrough for 2 hours but in another task only 5 minutes!

So, the selection of the particular glove and how it is used must be matched to the conditions prevailing during the execution of the particular task for which it is intended.

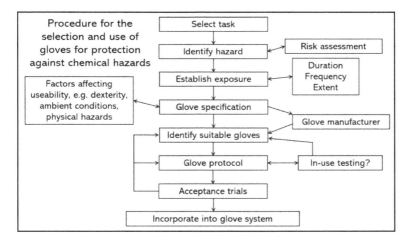

FIGURE 22.3 Example procedure for the selection and use of gloves for protection against chemical hazards. Printed with permission of the authors and EnviroDerm Services (UK), Ltd.

The next step in the process is to identify exactly what conditions the glove will encounter.

22.6.2 IDENTIFY HAZARD

Ideally, the glove will only be required to protect against the residual hazard identified in the risk assessment for that task. It is essential to ensure that the hazard is that which arises when one or more chemicals are used. This is rarely the same as the hazard stated on the safety data sheet(s). In the UK this has been recognized by the Health and Safety Executive, whose guidance on risk assessment states:

> *Employers should regard a substance as hazardous to health if it is hazardous in the form in which it may occur in the work activity. A substance hazardous to health need not be just a chemical compound, it can also include mixtures of compounds, micro-organisms or natural materials, such as flour, stone or wood dust.* (HSE ACoP)[6]

Good practice with risk assessment for skin exposure to chemicals in the workplace recognizes the limitations of safety data sheets and that many chemicals will not have been formally classified as hazardous but that in use may, if contact with the skin occurs, result in damage to the skin, or due to uptake through the skin to internal organs.

Furthermore, we generally purchase chemicals to use for a particular purpose. In doing so it is almost inevitable that they will undergo changes, and these can significantly alter the hazard that they present. Table 22.6 shows some of these.

These changes can have important implications on the level of performance of a glove such that the performance data given for the chemical, or each of the chemicals,

TABLE 22.6

Changes That Can Occur When Chemicals Are Used

- *Contamination*, e.g. in cleaning chemicals, solvents used for degreasing items
- *Reaction* between two or more chemicals, e.g. glass fiber moldings using epoxy resins, two-pack paints
- *Processes* that change the properties of the chemical, e.g. vulcanizing rubber
- *Oxidization* changing the chemical to include sensitizers
- *Heating* can both affect the properties of the chemical and cause the release of sensitizers, e.g. solder flux
- *Metabolization* within the skin, e.g. methanol can metabolize to formaldehyde, a sensitizer
- *Changes* to the chemical properties that occur over time, e.g. biocides that are formaldehyde releasers
- *Physical changes*, such as leaching of metals into metalworking fluid, grinding causing fine dust that can settle on the skin
- *Combinations* of these effects!

in the manufacturer's published data may have little in common with what will occur during the execution of the task.

Determining the real hazard can be a simple task or maybe one where the changes and their implications are not easily determined. A simple example is a solvent contained in a degreasing tank. This is only purely the solvent until the first article is degreased, whereupon it is a mixture of the solvent and what this has removed. Each further article degreased will change the composition of what is in the task. If the material removed from individual articles is different, then the hazard will also almost certainly vary, particularly since any glove failure could result in the wearer being exposed to something far more hazardous than the solvent itself.

22.6.3 ESTABLISH EXPOSURE

Having established the hazard, the next step should be to determine the extent to which the glove will be exposed. Keep in mind that the standard permeation breakthrough test is to total liquid exposure whereas the exposure during a task may be variable, ranging from light splash to full immersion. Furthermore, the condition of the chemical may vary during the execution of the task. It could start as a powder (where permeation would not be an issue), be diluted in a chemical, and then mixed with another. At each stage, the performance of the glove may change. Add to this the extent of the exposure and factors such as the temperature of the chemical, and identifying the extent of the exposure can be critical, as was indicated earlier in this chapter from the in-use tests. Some of the factors that one should identify and include when attempting to describe the nature of the exposure are shown in Table 22.7.

A detailed description of what happens to the chemical during the task will be useful when finally establishing what has been termed the "Glove specification" in Figure 22.3.

TABLE 22.7

Chemical and Exposure Factors to Consider When Identifying the Nature of the Hazard and Exposure

Condition of the Chemical	Nature of Exposure
• Solid	• Direct
• Powder (coarse, fine) or other particulates	• Limited area of the glove
• Liquid	• Occasional splash
• Aerosol	• Indirect
• Fume	• Handling contaminated objects
• Vapor	• Contact with persons or surfaces
• Gas	• Extensive
• Combinations of these	• Frequent splash
	• Short-term immersion
	• Long-term immersion

22.6.4   IDENTIFYING OTHER FACTORS

Having identified the nature of the hazard and exposure against which the glove will need to provide protection, it is now essential to consider other factors that will affect the type of glove that can be used for the task.

22.6.4.1   Dexterity

Firstly, there is a direct inverse relationship between the dexterity that the wearer will experience and the protection against the chemical afforded. Whereas from the protection aspects a particular glove may appear ideal, if the result is a glove where the wearer finds it difficult, even impossible, to carry out the task due to the level of dexterity required, the consequences are almost certain that the glove will not be worn, or a different glove affording the dexterity will be worn which will not provide the protection needed.

22.6.4.2   Physical Hazards

If gloves are to be used as protection against chemicals, then it is important that the integrity of the glove, and therefore the protection provided, is not impaired by physical damage to the glove. Thus it will be necessary to examine the application to establish whether physical damage is, or might be, a factor we need to take into consideration.

Damage can take the form of:

1. *Abrasion*: This reduces the effective thickness of the glove and thus reduces also the permeation breakthrough. Furthermore, if there is a degradation of the glove material, there will be less glove material to degrade and complete breakdown of the glove will occur more rapidly.

2. *Cuts*: Obviously, any cut will mean that the glove immediately ceases to protect the user.
3. *Punctures*: These may be so small that they are not immediately apparent to the wearer. Since the puncture by a sharp object may result also in a puncture of the skin, the potential for skin penetration may be significant.

Where physical damage is a possibility it may be necessary to double glove, i.e. to wear a suitable glove directly on the hand for chemical protection and a second glove on top to protect both glove and hand from physical damage. Gloves of cut-resistant material, such as Kevlar™, are available with a chemical protective coating. However, these are of limited help, since invariably the chemical-resistant coating is applied to the outside of the glove. Any physical damage will thus result in the destruction of the chemical barrier.

While abrasion and cuts are relatively easily dealt with by the use of a glove made of a cut-resistant material, these gloves rarely protect against pointed objects, such as needles. Special gloves do exist for the prevention of the so-called needle stick injury, but these tend to be both expensive and offer only limited dexterity.

When outer gloves from a cut-resistant material are used, it is important to consider the effect of the chemical on the material of this glove. Some cut-resistant materials degrade quickly if in contact with certain chemicals, and this could significantly reduce the level of protection from physical damage afforded, with an increased risk of damage to the chemical protective glove and thus contact between the skin and chemical. We need also to remember that once the outer glove has become contaminated with the chemical, it forms a reservoir ensuring ongoing contact between the chemical protective glove and the chemical itself, even if this is no longer occurring as part of the work.

22.6.4.3 Temperature

With temperature, we need to consider both general ambient temperature and the temperature of any object or chemical with which the glove will be in contact. Both can affect glove performance. Ambient temperature will influence the effect that wearing the occlusive glove will have on the wearer's skin.

22.6.4.4 Grip

Different glove materials will have different levels of friction. Particularly with liquids, this needs to be considered. The ideal glove from a chemical protection aspect may be unsuitable if when wet the wearer cannot adequately grip items as part of the task. One possibility here is to wear a second glove that provides the grip over the chemical protective glove. However, this will inevitably have some effect on dexterity.

22.6.4.5 Flexing and Stretching

In the in-use investigation, already referred to into glove performance under actual conditions of use, the effect of flexing and stretching became apparent because with snuggly fitting gloves permeation breakthroughs often first occurred on the knuckles of the fingers due to the stretching when objects were gripped. This was particularly the case where the thin, tightly fitting single-use gloves were worn.

22.6.4.6 Glove Specification

We should now be in a position to produce what we have termed a glove specification. This should list all the different parameters that we have identified that are relevant for the selection and use of the glove.

The aim of the glove specification is that it forms the basis on which we request a recommendation from one or more glove manufacturers as to which of the gloves from their range they would recommend and the performance that they expect that the glove will achieve, given the information in our specification.

Of course, in some situations, the information gained may indicate that the selection of the optimum glove and how this should be used is straightforward. However, even in such situations, it may be prudent to contact someone with specialist knowledge about gloves to ensure that there is not something we have overlooked.

22.6.4.7 Glove Manufacturer

Experience suggests that it is advisable to contact the glove manufacturer directly if possible. After all, they manufacture and place their products on the market, so presumably, they have carried out the appropriate tests to establish how their gloves perform. To achieve this, they will need either to have the appropriate test facilities themselves or an arrangement with an accredited test laboratory. Experience indicates clearly that many of those organizations selling gloves as part of general health and safety equipment have at best only a rudimentary knowledge of the complexities that selection and use bring with them.

22.6.5 IDENTIFY SUITABLE GLOVES

Once the recommendations from glove manufacturers are to hand, their content can be analyzed so that the most appropriate glove, or gloves, can be identified and a decision reached as to which glove, or gloves, should be selected. It is here that cost also enters our deliberations. It may well be that the optimum glove is expensive and a glove with shorter safe use time but considerably less costly may be a sensible choice.

One such example is a company that was manufacturing large objects made of resin-reinforced glass fiber. The nature of the objects was such that most of the lay-up was done manually. There was considerable potential for skin contact with the resin which contained both a solvent and skin sensitizers. The ideal glove was one manufactured from butyl. This would have lasted for a complete shift. However, the resin on the glove cured within 1 or 2 hours, rendering the glove useless. A nitrile glove would provide sufficient protection if changed at appropriate intervals, i.e. just before the resin cured to the state where the glove became unusable and would represent a considerable cost saving.

22.6.6 GLOVE PROTOCOL

We should now be in a position where we can create our glove protocol, i.e. a document that states which glove should be used, how often it should be changed, and any other relevant information relating to its use (e.g. the wearing of a second glove to protect against physical hazards). Once we have this, we may wish to ask the manufacturer of the glove selected for their opinion on our protocol.

22.6.7   In-Use Testing

In some circumstances, in particular, where we have any reservations about whether our assessment of actual in-use performance matches reality, we may decide it advisable to carry out in-use testing. This is particularly advisable where the consequences of glove failure could be acute and cause severe damage to the skin of the hands.

One method for in-use testing is the use of small activated carbon fiber pads (Permea-Tec, SKC) shown in Figure 22.4. These are usually attached to a single-use glove. A new glove of the type that it is proposed to be used for the task is then donned and work commenced. The hand most exposed to the chemicals is usually the test site; however, it may be desirable to test both hands. In the study already referred to, four pads were attached, three as shown in Figure 22.5 and one on the knuckle of the middle finger.

A new glove of the type proposed to be used for the task is then donned and work commenced.

At predetermined intervals, based on an interpretation of how quickly permeation breakthrough might occur, the work was stopped, the outer glove removed, and each of the pads detached and placed in a labeled, sealed plastic pouch. Fresh pads were

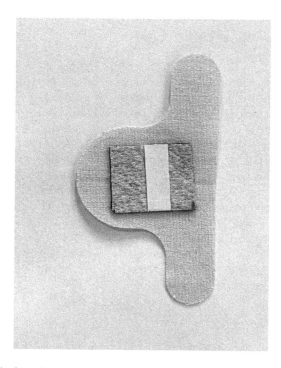

FIGURE 22.4   Activated carbon pad (Permea-Tec).

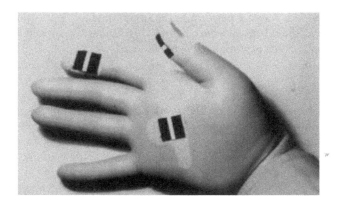

FIGURE 22.5 Pads located on hand for permeation testing.

attached, the protective glove redonned and work recommenced. This was repeated until it could be assumed that a permeation breakthrough would have occurred.

All pads are then analyzed to establish the point in time where the chemical is first detected on a pad. Experience indicates that this can vary substantially from task to task, even when the same chemical is used.

Based on the in-use testing, a modification to the glove use protocol may be indicated to establish a time that can be set for glove change ensuring a safety margin.

22.6.8 ACCEPTANCE TRIALS

Once it has been decided that the glove protocol is acceptable, then those using the gloves should be asked to test them to ensure that they can comfortably carry out the task for which the gloves are to be used. Feedback can be used to fine-tune our protocol.

22.6.9 INCORPORATION INTO GLOVE SYSTEM

We can now incorporate the glove protocol into our working practice for the selected task. Depending on how the health and safety management system is structured, it may be sensible to incorporate the glove use system into the general working procedure for the task.

For our glove system to be most effective, it is important to integrate it into our overall exposure control system and to consider other factors, e.g. working procedures, other health or exposure situations, and skin condition.

22.6.10 PROCUREMENT AND SUPPLY

Those responsible for the procurement and supply of gloves for chemical protection should have at least a basic understanding of how gloves work and why only the approved gloves should be purchased. There is abundant evidence that similar gloves from other suppliers may not perform to the same standard. If it is decided that an alternative glove should be introduced, then this should be subjected to the same procedure to ensure that performance is not reduced.

22.6.11   LOGISTICS

Those responsible for the storage and issuing of gloves should be provided with appropriate training so that they appreciate why only the approved gloves for a task should be issued. Allowing glove users to access gloves other than those selected for the specific task creates a risk that personal preference could result in inappropriate gloves being worn.

Gloves should always be stored in a manner that their performance will not be adversely affected. All gloves deteriorate over time, so it is recommended that excessive quantities not be held and that gloves are issued on a "first in—first out" basis.

Where used gloves have been actually or potentially contaminated with hazardous chemicals, they should be considered contaminated waste and disposed of accordingly.

22.6.12   TRAINING

Those affected by the provision and use of gloves for chemical protection must understand what this involves and why ensuring an effective system is important. The training that each receives needs to be matched to their role within the system. So, training will be different for those in procurement and logistics. The line managers responsible for compliance with good working practices will also need to understand their role and the reasons for this.

Those who will be wearing the gloves need a basic understanding of how gloves work and fail so that they can appreciate the need for compliance with the glove protocol. This must involve correct glove donning and particularly removal. Studies show that unless practical training in glove removal is provided, the percentage of those who, on removing their gloves, will contaminate their hands with what is on the outside of the glove, can reach as high as 100%. Even with training, it is unlikely that this problem can be completely eliminated. Any such contact will impair any benefit that has been achieved by wearing the gloves.

22.6.13   MONITORING FOR IMPACT ON THE SKIN

It should be recognized that should gloves fail to protect and chemicals become present inside the gloves, the condition of the skin inside the gloves will be a significant factor in the damage that can be caused by this breach. This is all the more important when we remind ourselves that wearing occlusive gloves for any length of time will result in hyperhydration and damage to the skin. This damage will vary among individuals and as a result of several different variables (length of time worn, ambient temperatures, time of day, etc.). Where gloves are worn for significant lengths of time, e.g. more than 25% of the work time, it would be advisable (and in some cases is a legal requirement) to have skin health surveillance in place. The minimum should include skin inspections, but it is possible to use skin measurements to better understand the condition of the skin and gain an appreciation for the effectiveness of the skin barrier. Measurements such as hydration, TEWL, pigmentation, and skin surface texture can all be used effectively for this purpose.

REFERENCES

1. ECHA. 2021. Combined effects of chemicals. European Chemicals Agency (ECHA). Available at: https://chemicalsinourlife.echa.europa.eu/combined-effects-of-chemicals.
2. Rawson, B.V., Cocker, J., Evans, P.G., Wheeler, J.P., and Akrill, P.M. 2005. Internal contamination of gloves: Routes and consequences. *Ann Occup Hyg* 49(6):535–541.
3. Oreskov, K.W., Søsted, H., and Johansen, J.D. 2015. Glove use among hairdressers: Difficulties in the correct use of gloves among hairdressers and the effect of education. *Contact Dermatitis* 72:6. DOI: 10.1111/cod.12336.
4. Cavanaugh, R. 2019. The dangers of dimethylmercury. *Chemistry World*, 19 February 2019.
5. Creta, M., Savoy, L., Duca, R.-D., Chu, W.K., Poels, K., Pan, J., Zheng, J., Godderis, L., Draper, M., and Vanoirbeek, J.A.J. 2021. An alternative method to assess permeation through disposable gloves. *J Hazard Mater* 411:125045. DOI: 10.1016/j.jhazmat.2021.125045.
6. HSE. 2013. *The Control of Substances Hazardous to Health Regulations: Approved Code of Practice and Guidance*, Sixth Edition. London: Health and Safety Executive.

23 Glove Selection for Work with Acrylates Including Those Cured by Ultraviolet, Visible Light, or Electron Beam

R.N. Phalen and D.M. Ceballos

CONTENTS

DOI: 10.1201/9781003126874-27

23.1   INTRODUCTION

Acrylates, including those cured by ultraviolet (UV), visible light, and electron beam (EB), are widely used in many occupational and industrial applications, including medicine (e.g., surgical sutures), dentistry (e.g., dentures), personal care (e.g., long-lasting nails), electronics, coatings, and printing.[1] One distinct advantage of acrylates is the replacement of solvent evaporation with reactive monomers that are incorporated into the polymer during a crosslinking phase, which can result in improved chemical and physical properties of the coating. The technical and economic advantages of this technology are increasingly recognized, and therefore the industrial use of these acrylates is rapidly growing, both in the number of applications and in tonnage.[2] A key element in the success of acrylates is that these are highly reactive molecules that allow for easy molding and fast drying. This, however, has dermatological consequences, as these acrylates may react with biomolecules in the skin, as well. This sometimes results in occupational dermatological disorders, mainly irritant contact dermatitis (ICD),[3–6] and allergic contact dermatitis (ACD).[7–10] Some may also be classified as skin sensitizers. Additionally, ACD could develop into immune-mediated responses such as occupational asthma.[11] Several acrylates such as acrylic acid and ethyl acrylate have National Institute for Occupational Safety and Health (NIOSH) skin notation denominations indicating that dermal care must be taken.[12] It must be noted that cured products are less associated with ICD and ACD. Instead, the reactive precursors or acrylate monomers are most associated with dermatitis.[1] Adequate industrial hygiene should therefore be ensured in every industrial use of acrylates. This should be integrated with proper risk assessment as well as management. Personal protection is an essential element in industrial hygiene. ACD has commonly been reported to affect the fingernails, fingers, hands, and forearms of workers.[1] Thus, protective gloves are necessary whenever workers handling products containing acrylates may be exposed to skin contact. Guidelines for the selection of adequate protective gloves for several types of occupational and industrial exposure situations are discussed.

23.2   GENERAL OVERVIEW OF ACRYLATES

23.2.1   CHEMISTRY[1,13,14]

Acrylates refer to a class of acrylic acids (Figure 23.1), and their esters are defined by a carboxylic acid group bound to a carbon–carbon double bond (vinyl group), which is involved in polymerization and the formation of plastics. Acrylates can be divided into two broad categories of products. The first category is resinous-type chemicals that give the basic properties to the final industrial application. These synthetic molecules, which

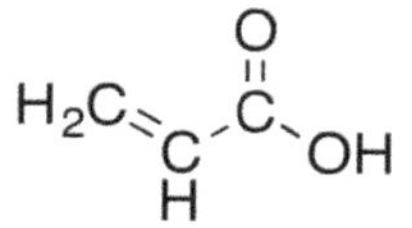

FIGURE 23.1   Acrylic acid.

generally are of medium-to-high viscosity (typically ranging from syrupy to nearly solid or purely solids), are referred to as *oligomers* in industry. The second category consists of reactive diluents that co-react with the oligomers into the final polymeric network upon curing. They are typically referred to as *monomers* or *MFAs* (multifunctional acrylates) in industry. Their viscosity ranges from watery to more viscous, but still easily pourable liquids. Although these names are not chemically correct, we use the terms oligomer and monomer as described above throughout this chapter.

23.2.1.1 Oligomers

In today's industrial practice, some five to ten different families of acrylate oligomers (molecules with few repeating units) are commercially available. The most widely used families are commonly referred to as epoxy acrylates, urethane acrylates, and polyester acrylates. They are typically manufactured in a relatively short synthetic route and sold as such or diluted in acrylate monomer for easier handling. As for most industrial applications, synthesis does not normally include washing, distilling, or other purification steps; these chemicals are rather complex mixtures of molecules with various molecular weights. Moreover, the final product typically contains lesser amounts of residual catalysts (all kinds of industrial catalysts are in use for their manufacture) and one or more inhibitors. Inhibitors are used to prevent polymerization during transport, storage, and the manufacture of industrial intermediates such as inks, coatings, or adhesives. The inhibitors are typically phenolic molecules, of which the two most widely used are hydroquinone and *p*-methoxyphenol.

The chemical composition of acrylate oligomers is normally not given on the label, the safety data sheet, or the technical data sheets. It is considered the technical knowledge of the acrylate oligomer manufacturer. This means that in most cases the chemical composition of a given acrylate oligomer is unique for a given manufacturer and considered proprietary information (e.g., a trade secret) and can only be divulged in private communication, often covered by secrecy or non-disclosure agreements.

The most important exception used in industrial volume is epoxy acrylates. This name, widely used in the industry, might be misleading to medical professionals. Epoxy acrylates are oligomers that are produced via the reaction of an epoxy resin with acrylic acid. In this reaction, the epoxy groups are converted into an α-hydroxy ester, and virtually zero residual epoxy groups can be detected in the final product.

For some specific industrial, medical, or dental applications, the oligomers are manufactured in a more controlled synthetic route to a purer product with narrow molecular weight distribution. Moreover, purification steps may be added to remove impurities such as catalysts and other low-molecular-weight chemicals that will not be incorporated into the polymer network upon cure and/or that might be of toxicological concern.

23.2.1.2 Monomers

More than 50 different acrylic monomers are commercially available and used industrially. They range from monofunctional acrylates (i.e., with one acrylic double bond) to difunctional acrylates (i.e., with two acrylic double bonds) and to multifunctional acrylates (i.e., with three, four, five, or six acrylic double bonds). Table 23.1 provides examples of these main groups of acrylates (acrylic resins or monomers)

TABLE 23.1

Examples of Acrylates (Acrylic Resins) Associated with Dermatitis and Contact Dermatitis (with Common Acronyms)

Monofunctional monomers:
- Ethyl acrylate (EA)
- 2-Ethylhexyl acrylate (2-EHA)
- Ethyl methacrylate (EMA)
- 2-Hydroxyethyl acrylate (2-HEA)
- 2-Hydroxyethyl methacrylate (2-HEMA)
- 2-Hydroxypropyl acrylate (2-HPA)
- 2-hydroxypropyl methacrylate (2-HPMA)
- Isobornyl acrylate (IBA)
- Methyl methacrylate (MMA)
- 2-Phenoxyethyl acrylate (2-PEA)

Difunctional monomers:
- Epoxy diacrylate (BIS-GA)
- Bisphenol A-diglycidyl methacrylate (BIS-GMA)
- Dipropyleneglycol diacrylate (DPGDA)
- Ethyleneglycol dimethacrylate (EGDMA)
- 1,6-Hexanediol diacrylate (HDDA)
- Tripropyleneglycol diacrylate (TPGDA)
- Triethyleneglycol dimethacrylate (TREGDMA)
- Urethane dimethacrylate (UEDMA or UDMA)

Multifunctional monomers:
- Pentaerythritol triacrylate (PETA)
- Trimethylolpropane triacrylate (TMPTA)
- Trimethylolpropane ethoxy triacrylate (TMPEOTA)

associated with dermatitis and contact dermatitis, which are discussed in this chapter. They can be divided roughly into two categories: the rather well-defined molecules with narrow molecular weight distribution and the so-called alkoxylated (i.e., ethoxylated and propoxylated) types. The former category is mostly referred to by an acronym, an abbreviation of their chemical name. The more widely used monomers in this category are the following:

TPGDA, tripropyleneglycol diacrylate
HDDA, 1,6-hexanediol diacrylate
TMPTA, trimethylolpropane triacrylate

Some in the second category, the alkoxylated monomers, are also referred to by an acronym, an abbreviation of their chemical name, e.g.:

GPTA, glyceryl propoxy triacrylate
TMPEOTA, trimethylolpropane ethoxy triacrylate

Acrylic monomers are manufactured in a multistep synthesis, including washing and distilling steps. Therefore, most of the starting materials like catalysts, acrylic acid, processing solvents, etc. are virtually absent in the final product. Nevertheless, acrylic monomers are still mostly rather complex mixtures. The reasons for this are multiple. One of the reasons may be a distribution of stereoisomers as in TPGDA. Another reason is a myriad of possible equilibrium reactions during manufacture, resulting in the distribution of the various possible by-products in addition to the main product. Yet another reason, specific for alkoxylated monomers, is the molecular weight distribution of the parent glycol as a result of multiple addition possibilities of ethylene or propylene oxide (ethylene oxide and propylene oxide are absent in industrially used acrylic monomers).

Finally, as for acrylic oligomers, acrylic monomers for some specific industrial, medical, and dental applications undergo added purification steps to remove low-molecular-weight chemicals that will not be incorporated into the polymer network upon cure and/or that are of toxicological concern.

23.2.2 INDUSTRIAL APPLICATIONS[1]

Acrylates in industrial applications are mostly used in coatings, inks, and adhesives. The main application areas are graphic arts, wood coatings, and miscellaneous applications. These graphic arts applications typically cover overprint varnishes and several types of printing inks, including offset, flexography, screen-printing, and letterpress. Wood coatings cover both liquid and powder coatings for wood parquet and furniture. The miscellaneous applications include optical fiber coatings, can and optical disk coatings, printing plates, resists, coatings and adhesives for electronic parts, and coatings for plastics. This list is far from being exhaustive. Further details can be found in textbooks,[15,16] at various sites on the Internet,[17,18] and a recent review.[1]

23.2.3 OTHER OCCUPATIONAL APPLICATIONS

Acrylates are also used in several occupations because of their unique sculpting, adhesive, and resistant properties, including medicine (e.g., orthopedic cement), dentistry (e.g., dental guards, dental prostheses, dental composites, sealants, and cement), and cosmetology (e.g., adhesives, acrylic nails, and long-lasting nail polish).[1]

The innovation in medicine of the last few decades has resulted in more uses of methacrylates in different medical procedures, which has increased the chances for medical personnel to be exposed to acrylates, especially methyl methacrylate (MMA).[19] Acrylate adhesives are, for example, extensively used in surgery as they are an important class of medical adhesives, with applications such as bone cement (i.e., methyl acrylate) as well as liquid skin or tissue sutures or wound-care products (i.e., cyanoacrylate).[19–21] Acrylates are also extensively used in surgical reconstruction or replacement of joints or on prosthetic limbs.[19,21]

In dentistry, different acrylate formulations are commonly used to construct dentures or temporary restorations, bone or teeth cement, and orthodontia.[22,23] The two-component acrylic resins used in dentistry typically use a mix of a powder and a liquid monomer solution containing different kinds of methacrylates, including

MMA.[22] The polymerization of methacrylates for dental applications, besides being initiated by mixing powder and liquid, can also be initiated by light or heating.[23] Besides the direct contact of the skin with the resins, acrylates in the air have also been suggested as another route of exposure in dentistry.[22]

Nowadays in cosmetology, many products use or contain acrylic ingredients.[24] For example, nail sculpting, including extensions and enhancements, is made of an applied acrylic mixture that becomes hard and inflexible so nails last. Acrylic nails, commonly known as fake nails or artificial nails, can be pre-sculpted or sculpted in situ.[22] Sculpted nails can use a two-component acrylic resin or UV-cured acrylic resin.[22] The two-component acrylic resins are made in the salon by mixing a powder and a liquid that react without the need of a UV lamp. The powdered polymer typically contains polymethyl methacrylate (PMMA) and a liquid monomer solution typically contains ethyl methacrylate (EMA). PMMA is a combination of two different monomers, such as EMA and MMA. However, many other acrylates have been used in cosmetology.[11,22,25] Another common source of acrylics in nail salons in recent years is the long-lasting nail polish, commonly known as gels, which do require an ultraviolet (UV) or light-emitting diode lamp for 2–3 min to cure. Lastly, cyanoacrylate or methacrylate glues are commonly used for placing pre-sculpted nail applications or extensions, applying nail art, fixing broken nails, or placing eyelash extensions.[22,23]

Because of the common use of acrylates in nail products, acrylates have been measured in the air of nail salons.[26] Although nail technicians' skin can be in direct contact with acrylates, acrylate traces were not measurable on the skin of the workers in a small study,[24] which is likely due to acrylates rapidly being absorbed into the skin or evaporated off the skin and also suggesting that the use of disposable chemically protective gloves is paramount in nail salons for the protection against acrylates.

Additionally, the ventilation in nail salons was shown to affect the air concentrations of acrylates. Ceballos et al.[26] documented significantly higher MMA air concentrations with higher airflow in the salons. It was likely that ventilation in the salon increased the rate of evaporation of the acrylic monomers or dispersed the acrylic powders while acrylic nail products were in use. Acrylates in the air could increase the potential for dermal uptake from the air and provide further justification for why it is important to use chemical protective gloves in the nail salon environment to protect the skin even when there is no direct contact.

23.3 DERMATOLOGICAL PROBLEMS WITH ACRYLATES IN INDUSTRIAL APPLICATIONS

23.3.1 EARLIER STUDIES

At the beginning of the use of acrylates in industrial applications, it was discovered that these chemicals may cause ICD and ACD. Decades ago, cases of ICD due to occupational exposure received relatively little attention in the literature. Most attention from a clinical perspective was given to cases of ACD.[27–40] The importance of studying the sensitizing potential of acrylates was recognized, and this challenge was picked up by two laboratories of clinics that had encountered cases of ACD due to occupational exposure: one from Bertil Magnusson in Sweden, and the other from Klaus Malten in the Netherlands. This resulted in two remarkable doctoral theses about the sensitizing potential of acrylates in the guinea pig maximization test by van der Walle[7,41,42] and Björkner.[8,43–45] The sensitizing capacity of acrylates was studied in other animal models as well.[46–51]

Later, also the occupational hygiene aspects of industrial use of acrylates were studied in Sweden.[9,10] This clearly showed that despite proper labeling and adequate safety data sheets showing the potential irritant and allergenic risks of exposure of unprotected skin to acrylates, the measures of industrial hygiene, including personal protective equipment, are sometimes still extremely poor in industry.

The irritancy of acrylates to the skin and eyes was recognized by the manufacturers of these chemicals as a limiting factor in the development of this technology at an early stage. This resulted in successful efforts to develop acrylates that are intrinsically much less irritant to the skin and eyes than the so-called first-generation acrylates.[52,53]

Several interesting statistical studies have been published about the clinical experience with occupational skin disorders due to acrylates.[54–59]

In addition, paresthesias in surgical, dental, and cosmetology settings have been documented.[60] Potential for phototoxicity associated with an added photo inhibitor has also been indicated.[29]

23.3.2 MORE RECENT STUDIES

In a recent review,[1] not many new developments on the irritant and corrosive properties of acrylate, methacrylate, and ethyl acrylate monomers were observed. In general, as the number of carbon atoms increases, the severity of skin and mucous membrane irritation decreases. Methacrylates have also been associated with respiratory tract irritation, rhinitis, and asthma in dental workers and nail technicians.

Sood and Taylor[61] reviewed 56 cases of acrylic reactions between 1988 and 2002, a follow-up from earlier work.[54] The sources of acrylic exposure included acrylic nails, dental materials, adhesives, and UV paint. The authors noted an increase in positive (meth)acrylate patch tests compared to a previous 10-year period. The highest number of reactions, in order of the number of positive reactions, was seen with ethylene glycol dimethacrylate (EGDMA), 2-hydroxyethyl methacrylate (2-HEMA), and 2-hydroxypropyl methacrylate (2-HPMA). They noted that EGDMA was a good marker for all the exposure groups. These results have been consistent with earlier patient studies,[57,59] as well as more recent reports.[62,63]

As seen in earlier studies, [57,59] ACD is more commonly associated with dental products, artificial nails, and adhesives containing methacrylates such as EGDMA, 2-HEMA, and 2-HPMA, compared to acrylates.[61–65]

23.3.2.1 Dental Acrylates

Common UV or light-cured composites for dental fillings and sealants include bisphenol A-diglycidyl methacrylate (BIS-GMA), triethyleneglycol dimethacrylate (TREGDMA), 2-HEMA, TMPTA, and sometimes methyl methacrylate (MMA; Figure 23.2).[66,67] The most common ACD reactions are to 2-HEMA and

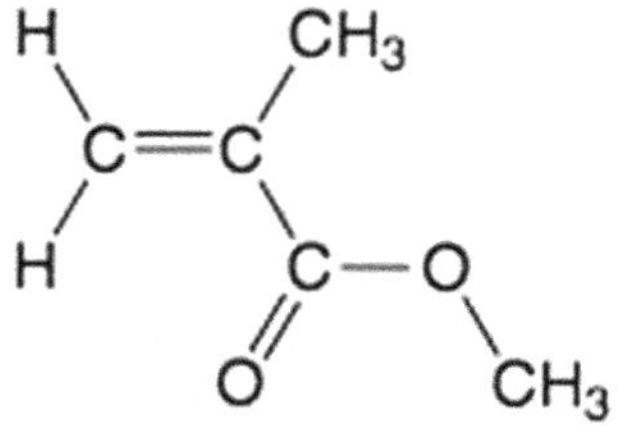

FIGURE 23.2   Methyl methacrylate (MMA).

TREGDMA;[62,65] however, reactions to 2-HPMA, THFMA, EMA, butanediol dimethacrylate (BUDMA), and urethane dimethacrylate (UDMA) are common among dental workers.[62] In the latter, cross-allergy to other methacrylates is suspected.

23.3.2.2   Cured Acrylic Nails and Long-Lasting Nail Polish

Acrylic nails, also known as artificial or sculptured nails, used to require a UV lamp to be cured although some formulations do not require UV or photo bonding.[22] However, "gel nails" do still require UV or light for curation. Acrylic nail products usually contain components similar to those used for dental bonding, including MMA, EMA, or 2-HEMA as primers, as well as the resins BIS-GMA, EGDMA, 2-HEA, 2-HPMA, and TREGDMA.[11,22,24,25,68] The most frequent allergens associated with ACD among nail technicians were 2-HEMA and 2-HPMA, and to a lesser extent EDGMA. [22,63,68–72]

ACD in sensitized patients is usually localized in contact areas, but it can also show in areas distant to direct contact.[68] Direct contact with acrylates typically includes the skin around the acrylic nails, fingers, and hands. Miao et al.[68] hypothesized that distant-to-direct-contact reactions, such as that in the eyelids or face, can be caused by acrylates in the salon air from monomer evaporation or airborne polymethacrylate dust (i.e., dust from powder ingredients or filling). However, the authors only studied four cases (three nail technicians of acrylic nails, and a customer of acrylic nails); thus it is possible too that patients touched their faces or eyelids unintentionally with acrylic-contaminated nails or hands. In all cases, symptoms resolved after removing acrylic nails and stopping work as a manicurist.

23.3.2.3   UV-Cured Acrylic Adhesives

ACD has been associated with UV-cured acrylic glues containing primarily acrylates[73–76] and orthopedic adhesives (i.e., bone cement) often containing MMA and a methacrylate polymer as a two-part system.[1] Limited evidence of ACD in orthopedic surgeons was observed. With UV-cured acrylic glues, ACD cases involved a variety of sensitivities, likely depending on the components of the products. The more common positive reactions were to 2-HEMA, 2-HPMA,[74,76] and EGDMA, but MMA, TREGDMA, and others were also noted. [73–76]

23.3.2.4   UV-Cured Inks, Paints, Varnishes, Lacquers, and Coatings

Occupational cases of ACD and phototoxicity have been observed in both the production and use of UV-cured inks, paints, varnishes, lacquers, and coatings.[29,34,43,44,59,65,77–79] A more recent report of ACD associated with UV-cured inks and paints includes continued sensitivity to epoxy diacrylate (BIS-GA),[65] as compared to earlier studies.[29,34,44,77]

23.3.2.5 Anaerobic Adhesives

Anaerobic adhesives are single-component liquid mixtures of acrylic esters that harden when confined between two metal surfaces under anaerobic conditions.[1] Some common examples include thread sealants (e.g., Loctite® Thread Sealant), thread locking agents (e.g., Loctite® Threadlocker or Anti-Seize), and custom gaskets (e.g., Permabond® Gasketmaker). Many of the components are similar to those of dental acrylates and other acrylate adhesives. For anaerobic adhesives, the most common occupational cases of ACD have been associated with the methacrylates 2-HEMA, 2-HPMA, EGDMA, and TREGDMA.[80–83] Sensitization to BIS-GA has also been reported.[65]

23.3.2.6 Two-Component Adhesives

Two-component acrylate adhesives contain acrylate or methacrylate monomers (part 1) and a hardener (part 2) that when combined polymerize under ambient conditions.[1] The few reported occupational cases of ACD have been associated with the methacrylates 2-HEMA, EGDMA, and MMA.[53,82]

23.3.2.7 Cyanoacrylates

Cyanoacrylate adhesives or glues contain esters of cyanoacrylic acid and rapidly polymerize in the presence of moisture in the air or on a surface but involve less cross-linking than other acrylate-based adhesives.[1] They are more commonly recognized as quick-bonding "instant adhesive" or "super glue." They are also used in surgery and for wound-care products,[1] such as Liquid Skin® and Dermabond®. Several recent cases of cyanoacrylate allergy have been reported in association with cosmetology (e.g., false eyelashes and press-on nails), as well as medical use of Dermabond®.[71]

23.3.2.8 Isobornyl Acrylate (IBA)

Isobornyl acrylate (IBA) is a low-molecular-weight acrylic monomer, common to several industrial and medical products.[71] It has been more recently associated with contact dermatitis and allergy secondary to medical devices, such as glucose monitors and insulin pumps.[83] This is an area of continued investigation and monitoring, especially given the growing use of these devices.

23.4 RESISTANCE OF PROTECTIVE GLOVES TO PERMEATION BY ACRYLATES

Rietschel et al.[84] performed *in vivo* and *in vitro* testing of natural rubber latex (NRL), chloroprene (neoprene), and nitrile gloves for protection against UV-curing urethane acrylate resin systems. The measurements of permeation rate and breakthrough times were done in non-standardized ways, and the exact composition of the acrylate products and glove types, including their thickness, was not specified. The study showed that nitrile rubber could provide adequate protection against UV-curing acrylate resin systems for an entire 8-h work shift and that the gloves should not be reused on the following day.

Using the ASTM method F 739-81, Huggins et al.[85] studied the permeation of a UV-curing urethane acrylate resin coating formulation and its individual acrylate components (a low-viscosity acrylate diluent of low molecular weight) used for optical fibers through latex rubber (probably both synthetic polyisoprene and NRL), chloroprene, and nitrile gloves. For acrylate components, breakthrough times of 75–145 min were measured for two nitrile gloves (thickness of about 0.3–0.4 mm), 130 min for a chloroprene glove (thickness of about 0.4 mm), and 30 min for a premium disposable surgical NRL glove (thickness of about 0.2–0.3 mm). For the whole coating formulation, the breakthrough times were significantly higher: for the nitrile gloves more than 480 min, for the chloroprene gloves 420 min, and for the latex rubber gloves 90 min. The study indicated, similarly to their earlier findings,[84] that nitrile gloves provided better protection than latex gloves to employees handling the UV-curing acrylate resin coating formulation or its components. Chloroprene gloves were not recommended, possibly because they tore easily under test conditions. For tasks requiring more dexterity and tactile sensation than nitrile gloves have, the premium NRL gloves could be used for short periods. Huggins et al.[85] also found that if some organic solvents, such as methyl ethyl ketone or methylene chloride, are used in conjunction with the low-molecular-weight acrylate component, other gloves would be necessary, because nitrile gloves are not compatible with the solvents.

Renard et al.[86] studied the permeation of three UV/EB-curing acrylate monomers (TMPTA, HDDA, and 2-EHA) through three rather thick glove materials (butyl rubber, NRL, and nitrile rubber) using ASTM method F 739-85 with modification for the solid collection medium. Permeation tests were conducted at 20 °C in a controlled temperature and humidity laboratory. The thickness of the gloves ranged from about 0.4 to 0.5 mm. The overall conclusions of this study were that the pure acrylate monomers did not permeate the butyl or the nitrile gloves in 480 min but did permeate NRL gloves. HDDA permeated NRL gloves in 60–120 min and TMPTA in 360–480 min. When 2-EHA and HDDA were tested in two mixtures (50% HDDA/50% 2-EHA and 25% HDDA/75% 2-EHA), the permeation occurred in 30–60 min and 120–180 min, respectively.

Munksgaard[87] and Mäkelä et al.[88,89] have studied the permeation of low-molecular-weight methacrylates used in dental care work through a range of thin disposable gloves. The Munksgaard[87] study was done with a non-standardized test system for 11 gloves made of polyvinyl chloride (vinyl, PVC), NRL, and some materials made of more than one polymer and probably comprising more than one layer. The methacrylates studied were 2-HEMA, TREGDMA, BIS-GMA, and urethane dimethacrylate (UEDMA). These are all methacrylates that are not used as UV/EB-curing acrylates in industrial applications but in dentistry only. In chemical structure, however, they closely resemble the UV/EB-curing acrylates used in industry. The breakthrough times obtained in this study for 2-HEMA ranged from less than 1 to 8 min, for TREGDMA from 1 to 9 min, and for BIS-GMA and UEDMA from 20 to more than 100 min.

Mäkelä and co-workers[88,89] studied the resistance of thin disposable and industrial gloves (e.g., NRL, nitrile, PVC, neoprene, and polyethylene) against small-molecular-weight methacrylates or their mixtures, i.e., MMA, 2-HEMA+TREGDMA (50%+50%) and 2-HEMA+ethanol (50%+50%), according to European standard EN 374-3 from 1994. Also, the influence of the use of double gloving on the permeation rate was studied.

The main conclusions of the first study of Mäkelä et al.[88] were as follows. The breakthrough times for double-layer glove materials were more than 1.5-fold the sum of the breakthrough times obtained when single layers were tested. Tests performed with the mixture of 2-HEMA and TREGDMA indicated that 2-HEMA passed the glove materials more quickly than TREGDMA in every test in which permeation was detected. The breakthrough times for common disposable PVC and NRL gloves were less than 10 min and for thicker disposable PVC and NRL gloves 10–16 min. The study also showed that chloroprene and good-quality nitrile glove material resulted in breakthrough times longer than 1 h, but another nitrile glove was permeated by 2-HEMA from the mixture in 14 min. The highest breakthrough time was obtained with double gloves of 4H® (Safety4, Denmark) (inner) and NRL (outer). Also, with double layers of polyethylene (inner) and NRL (outer) breakthrough was not obtained in 8 h. However, low permeation could be detected ($0.4\,|\mu g/cm^2$min) almost during the whole test period of 8 h, but the permeation rate of $1.0\ \mu g/cm^2/$ min was not exceeded, and thus the breakthrough time of the standard EN 374-3 was not reached. Tests performed with the mixture of 2-HEMA and ethanol showed that the 2-HEMA from the mixture passes the one-layered PVC, NRL, and nitrile glove materials in less than 4 min, but for chloroprene materials, the breakthrough times were more than 2 h.[89] 2-HEMA did not permeate double layers of 4H® or polyethylene under NRL glove from the 2-HEMA and ethanol mixture during the 8-h test period.

In the tests in which MMA was the test chemical, the breakthrough times for even double layers of PVC, NRL, nitrile, and polyethylene layer under NRL layer MMA were less than 5 min and less than 10 min for double layers of chloroprene.[89] Only multilayered 4H® gloves gave adequate protection against MMA.

Zwanenburg[90] used a slightly modified version of the ASTM Standard F 739-81 to test the resistance of three nitrile gloves against five widely used UV/EB-curing acrylates (2-PEA, HDDA, TPGDA, TMPTA, TMPEOTA). Dipropyleneglycol diacrylate (DPGDA) was not tested in the study, but its influence on glove materials was regarded to be similar to HDDA because of the close resemblance in chemical structures and molecular weights of these acrylate monomers. NRL, which has poor resistance against UV-curing acrylates according to earlier studies,[84–86] and excessively expensive gloves were not included in the study. The glove materials were tested for three typical work situations.

Andreasson et al.[91] evaluated the permeation of MMA, 2-HEMA, and triethylene glycol dimethacrylate (TEGDMA), with preparations in 30% water, acetone, or ethyl alcohol, using a Franz-type permeation cell. For MMA, the lag-breakthrough time (lag-BT) was 2 min or less for all the dental gloves tested (i.e., NRL, nitrile, PVC, and a polyethylene copolymer). An NRL and polyethylene-copolymer glove provided better protection for MMA in acetone or ethyl alcohol. The lag-BTs were generally longer for 2-HEMA (15–104 min in water) and TEGDMA (1–80 min in ethyl alcohol). A neoprene glove appeared to be the better choice for 2-HEMA and TEGDMA.

Lönnroth et al.[23,92] evaluated the permeability of 15 different types of dental and surgical gloves to acrylic monomers using EN 374-3 (discontinued). MMA permeated all the gloves within a BT of 2 min. A polyethylene glove provided >120 min BT protection for EGDMA and 1,4-butanediol dimethacrylate (1,4-BDMA), with BTs less than 10 min for a nitrile and surgical glove. Double gloving with a pre-treated water-rinsed synthetic rubber glove (inner) and NRL glove (outer) provided increased protection.

Nakamura et al.[93] evaluated the finger permeability of NRL, chloroprene, and PVC disposable dental gloves to MMA, 2-HEMA, TEGDMA, EGDMA, UDMA, and BIS-GMA. They found that BIS-GMA and UDMA did not permeate the gloves. All other monomers, MMA, 2-HEMA, TEGDMA, and EGDMA, permeated the glove fingers of all glove types within 10 min. PVC showed the highest overall permeability.

Tomas and Padmanabhan[94] evaluated the finger permeability of NRL, PVC, and neoprene gloves to MMA. The PVC gloves showed the highest permeability with the first detection at about 1 min and a 30-min mean concentration of 58 µL/ml. NRL gloves also showed a higher permeability with the first detection at about 1 min and a 30-min mean concentration of 43.5 µL/ml. The neoprene gloves were impermeable for up to 25 min and at 30 min the mean concentration was 5.6 µL/ml.

23.5 RECOMMENDATIONS FOR PROTECTIVE GLOVES FOR WORK WITH ACRYLATES

The recommendations for adequate protective gloves in work with acrylates are principally based on Zwanenburg's study,[90] which gives practical and applicable guidelines for companies where employees can be exposed to acrylates. In addition, consideration was provided for the earlier studies investigating the resistance of protective gloves against permeation of acrylates,[84–86] and dental materials.[87–90]

23.5.1 Brief Direct Contact with Acrylates without Organic Solvents

Thin good-quality disposable nitrile gloves at least 0.1 mm in thickness, such as Touch N Tuff brand gloves (Ansell Healthcare Inc., Red Bank, NJ; USA/Ansell Healthcare Europe, Brussels, Belgium), have been found suitable for workers with brief, direct contact with the acrylates without organic solvents and physical stress. These gloves are not recommended for situations where exposure to HDDA or DPGDA may occur. The gloves should not be used for more than 30 min after the first contact with the exposed acrylate on the glove surface.[90] The use of polyethylene gloves under NRL gloves probably also gives adequate protection against acrylates for short periods without simultaneous exposure to organic solvents or physical stress.[88] Gloves should never be used after any observed change in appearance (tearing, blisters, changes in color, dimensions, or flexibility). To avoid skin contact with acrylates on the glove surface, the gloves should be wiped clean with a piece of cloth or paper, before doffing. The paper or cloth should also be discarded with gloves. Reuse of the gloves is not allowed.

23.5.2   LONG-LASTING CONTACT WITH ACRYLATES WITHOUT ORGANIC SOLVENTS

Medium nitrile gloves at least 0.45 mm in thickness, such as Ultranitril 492 (MAPA Spontex, Inc., Columbia, TN; USA/MAPA Spontex, SNC, Neuilly-sur-Seine, France), are suitable for a few hours of contact to acrylates without simultaneous exposure to certain organic solvents, e.g., ketones, acetates, chlorinated hydrocarbons.[90] The gloves also tolerate some physical stress like the opening of a drum or using tools, but they are not suitable for situations where exposure to HDDA or DPGDA may occur. According to the results of this study, it seems safe to use these gloves up to 4 h after first contact with the acrylates, unless the gloves are damaged (tears, holes) or significantly changed in appearance. To avoid skin contact with acrylates on the glove surface, the gloves should be wiped clean with a piece of cloth or paper, before doffing. The paper or cloth should also be discarded with gloves. Reuse of the gloves is not allowed.

23.5.3   LONG-DURATION CONTACT WITH ACRYLATES WITH ORGANIC SOLVENTS

Thick unlined nitrile gloves at least 0.55 mm in thickness, such as Sol-Vex 37-667 (Ansell Protective Products), are recommended for a few hours' contact with acrylates in combination with a mixture of organic solvents, used in the cleaning of printing and coating equipment contaminated with acrylates.[90] Thick unlined chloroprene gloves would probably also be a good choice, but the material has not been tested against acrylates in organic solvents.[90] Nitrile gloves are not recommended for protection against ketones such as methyl isobutyl ketone, methyl ethyl ketone, acetone, or most other ketones, nor to acetates such as ethyl acetate or butyl acetate.[95] These solvents as well as chlorinated solvents should not be used for cleaning equipment or tools contaminated with acrylates. These gloves are not suitable for situations where exposure to HDDA or DPGDA, or acrylates labeled corrosive or toxic, especially in combination with organic solvents, may occur. For all other acrylates, these gloves seem to be safe to use up to 8 h (cumulative, starting from the first physical contact) with solvents or acrylates, unless they are physically damaged (tear or hole), or significantly changed in appearance. To avoid skin contact with acrylates on the glove surface, the gloves should be wiped clean with a piece of cloth or paper, before doffing.

23.5.4   HANDLING OF HDDA OR DPGDA WITH OR WITHOUT SOLVENTS

Thin and medium gloves are unreliable for handling HDDA, and probably DPGDA as well.[90] There are no studies on the resistance of thick nitrile gloves against

HDDA, but there is good reason to believe that HDDA will permeate thick nitrile gloves quickly, especially in situations where HDDA is handled simultaneously with organic solvents. The only gloves on the market that could protect against the chemicals are Barrier™ (Ansell Protective Products) and North Silver Shield™/4H® gloves (North Safety Products, Cranston, RI).[90,96] All of these are multilayer laminated gloves. They are thin (thickness of about 0.065 mm), but they give excellent protection against most chemicals. The gloves are rather stiff, however, and therefore not tactile. To improve dexterity, laminated gloves should be used under gloves made of nitrile rubber or NRL.[88] Although this has not been verified in any study, there is good reason to believe that laminated gloves give adequate protection against HDDA and DPGDA, even in combination with organic solvents (except halogenated hydrocarbons).

23.6   CONCLUSIONS

Several monomers or uncured acrylates are highly sensitizing chemicals that may cause ACD after skin contact. Other skin disorders including ICD may also develop upon exposure of the skin to monomers or uncured acrylates. To prevent sensitization and other skin hazards while working with acrylates in an industrial environment, skin exposure should be prevented. If technical or other available measures do not provide adequate skin protection, the use of protective gloves is necessary. Present guidelines on glove selection for work with acrylates are based on permeation studies conducted with acrylates since 1984.[84–90] The aim has been to give practical and applicable guidelines for companies where employees can be exposed to acrylates. Nitrile glove material seems to provide good resistance against acrylates in many situations where acrylates are handled. Thin gloves are suitable for short exposure only, thicker medium gloves provide protection for a few hours, and thick unlined nitrile gloves may give adequate protection when acrylates are handled in combination with organic solvents (except ketone, acetate, and chlorinated solvents). In the handling of multifunctional acrylates such as HDDA and DPGDA, only laminated multilayer gloves can be recommended.

Many of the cases from the literature mentioned in this chapter that documented skin sensitization reactions related to the use of acrylates in occupational settings acknowledged that patients are commonly also allergic to latex gloves and other sensitizers used in their work settings, such as isocyanates. It is thus important for an industrial hygienist deciding on protective gloves to use with an acrylic industrial application or an occupational physician treating a skin reaction, to do a comprehensive assessment of the workplace chemical hazards including the different sensitizer ingredients beyond acrylates so that co-exposures are considered in the final decision as necessary and when possible.

It is of utmost importance to emphasize that only reputable gloves should be used against potentially sensitizing chemicals such as acrylates. The glove suppliers should be able to confirm that their products give the same level of protection as the gloves recommended in Sections 23.4 and 23.5.

ACKNOWLEDGMENTS

The authors express their gratitude to the previous authors of this chapter (Rob Zwanenburg, Ritta Jolanki, Erja A. Mäkelä, and Tuula Estlander), as well as RadTech Europe and RadTech North America for funding a critical study,[90] summarized in Section 23.4, and for the free use of the data generated therein. We would also like the thank Dr James Taylor, MD, at Cleveland Clinic, for his valuable review and feedback on this chapter.

REFERENCES

1. Aalto-Korte, K. 2017. Acrylic resins, in *Kanerva's Occupational Dermatology*, John, S.M., Johansen, J.D., Rustemeyer, T., Elsner, P., and Maibach, H.I., Eds., Vol 1. Heidelberg: Springer. DOI: 10.1007/978-3-319-40221-5_50-2.
2. Knight, R. 1991. UV curing equipments and applications, in *Markets and Curing Equipment*, Dufour, P., Pincus, A., Tanihata, A., Skelhorne, G., and Knight, R., Eds., Vol 1. London: SITA Technology, 159–269.
3. Cavelier, C., Jelen, G., Hervé-Bazin, B., and Foussereau, J. 1981. Irritation et allergie aux acrylates et methacrylates. *Ann Dermatol Venereol (Paris)* 108:59–66.
4. Lovell, C.R., Rycroft, R.C.G., and Williams, D.M.J. 1985. Contact dermatitis from the irritancy (immediate and delayed) and allergenicity of hydroxypropyl acrylate. *Contact Dermatitis* 12:117–118.
5. Malten, K.E., den Arend, J.A.C.J., and Wiggers, R.E. 1979. Delayed irritation: Hexanediol diacrylate and butanediol diacrylate, *Contact Dermatitis* 5:178–184.
6. Nethercott, J.R. 1988. Dermatitis in the printing industry. *Dermatol Clin* 6:61–66.
7. van der Walle, H.B. 1982. *Sensitizing Potential of Acrylic Monomers in Guinea Pigs.* Thesis, Nijmegen: Radboud University, pp.119.
8. Björkner, B. 1984. The sensitizing capacity of multifunctional acrylates in the guinea pig. *Contact Dermatitis* 4:236–246. DOI: 10.1111/j.1600-0536.
9. Nylander-French, L.A. 1994. *Identification of Risk to Workers in the Ultraviolet Radiation Curing Wood Surface Coating Industry.* Doctoral thesis, Stockholm, Sweden: Royal Institute of Technology.
10. Surakka, J. 2000. *Dermal Exposure to UV-Radiation and UV-Curable Acrylate Coatings in the Wood Working Industry.* Doctoral thesis, Luleå, Sweden: Luleå University of Technology.
11. Sauni, R., Kauppi, P., Alanko, K., Henriks-Eckerman, M.L., Tuppurainen, M., and Hannu, T. 2008. Occupational asthma caused by sculptured nails containing methacrylates. *Am J Ind Med* 51(12):968–974. DOI: 10.1002/ajim.20633.
12. NIOSH. 2022. *NIOSH Skin Notations.* Washington, DC: National Institute for Occupational Safety and Health (NIOSH). Available at: https://www.cdc.gov/niosh/topics/skin/skin-notation_profiles.html.
13. Oldring, P.K.T., Ed. 1991. *Chemistry and Technology of UV & EB Formulation for Coatings, Inks and Paints.* London: SITA Technology.
14. Webster, G., Ed. 1997. *Chemistry and Technology of UV and EB Formulation for Coatings, Inks and Paints: Prepolymers and Reactive Diluents for UV and EB Curable Formulations.* London: Wiley-SITA.
15. Brack, K., and Braddock, J., Eds. 1999. *Radiation-Curable Coatings, Adhesives, and Inks: Technology and Practical Applications.* Lancaster, PA: Technomic Publishing.
16. Neckers, D.C. 1999. *Chemistry and Technology of UV and EB Formulation for Coatings, Inks and Paints: UV and EB at the Millennium.* London: Wiley-SITA.

17. RadTech Europe. 2021. http://www.radtech-europe.com/.
18. RadTech North America. 2021. http://www.radtech.org/.
19. Walters, G.I., Robertson, A.S., Moore, V.C., and Burge, P.S. 2017. Occupational asthma caused by acrylic compounds from SHIELD surveillance (1989–2014). *Occup Med* 67(4):282–289. DOI: 10.1093/occmed/kqx036.
20. Sierra, D.H., and Saltz, R. 1998. *Surgical Adhesives & Sealants: Current Technology and Applications.* Lancaster, PA: Technomic Publishing (CRC Press).
21. Leggat, P.A., Smith, D.R., and Kedjarune, U. 2009. Surgical applications of methyl methacrylate: A review of toxicity. *Arch Environ Occup Health* 64(3):207–212. DOI: 10.1080/19338240903241291.
22. Minamoto, K. 2014. Allergic contact dermatitis from two-component acrylic resin in a manicurist and a dental hygienist. *J Occup Health* 56(3):229–234. DOI: 10.1539/joh.13-0244-cs.
23. Lönnroth, E.C., and Eystein Ruyter, I. 2003. Resistance of medical gloves to permeation by methyl methacrylate (MMA), ethylene glycol dimethacrylate (EGDMA), and 1,4-butanediol dimethacrylate (1,4-BDMA). *Int J Occup Saf Ergon* 9(3):289–299. DOI: 10.1080/10803548.2003.11076569.
24. Kalenge, S., Kirkham, T.L., Nguyen, L.V., Holness, D.L., and Arrandale, V.H. 2021. Skin exposure to acrylates in nail salons. *Ann Work Expo Health* 65(2):162–166. DOI: 10.1093/annweh/wxaa063.
25. Kanerva, L., Lauerma, A., Estlander, T., Alanko, K., Henriks-Eckerman, M.L., and Jolanki, R. 1996. Occupational allergic contact dermatitis caused by photobonded sculptured nails and a review of (meth) acrylates in nail cosmetics. *Am J Contact Dermat* 7(2):109–115.
26. Ceballos, D.M., Craig, J., Fu, X., Jia, C., Chambers, D., Chu, M.T., et al. 2019. Biological and environmental exposure monitoring of volatile organic compounds among nail technicians in the Greater Boston area. *Indoor Air* 29(4):539–550.
27. Magnusson, B., and Mobacken, H. 1972. Allergic contact dermatitis from acrylate printing plates in a printing plant. *Berufsdermatosen* 20:138.
28. Emmett, E.A. 1977. Contact dermatitis from polyfunctional acrylic monomers. *Contact Dermatitis* 3:245–248.
29. Emmett, E.A. 1977. Allergic contact dermatitis from ultraviolet cured inks. *J Occup Med* 19:113–115.
30. Malten, K.E. 1977. Contact sensitization to Letterflex urethane photopolymer mixture used in printing. *Contact Dermatitis* 3:115–121.
31. Malten, K.E., and Seutter, E. 1984. Contact dermatitis from acrylated resins in UV ebecryl printing ink. *Contact Dermatitis* 11:56–58.
32. Nethercott, J.R. 1978. Skin problems associated with multifunctional acrylic monomers in ultraviolet curing inks. *Br J Dermatol* 98:541–552.
33. Nethercott, J.R. 1981. Allergic contact dermatitis due to an epoxy acrylate. *Br J Dermatol* 104:697–703.
34. Nethercott, J.R., Jakubovic, H.R., Pilger, C., and Smith, J.W. 1983. Allergic contact dermatitis due to urethane acrylate in ultraviolet cured inks. *Br J Ind Med* 40:241–250.
35. Nethercott, J.R., Gupta, S., Rosen, C.I., Enders, L.J., and Piger, C.W. 1984. Tetraethylene glycol diacrylate. A cause of delayed cutaneous irritant reaction and allergic contact dermatitis. *J Occup Med* 26:513–516.
36. Nethercott, J.R., and Nosal, R. 1986. Contact dermatitis in printing tradesmen. *Contact Dermatitis* 14:280–287.
37. Nethercott, J.R. 1988. Dermatitis in the printing industry. *Dermatol Clin* 6:61–66.
38. Widström, L. 1982. Contact allergy to acrylate monomer in a printing plate. *Contact Dermatitis* 8:68–80.

39. Pedersen, N.B., Senning, A., and Nielsen, A.O. 1983. Different sensitising acrylic monomers in Napp® printing plate. *Contact Dermatitis* 9:459–464.

40. Wahlberg, J.E. 1983. Contact sensitivity to Napp® printing plates secondary to a relapsing hand dermatitis. *Contact Dermatitis* 9:239.

41. van der Walle, H.B., Klecak, G., Geleick, H., and Bensink, T. 1982. Sensitizing potential of 14 mono(meth)acrylates in the guinea pig. *Contact Dermatitis* 8:223–235.

42. van der Walle, H.B., Waegemaekers, Th., and Bensink, T. 1983. Sensitizing potential of 12 di(meth)acrylates in the guinea pig. *Contact Dermatitis* 9:10–20.

43. Björkner, B. 1980. Allergenicity of trimethylol propane triacrylate in ultraviolet curing inks in the guinea pig. *Acta Derm Venereol* 60:528–531.

44. Björkner, B., Dahlquist, I., and Fregert, S. 1980. Allergic contact dermatitis from acrylates in ultraviolet curing inks. *Contact Dermatitis* 6:405–409.

45. Björkner, B., and Niklasson, B. 1984. Influence of the vehicle on elicitation of contact allergic reactions to acrylic compounds in the guinea pig. *Contact Dermatitis* 11:268–278.

46. Parker, D., and Turk, J.L. 1983. Contact sensitivity to acrylate compounds in guinea pigs. *Contact Dermatitis* 9:55–60.

47. Parker, D., Long, P.V., Bull, J.E., and Turk, J.L. 1985. Epicutaneous induction of tolerance with acrylates and related compounds. *Contact Dermatitis* 12:146–154.

48. Basketter, D.A., and Scholes, E.W. 1992. Comparison of the local lymph node assay with the guinea-pig maximization test for the detection of a range of contact allergens. *Food Chem Toxicol* 30:65–69.

49. Arimura, M., Yokozeki, H., Katayama, I., Nakmura, T., Masuda, M., and Nishioka, K. 1998. Experimental study for the development on an *in vitro* test for contact allergens. *Arch Allergy Immunol* 115:228–234.

50. Hayes, B.B., and Meade, B.J. 1999. Contact sensitivity to selected acrylate compounds in B6C3F1 mice: Relative potency, cross reactivity and comparison of test methods. *Drug Chem Toxicol* 22:491–506.

51. Andrews, L.S., and Clary, J.J. 1986. Review of the toxicity of multifunctional acrylates. *J Toxicol Environ Health* 19:149–164.

52. Sinka, J.V., Higbie, F.A., and Lieberman, R.A. 1984. *Radiation-Hardenable Diluents.* Eur. Pat. Appl. 0 062 807 B1.

53. Bergvall, G. 1996. *Acrylate Monomer Having a Reduced Primary Irritation Index and a Method of Making Same.* U.S. Patent 5,543,557.

54. Taylor, J.S. 1989. Acrylic reactions — Ten-years experience, in *Current Topics in Contact Dermatitis*, J.P. Frosch et al., Eds. Berlin: Springer-Verlag, 346–351.

55. Kanerva, L., Estlander, T., Jolanki, R., and Tarvainen, K. 1995. Statistics on allergic patch test reactions caused by acrylate compounds, including data on ethyl methacrylate. *Am J Contact Dermatitis* 6:75–77.

56. Kanerva, L., Jolanki, R., and Estlander, T. 1997. 10 years of patch testing with the (meth)acrylate series. *Contact Dermatitis* 37:255–258.

57. Tucker, S.C., and Beck, M.H. 1999. A 15-year study of patch testing to (meth)acrylates. *Contact Dermatitis* 40:278–279.

58. Livesley, E., Rushton, L., English, J., and Williams, H. 2000. The prevalence of occupational dermatitis in the UK printing industry. Poster at *5th ESCD*, Amsterdam.

59. Geukens, S., and Goossens, A. 2001. Occupational contact allergy to (meth)acrylates. *Contact Dermatitis* 44:153–159.

60. Rodrigues-Barata, A.R., Gomez, L.C., Arceo, J.E., and Barco, L. 2015. Occupational sensitization to acrylates with paresthesias. *Dermatitis* 26(2):103–104.

61. Sood, A., and Taylor, J.S. 2003. Acrylic reactions: A review of 56 cases. *Contact Dermatitis* 48(6):346–347. DOI: 10.1034/j.1600-0536.2003.00148.x.

62. Aalto-Korte, K., Alanko, K., Kuuliala, O., and Jolanki, R. 2007. Methacrylate and acrylate allergy in dental personnel. *Contact Dermatitis* 57(5):324–330. DOI: 10.1111/j.1600-0536.2007.01237.x.

63. Teik-Jin Goon, A., Bruze, M., Zimerson, E., Goh, C.L., and Isaksson, M. 2007. Contact allergy to acrylates/methacrylates in the acrylate and nail acrylics series in southern Sweden: Simultaneous positive patch test reaction patterns and possible screening allergens. *Contact Dermatitis* 57(1):21–27. DOI: 10.1111/j.1600-0536.2007.01151.x.

64. Goon, A.T., Isaksson, M., Zimerson, E., Goh, C.L., and Bruze, M. 2006. Contact allergy to (meth)acrylates in the dental series in southern Sweden: Simultaneous positive patch test reaction patterns and possible screening allergens. *Contact Dermatitis* 55(4):219–226. DOI: 10.1111/j.1600-0536.2006.00922.x.

65. Aalto-Korte, K., Jungewelter, S., Henriks-Eckerman, M.L., Kuuliala, O., and Jolanki, R. 2009. Contact allergy to epoxy (meth)acrylates. *Contact Dermatitis* 61(1):9–21. DOI: 10.1111/j.1600-0536.2009.01574.x.

66. Henriks-Eckerman, M.L., Suuronen, K., Jolanki, R., and Alanko, K. 2004. Methacrylates in dental restorative materials. *Contact Dermatitis* 50(4):233–237. DOI: 10.1111/j.0105-1873.2004.00336.x.

67. Craig, R.G., Welker, D., Rothaut, J., Krumbholz, K.G., Stefan, K-P., Dermann, K., et al. 2006. Dental materials, in *Ullmann's Encyclopedia of Industrial Chemistry*, Ley, C. Ed., Wiley Online Library. https://onlinelibrary.wiley.com/doi/book/10.1002/14356007.

68. Maio, P., Carvalho, R., Amaro, C., Santos, R., and Cardoso, J. 2012. Allergic contact dermatitis from sculptured acrylic nails: Special presentation with an airborne pattern. *Dermatol Reports* 4(1):e6. DOI: 10.4081/dr.2012.e6.

69. Constandt, L., Hecke, E.V., Naeyaert, J.M., and Goossens, A. 2005. Screening for contact allergy to artificial nails. *Contact Dermatitis* 52(2):73–77. DOI: 10.1111/j.0105-1873.2005.00496.x.

70. Lazarov, A. 2006. Sensitization to acrylates is a common adverse reaction to artificial fingernails. *J Eur Acad Dermatol Venereol* 21(2):169–174. DOI: 10.1111/j.1468-3083.2006.01883.x.

71. Voller, L.M., and Warshaw, E.M. 2020. Acrylates: New sources and new allergens. *Clin Exp Dermatol* 45:277–283. DOI: 10.1111/ced.14093.

72. Raposo, I., Lobo, I., Amaro, C., Lobo, M.L., Melo, H., Parente, J., et al. 2017. Allergic contact dermatitis caused by (meth)acrylates in nail cosmetic products in users and nail technicians - A 5-year study. *Contact Dermatitis* 77(6):356–359. DOI: 10.1111/cod.12817.

73. Whittington, C.V. 1981. Dermatitis from UV acrylate in adhesive. *Contact Dermatitis* 7(4):203–204. DOI: 10.1111/j.1600-0536.1981.tb04044.x.

74. Brooke, R.C., and Beck, M.H. 2002. A new source of allergic contact dermatitis from UV-cured (meth)acrylate adhesive. *Contact Dermatitis* 47(3):179–180. DOI: 10.1034/j.1600-0536.2002.47030815.x.

75. Kiec-Swierczynska, M., Krecisz, B., Swierczynska-Machura, D., and Zaremba, J. 2005. An epidemic of occupational contact dermatitis from an acrylic glue. *Contact Dermatitis* 52(3):121–125. DOI: 10.1111/j.0105-1873.2005.00527.x.

76. Minamoto, K., and Ueda, A. 2005. Occupational allergic contact dermatitis due to ultraviolet-cured acrylic glue. *J Occup Health* 47(4):340–342. DOI: 10.1539/joh.47.340.

77. Jolanki, R., Kanerva, L., Estlander, T., and Tarvainen, K. 1994. Concomitant sensitization to triglycidyl isocyanurate, diaminodiphenylmethane and 2-hydroxyethyl methacrylate from silk-screen printing coatings in the manufacture of circuit boards. *Contact Dermatitis* 30(1):12–15. DOI: 10.1111/j.1600-0536.1994.tb00721.x.

78. Jolanki, R., Kanerva, L., and Estlander, T. 1995. Occupational allergic contact dermatitis caused by epoxy diacrylate in ultraviolet-light-cured paint, and bisphenol A in dental

composite resin. *Contact Dermatitis* 33(2):94–99. DOI: 10.1111/j.1600-0536.1995. tb00508.x.

79. Goossens, A., Coninx, D., Rommens, K., and Verhamme, B. 1998. Occupational dermatitis in a silk-screen maker. *Contact Dermatitis* 39:40–42.
80. Condé-Salazar, L., Guimaraens, D., and Romero, LV. 1988. Occupational allergic contact dermatitis from anaerobic acrylic sealants. *Contact Dermatitis* 18(3):129–132. DOI: 10.1111/j.1600-0536.1988.tb04497.x.
81. Holme, S.A., and Statham, B.N. 2000. A cluster of 6 cases of occupational allergic contact dermatitis from (meth)acrylates. *Contact Dermatitis* 43(3):179–180.
82. Aalto-Korte, K., Alanko, K., Kuuliala, O., and Jolanki, R. 2008. Occupational methacrylate and acrylate allergy from glues. *Contact Dermatitis* 58(6):340–346. DOI: 10.1111/j.1600-0536.2008.01333.x.
83. Herman, A., de Montjoye, L., Tromme, I., Goossens, A., and Baeck, M. 2018. Allergic contact dermatitis caused by medical devices for diabetes patients: A review. *Contact Dermatitis* 79(6):331–335. DOI: 10.1111/cod.13120.
84. Rietschel, R., Huggins, R., Levy, N., and Pruitt, P.A. 1984. *In vivo* and *in vitro* testing of gloves for protection against UV-curable acrylate resin systems. *Contact Dermatitis* 11:279–282.
85. Huggins, R., Levy, N., and Pruitt, P.M. 1987. Testing of gloves for permeability to UV-curable acrylate coatings. *Am Ind Hyg Assoc J* 48:656–659.
86. Renard, E.P., Goydan, R., and Stolki, T. 1992. Permeation of multifunctional acrylates through selected protective glove materials. *Am Ind Hyg Assoc J* 53:117–123.
87. Munksgaard, E.C. 1992. Permeability of protective gloves to (di)methacrylates in resinous dental materials. *Scand J Dent Res* 100:189–192.
88. Mäkelä, E., Väänänen, V., Alanko, K., Jolanki, R., Estlander, T., and Kanerva, L. 1999. Resistance of disposable gloves to permeation by 2-hydroxyethyl methacrylate and triethyleneglycol dimethacrylate. *Occup Hyg* 5:121–129.
89. Mäkelä, E., Jolanki, R., Väänänen, V., Estlander, T., and Alanko, K. 2003. Kertakäyttökäsi- neiden metakrylaattiläpäisevyys [Methacrylate permeation through disposable gloves]. *Suomen Hammaslääkärilehti* [*Finnish Dental Journal*] 10:356–363 (in Finnish with English summary).
90. Zwanenburg, R.C.W. 2000. Adequate protective gloves for working with UV/EB-curing acrylates, in *Proceedings of RadTech Berlin*. Also published at the sites of RadTech Europe: http://www.radtech-europe.com/, RadTech North America: http://www.radtech.org/ and CEPE: http://www.cepe.org.
91. Andreasson, H., Boman, A., Johnsson, S., Karlsson, S., and Barregård, L. 2003. On permeability of methyl methacrylate, 2-hydroxyethyl methacrylate and triethyleneglycol dimethacrylate through protective gloves in dentistry. *Eur J Oral Sci* 111(6):529–535. DOI: 10.1111/j.0909-8836.2003.00070.x.
92. Lönnroth, E.C., Wellendorf, H., and Ruyter, E. 2003. Permeability of different types of medical protective gloves to acrylic monomers. *Eur J Oral Sci* 111(5):440–446. DOI: 10.1034/j.1600-0722.2003.00064.x.
93. Nakamura, M., Oshima, H., and Hashimoto, Y. 2003. Monomer permeability of disposable dental gloves. *J Prosthet Dent* 90(1):81–85. DOI: 10.1016/s0022-3913(03)00178-1.
94. Tomas, S., and Padmanabhan, T.V. 2009. Methyl methacrylate permeability of dental and industrial gloves. *New York State Dental J* 75(4):40–42.
95. Forsberg, K., and Mansdorf, S.Z. 2014. *Quick Selection Guide to Chemical Protective Clothing*, 6th ed. New York: Van Nostrand Reinhold.
96. North. 2001. *Silver Shield/4H Chemical Protection Guide*. Netherlands: North Safety Products. Available at https://www.northsafety.com.

24 Chemical Permeation through Disposable Gloves

D.M. Ceballos and R.N. Phalen

CONTENTS

24.1 INTRODUCTION

Chemical protective gloves are often thought to be the thick, heavy-duty gloves used in the chemical industry or laboratories in the handling of highly hazardous chemicals, but disposable gloves can also be used to protect against incidental contact with chemicals. Disposable gloves are usually thinner and allow for work tasks that require high dexterity. Disposal gloves are also used when trying to avoid cross-contamination or to secure antiseptic work conditions. Such tasks are routine in healthcare and laboratories, but they can also be found in many other workplaces. In particular, disposable gloves may be used when the user is not immersing hands

DOI: 10.1201/9781003126874-28

inside the chemicals, and any potential contact with the hazardous substance may be brief or indirect. In these cases of inadvertent and incidental contact, the disposable glove would be promptly removed and/or replaced. However, selecting disposable gloves to protect against chemicals can be difficult.

Many chemicals already permeate thick industrial gloves, so thin disposable gloves made commonly from the same materials are permeated even more rapidly. Disposable gloves also break more easily under chemical or mechanical stress and, in a departure from thicker gloves, holes or other defects may be more prominent. Further, the variability among different brands and manufacturers of disposable gloves creates some unpredictability related to chemical protection with the same material and thickness glove.[1] For certain high-hazard chemicals, only information on thick industrial gloves may be available, although glove manufacturers' chemical compatibility charts and published scientific studies are including more information on the permeation of disposable gloves. Chemical permeation described in this chapter is usually measured through the detection of the breakthrough time (BT) and the steady-state permeation rate (SSPR) of the chemical through the glove.[1]

24.2   FINDING INFORMATION

According to legislation in Europe, the suppliers of chemical protective gloves must be able to provide information on the efficacy of the protection.[2] Still, information on the chemical protective properties of disposable gloves is often difficult to find. This is because the variety of the chemicals used in permeation tests does not directly correspond to the numerous chemicals in use, and only gloves that are claimed to have protective properties against chemicals are often tested. Some of the disposable gloves are certified for chemical protection, but some are certified for healthcare use, or they are meant for technical tasks in which the risks of chemical contact are minimal.[2,3]

For some workplaces finding appropriate gloves may be facilitated by certain certifications. For example, some disposable chemical protective gloves are certified for healthcare purposes under different names such as "medical gloves," "examination gloves," "patient examination gloves," "surgeon's gloves," and "tested for use with [name of the chemotherapeutic drug(s)]," among others.[4] The use of the information on the certified protective product for healthcare gloves, or the use of the protective product in healthcare, may not be the perfect way of handling the matter and may not be possible for all industries, but sometimes it is useful.

Workers risking skin contact with hazardous chemicals should wear chemical protective gloves conforming to the directive or regulation on personal protective equipment (PPE).[5,6] But glove users, or the health and safety professionals advising users, often have to find relevant glove permeation information from the glove suppliers or in the scientific literature. Despite information on glove permeation being available, selecting gloves based on published information is not easy. Challenges may include that the tests have employed different methods or reporting or that the glove materials differ from the materials that the user of the gloves can find. This chapter will discuss the different methods that are commonly used for testing the chemical permeation of disposable gloves. However, permeation information often concerns specific gloves tested with specific chemicals; therefore, broad generalizations must be avoided, although sometimes professionals need to make decisions with the best available information.

In the literature, several groups of chemicals that have been used in glove permeation testing can easily be distinguished: disinfectants, isocyanate compounds, cytostatic drugs, solvents, and acrylic compounds.[7–9] This chapter will describe the first four groups as well as other chemicals, mixtures, and formulations, and Chapter 23 described in depth how to choose protective gloves for acrylates and acrylic compounds.

24.3 TEST METHODS

There are several similar standard tests for measuring the permeation of chemicals through protective gloves or other protective materials. The most commonly used methods are the American standard ASTM F 739 and the European standards EN 374-1 and EN 16523-1.[10–12] They both use a similar test cell with two chambers: a flow-through chamber for the collection medium and a chamber with an inlet for a test chemical (Figure 24.1). A sample of the protective material being studied is clamped between the chambers. The permeation of a test chemical is measured periodically from the flow of the collection medium. Methods of analytical chemistry such as chromatography and spectrometry are used; the collecting medium is usually nitrogen, purified air, or water.

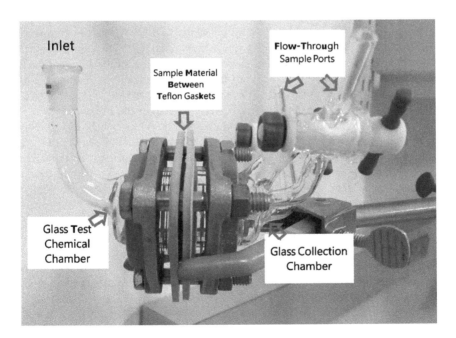

FIGURE 24.1 ASTM-type chemical permeation cell showing the glass chemical challenge chamber and inlet, sample interface where the material is placed between two Teflon gaskets, and the glass collection chamber with flow-through ports for continuous sampling.

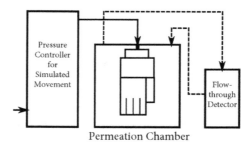

Permeation Chamber

FIGURE 24.2   Example of a whole glove permeation test set-up with a permeation chamber (the glove is inverted for testing), a pump-driven flow-through detector, and a pressure controller for simulated movement.

The test is carried out for the time specified in the standard or until a specified permeation rate is exceeded. BT is used as the criterion of the resistance to permeation. The BT is the time between the application of the test chemical onto the outer surface of the sample material and the detection of the test chemical permeating the material at a specified rate (in $\mu g/cm^2/min$). The major differences in the standards are discussed elsewhere in this book, as well as in a review by Banaee and Que Hee.[13]

The reason for using standard tests is the need for comparable results between all the glove products tested in the different laboratories. When tested with different methods, the results deviate or they may be in such a format that the comparison of gloves between different studies is impossible. The reported chemical permeation testing methods for disposable gloves are variable. In addition, some of the test methods discussed in this chapter do not follow standardized test methods, which include whole glove testing (Figure 24.2), the use of an inverted glove fingertip, and *in vivo* test methods.[14–17] In these kinds of methods neither the exposed area of the glove, the determination limit for the chemical, nor the rate at which the collection medium changes are often normalized for comparison to the methods in other studies. Connor's research group has developed an assay to quantify the permeability of cytostatic drugs.[18,19] In the assay, an inverted glove fingertip is secured over the mouth of a sterile glass vial containing the test chemical. The vial is then placed upside down into one well of a sterile plastic 24-well cell plate. The well contains an absorbent paper disc saturated with sterile water. A weight is placed on top of the vials to ensure close contact. The test is carried out for a previously determined time at 37 °C. As a detection method, mutagenicity testing, color detection, or liquid chromatography can be used. An *in vivo* method for studying glove permeability by allergens has been developed by Andersson and Bruze.[20] The results of these studies are also presented elsewhere in this book.

24.4   DISINFECTANTS

The use of disinfectants is widespread in healthcare for cleaning surfaces and objects, sterilizing instruments, and skin disinfection. Gloves are to be used for preventing contact with disinfectants, as they may cause allergic and irritant reactions.[21-25] Common agents in disinfectants are ethyl alcohol, 2-propyl alcohol (isopropyl alcohol), formaldehyde, glutaraldehyde, chlorhexidine gluconate, hydrogen peroxide, peracetic acid, and povidone-iodine. The use of hydro-alcoholic gels with gloves, and its relevance to infection control and COVID-19, are discussed further in Chapter 27.

24.4.1 CHEMICAL PERMEATION STUDIES

A past study evaluated the permeation of common hospital chemicals through surgical single-layered and double-layered natural rubber (NR) and single-layered chloroprene gloves with standard methods EN 374 and ASTM F 739.[26,27] The gloves did not exhibit permeation for potassium hydroxide (45%), sodium hypochlorite (13%), or hydrogen peroxide (30%). Furthermore, neither glutaraldehyde, chlorhexidine digluconate, nor iodine in the studied commercial disinfectant solutions permeated the gloves. Slight permeation of peracetic acid (0.35%) and acetic acid (4%) from a disinfectant agent was observed through single-layered NR materials.

Clear evidence of formaldehyde permeation was detected through single-layered NR gloves, in which the ASTM BTs were 17–67 min, but the permeation rates were not high enough for the breakthrough to have occurred according to the EN standard.[26] When tested with 70% isopropyl alcohol, the thin (0.22–0.28 mm) NR materials yielded BTs of 4.6–9.1 min with both standards.[28] For the thicker and double-layered NR gloves and the chloroprene gloves, the EN BTs were from 21 min to more than 240 min and the ASTM BTs from 12 to 103 min.

In contrast to these results, permeation of hydrogen peroxide (7.5%) through polyvinyl chloride (PVC, vinyl) and NR examination gloves has been reported to occur in less than 30 min.[29] The testing of NR gloves was discontinued after 3 h because the permeation rate had been accelerating at a rate too high to be meaningful. One of the probable reasons for the differences between the results in the two studies may be found in the glove thicknesses and materials: the thinnest gloves used in this study are double the thickness of the gloves examined in the other study. The compendium of permeation indices presents one BT of 150 min for NR gloves with a thickness of 0.15 mm; the other BTs for NR gloves (0.15–0.73 mm) are >360 min or >480 min, which means that permeation has not been detected.[30] In the compendium there are no published data on surgical chloroprene gloves, but BTs from 5 to >480 min are reported for industrial chloroprene glove materials.

Earlier, Schwope et al.[31] described methods for detecting the permeation of formaldehyde through disposable gloves. The BTs ranged from 1 to 15 min for NR and chloroprene gloves. In the permeation index compendium, the BTs for disposable glove materials tested with formaldehyde vary a great deal (from 4 to >360 min).[30]

Lehman et al.[32] have observed that the permeation of dilute glutaraldehyde through examination of NR or Tactylon® gloves was nil or very low after 4 h of testing if the glove samples are not stretched. Mellström et al.[33] have also tested the permeation of glutaraldehyde from a disinfectant through thin NR, PVC, and polyethylene (PE) gloves, and no evidence of glutaraldehyde permeation was detected.

On the other hand, Jordan et al.[34] have reported that a 2% glutaraldehyde solution can permeate rather thin NR gloves in 45 min.

Alongside glutaraldehyde, Mellström et al.[33] studied the permeability of isopropyl alcohol, ethyl alcohol, and p-chloro-m-cresol. For 1 h, NR, PVC, and PE glove materials were found to provide acceptable protection against p-chloro-m-cresol along with glutaraldehyde. Isopropyl alcohol and ethyl alcohol permeated NR and PVC gloves in less than 10 min. The PE gloves were of variable quality, and the BT ranged from 4 to >240 min for the alcohols.

A more recent study evaluated the permeation of ethyl alcohol through disposable NR, nitrile, and PVC exam gloves.[35] The whole-glove study evaluated the effect of simulated hand movement on permeation. Regardless of movement, the PVC glove had the lowest BT (about 1 min), as compared to NR (2–3 min) and nitrile (8–11 min), but PVC was less affected by movement overall. The cumulative amount permeated after 30 min was the highest for PVC, followed by NR, and then nitrile. However, none of the disposable exam gloves provided more than 12 min of BT protection against ethyl alcohol, on average.

Similar results were obtained for 37 disposable nitrile exam gloves evaluated for permeation of ethyl alcohol.[36] On average, the BT was 14 min (±6 min) and ranged from 7 to 20 min. Much of the variability in BT was attributed to differences in the formulations, such as acrylonitrile content and the amount of carboxylation of the base polymer, as well as extractible oils or plasticizer content.

24.4.2 Recommendations

Ordinary disposable gloves made of NR or PVC provide sufficient protection against occasional splashes of disinfectants.[9] Alcohols and formaldehyde rapidly permeate these gloves, and thus the contaminated gloves must be readily replaced, and hands must be washed. In continuous contact, even dilute glutaraldehyde and concentrated hydrogen peroxide permeate through the thin examination gloves. For prolonged handling of alcohols, aldehydes, concentrated peracetic acid solution, or concentrated hydrogen peroxide, only gloves with at least a twofold chemical-specific BT compared to the work period should be used. Chlorhexidine digluconate or povidone-iodine is not likely to permeate the intact gloves.

24.5 ISOCYANATE COMPOUNDS

The need to test the permeation of isocyanates compounds through disposable gloves has arisen from isocyanates being a skin sensitizer and causative agent for allergic contact dermatitis.[37–40] Isocyanate compounds are used in several industries beyond the collision repair industry and construction, as well as in many products and applications, e.g., in foams, bed liners, adhesives, insulation, varnishes, and isocyanate paints.[41,42] Figure 24.3 shows an example of the PPE worn by a worker using an isocyanate. Isocyanates include diisocyanates both in monomer and polymer forms. Monomer diisocyanates include methylenebis (phenyl isocyanate) (MDI), toluene diisocyanate (TDI), and hexamethylene diisocyanate (HDI), followed by

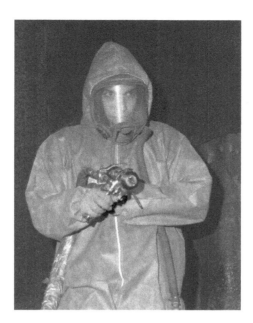

FIGURE 24.3 Worker wearing a protective suit and disposable gloves for spray application containing an isocyanate. Adapted from DHHS (NIOSH) Publication No. 2008-109, National Institute for Occupational Safety and Health (Public Domain).

less common naphthalene diisocyanate (NDI), methylene bis-cyclohexylisocyanate (HMDI) (hydrogenated MDI), and isophorone diisocyanate (IPDI). Examples of widely used polyisocyanates include HDI biuret and HDI isocyanurate.

24.5.1 CHEMICAL PERMEATION STUDIES

Isocyanates permeation was first tested as recently as 2010 because traditional permeation methods were not appropriate for measuring reactive polymerizing chemicals that require a derivatization solution to be captured.[43] Ceballos et al.[43] developed a permeation panel to test the permeation of isocyanates in solvent-based autobody paint formulations typically used in the collision repair industry against NR (i.e., latex) disposable gloves commonly used by spray painters. This new method concluded that monomers HDI and IPDI permeated through the (0.10–0.13 mm) latex glove material under typical glove use conditions (30 min). The latex glove material exhibited immediate breakthrough, with a permeation rate of 2.9 ng/min/cm^2 (equivalent to 0.0029 µg/cm^2/min). The oligomeric forms of HDI and IPDI did not permeate the latex glove material. The same authors automatized the permeation panel with a reciprocator arm to provide more permeation data and test different types of gloves commonly used by spray painters.[44] Disposable nitrile gloves were found to be more protective against isocyanates compared to latex (both 5 mil or 0.13 mm thickness). However, 13 mil or 0.33 mm butyl rubber gloves were the only glove that adequately protected against isocyanates (both HDI and IPDI) during the testing period, which are non-disposable chemical protective gloves usually recommended by the paint manufacturers and rarely used by spray painters (due in part to the higher cost and comfort issues). Both NR and nitrile gloves were heavily used by spray painters because of the need for high dexterity during the painting of automobiles.[44] The authors recommended the use of disposable nitrile gloves that are thicker than 5 mil or 0.13 mm.

Since the first publication on isocyanate permeation, several other methods and tests have been published to cover different isocyanates of interest and to address the use of isocyanates in other applications beyond spray painting. For example, in construction, MDI and its polymers are used in thermal insulation of windows, the coating of roofs or floors, and sewer relining. Makela et al. [45] studied permeation of pure monomer 4,4′-MDI through eight glove materials with a method derived from the EN 374-3 and ASTM F 739 standards. All tested materials permeated in less than 480 min (range: 23–406 min). NR (0.53 mm), thick (1.7 mm) PVC, neoprene-NR (0.78 mm), and nitrile rubber of various thicknesses (0.10–0.96 mm) provided affordable chemical protection with a BT of over 75 min. This study emphasizes that even small amounts of the monomer permeating the gloves are a concern for users given the high skin toxicity specific to these chemicals. Later, the same research group developed a different method to test gloves against MDI by measuring penetration rather than permeation and further concluded that both NR and nitrile disposable gloves were acceptable for brief uses of MDI.[46] Thus, use of disposable NR and nitrile gloves should only be used for inadvertent and incidental contact, in which contaminated gloves are promptly discarded and/or replaced.

Glove permeation of MDI, including 4,4′-MDI, 2,4′-MDI, 2,2′-MDI, and 4,4′-MDI, from spray polyurethane foam formulations, has also been tested recently.[47] Disposable NR gloves (0.07 mm thickness) permeated more than nitrile (0.07 mm) or PVC gloves (0.07 mm). Polyurethane anticorrosive coatings containing either MDI or HDI isocyanates were also tested, and nitrile was determined as superior to NR gloves; nitrile gloves were not permeated until after 15 min.[48] No oligomeric isocyanates permeated the disposable gloves.

24.5.2 RECOMMENDATIONS

Small molecular isocyanate compounds permeate common disposable NR (i.e., latex) gloves rapidly. Polyisocyanates or the oligomeric form of the isocyanates did not permeate the disposable gloves. For adequate protection, it is important to find workplace controls that lessen the handling of these chemicals. Against isocyanates, there are a few protective glove alternatives, such as butyl and neoprene, recommended by the manufacturers of paints and other isocyanate products. However, new studies have suggested that the use of disposable nitrile gloves may provide adequate protection for brief incidental contact, and with thicker nitrile gloves better than thin ones. However, glove labels with information on the material type and thickness should be ideally checked to guarantee adequate gloves for isocyanates are chosen. Blue or purple may not always mean nitrile as disposable gloves now come in many colors and presentations, and brands are no longer consistent in matching the glove color to a material as they did in the early years of the production of disposable gloves. Ceballos et al.[44] documented how some car painters, for example, have gotten confused when choosing gloves in recent years because they were buying "nice blue thick gloves" that were very elastic and thought were nitrile based on the color but resulted being NR gloves instead.

24.6 CYTOSTATIC DRUGS

Many cytostatic drugs are genotoxic carcinogens against which the healthcare personnel must protect themselves carefully.[49,50] Besides their toxic properties, some of these drugs are sensitizers,[51–53] or they can cause acute skin injuries.[49] Skin is reported to be an important exposure route for these drugs, even if the personnel use gloves, hairnets, and special clothing.[54–56]

Banaee and Que Hee[57] provide a more recent and thorough review of the permeation of healthcare gloves by cytostatics (e.g., antineoplastic, cytotoxic, chemotherapeutic, and chemotherapy drugs), which are typically nonvolatile solids dissolved in solution for injection, topical delivery, or taken orally. Due in part to the inherent hazards to normal cells and tissues associated with these drugs, special attention has been focused on protecting healthcare workers against dermal exposures to cytostatics. Beginning in 2005, and recently updated in 2019, ASTM International established ASTM D 6978,[58] *Standard Practice for Assessment of Resistance of Medical Gloves to Permeation by Chemotherapy Drugs*, to aid in the selection of medical gloves and materials (e.g., gowns) resistant to the permeation of cytostatics. The standardized assessment is based on the permeation BT of at least nine chemotherapy drugs, as a worst-case scenario, and designed to encompass a range of chemotherapy drugs. The seven required cytostatics include carmustine, cyclophosphamide, doxorubicin hydrochloride, fluorouracil, etoposide, paclitaxel, and thiotepa. In contrast to ASTM F 739, EN 374, and EN 16523-1,[10–12] ASTM D 6978 permeation testing is conducted for 240 min (versus 480 min), at 35°C (versus ambient lab conditions), using the thinnest part of the glove, and with a lower permeation level of 0.01 μg/cm^2/min for BT.[58] As a result, ASTM D 6978 is a more sensitive permeation test than other standardized permeation methods.

One general observation that can be made for chemotherapy gloves labeled as meeting ASTM D 6978 is that they are often thicker than normal exam gloves. Prior observations in the literature have indicated that thicker gloves, as well as double gloving, have been more effective against chemotherapy agents.[57]

24.6.1 EARLIER CHEMICAL PERMEATION STUDIES

Several studies have dealt with the permeation of cytostatic drugs through disposable gloves. Although most of the test results do not show any permeation, in all of the studies at least one of the drugs has permeated one of the tested glove materials. Common NR or PVC examination gloves fail to provide adequate protection in many studies. Mader et al.[14] have divided some cytostatic drugs into groups of rapidly permeating, slowly permeating, and nonpermeating drugs. The rapidly permeating drugs were mitoxantrone and carmustine (BCNU), and the slowly permeating drugs were cyclophosphamide and bleomycin. Nonpermeating drugs were methotrexate, arabinosyl-cytosine, 5-fluorouracil, adriamycin, 4'-O-tetrahydropyranyladriamycin, vincristine, etoposide, and cisplatin. Further investigation and explanation of this are provided in the next section.

Connor's research group has studied the permeation of cytostatic drugs since 1984.[18,19,59] In their early works with Laidlaw,[60] they found that glove thickness is a major determinant of permeability. They reported that thin PVC gloves were permeated by all 20 tested drugs. Surgical gloves were permeable by only carmustine, thiotepa, and mechlorethamine hydrochloride. In addition to these drugs, cyclophosphamide permeated NR examination gloves. Thick PVC gloves were permeable to six drugs. NR and PVC examination gloves have also been proved permeable to fluorouracil and methotrexate.[61]

In 1992, Dinter-Heidorn and Carstens[15] were unable to show that gloves meant for handling cytostatic drugs could provide adequate protection against permeation by carmustine. The liquid chromatographic test method showed permeation to begin in 5–15 min from the start of the tests. Raster electron microphotography also revealed pores and fissures in intact and dilated gloves. Connor[62] obtained similar results in 1995, when he tested NR and styrene-ethylene-butadiene rubber gloves, all of which were recommended by the manufacturers for the handling of cytostatic drugs. He observed the permeation of 5-fluorouracil through NR examination gloves (0.46 mm) and the permeation of carmustine through other NR examination gloves (0.22–0.45 mm). Doxorubicin, cyclophosphamide, and cisplatin did not permeate any of the glove materials. In 1999, the situation seemed better: Singleton and Connor[19] reported that gloves especially intended for handling cytostatic drugs provide protection against carmustine, etoposide, and paclitaxel. In their test, 11 test glove types were made of NR and 3 were nitrile rubber. All the nitrile rubber materials did not prove quite as good protection as the NR material against etoposide.

In 1999, Connor[59] also reported on the protection provided by nitrile rubber examination gloves, NR examination gloves, polyurethane surgical gloves, and neoprene surgical gloves against 18 cytostatic drugs. Permeation was detected only occasionally in the tests. The permeability could have been caused by weak points in the materials. Connor emphasized that these results cannot be generalized to all the gloves with the same material name, and he discussed the effect of the material thickness on the results. Also, Gross and Groce[63] have reported that disposable nitrile rubber provides protection against carmustine. Furthermore, Slevin et al.[64] have studied alternative glove materials by adding industrial gloves to the PVC and NR examination gloves and surgical gloves. Again, examination gloves proved to be the worst choice for protection. An NR material with chloroprene (NR-CR) and a thick nitrile rubber material were better against daunomycin than the rest of the materials. Surgical NR gloves (0.25 mm) were approximately as good as nitrile rubber gloves (0.58 mm) and NR-CR gloves (0.44 mm) against vincristine, cytosine arabinoside, and methotrexate. The thick nitrile rubber gloves were the best against cyclophosphamide, while all the other glove materials displayed similar permeation.

European standard EN 396 (possibly misreported; EN 374) has been used by Mellström et al.[65] in a permeation study with cytostatic drugs. For carmustine, the tests resulted in standard BTs of about 80 min for NR gloves (0.21 mm) and PVC gloves. Carmustine started to permeate also ethyl methacrylate gloves and thicker NR gloves (0.32 mm) in 30 min, but the permeation rate (1.0 µg/min/cm^2) required by the standard for the detection of the BT was not reached during the 3-h testing time. All the tested gloves proved to provide protection against etoposide, bleomycin, mitoxantrone, and cyclophosphamide.

Mellström et al.[65] also showed that a 10-min treatment of the gloves with ethyl alcohol did not increase the permeation of NR gloves by carmustine. A study by Connor and Xiang[66] in 2000 showed that 5 min contact with 70% isopropyl alcohol did not increase the permeation of carmustine, cyclophosphamide, fluorouracil, doxorubicin, thiotepa, or cisplatin through NR or nitrile rubber glove material. Thus, disinfection with ethyl alcohol or isopropyl alcohol solution does not affect the exposure of healthcare workers to these cytostatic agents.

According to Colligan and Horstman[67] surgical NR gloves provide the greatest resistance to permeation by cyclophosphamide and 5-fluorouracil when compared to PVC and NR examination gloves. In their study, all three materials showed good resistance to permeation by doxorubicin, and methotrexate did not show any permeation. Flexing the glove materials during the test to simulate an occupational setting did not shorten the BTs significantly.

Double gloving seems to be beneficial for protection against cytostatic drugs. Mellström[65] stated this in 1996 after tests with carmustine and different kinds of double layers of glove materials. Klein et al.[68] showed that thiotepa and cyclophosphamide permeated single-layered NR and chloroprene rubber surgical gloves slightly, but double-layered NR gloves were not permeable to any of the studied drugs: amsacrine, cisplatin, cyclophosphamide, doxorubicin hydrochloride, 5-fluorouracil, disodium methotrexate, paclitaxel, thiotepa, and vincristine sulfate.

24.6.2 MORE RECENT CHEMICAL PERMEATION STUDIES

Some more recent studies are included in the abovementioned review by Banaee and Que Hee.[57] Wallemacq et al.[69] evaluated the permeation of 13 cytotoxic agents through NR, neoprene, nitrile, and PVC exam-type gloves under dynamic conditions. They found the PVC glove to provide the least protection against permeation and that carmustine permeated most of the materials within 1 h. In a similar study,[70] with 17 antineoplastic drug solutions and the addition of an alcohol pretreatment, the NR, neoprene, nitrile, and synthetic polyisoprene gloves all exceeded ASTM F 739 and EN 374 limits for BT. However, two of the NR gloves exceeded the ASTM D 6978 limit for BT for carmustine. Studies evaluating doxorubicin and epirubicin[71-72] found that NR and nitrile gloves resisted permeation under neutral pH and ambient temperature conditions. However, permeation was detected for the nitrile gloves under acidic pH conditions. Oriyama et al.[73] evaluated cyclophosphamide, doxorubicin hydrochloride, etoposide, fluorouracil, and paclitaxel against NR, chlorinated NR, and nitrile disposable exam gloves. As per the ASTM D 6978 criterion for BT, the nitrile glove resisted permeation, whereas cyclophosphamide and fluorouracil permeated the NR gloves. Krzeminska et al.[74] evaluated docetaxel (with 25% ethyl alcohol), doxorubicin, and fluorouracil in isotonic solutions against NR, neoprene, and nitrile gloves. As per EN 16523-1 criterion for BT, three glove materials resisted permeation of all three cytostatics and greater than 8 h for doxorubicin and fluorouracil. The ethyl alcohol in docetaxel was noted to accelerate permeation, especially with layered protective clothing materials that were also tested alongside the gloves.

Nalin et al.[75] evaluated the permeation of 27 chemotherapy drugs on 15 surgical and examination gloves using a simulated-dynamic testing method at 37 or 43 °C for up to 30 min of permeation resistance. All the gloves were below the EN 16523-1 criterion for BT after 30 min. However, several of the nitrile exam gloves exceeded the ASTM D 6978 criterion for BT after 30 min for busulfan (five gloves), carmustine (four gloves), and thiotepa (two gloves). Many of these nitrile gloves were from a single brand/manufacturer. Five surgical gloves made of polychloroprene, polyisoprene, or NR also exceeded the ASTM D 6978 criterion for BT after 30 min exposure to carmustine and thiotepa. The authors noted that the lower molecular weight, hydrogen bond donor, and topographical polar surface area contributed to the higher permeation of busulfan, carmustine, and thiotepa. In addition, double gloving helped reduce chemical permeation to an acceptable level in these cases.

Oriyama et al.[76] evaluated the permeation of ten antineoplastic agents against nitrile examination gloves with a focus on the physicochemical properties of the agents. They found that the molecular weight and LogP values were predictive of permeation. Higher permeation rates, in excess of the ASTM D 6978 criterion for BT, were observed for agents with a molecular weight <500 daltons and LogP greater than −1. This included carboplatin, carmustine, cyclophosphamide, fluorouracil, and ifosfamide, with the first four being consistent with the findings of Wallemacq et al.[69]

24.6.3 Recommendations

Glove recommendations against cytostatic drugs include double gloving and, in prolonged work, changing gloves every 30 min.[8,57,61,65,68] Hands should be washed before putting on the gloves and after the handling of the cytostatic drugs. In case of glove breakage, the gloves must be immediately disposed of, the hands must be washed thoroughly, and new gloves have to be put on. It is worth noting that the bottles and packages of cytostatic drugs are often contaminated.[77] Furthermore, the surfaces on which the drugs are diluted or otherwise handled may be contaminated despite careful cleaning. The handling of cytostatic drugs necessitates careful planning of the work methods and premises for which many agencies and groups continue to update.[78-81] Aside from the critical procedural, engineering, administrative, and work practice controls needed when handling cytostatic drugs, greater assurance can be obtained with the use of gloves evaluated and adhering to the ATSM D 6978 standard. Lastly, it is also of importance to ensure specific permeation testing is provided for cytostatic drugs with a lower molecular weight, higher lipophilicity (LogP), and/or low hydrogen donor status.

24.7 SOLVENTS

Millions of workers are exposed to solvents.[82] Solvents can have an irritant and degreasing effect on the skin, and many solvents can also permeate the skin and enter the blood circulation.[83] Therefore, gloves are commonly used when handling solvents, handling materials made with solvents, or processes that use solvents. Solvents usually refer to a wide variety of chemicals, including alcohols, organic solvents such as aliphatic and aromatic hydrocarbons, and gasoline among many others.[84] Solvents are widely used in many applications such as paints, varnishes, lacquers, paint removers, plastics, adhesives, textiles, printing inks, rubber products, and waxes.[84] However, permeation measurements of solvents can be challenging because solvents can often degrade the quality of disposable gloves in a short time.[85]

24.7.1 CHEMICAL PERMEATION STUDIES

Solvent permeation studies have been published since the early 2000s, likely due to improvements in the sensitivity of analytical chemistry laboratory methods for solvent analysis. For example, nitrile disposable gloves (0.63 ± 0.03 mm) were tested against several pure organic solvents using the ASTM F 739 method.[86] Chao et al.[86] used the solvent's SSPR to calculate an effective diffusion coefficient. Solvents through nitrile gloves had effective diffusion coefficients that were inversely correlated to the molecular weight of the compounds, in the following order: benzene > toluene > ethyl benzene > xylene > styrene. While benzene and toluene first permeated (i.e., BT) at approximately 30 min, the other solvents permeated through nitrile gloves after about an hour, which meant that the physicochemical properties of the solvent were a good predictor of permeation rates. In a follow-up study, nitrile gloves (0.63 ± 0.03 mm) were compared with neoprene/NR gloves (0.72 ± 0.05 mm) and determined to be better at protecting against benzene, toluene, and styrene, with the greatest difference regarding benzene—specifically, nitrile gloves had a breakthrough of approximately 10 min, while neoprene/NR gloves had a breakthrough of approximately 5 min.[87]

Disposable thin nitrile gloves (0.34 mm) have also been tested against solvents in contrast to neoprene and butyl rubber using an AMK chemical permeation test cell (AMK Glass, Inc.).[88] Acetone, for example, had a BT of about 5.5 min and an SSPR of approximately 3000 µg/min/cm^2, and although these nitrile gloves are considered disposable, they were not significantly affected by several thermal decontamination cycles. Most surprising was that butyl gloves, when tested against toluene, had a larger change in decreasing performance after several thermal decontamination cycles compared to nitrile—specifically, nitrile gloves BT for toluene of approximately 20 min did not change significantly while SSPR increased from about 250–300 µg/min/cm^2, and butyl gloves BT for toluene changed from approximately 6–3 min while SSPR increased from about 800–1000 µg/min/cm^2.

Disposable nitrile gloves of different thicknesses have also been tested using a robotic hand and found protective within 5–30 min against limonene, which is a low volatile solvent commonly used as a fragrance.[89] Variability within disposable nitrile gloves has been documented when testing for solvents by Brown et al.[90] The polarity of the solvent can play a role in glove performance, with disposable nitrile gloves providing increased protection with an increase in solvent polarity—nitrile performed better with cyclohexanol than with cyclohexane as the alcohol is more polar. However, many solvents have not been tested on disposable gloves using permeation methods.

24.7.2 RECOMMENDATIONS

Health and safety professionals must be cautious when selecting disposable gloves for chemical protection against solvents. Appropriate work with solvents often must exclude any possibility of direct skin contact. In general, gloves should be used only as a safety measure against accidental splashes and, after use or contamination, the gloves are promptly discarded. Selection should be based on the available chemical permeation data for the product, especially when skin protection is critical.[1] If gloves must be used for prolonged solvent contact, then the imperviousness should first be checked by the glove manufacturer. The glove-specific BT for the solvent should be at least double the work period—as solvents can degrade disposable gloves. [85,91] Gloves best suitable for protecting against solvents are usually well-tested industrial chemical protective gloves, which have available chemical permeation data and detailed instructions for the users. Even though disposable gloves may still be adequate, selecting the thinnest disposable gloves are seldom an adequate choice for protection against most hazardous solvents or immersion work conditions. Disposable gloves made of synthetic rubber materials (e.g., nitrile, butyl, and chloroprene rubber or neoprene) are often less permeable to solvents than NR (i.e., latex) and PVC gloves. Thankfully nowadays there are many types and thicknesses of disposable gloves available, including neoprene, which makes opting for disposable gloves when handling solvents easier compared to a few decades ago.

It must be noted that some manufacturers or suppliers may not test their products and instead provide generic ratings based on available data in the literature or from other sources. Given the observed wide variation in the chemical permeation of solvents for different brands of disposable nitrile gloves,[36,90] reliance on generic chemical resistance ratings is not a recommended practice, especially when skin protection is critical.

24.8 OTHER CHEMICALS, MIXTURES, AND FORMULATIONS

The testing of gloves against all chemicals is not always necessary or possible. The decision to test includes the estimation of the harmfulness and the toxicity of the chemical, how it is used, and its probable ability to permeate glove materials. However, new chemicals are being produced every year and chemical glove permeation information may not be easily found. Chemicals that are not likely to be tested include those that do not permeate common glove materials, for example, ionic or large molecular compounds, as long as they cannot degrade the glove materials.[14]

On the other hand, some other chemicals will not be tested because they might permeate the gloves so fast that a measurement is not feasible, or the chemical might damage the testing system. Rarely used chemicals may also not be routinely tested. Finally, testing might not have been done because the testing laboratory may have considered the testing too hazardous for its personnel.

Of the chemicals tested, permeation information of disposable gloves may be found for chemicals beyond disinfectants, isocyanates, solvents, and chemotherapeutic compounds such as acrylates, amines, polychlorinated biphenyls, and oils, among others. Permeation information is also now more available for mixtures of chemicals and commercial formulations. Permeation studies for mixtures and formulations are extremely important as they reflect real-life scenarios, and typical permeation information for pure chemicals is not always predictive of permeation behavior within a mixture or formulation.[92] Regardless, this research area is nascent, and only a few studies have been published with solvent mixtures, autobody paints, and metalworking fluids, among a few others.

Aniline, an aromatic amine, has been detected to permeate thin PVC gloves in 4–9 min, thin NR gloves in 8 min, and thin nitrile gloves in 3 min by using amine adsorptive pads.[93] Studying the permeation of aromatic amines through glove materials was already started in 1977.[94]

The glove permeability of several nitrosamines as 0.136 M solutions in dichloromethane, acetone, ethanol, and water has been studied by Sansone and Tewari.[95] Nitrosamines in dichloromethane and acetone rapidly permeated the tested glove materials, but clear permeation was also detected for nitrosamines in ethanol and water. Thin PVC materials were reported to provide the worst protection.

Synthetic glove materials, nitrile rubber, and chloroprene rubber afford protection sometimes when PVC and NR do not.[96] A disposable glove brand made of nitrile rubber has, for example, a BT of 41 min against triethylamine. Nitrile is also protective regarding substituted silanes and siloxanes—13 mil or 0.33 mm nitrile gloves protected from 20 min to 8 h or more depending on the chemical or the presence of methanol.[97] Nitrile has also been reported as protective against hair dyes used in hairdressing as well as hair dyes in ethanol and hydrogen peroxide solutions; however, 0.14 mm nitrile gloves should be changed frequently as in some instances BT occurred a little longer than an hour.[98,99]

Nitrile glove material seems to provide good resistance against acrylates in many situations where UV/EB-curing acrylates are handled such as in dental offices, nail salons, or other workplaces—although the thickness is critical in determining how long disposable gloves may be used, especially when handled in combination with organic solvents.[100] More on acrylates are included in Chapter 23.

It is crucial to be aware that the permeation of some highly toxic chemicals through disposable gloves can be efficient and rapid. One provided example on the subject is tragic. Dr Karen Wetterhahn, a toxicologist, died in 1997 of mercury poisoning after 15 months had passed from a work task in which she transferred a small amount of dimethyl mercury to a nuclear magnetic resonance (NMR) tube while wearing disposable NR gloves.[101] Effective chemical protective gloves existed at the time and could have saved her life. Another example of hazardous materials includes polychlorinated biphenyls and their solutions and the use of surgical NR gloves that have been rated as providing poor protection.[102]

Concerning mixtures of chemicals, nitrile gloves showed protective qualities against solvent mixtures of benzene, toluene, ethylbenzene, and p-xylene using the ASTM F 739 method.[92] Solvents within a mixture had a shorter BT than their pure form.[92] The larger differences in solubility parameter between a solvent mixture and glove resulted in a lower permeation rate.

The mixture of solvents N,N-dimethylformamide (DMF) and methyl ethyl ketone (MEK), hazardous chemicals commonly used in the synthetic leather industries have been tested against neoprene gloves (0.75 mm thickness) using the ASTM F 739 cell.[103] MEK had a shorter BT (approximately 34.5 min) compared to DMF (45 min) for the neoprene gloves. Decontamination of the gloves by heating at 70 or 100 °C showed that the gloves had a similar protective effect as that of new gloves.

When working in machine shops, to prevent exposure to metal-working fluids, well-fitted disposable gloves are often needed to avoid additional safety hazards to hands around moving parts. It is well known that nitrile rubber is not permeated by oils, and thus disposable nitrile gloves are commonly used in machine shops or for car repair.[104] A metalworking fluid was tested on four types of glove materials using a gravimetric method and the ASTM F 739 method by Xu and Que Hee.[105] With perfluorohexane as the collection solvent in the permeation method, the metalworking fluid permeated through the gloves after 8 h and was better for nitrile gloves compared to PVC, chloroprene, or NR, although the relative ranking of the gloves was the same.[105] However, the universe of different metalworking fluids has not been tested, and professional judgment should be used when deciding on a disposable glove when using different mineral oil-based metalworking fluid formulations.

Gasoline, diesel, and biofuels (bioethanol 85%, biodiesel 20%) were tested using the ASTM F 739 method on three thin disposable gloves including 0.14 mm NR, 0.11 mm nitrile, and 0.14 mm PVC.[106] Gasoline had the highest permeation rate among the four fuels. NR gloves broke during testing against gasoline, while PVC BT of less than a minute (permeation rate of 12.2 sg/min/cm^2) and nitrile BT of 2.1 min (permeation rate of >63.3 sg/min/cm^2). Nitrile also performed better than NR and PVC for the other three fuels, with nitrile protecting against diesel fuel for at least 92.6 min.

NR (4 mil or 0.108 ± 0.001 mm) and nitrile (5 mil or 0.128 ± 0.001 mm) gloves were tested against an autobody paint formulation for solvent protection using a permeation panel with a charcoal cloth to collect the solvents that passed through the gloves in time.[85] The paint formulation contained ketones, acetates, and aromatics. Neither glove provided adequate protection; however, NR allowed 6–10 times the transport of solvents relative to nitrile for the key eight-solvent components: methyl ethyl ketone, toluene, styrene, ethylbenzene, xylene isomers, and 2-heptanone.

As mentioned in the permeation studies for solvent-based isocyanate formulations in this chapter, autobody paint has been tested against disposable gloves used by spray painters providing evidence that butyl and nitrile gloves are superior to NR gloves, with thicker products better than thinner ones.[43,44,85] However, the universe of autobody paints was not tested, and professional judgment should be used when deciding on disposable gloves for this or other workplaces using diisocyanates and solvent-based paint formulations. Other studies on isocyanate monomers such as MDI permeating from spray polyurethane formulations or polyurethane anticorrosive coatings also suggest that nitrile disposable gloves were better than NR.[47,48]

Seven paint stripping formulations were tested against gloves by Stull et al.[91] after passing degradation resistance screening tests to measure permeation with the ASTM F 739 method for continuous contact and the ASTM F 1383 for intermittent contact. Plastic laminate (2.7 mil or 0.069 mm) and butyl rubber (16 mil or 0.41 mm) were the most effective gloves against the majority of paint stripping formulations.[91] Non-disposable NR (30 mil or 0.76 mm) gloves showed rapid permeation (<15 min) for solvent-based paint strippers, while BTs were greater than 2 h for dibasic ester-based paint strippers. More gloves resisted permeation by N-methyl-2-pyrrolidone and dibasic ester-based paint strippers than conventional solvent products such as methylene chloride, methanol, isopropanol, acetone, and toluene. However, more readily available disposable thinner gloves were not tested. These results were consistent with those of Zellers and Sulewiski,[107] where butyl gloves were more protective than NR gloves even at different temperatures.

Another example of formulations tested on disposable gloves includes the case of widely used epoxy resins and diamine hardeners.[46] Both nitrile, a nitrile–NR–neoprene blend known as "rubber blend," and PVC gloves were tested using an experimental method with different formulations and found to be appropriate if changed frequently (less than every 10 min ideally).

24.9 CONCLUSIONS

Disposable gloves are personal protective equipment that should be considered only as a last resort, or a last line of defense, in terms of dermal protection. Gloves should always be used when chemicals are handled, and other workplace controls fail to provide sufficient dermal protection. Minor risks can sometimes be averted by using disposable gloves that are disposed of often or immediately after first contact with the chemical, but it is necessary to know what polymer type and thickness of gloves can give protection against the chemicals used, as well as how long the gloves should be used to provide adequate protection. Further, glove labels with information on the material type and thickness should be ideally checked to guarantee adequate gloves are selected. Blue color may not mean it is a nitrile material, as disposable gloves now come in many colors and presentations and brands are not as consistent anymore on matching the glove color to a certain material, as they did in the early years of disposable gloves.

Chemical resistance and permeation information for disposable gloves has become more and more available. However, if no information is available from the manufacturers and distributors of gloves or in the peer review literature, then it is prudent to use thicker, chemical protective gloves instead. This is especially the case for chemical mixtures or formulations, in which the gloves may fail sooner than expected compared with pure substances alone. Regardless of having chosen the best protective disposable gloves for a certain work task, the users should always inspect gloves during donning, as disposable gloves are prone to holes and other imperfections that can jeopardize protection. Users must also observe gloves for signs of chemical action, such as color change, swelling, cracking, or deformation, as those signs would indicate that the gloves are degrading and not providing needed chemical resistance.

ACKNOWLEDGMENTS

Thanks to Boston University graduate student Paavni Sangal for her assistance with the literature review and bibliography for this chapter.

REFERENCES

1. Phalen, R.N., Dubrovskiy, A.V., Brown, B.C., Gvetadze, A.R., Bustillos, M., and Ogbonmwan, J. 2020. Chemical permeation of similar disposable nitrile gloves exposed to volatile organic compounds with different polarities. Part 2. Predictive polymer properties. *J Occup Environ Hyg* 17(4):172–180.
2. Council of the European Communities. 1989. Council directive 89/686/EEC of 21 December 1989 on the approximation of the laws of the Member States relating to personal protective equipment. *Off J Eur Commun* L 399:18.
3. Council of the European Communities. 1989. Council directive 93/42/EEC of 14 June 1993 concerning medical devices. *Off J Eur Commun* L 169:0001-0043.
4. FDA. 2020. *Medical Glove Guidance Manual*. Washington, DC: U.S. Food and Drug Administration (FDA). Available from https://www.fda.gov/regulatory-information/search-fda-guidance-documents/medical-glove-guidance-manual.
5. Council of the European Communities. 1989. Council directive 89/656/EEC of 30 November 1989 on the minimum health and safety requirements for the use by workers of personal protective equipment at the workplace. *Off J Eur Commun* L 393:18.
6. OSHA. 2020. *Personal Protective Equipment*. Washington, DC: Occupational Safety and Health Administration (OSHA), U.S. Department of Labor. Available from https://www.osha.gov/pls/publications/publication.athruz?pType=Industry&pID=158.
7. OSHA. 2020. *Dermal Exposure Control and Prevention*. Washington, DC: Occupational Safety and Health Administration (OSHA), U.S. Department of Labor. Available from https://www.osha.gov/dermal-exposure/control-prevention.
8. Mellstrom, G.A. 1996. The value and limitations of protective gloves in medical health service: part II. *Dermatol Nurs* 8:287.
9. Mellström, G.A., and Boman, A. 2000. Protective gloves, in *Handbook of Occupational Dermatology*, L. Kanerva, P. Eisner, J.E. Wahlberg, and H.I. Maibach, Eds. Berlin: Springer.
10. ASTM International. 2020. *ASTM F739-20, Standard Test Method for Permeation of Liquids and Gases Through Protective Clothing Materials under Conditions of Continuous Contact*. West Conshohocken, PA: ASTM International.
11. European Committee for Standardization (CEN). 2016. *EN 374-1:2016 Protective Gloves against Dangerous Chemicals and Micro-Organisms. Part 1: Terminology and Performance Requirements for Chemical Risks*. Brussels: European Committee for Standardization (CEN).
12. European Committee for Standardization (CEN). 2018. *EN 16523-1:2018 Determination of Material Resistance to Permeation by Chemicals - Part 1: Permeation by Potentially Hazardous Liquid Chemicals under Conditions of Continuous Contact*. Brussels: European Committee for Standardization (CEN).

13. Banaee, S., and Que Hee, S.S. 2019. Glove permeation of chemicals: The state of the art of current practice, Part 1: Basics and the permeation standards. *J Occup Environ Hyg* 16(12):827–839.

14. Mader, R.M., Rizovski, B., Steger, G.G., Moser, K., Rainer, H., and Dittrich, C. 1991. Permeability of latex membranes to anti-cancer drugs. *Int J Pharm* 68:151.

15. Dinter-Heidorm, H., and Carstens, G. 1992. Comparative study on protective gloves for handling cytotoxic medicines: a model study with carmustine. *Pharm Weekblad Sci Ed* 14:180.

16. Darre, E., Vedel, P., and Jensen, J.S. 1987. Skin protection against methylmethacrylate. *Acta Orthop Scand* 58:236.

17. Munksgaard, E.C. 1992. Permeability of protective gloves to (di)methacrylates in resinous dental materials. *Scand J Dent Res* 100:189.

18. Connor, T.H., Laidlaw, J.L., Theiss, J.C., Anderson, R.W., and Matney, T.S. 1984. Permeability of latex and polyvinyl chloride gloves to carmustine. *Am J Hosp Pharm* 41:676.

19. Singleton, L.C., and Connor, T.H. 1999. An evaluation of the permeability of chemotherapy gloves to three cancer chemotherapy drugs. *Oncol Nurs Forum* 26:1491.

20. Andersson, T., and Bruze, M. 1999. In vivo testing of the protective efficacy of gloves against allergen-containing products using an open chamber system. *Contact Dermatitis* 41:260.

21. Timmer, C. 2000. Antimicrobials and disinfectants, in *Handbook of Occupational Dermatology*, Kanerva, L., Eisner, P., Wahlberg, J.E., and Maibach, H.I., Eds. Berlin: Springer.

22. Heinemann, C., Sinaiko, R., and Maibach, H.I. 2002. Immunological contact urticaria and anaphylaxis to chlorhexidine: overview. *Exog Dermatol* 1:186.

23. Jensen, O. 1981. Contact allergy to propylene oxide and isopropyl alcohol in a skin disinfectant swab. *Contact Dermatitis* 7:148.

24. Ojajärvi, J., Mäkelä, P., and Rantasalo, I. 1977. Failure of hand disinfection with frequent hand washing: a need for prolonged field studies. *J Hyg (Cambridge)* 79:107.

25. Packham, C.L. 1998. *Essentials of Occupational Skin Management*. Southport, UK: Limited Edition Press.

26. Mäkelä, E.A., Vainiotalo, S., and Peltonen, K. 2003. The permeability of surgical gloves to seven chemicals commonly used in hospitals. *Ann Occup Hyg* 47:313.

27. Mäkelä, E.A. 2003. The permeability of surgical gloves to chemicals commonly used in hospitals. Paper presented at *First World Congress on Work-Related and Environmental Allergy (1st WOREAL)*. Helsinki, July 9–12.

28. Mäkelä, E.A., Vainiotalo, S., and Peltonen, K. 2003. Permeation of 70% isopropyl alcohol through surgical gloves: comparison of the standard methods ASTM F 739 and EN 374. *Ann Occup Hyg* 47:305.

29. Monticello, M.V., and Gaber, D.J. 1999. Glove resistance to permeation by a 7.5% hydrogen peroxide sterilizing and disinfecting solution. *Am J Infect Control* 27:364.

30. Forsberg, K., and Keith, L.H. 1999. *Chemical Protective Clothing — Performance Index*, 2nd ed. New York: John Wiley & Sons.

31. Schwope, A., Costas, P.P., Mond, C.R., Nolen, R.L., Conoley, M., Garcia, D.B., Walters, D.B., and Prokopetz, A.T. 1988. Gloves for protection from aqueous formaldehyde: permeation resistance and human factors analyses. *Appl Ind Hyg* 3:167.

32. Lehman, P.A., Franz, T.J., and Guin, J.D. 1994. Penetration of glutaraldehyde through glove material: Tactylon versus natural rubber latex. *Contact Dermatitis* 30:176.

33. Mellström, G.A., Lindberg, M., and Boman, A. 1992. Permeation and destructive effects of disinfectants on protective gloves. *Contact Dermatitis* 26:163.

34. Jordan, S.L., Stowers, M.F., Trawick, E.G., and Theis, A.B. 1996. Glutaraldehyde permeation: choosing the proper glove. *Am J Infect Control* 24:67.

35. Phalen, R.N., Le, T., and Wong, W.K. 2014. Changes in chemical permeation of disposable latex, nitrile, and vinyl gloves exposed to simulated movement. *J Occup Environ Hyg* 11(11):716–721. DOI: 10.1080/15459624.2014.908259.

36. Phalen, R.N., and Wong, W.K. 2015. Polymer properties associated with chemical permeation performance of disposable nitrile rubber gloves. *J of Applied Polymer Sci* 132(6):41449. DOI: 10.1002/app.41449.

37. Anderson, R. 2006. *Your Lungs, Your Skin, Your Life.* Available from https://www.bodyshopbusiness.com/your-lungs-your-skin-your-life/.

38. Bello, D., Herrick, C.A., Smith, T.J., et al. 2007. Skin exposure to isocyanates: reasons for concern. *Environ Health Perspect* 115(3):328–335.

39. NIOSH. 2014. *NIOSH Skin Notation Profiles: Methyl Isocyanate.* Washington, DC: National Institute for Occupational Safety and Health (NIOSH), Centers for Disease Control and Prevention. Available from https://www.cdc.gov/niosh/docs/2014-145/.

40. NIOSH. 2014. *NIOSH Skin Notation Profiles: Isophorone Diisocyanate.* Washington, DC: National Institute for Occupational Safety and Health (NIOSH), Centers for Disease Control and Prevention. Available from https://www.cdc.gov/niosh/docs/2014-148/.

41. OSHA. 2021. *Isocyanates.* Washington, DC: Occupational Safety and Health Administration (OSHA), U.S. Department of Labor. Available from https://www.osha.gov/isocyanates.

42. NIOSH. 2021. *Isocyanates.* Washington, DC: National Institute for Occupational Safety and Health (NIOSH), Centers for Disease Control and Prevention. Available from https://www.cdc.gov/niosh/topics/isocyanates/default.html.

43. Ceballos, D.M., Yost, M.G., Whittaker, S.G., Reeb-Whitaker, C., Camp, J., and Dills, R. 2010. Development of a permeation panel to test dermal protective clothing against sprayed coatings. *Ann Occup Hyg* 55(2):214–27.

44. Ceballos, D., Reeb-Whitaker, C., Glazer, P., Murphy-Robinson, H., and Yost, M. 2014. Understanding factors that influence protective glove use among automotive spray painters. *J Occup Environ Hyg* 11(5):306–313.

45. Mäkelä, E.A., Henriks-Eckerman, M.L., Ylinen, K., Vuokko, A., and Suuronen, K. 2014. Permeation tests of glove and clothing materials against sensitizing chemicals using diphenylmethane diisocyanate as an example. *Ann Occup Hyg* 58(7):921–930.

46. Henriks-Eckerman, M.L., and Mäkelä, E. 2015. A new penetration test method: protection efficiency of glove and clothing materials against diphenylmethane diisocyanate (MDI). *Ann Occup Hyg* 59(2):221–231.

47. Mellette, M.P., Bello, D., Xue, Y., Yost, M., Bello, A., and Woskie, S. 2018. Testing of disposable protective garments against isocyanate permeation from spray polyurethane foam insulation. *Ann Work Expo Health* 62(6):754–764.

48. Mellette, M.P., Bello, D., Xue, Y., Yost, M., Bello, A., and Woskie, S. 2019. Evaluation of disposable protective garments against isocyanate permeation and penetration from polyurethane anticorrosion coatings. *Annals of Work Exposures and Health* 63(5):592–603.

49. Knowles, R.S., and Virden, J.E. 1980. Handling of injectable antineoplastic agents. *Br Med J* 30:589.

50. Sessink, P.J., Cerná, M., Rössner, P., Pastorková, A., Bavarová, H., Franková, K., Anzion, R.B., and Bos, R.P. 1994. Urinary cyclophosphamide excretion and chromosomal aberrations in peripheral blood lymphocytes after occupational exposure to antineoplastic agents. *Mutat Res* 309:193.

51. Knowles, S.R., Gupta, A.K., Shear, N.H., and Sauder, D. 1995. Azathioprine hypersensitivity-like reactions — A case report and a review of the literature. *Clin Exp Dermatol* 20:353.

52. Jolanki, R., Alanko, K., Pfäffli, P., Estlander, T., and Kanerva, L. 1997. Occupational allergic contact dermatitis from 5-chloro-1-methyl-4-nitroimidazole. *Contact Dermatitis* 36:53.

53. Lauerma, A.I., Koivuluhta, M., and Alenius, H. 2001. Recalitrant allergic contact dermatitis from azathioprine tablets. *Contact Dermatitis* 44:129.

54. Sessink, P.J., Van de Kerkhof, M.C., Anzion, R.B., Noordhoek, J., and Bos, R.P. 1994. Environmental contamination and assessment of exposure to antineoplastic agents by determination of cyclophosphamide in urine of exposed pharmacy technicians: is skin absorption an important exposure route? *Arch Environ Health* 49:165.

55. Kromhout, H., Hoek, F., Uitterhoeve, R., Huijbers, R., Overmars, R.F., Anzion, R., and Vermeulen, R. 2000. Postulating a dermal pathway for exposure to anti-neoplastic drugs among hospital workers. Applying a conceptual model to the results of three workplace surveys. *Ann Occup. Hyg* 44:551.

56. Ensslin, A.S., Stoll, Y., Pethran, A., Pfaller, A., Römmelt, H., and Fruhmann, G. 1994. Biological monitoring of cyclophosphamide and ifosfamide in urine of hospital personnel occupationally exposed to cytostatic drugs. *Occup Environ Med* 51:229.

57. Banaee, S., and Que Hee, S.S. 2019. Glove permeation of chemicals: The state of the art of current practice, Part 2: Research emphases on high boiling point compounds and simulating the donned glove environment. *J Occup Environ Hyg* 17(4):135–164. DOI: 10.1080/15459624.2020.1721509.

58. ASTM International. 2019. *ASTM D6978-05(2019), Standard Practice for Assessment of Resistance of Medical Gloves to Permeation by Chemotherapy Drugs.* West Conshohocken, PA: ASTM International.

59. Connor, T.H. 1999. Permeability of nitrile rubber, latex, polyurethane and neoprene gloves to 18 antineoplastic drugs. *Am J Health Syst Pharm* 56:2450.

60. Laidlaw, J.L., Connor, T.H., Theiss, J.C., Anderson, R.W., and Matney, T.S. 1984. Permeability of latex and polyvinyl chloride gloves to 20 antineoplastic drugs. *Am J Hosp Pharm* 41(12):2618.

61. Stoikes, M.E., Carlson, J.D., Farris, F.F., and Walker, P.R. 1987. Permeability of latex and polyvinyl chloride gloves to fluorouracil and methotrexate. *Am J Hosp Pharm* 44:1341.

62. Connor, T.H. 1995. Permeability testing of glove materials for use with cancer chemotherapy drugs. *Oncology* 52:256.

63. Gross, E.R., and Groce, D.F. 1998. An evaluation of nitrile gloves as an alternative to natural rubber latex for handling chemotherapeutic agents. *J Oncol Pharm Pract* 4:165.

64. Slevin, M.L., Ang, L.M., Johnston, A., and Turner, P. 1984. The efficiency of protective gloves used in the handling of cytotoxic drugs. *Cancer Chemother. Pharmacol* 12:151.

65. Mellström, G.A., Johansson, S., and Nyhammar, E. 1996. Barrier effect of gloves against cytostatic drugs, in *Prevention of Contact Dermatitis*, Eisner, P., Lachapelle, J.M., Wahlberg, J.E., and Maibach, H.I., Eds. Basel: Karger. *Curr Probl Dermatol* 25:163.

66. Connor, T.H., and Xiang, Q. 2000. The effect of isopropyl alcohol on the permeation of gloves exposed to antineoplastic agents. *J Oncol Pharm Pract* 6:109.

67. Colligan, S.A., and Horstman, S.W. 1990. Permeation of cancer chemotherapeutic drugs through glove materials under static and flexed conditions. *Appl Occup Environ Hyg* 5:848.

68. Klein, M.,, Rau, S., Samev, N., and Carstens, G. 1999. Protection offered by selected medical gloves made of either latex or a synthetic elastomer against exposure to nine cytotoxic agents. *Environ Health Persp* 5:152.

69. Wallemacq, P.E., Capron, A., Vanbinst, R., Boeckmans, E., Gillard, J., and Favier, B. 2006. Permeability of 13 different gloves to 13 cytotoxic agents under controlled dynamic conditions. *Am J Health-System Pharm* 63(6):547–556. DOI: 10.2146/ajhp050197.

70. Capron, A., Destree, J., Jacobs, P., and Wallemacq, P. 2012. Permeability of gloves to selected chemotherapeutic agents after treatment with alcohol or isopropyl alcohol. *Am J Health-System Pharm* 69(19):1665–1670. DOI: 10. 2146/ajhp110733.

71. Boccellino, M., Pedata, P., Castiglia, L., La Porta, R., Pieri, M., Quagliuolo, L., Acampora, A., Sannolo, N., and Miraglia, N. 2010. Doxorubicin can penetrate nitrile gloves and induces apoptosis in keratinocytes cell line. *Toxicol Lett* 197(2):61–68. DOI: 10.1016/j.toxlet.2010.04.026.

72. Pieri, M., Quagliuolo, L., La Porta, R., Silvestre, A., Miraglia, N., Pedata, P., Acampora, A., Castiglia, L., Sannolo, N., and Boccellino, M. 2013. Epirubicin permeation of personal protective equipment can induce apoptosis in keratinocytes. *J Expo Sci Environ Epidemiol* 23(4):428–434. DOI: 10.1038/jes.2012.38.

73. Oriyama, T., Yamamoto, T., Yanagihara, Y., Nara, K., Abe, T., Nakajima, K., Aoyama, T., and Suzuki, H. 2017. Evaluation of the permeation of antineoplastic agents through medical gloves of varying materials and thicknesses and with varying surface treatments. *J Pharm Health Care Sci* 3(1):13. DOI: 10.1186/s40780-017-0082-y.

74. Krzeminska, S., Posniak, M., and Szewczynska, M. 2018. Resistance of gloves and protective clothing materials to permeation of cytostatic solutions. *Int J Occup Med Environ Health* 31(3):341–350. DOI: 10.13075/ijomeh.1896.01140.

75. Nalin, M., Hug, G., Boeckmans, E., Machon, C., Favier, B., and Guitton, J. 2021. Permeation measurement of 27 chemotherapy drugs after simulated dynamic testing on 15 surgical and examination gloves: A knowledge update. *J Oncol Pharm Pract* 27(6):1395–1408. DOI: 10.1177/1078155220950423.

76. Oriyama, T., Yamamoto, T., Nara, K., Kawano, Y., Nakajima, K., Suzuki, H., and Aoyama, T. 2020. Prediction of the permeability of antineoplastic agents through nitrile medical gloves by zone classification based on their physicochemical properties. *J Pharm Health Care Sci* 6:23. DOI: 10.1186/s40780-020-00179-3.

77. Hämeilä, M., Aaltonen, K., Santonen, T., Hesso, A., Tornaeus, J., Järviluoma, E., and Peltonen, K. 2003. *Altistuminen solunsalpaajille apteekki ja hoitotyössä* [Occupational exposure to cytostatic drugs in pharmaceutical and healthcare work, in Finnish]. Työterveyslaitos, Helsinki: Finnish Institute of Occupational Health.

78. Easty, A.C., Coakley, N., Cheng, R., Cividino, M., Savage, P., Tozer, R., and White, R.E. 2015. Safe handling of cytotoxics: Guideline recommendations. *Curr Oncol* 22(1):e27–e37. DOI: 10.3747/co.21.2151.

79. Connor, T.H. 1993. An evaluation of the permeability of disposable polypropylene-based protective gowns to a battery of cancer chemotherapy drugs. *Appl Occup Environ Hyg* 8:785.

80. Laidlaw, J.L., Connor, T.H., Theiss, J.C., Anderson, R.W., and Matney, T.S. 1985. Permeability of four disposable protective-clothing materials to seven antineoplastic drugs. *Ant J Hosp Pharm* 42:2449.

81. OSHA. 2021. *Controlling Occupational Exposure to Hazardous Drugs*. Washington, DC: Occupational Safety and Health Administration (OSHA), U.S. Department of Labor. Available from https://www.osha.gov/hazardous-drugs/controlling-occex.

82. OSHA. 2021. *Solvents*. Washington, DC: Occupational Safety and Health Administration (OSHA), U.S. Department of Labor. Available from https://www.osha.gov/solvents.

83. Fiserova-Bergerova, V., Pierce, J.T., and Droz, P.O. 1990. Dermal absorption potential of industrial chemicals: Criteria for skin notation. *Am J Ind Med* 17:617.

84. NIOSH. 2021. *Organic Solvents.* Washington, DC: National Institute for Occupational Safety and Health (NIOSH), Centers for Disease Control and Prevention. Available from https://www.cdc.gov/niosh/topics/organsolv/default.html.

85. Trans, J.Q., Ceballos, D.M., Dills, R.L., Yost, M.G., and Morgan, M.S. 2012. Transport of a solvent mixture across two glove materials when applied in a paint matrix. *Arch Environ Contam Toxicol* 63(1):169–176.

86. Chao, K.P., Lee, P.H., and Wu, M.J. 2003. Organic solvents permeation through protective nitrile gloves. *J Hazard Mater* 99(2):191–201.

87. Chao, K.P., Wang, V.S., and Lee, P.H. 2004. Modeling organic solvents permeation through protective gloves. *J Occup Environ Hyg* 1(2):57–61.

88. Gao, P., El-Ayouby, N., and Wassell, J.T. 2005. Change in permeation parameters and the decontamination efficacy of three chemical protective gloves after repeated exposures to solvents and thermal decontaminations. *Am J Ind Med* 47(2):131–143.

89. Banaee, S., and Que Hee, S.S. 2017. Permeation of limonene through disposable nitrile gloves using a dextrous robot hand. *J Occup Health* 59(2):131–138.

90. Brown, B.C., Dubrovskiy, A., Gvetadze, A.R., and Phalen, R.N. 2020. Chemical permeation of similar disposable nitrile gloves exposed to volatile organic compounds with different polarities: Part 1: Product variation. *J Occup Environ Hyg* 17(4):165–171.

91. Stull, J.O., Thomas, R.W., and James, L.E. 2002. A comparative analysis of glove permeation resistance to paint stripping formulations. *Am Ind Hyg Assoc J* 63(1):62–71.

92. Chao, K.P., Hsu, Y.P., and Chen, S.Y. 2008. Permeation of aromatic solvent mixtures through nitrile protective gloves. *J Hazard Mater* 153(3):1059–1066.

93. Vo, E. 2000. A quantitative study of aromatic amine permeation through protective gloves using amine adsorptive pads. *Am Ind Hyg Assoc J* 61:837.

94. Weeks, Jr., R.W., and Dean, B.J. 1977. Permeation of methanolic aromatic amine solutions through commercially available glove materials. *Am Ind Hyg Assoc J* 38:721.

95. Sansone, E.B., and Tewari, Y.B. 1978. The permeability of laboratory gloves to selected nitrosoamines, in *Environmental Aspects of N-Nitroso Compounds*, E.A. Walker, Ed. Lyon: International Agency for Research on Cancer.

96. Ansell Edmont. 1997. *TNT Thin Nitrile Technology, Product Information Data Sheet.* Aalst, Belgium: Ansell Edmont Industrial, Inc.

97. Nelson, G.O., Priante, S.J., Strong, M., Anderson, D., and Fallon-Carine, J. 2000. Permeation of substituted silanes and siloxanes through selected gloves and protective clothing. *Am Ind Hyg Assoc J* 61(5):709–714.

98. Lind, M.L., Johnsson, S., Meding, B., and Boman, A. 2007. Permeability of hair dye compounds p-phenylenediamine, toluene-2,5-diaminesulfate and resorcinol through protective gloves in hairdressing. *Ann Occup Hyg* 51(5):479–485.

99. Lee, H.S., and Lin, Y.W. 2009. Permeation of hair dye ingredients, p-phenylenediamine and aminophenol isomers, through protective gloves. *Ann Occup Hyg* 53(3):289–296.

100. Munksgaard, E.C. 2000. Permeability of protective gloves by HEMA and TEGDMA in the presence of solvents. *Acta Odontol Scand* 58:57.

101. Blaynye, M.B. 2001. The need for empirically derived permeation data for personal protective equipment: the death of Dr. Karen Wetterhahn. *Appl Occup Environ Hyg* 16:233.

102. Stampfer, J.F., McLeod, M.J., Betts, M.R., Martinez, A.M., and Berardinelli, S.P. 1984. Permeation of polychlorinated biphenyls and solutions of these substances through selected protective clothing materials. *Am Ind Hyg Assoc J* 45:634.

103. Chao, K.P., Wang, P., Chen, C.P., and Tang, P.Y. 2011. Assessment of skin exposure to N,N-dimethylformamide and methyl ethylketone through chemical protective gloves and decontamination of gloves for reuse purposes. *Sci Total Environ* 409(6):1024–1032. DOI: 10.1016/j.scitotenv.2010.11.034.

104. Mäkelä, E.A., and Tammela, E. 2000. *Suojakäsineiden hankinta, valinta ja käyttö autoalalla* [Purchase, selection and usage of protective gloves in the field of vehicle repairing, in Finnish]. Study Report for Centre for Occupational Safety. Helsinki: Finnish Institute of Occupational Health.
105. Xu, W., and Que Hee, S.S. 2007. Permeation of a straight oil metalworking fluid through disposable nitrile, chloroprene, vinyl, and latex gloves. *J Hazard Mater* 147(3):923–929.
106. Chin, J.Y., and Batterman, S.A. 2010. Permeation of gasoline, diesel, bioethanol (E85), and biodiesel (B20) fuels through six glove materials. *J Occup Environ Hyg* 7(7):417–428.
107. Zellers, E.T., and Sulewski, R. 1993. Modeling the temperature dependence of N-methylpyrrolidone permeation through butyl- and natural-rubber gloves. *Am Ind Hyg Assoc J* 54(9):465–479.

25 The Selection and Use of Gloves against Pesticides

J.B. Nielsen and R.N. Phalen

CONTENTS

DOI: 10.1201/9781003126874-29

25.1 INTRODUCTION

Pesticides are developed with the purpose of being toxic to weeds (herbicides), fungi (fungicides), or insects (insecticides). The majority of them are, however, also to some extent toxic to humans. The toxicity profile of pesticides as a group varies and covers a wide range of potencies, bioavailabilities (the degree to which they will be absorbed through the skin), and endpoints from irritation and allergy to neurotoxicity and cancer.

Except for specific crops in confined areas, the use of pesticides is probably unavoidable in maintaining sufficient outcomes to cover the demand for food and other consumer products worldwide. The pragmatic preventive strategy is therefore to use pesticides with the lowest human toxicity and to reduce exposure as much as possible.

A range of older pesticides with high toxicities has been banned in several countries but is still used in other countries where cost effectiveness outplays human and ecological risk evaluations. Thus, primary prevention through substitution is moving only slowly forward, and prevention of human toxicity due to pesticides will still have to focus on exposure reduction. Legislative regulations have over the years reduced occupational exposure through inhalation considerably, and dermal exposure is now in many occupational settings of equal importance or even the dominating route of exposure to pesticides.[1–3]

25.2 DERMAL EXPOSURE TO PESTICIDES

Pesticides are used in the production of fruits, vegetables, grain crops, ornamental flowers, and plants, and in some areas of the world also for farm animals (e.g., sheep dipping), which generate diverse exposure scenarios from the frequent, specialized indoor use by skilled workers in confined areas of greenhouses to the less frequent use in outdoor production facilities. The different intensities may be illustrated by the fact that one study demonstrated that the average Danish ornamental greenhouse is treated with pesticides or growth retardants more than 50 times a year compared to conventional farmland, only being treated two to three times a year.[4] A frequent use of pesticides will have obvious implications for the possibility of reducing exposure through the use of long reentry intervals.

Occupational exposure to pesticides may occur during production, mixing, and loading of concentrated sales formulations, distribution and handling of diluted pesticides, and through reentry activities. The different tasks are characterized by causing a combination of short-term exposure (splashes, etc.) to concentrated formulations and medium- to long-term exposures to lower concentrations of pesticides or residues remaining on stems, leaves, or topsoil after treatment. Adherence to established reentry times can help minimize exposures in the latter.

A recurrent problem using tertiary prevention (i.e., use of gloves or other personal protective equipment [PPE]) is the lack of compliance with regulations among exposed individuals.[5–10] Thus, the use of a specified type of glove may work in some more temperate areas of the world, whereas the same gloves cannot be worn with comfort in warmer, more humid areas. Thus, recommendations on the use of specified gloves will also have to be considered. Another important caveat is that the employer not only has to buy the gloves but also educate/instruct the employees as to why, when, how, and for how long they have to use the gloves. Otherwise, tertiary prevention will not work.

In summary, working with pesticides is by definition hazardous, given the toxicity profile of most pesticides. Prevention must therefore concentrate on informing users about the hazard and about ways to reduce the risk. Gloves have repeatedly been demonstrated to significantly reduce the exposure to and toxic effects of pesticides.[1,2,7,9–11] In a thorough review, gloves and other forms of protective clothing have been shown to provide effective protection against a variety of dermal hazards, including pesticides.[12] Protection factors were 88% on average for gloves and 90% on average for suits. An important preventive aspect is, however, the correct selection and use of gloves. Thus, each exposure scenario has its distinctive characteristics that will influence recommendations regarding the selection and use of protective gloves to minimize dermal exposure.

25.3 COMFORT AND USE OF GLOVES

Comfort and resistance toward penetration of toxicants are two of the key issues that influence the choice and ultimately use of gloves in a given situation. The longer the time people have to wear gloves, the higher the demands for comfort. The higher the concentrations of the pesticides people have to handle, the higher the risk for toxicity, and the higher the demand for resistance to penetration. Unfortunately, both factors are not always fulfilled in one type of glove, and if so then at a price that often makes the gloves unrealistic for many practical settings, especially in many developing countries. Ideally, workers should always use the glove that gives maximal protection. As this glove is not necessarily the glove with maximal comfort, we have a difficult choice: Should we recommend a glove that gives maximal protection but is not used to the desired degree due to a lack of comfort, or should we recommend a glove with suboptimal penetration characteristics but with a comfort that will give satisfying compliance with the use of gloves? The choice should rely on knowledge of the specific pesticides used and the exposure scenarios.

The existence of reusable gloves complicates the situation further as one may afford higher quality (to a higher price) if the gloves are used repeatedly. This choice does, however, also come with a price as discussed later (Section 25.9), as there will be a relevant risk for secondary exposure due to a lack of sufficient donning and doffing skills among the glove users.

25.4 EXPOSURE SCENARIOS

25.4.1 MIXING AND LOADING

Pesticides are normally delivered from the producer to the end user in concentrations that by far exceed the concentrations used for the treatment of crops or animals. During the mixing and loading of pesticides, there is a potential for exposure to concentrated pesticides. The exposure will most often be characterized by being an occasional short-term exposure, e.g., splashes. An uncontrolled splash may, however, affect skin areas on the forearm not covered by traditional short gloves. Further, even short-term exposure to concentrated pesticides may impose a significant risk of toxicity. The short-term exposure to potential high concentrations, therefore, suggests that there should be a focus on resistance and coverage of forearms as well as hands and an acceptance of slightly lower comfort. These gloves are often reused several times, and it is extremely important that cleaning of gloves after use, as well as storage, assures that contamination of the inside of the gloves is avoided (discussed in Section 25.9). Otherwise, the use of these gloves becomes a false guarantee against exposure to pesticides.

25.4.2 DISTRIBUTION

The distribution of pesticides may involve automatic spraying, spraying from person-driven vehicles, hand-carried spraying, or watering systems. Worth noting is that the distribution of pesticides may cause very significant dermal exposure to large parts of the body besides the hands, as well as pulmonary exposure. In these cases, gloves will only be part of the preventive effort to reduce body dose. The distribution of pesticides involves varying exposure times to varying concentrations of pesticides with varying toxicities. However, the concentrations will not be expected to cause acute toxicity following accidental short-term exposures. Therefore, the focus must be on avoiding long-term dermal contact with pesticides. This implies the use of gloves at all times during spraying operations, which again requires a certain degree of comfort if good compliance should be attained. For workers to comply with the last recommendation, a glove with high comfort is needed—a situation that may incur a compromise with the demand for maximal protection capacity. Physical, as well as chemical, durability may, however, be a problem with these types of gloves, and very often the recommendation will be to change gloves with shorter intervals and avoid reusing these essentially disposable gloves.

25.4.3 REENTRY

Reentry exposure occurs when workers enter areas recently treated with pesticides. Depending on crops and specific work tasks, workers may have dermal exposure to pesticide residues deposited on leaves, stems, flowers, or soil. The pesticides will stay on the plants or the topsoil for varying periods depending on chemical stability, stability against sunlight, and metabolism of the active ingredient. The concentrations will, however, be considerably lower than during mixing and loading, although the exposure duration may be an entire working day. Some of the handling procedures may require a certain degree of dexterity that may be difficult to obtain with all glove types and materials. As exposure occurs with varying intensity of time and concentration, and as workers may not always know when they are exposed, recommendations will follow two lines. The first is to avoid exposure by defining reentry intervals that will allow the pesticide to wash off or degrade before workers handle the pesticide-treated crop. The second is to use gloves whenever handling plants recently treated with pesticides with an appreciable potential for dermal absorption. For workers to comply with the last recommendation, a glove with a high comfort is needed—a situation that again may incur a compromise with the demand for maximal protection capacity. Physical, as well as chemical, durability may, however, be a problem with these types of gloves, and very often the recommendation will be to change gloves with shorter intervals and avoid reusing these essentially disposable gloves.

25.4.4   NON-OCCUPATIONAL USE

Exposure to pesticides occurs in occupational as well as non-occupational settings. The two settings differ in important ways. The occupational setting is most often regulated by occupational health authorities with requirements on training and education and the use of PPE in different and specified exposure scenarios. In contrast, protection against dermal exposures during non-occupational use, e.g. home-gardening, is left to the consumer, who is dependent on the available written product labeling, which often lacks information on the proper use of PPE. A stronger incentive or legislation may be needed to further the inclusion of this information in the product labeling for the end user. Further, users may not be aware that different pesticides have different penetration characteristics through gloves.[13] Information on the use of gloves will need to be clear and simple: (1) use disposable nitrile gloves, (2) replace them after each use or after 2–3 h, whatever comes first, and (3) wash hands and affected areas of the body following contact, use, and before eating. Eventually, dermatologists should be aware that some skin diseases may worsen due to the prolonged use of gloves as they cause a strong occlusion of the hands (see Chapter 19 for more information).

25.5   IMPORTANT DETERMINANTS DESCRIBING PENETRATION CHARACTERISTICS OF GLOVES

Agricultural chemicals may cause severe acute toxicity after short-term exposure to high concentrations, but equally important are the long-term effects observed after prolonged exposure to lower doses. The selection of the best glove is therefore an integrated evaluation of different glove characteristics such as comfort, durability, and penetration characteristics.

Penetration characteristics may be described using breakthrough time and penetration rate. Breakthrough time is one of the most widely used parameters to judge the quality of a glove. The breakthrough time describes the time between the onset of exposure and until the first measurable amount of pesticide emerges on the inside of the glove. Breakthrough times ranging from less than 15 min and up to more than 24 h have been reported for different pesticides through different glove materials.[14–22] The resistance of a specific glove material against penetration will depend on pesticide,[14–22] as well as formulation.[3,15,18,20,22,23] The breakthrough time will, however, not say anything about the amount of pesticide absorbed into the glove as a potential reservoir for later penetration (if the gloves are used again) or the penetration rate after breakthrough time.

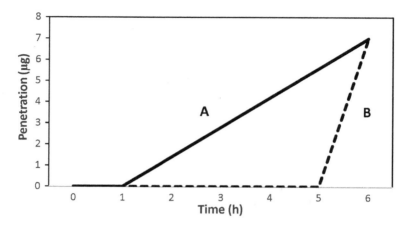

FIGURE 25.1   Penetration of two pesticides (A and B) through a glove. Penetration of A and B after 6 h are identical, but different breakthrough times and penetration rates are observed.

Penetration rates may be described directly as the total amount of a pesticide penetrating a glove within a specified time from onset of exposure,[2,15] as penetration rate after breakthrough, or indirectly as choline esterase activity in the receptor chamber after a specified exposure time to a choline esterase inhibitor (e.g., organophosphates or carbamates).[24,25] This information is, however, not very useful without knowledge of the breakthrough time from the same experiment. As illustrated in Figure 25.1, two gloves may have identical penetration rates observed over a 6-h period, but definitively different penetration characteristics. Thus, if the expected exposure time was 4 h, glove B would definitively be preferred. Therefore, any quantitative information on penetration must be supplemented by information on breakthrough time.

- If gloves are disposable, information on breakthrough time is sufficient to make a safe choice.
- Ideally, gloves should be changed whenever exposure time approaches the breakthrough time.
- If exposure continues after the breakthrough time, information on penetration rates must be included in the safety evaluation.
- If the same gloves are used several times (with or without washing/cleansing), information on penetration rates as well as information on the extent to which a possible reservoir will affect penetration characteristics must be included in the safety evaluation.

25.6   PERMEATION OF PESTICIDES THROUGH GLOVES

25.6.1   CARBAMATES

Data on penetration characteristics for these insecticides through gloves were identified for carbaryl, methomyl, sulfallate, methiocarb, and pirimicarb.[3,19,26–29] When carbaryl was tested for permeation breakthrough time using two alternative test procedures, PVC (polyvinyl chloride), nitrile butyl rubber, natural rubber, and Neoprene® (registered trademark of DuPont) all demonstrated breakthrough times exceeding 8 h.[19] Likewise, gloves made of butyl rubber, nitrile, or Viton® (registered trademark of DuPont) demonstrated breakthrough times against sulfallate exceeding 8 h, whereas Neoprene gloves offered complete resistance for 4 h only.[27] In two separate studies on chemical resistance and structural integrity, Raheel and Dai concluded that nitrile, butyl, and Viton exhibited a higher level of chemical and penetration resistance than did latex/natural rubber or PVC gloves.[28,29] Gloves made of polyethylene were penetrated by methomyl within 15 min.[26] A comparison of the penetration of pirimicarb and methiocarb through latex or nitrile gloves demonstrated that during an 18-h observation period, latex gloves reduced penetration of both carbamates by 50%, whereas the nitrile glove offered more than 90% protection against pirimicarb penetration.[3]

Generally, gloves made of nitrile, butyl rubber, and Viton appeared to offer the best protection against carbamates, though Neoprene also demonstrated long breakthrough times in one study.

25.6.2 PYRETHROIDS

Data on penetration characteristics for these insecticides through gloves were identified for cypermethrin, permethrin, and tefluthrin.[14,16,17,30] Breakthrough time for tefluthrin (as a granular pesticide) through gloves made of nitrile, Neoprene, or barrier laminate (Silver Shield™, trademark of Siebe North, Inc.) was above 24 h.[16] However, with increasing exposure time, increasing amounts of pesticide remained attached to or absorbed into the glove made of barrier laminate, and it was concluded that barrier laminate should be regarded as a single-use material, as gloves made of this material could not be cleaned.[30] Butyl rubber gloves demonstrated breakthrough times exceeding 8 h for cypermethrin.[17] In a study comparing the potential exposure (on the outside of the glove) with the actual exposure (on the inside of the glove), protection factors of 470, 200, and 96 against penetration of permethrin were obtained for two nitrile and one PVC glove, respectively. Thus, during a 20-min well-defined work schedule, the penetration of permethrin through gloves worn by volunteers was reduced to between 0.2% (nitrile) and 1% (PVC) of the potential exposure.[14]

Generally, the gloves made of nitrile, Neoprene, barrier laminate, butyl rubber, and PVC all demonstrated good protection against penetration of these pyrethroids, though one study suggested that barrier laminate (Silver Shield™) should be used only as a single-use material.[30]

25.6.3 ARYLOXYALCANOIC ACIDS (PHENOXY HERBICIDES)

Data on penetration characteristics for this group of herbicides through gloves were identified for 2,4-D and 4-chloro-2-methylphenoxyacetic acid (MCPA).[17–20,23] The permeation of two undiluted formulations of MCPA, one salt, and one ester was tested on four glove types.[20] There was no permeation of the salt formulation during a 24-h test period, but the ester formulation penetrated all four glove types (Viton, natural rubber, Neoprene, nitrile) with breakthrough times between 15 h (natural rubber and Neoprene) and 24 h (nitrile), and permeation rates for Neoprene exceeding the other glove materials with a factor of 3–7.[20] The nitrile gloves had the longest breakthrough time and the lowest permeation rate.[20]

Breakthrough times for 2,4-D through gloves made of nitrile, PVC, butyl, natural rubber, or Neoprene all exceeded 8 h,[17,19] although Harville and Que Hee note that Neoprene gloves were permeated much more than nitrile gloves.[23] Further, differences in glove permeation between two types of nitrile gloves (lined/unlined) and between different pesticide formulations were observed, stressing the difficulties of extrapolating penetration characteristics between pesticide formulations and even between gloves made of identical materials.[17,18,23]

Generally, all tested glove materials demonstrated good protection against these herbicides, although gloves made of nitrile offered the longest breakthrough time and the lowest permeation rate after breakthrough.

25.6.4 ORGANOCHLORINES

Only two studies on penetration characteristics for this group of insecticides through gloves were identified.[15,18] A study using DDT demonstrated that the penetration through nitrile butyl rubber during a 24-h study period was insignificant.[18] The second study used endosulfan (endosulfan, 34%, in xylene, 57%) as a test substance.[15] This study reported breakthrough times for seven glove materials (natural rubber, Neoprene, polyethylene, PVC, butyl rubber, Silver Shield™, nitrile) that, except for Neoprene (30–60 min), were in the region of 15 min.[15] The authors, however, did not clarify to what extent the formulation with 57% xylene affected the experimental outcome. A comparison of the quantity of endosulfan penetrating the gloves in an 8-h test period demonstrated that 10–100 times less endosulfan penetrated gloves made of Silver Shield™ and nitrile gloves than gloves made of the other materials.[15] The authors conclude that gloves made of nitrile rubber or Silver Shield™ were the most resistant to permeation, whereas natural rubber and polyethylene gloves were the least resistant.

Generally, the literature is scarce but suggests that breakthrough times for these insecticides may be very short, irrespective of glove material, but that gloves made of Silver Shield™ or nitrile are the most resistant.

25.6.5 ORGANOPHOSPHATES

Data on penetration characteristics for these insecticides through gloves were identified for azinphos-methyl, diazinon, ethyl parathion, malathion, methyl parathion, monocrotophos, tricresyl phosphate, and terbufos.[15,16,18,24,25,31,32] Breakthrough time for terbufos (tested as a granular pesticide) through gloves made of nitrile, Neoprene, or barrier laminate (Silver Shield™) was above 24 h. However, with increasing exposure time, increasing amounts of pesticide remained attached to or absorbed into the glove made of Neoprene.[16] Cotton gloves as well as 100% polypropylene gloves significantly reduced the penetration of the organophosphates azinphos-methyl and malathion in an *in vitro* epidermal test system but did not prevent penetration during the 4-h observation period,[24,25] thus demonstrating a breakthrough time through these glove materials less than 4 h. Use of a laminate-type glove (4H™, trademark of Safety4 A/S) increased breakthrough time for malathion and glyphosate (Round Up®) to above 4 h.[32] Gloves made of polyester or nylon did not offer any relevant protection against penetration of azinphos-methyl.[24] When applied in the commercial formulation, the penetration of diazinon through gloves made of nitrile butyl rubber was insignificant during a 24-h observation period.[18] Breakthrough times as well as the connected relative permeations after breakthrough have been reported for some organophosphates (summarized in Table 25.1 with data from References).[15,31]

Neither of the glove materials performed very well against monocrotophos, with Neoprene and Silver Shield™ gloves demonstrating the lowest relative permeation (Table 25.1). Likewise, methyl parathion penetrated most glove materials with short breakthrough times and significant quantitative permeation (Table 25.1). For ethyl parathion, nitrile, PVC, butyl rubber, and Silver Shield™, all demonstrated reasonable breakthrough times with butyl rubber and nitrile as the best overall glove material when data on relative permeation is also considered (Table 25.1). Nitrile and PVC were the only glove materials tested with acceptable penetration characteristics against tricresyl phosphate (Table 25.1).

The data presented illustrate the diversity in penetration characteristics even within a single group of pesticides. None of the glove materials offered very good protection against all tested organophosphates. But, in general, the gloves made of nitrile, butyl rubber, and Silver Shield™ were the most resistant to permeation. Natural rubber, polyethylene, and cotton were the least resistant even though they did reduce quantitatively the penetration of pesticides.

TABLE 25.1

Breakthrough Times and Relative Permeation of Four Organophosphates through Seven Glove Materials

	Monocrotophos		Methyl Parathion		Ethyl Parathion		Tricresyl Phosphate	
	BT (h)	RP	BT (h)	RP	BT (h)	RP	BT (h)	RP
Natural rubber	4–6	++	$<^1/_2$	+++	1–2	+	<1	+
Nitrile	1–2	++	1–2	++	6–8	0	>6	0
Neoprene	3–4	+	1–2	+++	3–4	+	$<^1/_2$	+++
Polyethylene	—	—	$<^1/_2$	+++	$<^1/_2$	+++	—	—
PVC	$<^1/_2$	++	$<^1/_2$	+++	4–6	+	>6	+
Butyl rubber	—	—	3–4	++	>8	0	—	—
Silver Shield™	$<^1/_2$	+	$<^1/_2$	++	4–6	+	—	—

BT—breakthrough time; RP—relative permeation.
Source: Data summarized from References.[15,31]

25.6.6 FUNGICIDES (WETTABLE POWDERS)

Data on penetration characteristics for these wettable powder fungicides through gloves were identified for benomyl, captan, chlorothalonil, and folpet.[33–36] Based on breakthrough times, Sol-Vex Nitrile gloves provided at least 4 h of protection against benomyl (tested as a concentrated emulsion), whereas a thinner disposable nitrile glove provided less than 4 h of protection.[35] The breakthrough times for Sol-Vex and a disposable nitrile glove were less than 4 h for folpet (as a concentrated emulsion), but similarly, the permeation rate was significantly lower for the thicker Sol-Vex product.[36] Similar results were observed for chlorothalonil (tested as a solid and emulsion), in which Sol-Vex provided additional protection.[34] The breakthrough time for a disposable nitrile glove was less than 2 h for captan (as a concentrated emulsion).[33] Thus, nitrile gloves have been shown to provide a limited level of protection against these fungicides, with the thicker Sol-Vex gloves providing additional chemical resistance to breakthrough and permeation. Given the low breakthrough times, irrespectively of glove type, gloves should be replaced every 2 h or whenever contaminated.

25.6.7 FUMIGANTS

Data on penetration characteristics for these fumigants through gloves were identified for chloropicrin and Telone® (active ingredient 1,3-dichloropropene).[37,38] The studies both concluded that disposable nitrile, nitrile Sol-Vex, and laminated Silver Shield™ gloves were degraded and/or did not provide adequate chemical resistance. They concluded that Viton gloves are recommended for 1,3-dichloropropene based on published data by the glove manufacturer, which is supported by a published chemical resistance guide for 1,3-dichloropropene showing polyvinyl alcohol and Viton providing greater than 8 h of protection.[39] However, supporting data for chloropicrin was not found in the literature.

25.7 RESISTANCE OF GLOVES TO PENETRATION OF PESTICIDES

25.7.1 POLYETHYLENE GLOVES

Data on the penetration of polyethylene gloves were identified for organochlorines, organophosphates, and carbamates, as well as a carrier solvent. All data demonstrated breakthrough times of less than 15 min and relatively large penetration rates.[15,21,26] Gloves made of polyethylene cannot generally be recommended as protection against pesticide exposure.

25.7.2 LATEX/NATURAL RUBBER

Data on the penetration of gloves made of latex/natural rubber were identified for most main groups of pesticides, as well as a carrier solvent.[3,15,19–22,28,29,31] Except for the carbamate carbonyl and 2,4-D studied by Moody and Ritter,[19] the breakthrough times reported were around 30 min with considerable penetration rates after breakthrough. However, Moody and Ritter used the carbamate carbonyl as a dry powder, which will potentially affect penetration characteristics. A recent field study on greenhouse workers using latex gloves during reentry activities demonstrated a breakthrough time for the fungicide Amistar® (a strobilurin analog) of less than 2 h.[40] Most authors do not recommend gloves made of latex/natural rubber against pesticides, given that alternatives exist.

25.7.3 PVC

PVC was reported to have breakthrough times above 6 h for 2,4-D, tricresyl phosphate, as well as pentachlorophenol.[19,22,31] For the remaining pesticides reported to penetrate the PVC material, breakthrough times were low and/or penetration rates relatively high and the glove material generally offered limited protection against penetration of pesticides at a level similar to latex/natural rubber.[14,15,21,28,29]

25.7.4 NEOPRENE

Except for the organophosphates parathion (ethyl- and methyl-) and monocrotophos, endosulfan, and pentachlorophenol,[15,31] breakthrough times through Neoprene materials were generally more than 8 h, and penetration rates relatively low. Data were reported on a carbamate, a triazine, several organophosphates, a pyrethroid, and two aryloxyalcanoic acids.[2,16,19,20,23,28,29,31] The authors conclude that Neoprene gloves offer good protection against exposure to the latter pesticides.

25.7.5 SILVER SHIELD™/LAMINATE

Studies on five different pesticides (terbufos, tefluthrin, pentachlorophenol, 2,4-D, and ethyl parathion) and two carrier solvents (hydrocarbons and xylenes) demonstrated that laminates offer good protection against exposure.[15,16,21,23,30] In one study, however, monocrotophos, endosulfan, and methyl parathion penetrated the Silver Shield™ material within 30 min.[15] Further, Guo et al.[30] characterized barrier laminate as a single-use material, as a glove made of this material could not be cleaned. However, the extent to which the pesticide remaining on the gloves after cleaning will eventually be available for penetration was not demonstrated. Thus, Silver Shield™ material offers protection that varies with the pesticide, and the use of gloves made of the material requires a continued focus on which pesticide is used.

25.7.6 NITRILE

Data were collected on penetration characteristics of 20 pesticides and 4 carrier solvents through gloves made of nitrile.[3,14–16,18–23,28,31,40] All but one study concluded that nitrile gloves offered good protection against exposure to the pesticides tested. In most studies, the breakthrough time, when reported, was above 8 h. One study reported breakthrough times for methyl parathion, endosulfan, and monocrotophos through nitrile gloves of less than 30 min but concluded that in comparison with other glove materials, nitrile (and Silver Shield™) offered the best protection also against these pesticides.[15] Thus, all studies included in this evaluation concluded that nitrile gloves offer good protection against exposure to pesticides.

25.7.7 ADDITIONAL CONSIDERATIONS

The selection of a glove material that provides a longer breakthrough time and lower permeation rate for the pesticide of concern is important. However, recent studies have shown significant inter-variability between gloves made of the same material but from different producers. One study found breakthrough times ranging from about 30 min up to 7 h for a captan (fungicide) formulation through various disposable nitrile gloves.[41] The permeation rate also varied by as much as 200-fold. Later studies with common solvents showed similar results.[42–44] All four of these aforementioned studies attributed variation in glove formulation (e.g., acrylonitrile content, plasticizer content, etc.) and/or thickness to these observed differences in chemical resistance. Thus, when critical, selection should be based on available chemical permeation data, instead of generic chemical resistance charts.

Additionally, intra-variability between disposable nitrile glove lots from the same producer and in-use conditions such as hand movement and skin temperatures different from laboratory conditions has resulted in unfavorable changes in both expected breakthrough times and permeation rates.[45–48] This further supports the notion that disposable gloves are designed for incidental contact and not continuous contact, as well as for immediate disposal and replacement of soiled disposable gloves.

25.8 PESTICIDE FORMULATIONS

Pesticides are seldom used as neat compounds. As liquids, they are used as salts or esters and dissolved in different solvents, solubilizers, and detergents. The purpose is often to assure that the pesticide may be dissolved and distributed homogeneously in an aqueous solution but still have sufficient lipophilicity to easily penetrate the outer barrier of a target organism.

The chemical form of the pesticide appears to be of some importance. For example, 4-chloro-2-methylphenoxyacetic acid (MCPA) had no appreciable permeation through gloves of natural rubber, Neoprene, nitrile, or Viton coated Neoprene when used in a salt formulation, whereas MCPA permeated through the same four glove materials with reduced lag-times when applied in an ester form.[20]

The different solvents, detergents, and solubilizers used in the final end-use formulations will, however, and probably to a larger degree, also affect the penetration of the active ingredients through different glove materials.[20,23] A study on pentachlorophenol demonstrated that if pentachlorophenol was dissolved in diesel oil, as previously recommended for long-term preservation of wood, instead of the use of pentachloro phenate in water, the breakthrough time through vinyl examination gloves was reduced from 5 h to 30 s, and the breakthrough time through latex/Neoprene gloves was reduced from 8 h to approximately 1 h.[22] Likewise, neither DDT, 2,4-D, nor diazinon penetrated nitrile gloves significantly during a 24-h observation period when applied in their commercial formulations, whereas the same pesticides in an acetone formulation penetrated the nitrile glove within a few hours.[18] Apparently, the more lipophilic and the higher the concentration of the carrier solvent, the more rapidly the active ingredient permeates the protective glove.[15] Detergent may, however, not always increase the penetration of the active ingredient. Thus, a study on penetration of pirimicarb and paclobutrazol through latex or nitrile gloves demonstrated that the detergent nonylphenol ethoxylate slightly decreased the penetration of the active ingredients through the glove and underlying skin.[3] The available open literature on the influence of formulations on penetration characteristics is limited, and data is often equivocal. As several studies have demonstrated how penetration characteristics of active ingredients may dramatically change depending on the formulation, there is a clear need for more research and more published data on this area.

25.9 USE OF GLOVES AFTER STORAGE, WASHING, OR CLEANSING

Information on storage conditions and shelf life of gloves is seldom available to the end user. Although most glove users know from experience that the structural integrity of some glove materials, i.e., latex, changes with time, information on how penetration characteristics change over time is lacking. Storage condition also needs to be addressed. One study demonstrated that even short-term storage (10 days) at -3 °C significantly decreases flexural rigidity (nitrile gloves) as well as puncture resistance (latex, natural rubber, Neoprene, nitrile gloves).[29] Further, exposure of gloves to intensive UV light for days may for some pesticides affect the resistance toward permeation through the glove.[49]

Based on these observations, a reasonable request to the glove producers would be to include information on shelf life and, if necessary, specific recommendations regarding storage conditions.

Reusable gloves are used extensively, and glove manufacturers often describe how to clean the used gloves. However, some studies demonstrate the presence of pesticide residues in the glove material after cleansing. Thus, clean-up procedures reduced contamination of the outside of nitrile and Neoprene gloves, but experimental evidence demonstrated that these materials retained residues after cleanup.[30] Further, barrier laminate was suggested as a single-use material as gloves made of this material could not be cleaned.[30] A reservoir effect within the glove has also been demonstrated regarding 2,4-D, DDT, and diazinon as significant amounts of pesticides could be extracted from the gloves after washing.[18] Whether this reservoir of pesticide would have been available for subsequent penetration and ultimately absorption was not studied. If this problem is not given sufficient research attention, we may have to conclude that it is better to use disposable gloves only—and dispose of them after use.

Taking off the gloves is an exposure that is often underestimated. However, one study demonstrated that when optimal gloves were used, as much as 50% of the total pesticide exposure during a working day occurred when the users changed gloves.[40] Interindividual variation was significant,[40] and the observation stresses the importance of hygiene and education regarding not only the correct use but also disposal of gloves.

Reuse of gloves also requires a strong focus on the personal hygiene aspect. Simple observations of workers putting on and taking off protective gloves indicate the potential for hand exposure.[6] When people take off dirty gloves, it is difficult to avoid touching the glove exterior, and a recently published survey demonstrates that protective gloves were nearly always found to be contaminated inside.[6] Inside contamination of gloves generates an exposure situation between the skin and the glove that may be characterized as being occluded, which might potentially enhance dermal penetration of those pesticides that end up here. Research on this topic is lacking as most experimental procedures involve penetration through a glove membrane only. Few studies have used experimental procedures with a glove on top of a dermal membrane,[3,25] but the extent to which this semi-occluded exposure will enhance penetration through the human skin is not addressed.

Further, practical experience tells us that disposable gloves are also sometimes reused. This is against the intended use, will not assure sufficient protection, and points to one of the main problems with a preventive strategy using gloves to eliminate pesticide exposure.

The problem is proper training, education, and compliance with regulations for use of gloves. Eighty-seven percent of male coffee farmworkers from The Dominican Republic did not use gloves at all,[50] only but 11% of cotton workers in South Pakistan used gloves to avoid exposure.[51] Same in Thailand,[52] and Uganda.[53] A Brazilian study showed that less than 20% of workers used masks, impermeable clothes, or gloves during pesticide application.[54]

General guidelines do exist on relevant training topics:

- Reading the pesticide product label carefully and following instructions
- Proper donning and doffing of gloves
- Washing reusable rubber glove products immediately following contamination or use
- Proper use, care, and cleaning/decontamination of reusable products
- Inspection of gloves for signs of degradation (e.g., discoloration, cracking, brittle/stiffness, etc.) and excessive wear
- Immediate disposal and replacement of soiled disposable gloves, designed for incidental contact and not continuous contact
- Washing hands and affected areas of the body following pesticide contact, after use, and before eating

But, a major challenge will be that a large fraction of the end users is most probably not able to read and appreciate the more traditional ways of communicating risk. Health literacy is a true challenge. More than 25% of the European population has low health literacy. This calls for more novel ways of communicating risk as well as the use of PPE. In other areas of society use of small videos, you-tube, podcast, etc., which works on a mobile phone, have proven beneficial in communicating information to citizens. Presently, this path has not been taken by either producers or distributors, as well as legislators responsible for offering enough and accessible knowledge on the correct use of gloves.

If workers, despite receiving and understanding recommendations to use gloves, do not use gloves, it is not ideal, but at least the workers will probably know that they are potentially exposed and it is hoped will act accordingly. A worse situation is actually if workers assume that they are protected against pesticide exposure by the gloves they are wearing, when not protected—because of wrong glove material, gloves with damaged structural integrity, or gloves contaminated from previous use. A situation with workers feeling safe, and acting as if protected without being protected, is unacceptable. This is why education, training, and supervision are almost as important elements in the preventive strategy to reduce exposure as the correct glove for the relevant task.

REFERENCES

1. Aprea, C., Sciarra, G., Lunghini, L., Centi, L., and Ceccarelli, F. 2001. Evaluation of respiratory and cutaneous doses and urinary excretion of alkylphosphates by workers in greenhouses treated with omethoate, fenitrothion, and tolclofos-methyl. *Am Indust Hyg Assoc J* 62 (1):87–95.
2. Cessna, A.J., and Grover, R. 2002. Exposure of ground-rig applicators to the herbicide bromoxynil applied as a 1:1 mixture of butyrate and octanoate. *Arch Environ Contam Tox* 42 (3):369–382.
3. Nielsen, J.B., and Andersen, H.R. 2001. Dermal in vitro penetration of methiocarb, paclobutrazol, and pirimicarb: Effect of nonylphenolethoxylate and protective gloves. *Environ Health Persp* 109 (2):129–132.
4. Andersen, H.R., and Nielsen, J.B. 2001. A Danish survey on use of pesticides and gloves in ornamental greenhouses. Denmark (unpublished report).
5. Cattani, M., Cena, K., Edwards, J., and Pisaniello, D. 2001. Potential dermal and inhalation exposure to chlorpyrifos in Australian pesticide workers. *Ann Occup Hyg* 45 (4):299–308.
6. Garrod, A.N.I., Phillips, A.M., and Pemberton, J.A. 2001. Potential exposure of hands inside protective gloves—A summary of data from non-agricultural pesticide surveys. *Ann Occup Hyg* 45 (1):55–60.
7. Gomes, J., Lloyd, O.L., and Revitt, D.M. 1999. The influence of personal protection, environmental hygiene and exposure to pesticides on the health of immigrant farm workers in a desert country. *Int Arch Occup Environ Health* 72 (1):40–45.
8. Mekonnen, Y., and Agonafir, T. 2002. Pesticide sprayers' knowledge, attitude and practice of pesticide use on agricultural farms of Ethiopia. *Occup Med* 52 (6):311–315.
9. Nielsen, J.B., and Andersen, H.R. 2002. Cholinesterase activity in female greenhouse workers—Influence of work practices and use of oral contraceptives. *J Occup Health* 44 (4):234–239.
10. Perry, M.J., and Layde, P.M. 1998. Sources, routes, and frequency of pesticide exposure among farmers. *J Occup Environ Med* 40 (8):697–701.
11. Harris, S.A., Sass-Kortsak, A.M., Corey, P.N., and Purdham, J.T. 2002. Development of models to predict dose of pesticides in professional turf applicators. *J Exposure Sci Environ Epidem* 12 (2):130–144.
12. Oltmanns, J., Kaiser, E., Heine, K., Schneider, K., Hesse, S., and Hahn, S. 2016. *Effectiveness of Personal Protective Equipment against Dermal Exposure – A Comparative Survey.* Dortmund, Germany: Federal Institute for Occupational Safety and Health.

13. Beránková, M., Hojerová, J., and Peráčková, Z. 2017. Estimated exposure of hands inside the protective gloves used by non-occupational handlers of agricultural pesticides. *J Exposure Sci Environ Epidem* 27 (6):625–631.

14. Creely, K.S., and Cherrie, J.W. 2001. A novel method of assessing the effectiveness of protective gloves—results from a pilot study. *Ann Occup Hyg* 45 (2):137–143.

15. Ehntholt, D.J., Cerundolo, D.L., Bodek, I., Schwope, A.D., Royer, M.D., and Nielsen, A.P. 1990. A test method for the evaluation of protective glove materials used in agricultural pesticide operations. *Am Indust Hyg Assoc J* 51 (9):462–468.

16. Guo, C., Stone, J., Stahr, H.M., and Shelley, M. 2001. Effects of exposure time, material type, and granular pesticide on glove contamination. *Arch Environ Contam Tox* 41 (4):529–536.

17. Krzemińska, S., and Szczecińska, K. 2001. Proposal for a method for testing resistance of clothing and gloves to penetration by pesticides. *Ann Ag Environ Med* 8 (2):145–150.

18. Moody, R.P., and Nadeau, B. 1994. Nitrile butyl rubber glove permeation of pesticide formulations containing 2, 4-D-amine, DDT, DEET, and Diazinon. *Bull Environ Contam Tox* 52 (1):125–130.

19. Moody, R.P., and Ritter, L. 1990. Pesticide glove permeation analysis: Comparison of the ASTM F739 test method with an automated flow-through reverse-phase liquid chromatography procedure. *Am Indust Hyg Assoc J* 51 (2):79–83.

20. Purdham, J.T., Menard, B.J., Bozek, P.R., and Sass-Kortsak, A.M. 2001. MCPA permeation through protective gloves. *Appl Occup Environ Hyg* 16 (10):961–966.

21. Schwope, A.D., Goydan, R., Ehntholt, D., Frank, U., and Nielsen, A.P. 1992. Permeation resistance of glove materials to agricultural pesticides. *Am Indust Hyg Assoc J* 53 (6):352–361.

22. Silkowski, J.B., Horstman, S.W., and Morgan, M.S. 1984. Permeation through five commercially available glove materials by two pentachlorophenol formulations. *Am Indust Hyg Assoc J* 45 (8):501–504.

23. Harville, J., and Que Hee, S.S. 1989. Permeation of a 2, 4-D isooctyl ester formulation through neoprene, nitrile, and Tyvek® protection materials. *Am Indust Hyg Assoc J* 50 (8):438–446.

24. Keeble, V.B., Correll, L., and Ehrich, M. 1993. Evaluation of knit glove fabrics as barriers to dermal absorption of organophosphorus insecticides using an in vitro test system. *Toxicology* 81 (3):195–203.

25. Keeble, V.B., Correll, L., and Ehrich, M. 1996. Effect of laundering on ability of glove fabrics to decrease the penetration of organophosphate insecticides through in vitro epidermal systems. *J Appl Tox* 16 (5):401–406.

26. DuPont, Co. 2018. *DuPont Permeation Guide: Tychem and Tyvex.* Wilmington, DE: DuPont Co.

27. Keith, L.H., Conoly, M., Nolen, R.L., Walters, D.B., and Prokopetz, A.T. Chemical permeation and degradation data from the National Toxicology Program measured by Radian Corporation. Austin, TX (unpublished report).

28. Raheel, M., and Dai, G.X. 1997. Chemical resistance and structural integrity of protective glove materials. *J Environ Sci Health Part A* 32 (2):567–579.

29. Raheel, M., and Dai, G.X. 2002. Viability of textile systems for hand and body protection: Effects of chemical interaction, wear, and storage conditions. *Bull Environ Contam Tox* 69 (2):164–172.

30. Guo, C., Stone, J., Stahr, H.M., and Shelley, M. 2002. Cleanup of gloves contaminated with granular terbufos and tefluthrin. *Arch Environ Contam Tox* 42 (3):383–388.

31. Ansell. 2008. *Chemical Resistance Guide: Permeation and Degradation Data,* 8th Edition. Red Bank, NJ: Ansell Healthcare. Available at www.ansellpro.com.

32. North. 2001. *Silver Shield®/4H® Chemical Protection Guide.* Cranston, RI: North Safety Products. Available at: www.northsafety.com.
33. Phalen, R.N., and Que Hee, S.S. 2003. Permeation of captan through disposable nitrile glove. *J Haz Mater* 100 (1–3):95–107.
34. Que Hee, S.S., and Zainal, H. 2010. Permeation of chlorothalonil through nitrile gloves: Collection solvent effects in the closed-loop permeation method. *J Haz Mater* 179 (1–3):57–62.
35. Zainal, H., and Que Hee, S.S. 2006. Nitrile glove permeation of benomyl. *Arch Environ Contam Tox* 50 (3):429–436.
36. Zainal, H., and Que Hee, S.S. 2003. Folpet permeation through nitrile gloves. *Appl Occup Environ Hyg* 18 (9):658–668.
37. Zainal, H., and Que Hee, S.S. 2005. Permeation of Telone EC™ through protective gloves. *J Haz Mater* 124 (1–3):81–87.
38. Zainal, H., and Que Hee, S.S. 2006. Permeation of Telone C-35 EC™ and chloropicrin through protective gloves. *J Appl Polymer Sci* 100 (1):18–25.
39. Forsberg, K., Van den Borre, A., Henry III, N., and Zeigler, J.P. 2020. *Quick Selection Guide to Chemical Protective Clothing.* Hoboken, NJ: John Wiley & Sons.
40. Kirknel, E., and Sjelborg, P. 2003. *Handskers beskyttelsesevne ved arbejde med pesticider I jordbrugene, samt modeler for håndeksponering* [in Danish with English summary]. Copenhagen, Denmark: Danish Environmental Protection Agency.
41. Phalen, R.N., Hee, Q., Xu, S.S., and Wong, W.K. 2007. Acrylonitrile content as a predictor of the captan permeation resistance for disposable nitrile rubber gloves. *J Appl Polymer Sci* 103 (3):2057–2063.
42. Brown, B.C., Dubrovskiy, A., Gvetadze, A.R., and Phalen, R.N. 2020. Chemical permeation of similar disposable nitrile gloves exposed to volatile organic compounds with different polarities: Part 1: Product variation. *J Occup Environ Hyg* 17 (4):165–171.
43. Phalen, R.N., Dubrovskiy, A.V., Brown, B.C., Gvetadze, A.R., Bustillos, M., and Ogbonmwan, J. 2020. Chemical permeation of similar disposable nitrile gloves exposed to volatile organic compounds with different polarities Part 2. Predictive polymer properties. *J Occup Environ Hyg* 17 (4):172–180.
44. Phalen, R.N., and Wong, W.K. 2015. Polymer properties associated with chemical permeation performance of disposable nitrile rubber gloves. *J Appl Polymer Sci* 132 (6):41449. https://doi.org/10.1002/app.41449
45. Banaee, S., and Que Hee, S.S. 2020. Glove permeation of chemicals: The state of the art of current practice—Part 2. Research emphases on high boiling point compounds and simulating the donned glove environment. *J Occup Environ Hyg* 17 (4):135–164.
46. Phalen, R.N., and Que Hee, S.S. 2008. A moving robotic hand system for whole-glove permeation and penetration: Captan and nitrile gloves. *J Occup Environ Hyg* 5 (4):258–270.
47. Phalen, R.N., Le, T., and Wong, W.K. 2014. Changes in chemical permeation of disposable latex, nitrile, and vinyl gloves exposed to simulated movement. *J Occup Environ Hyg* 11 (11):716–721.
48. Phalen, R.N., and Wong, W.K. 2012. Chemical resistance of disposable nitrile gloves exposed to simulated movement. *J Occup Environ Hyg* 9 (11):630–639.
49. Ismail, I., Gaskin, S., Pisaniello, D., and Edwards, J.W. 2018. Organophosphorus pesticide exposure in agriculture: Effects of temperature, ultraviolet light and abrasion on PVC gloves. *Indust Health* 56 (2):166–170.
50. Hutter, H.-P., Khan, A.W., Lemmerer, K., Wallner, P., Kundi, M., and Moshammer, H. 2018. Cytotoxic and genotoxic effects of pesticide exposure in male coffee farmworkers of the Jarabacoa Region, Dominican Republic. *Int J Environ Res Public Health* 15 (8):1641.

51. Memon, Q. Ul A., Wagan, S.A., Chunyu, D., Shuangxi, X., Jingdong, L., and Damalas, C.A. 2019. Health problems from pesticide exposure and personal protective measures among women cotton workers in southern Pakistan. *Sci Total Environ* 685:659–666.
52. Kongtip, P., Nankongnab, N., Mahaboonpeeti, R., Bootsikeaw, S., Batsungnoen, K., Hanchenlaksh, C., Tipayamongkholgul, M., and Woskie, S. 2018. Differences among Thai agricultural workers' health, working conditions, and pesticide use by farm type. *Ann Work Exposures Health* 62 (2):167–181.
53. Okonya, J.S., and Kroschel, J. 2015. A cross-sectional study of pesticide use and knowledge of smallholder potato farmers in Uganda. *BioMed Res Intern* 2015:759049. https://doi.org/10.1155/2015/759049
54. Recena, M.C.P., Caldas, E.D., Pires, D.X., and Pontes, E.R.J.C. 2006. Pesticides exposure in Culturama, Brazil—knowledge, attitudes, and practices. *Environ Res* 102 (2):230–236.

26 Gloves as Protection against Microbial Contamination

R.N. Phalen

CONTENTS

26.1 INTRODUCTION

Gloves, in healthcare referred to as medical gloves, can protect from cross-contamination with microorganisms as well as from adverse skin reactions caused by wet work and chemical contact.

26.2 PROTECTION AGAINST MICROORGANISMS

Contact contamination via the hands is the most important route of transmission for healthcare-associated infections. Contact contamination from an infected wound, cuticle infections (paronychia), or other kinds of local infections is the greatest risk, but indirect contact contamination is also of great importance. This has been known since the days of Semmelweis.[1] *Staphylococcus aureus*, *Klebsiella*, and many other species are also spread by this route as are many viruses, e.g., RS-virus (respiratory syncytial virus), rhinovirus, and adenovirus.

Protective gloves, proper hand hygiene, and additional personal protective equipment (PPE) are important considerations with many of the infections common to healthcare settings, such as:[2]

- The bloodborne pathogens hepatitis C virus (HCV), hepatitis B virus (HBV), and human immunodeficiency virus (HIV), in which exposures are often associated with sharps or needle puncture injuries

DOI: 10.1201/9781003126874-30

- Contact with hepatitis A virus-infected patients via fecal-oral contamination
- Contact with the saliva and respiratory secretions of patients infected with rabies
- Contact with primary and secondary stage lesions of patients infected with syphilis, as well as the secretions of children with congenital syphilis

The provision of adequate PPE, training on its use, and proper hand hygiene are critical components of the US Occupational Safety and Health Administration Bloodborne Pathogen Standard (29 CFR 1910.1030).[3] The US Centers for Disease Control and Prevention (CDC) provide guidelines on hand hygiene, including the use of alcohol-based hand rubs or hand washing with soap and water before and after coming in contact with a patient, contacting contaminated surfaces, or performing an aseptic procedure.[3,4] This includes hand hygiene immediately after glove removal. The World Health Organization (WHO) also provides detailed guidelines on hand hygiene for healthcare workers and surgeons, which includes additional hand hygiene products or preparations.[5]

26.2.1 SURGERY

Gloves were first introduced into surgery to protect operating-room nurses from corrosive disinfectants at the end of the 19th century.[6] They are still used for that purpose in operative theaters as well as wards and laboratories. Gloves can also reduce the spread of microorganisms from personnel to the patient during surgical procedures. Disinfecting the hands of operating personnel prior to surgical procedures has long been recommended to reduce not only the transient but also the resident skin flora of microorganisms. Preoperative hand disinfection is practiced even when sterile gloves are used, as the gloves are often lacerated or torn during the surgical procedure. Hand sweat with resident skin flora organisms has been shown experimentally to permeate to the outside of the glove and in doing so contaminate the wound being operated on. If scrubbed surgical staff follows the routines for preoperative hand disinfection, no increased infection rates have been shown following leakage.[7]

In response to the COVID-19 pandemic, Dexter et al.[8] provided additional recommendations for operating-room hygiene, infection control, and management. They include important considerations, such as preoperative skin preparation, double-gloving, environmental cleaning using disinfectants and UV-C, and PPE (e.g., N95 mask, gown, gloves, and eye protection). As previously mentioned, many of these similar recommendations have been made by the CDC (https://www.cdc.gov/) and WHO (https://www.who.int/) in response to the COVID-19 pandemic.

26.2.2 PATIENT CARE

With patient care, such as the changing of wound dressings or diapers, handling bedpans, urinals, etc., medical gloves may prevent cross-contamination by reducing soiling of the hands. Gloves are used to markedly reduce the number of microorganisms that reach the hands so that the hand disinfectant will be able to reduce the rest.

The importance of the protective glove in reducing indirect contact contamination between patients is well documented for both bacteria and viruses.[9]

Gloves offer little protection to the patient if a healthcare worker has a skin infection on the hand. To put a glove or finger stall on a finger with paronychia is seldom an effective way to avoid cross-contamination, either with MRSA (methicillin-resistant *S. aureus*) or beta-hemolytic group A streptococci.

Gloves must be changed between attending patients; otherwise, there is a self-evident risk for cross-contamination, e.g., with *S. aureus*, enterococci, or *Acinetobacter* sp.[10] Gloves are easily torn and the hands may be contaminated while removing the gloves as well. For that reason, the hands must be disinfected even if gloves have been used during patient care. Gloves should not be disinfected and reused.

In the early stages of the COVID-19 pandemic, a global shortage of disposable medical gloves occurred, resulting in the CDC and others issuing crisis capacity strategies involving the disinfection and extended use of these gloves. The CDC issued *Strategies for Optimizing the Supply of Disposable Medical Gloves*,[11] which included the disinfection and extended use of disposable medical gloves during extreme shortages. Reuse and repeated donning and doffing were not recommended, and visibly soiled or damaged gloves were to be promptly discarded. For disinfection, up to six repeated treatments with an alcohol-based hand rub (ABHR) or ten treatments with soap and water were recommended. As an alternative, and based on limited data, up to ten repeated treatments with dilute bleach (e.g., 0.1% sodium hypochlorite) could be considered. Additional research on the effects of repeated disinfection on glove integrity has since been published,[12-19] which indicates that these recommendations will need to be revisited and updated in the event of a future crisis involving glove shortages. Research is ongoing at this time. Some of this research is discussed in this chapter and other chapters in this book (see Chapter 30).

In a recent review by Picheansanthian and Chotibang,[20] compliance with the use of gloves is low and there is inadequate or conflicting evidence that gloves use influences hand hygiene among healthcare workers. Thus, improving glove compliance is not an optimal strategy to improve hand hygiene compliance. Effective strategies for hand hygiene compliance among healthcare workers include education, observation, providing adequate supplies, improving access to supplies, and via administrative directives.[21] Effective strategies for PPE compliance include increasing the perception of risk among healthcare staff, addressing workload issues to reduce fatigue and time constraints impacting glove use, providing adequate training and education, and providing adequate PPE supplies.[22,23]

Gloves are also used to reduce the risk for transmission of bloodborne infections from patients to personnel and between patients. This has been well documented in hepatitis outbreaks in the 1960s among dialysis patients and cross-country runners. The glove material used at that time was probably natural rubber latex (NRL). Protection from inoculation is also well documented both for NRL and polyvinyl chloride (PVC), as the gloves can significantly reduce the delivered blood volume with needle sticks.[24] Unused medical gloves made of these materials are effective barriers against, e.g., HIV.[25] Occupational safety guidelines in most countries recommend or mandate gloves to be worn during all patient-care activities that may involve exposure to blood or body fluids that may be contaminated with blood. Gloves can provide a protective effect and should be worn whenever needles are handled.[24]

26.3 BARRIER INTEGRITY OF GLOVES

The barrier integrity of new and used gloves to penetration of blood and viruses is covered extensively in Chapter 11. This includes standard tests such as the 1000 mL water leak test and established acceptable quality levels (AQLs) for single-use medical gloves and surgical gloves. As of 2008, the US Food and Drug Administration, under 21 CFR 800.20, has established an appropriate AQL at 1.5 for surgeons' gloves and 2.5 for patient examination gloves.[26] The ASTM International Standard ASTM D 5151, *Standard Test Method for Detection of Holes in Medical Gloves*, also implements an equivalent 1000 mL water leak test method.[27] The European Union has an equivalent 1000 mL water leak test for single-use medical gloves: EN-455-1, *Medical gloves for single use - Part 1: Requirements and testing for freedom from holes*, with an established AQL of 1.5.[28] Some glove manufacturers and standard-setting organizations may establish more stringent AQLs, providing an added level of quality assurance and barrier protection to end users.

A viral penetration test for elastomeric materials using a bacteriophage as a surrogate for HBV, HCV, and HIV is available with ASTM F 1671.[29] The method is based on the use of the ASTM F 903 penetration test cell, which is used for measuring the resistance of chemical protective clothing materials to penetration by liquids. A screening test, ASTM F 1670 that evaluates penetration of synthetic blood using the same test cell, is recommended. It must be noted that these standardized methods can only test a swatch of the material. Chapter 11 provides a more robust discussion on the topic and provides alternative methods available in the literature.

The resistance to punctures and needle sticks, which could compromise barrier effectiveness, is covered under additional standards. ASTM F 1342, *Standard Test Method for Protective Clothing Material Resistance to Puncture*, is designed to determine the puncture resistance of protective articles to rounded or blunt probes.[30] EN 388 has a similar standard. For hypodermic needles, ASTM F 2878, *Standard Test Method for Protective Clothing Material Resistance to Hypodermic Needle Puncture*, is available.[31] Performance rankings based on these ASTM standard test methods are available under the American National Standards Institute/International Safety Equipment Association (ANSI/ISEA) standard ANSI/ISEA 105.[32] The ANSI/ISEA standard establishes performance levels for several factors and is covered in more detail in Chapter 6. EN 388 also provides a performance ranking scale. Additionally, the National Fire Protection Association (NFPA) standard NFPA 1999 indicates a minimum requirement for puncture resistance when tested according to ASTM F 1342.[33]

These standards can aid in the selection of an appropriate glove product for use in a variety of healthcare settings. Most glove manufacturers will test, label, and market their products as attaining one or more of these standards.

26.4 EFFECTS OF CHEMICALS COMMONLY USED IN MEDICAL CARE

In many healthcare-associated procedures, gloves are used not only to prevent cross-contamination of microorganisms but also to give protection against frequently handled chemicals: disinfecting and cleaning agents (Chapter 24), laboratory chemicals (Chapter 24), antineoplastic agents (Chapter 24), other pharmaceuticals, and thermosetting plastics in orthopedic surgery and dentistry (Chapter 23). The highest demands are put on gloves for long-term use, not only for comfort and fit but also when mechanical abrasion or chemical exposure may reduce their barrier properties. Testing of glove materials is mostly performed on unused gloves, as required by European Committee for Standardization (CEN), International Organization for Standardization (ISO), and ASTM International standards. The effect of wear and tear, aging, and exposure to disinfectants is not usually tested. Studies on used surgical gloves show that, even though polymer defects occur in unused gloves at a rate up to 3%, mechanical damage to gloves during operations is four times as common.[34]

Contact with chemicals during the use of medical gloves is as common as mechanical strain. Disinfectants, mostly containing alcohol, are used routinely for the disinfection of skin and medical products. When medical gloves are used in performing work tasks that involve contact with chemicals and pharmaceuticals, it is important to note that medical gloves are usually not tested according to ASTM F 739, EN/ISO 6529, or any other standard method for chemical permeation. It is necessary to consider what level of protection is needed in every situation involving that type of exposure. For example, acrylates used in dentistry and orthopedic surgery may permeate medical gloves within a few minutes and so may cytostatics such as carmustine.[35]

Standard test methods ASTM F 739 and EN 374 were compared by assessing the permeation of 70% isopropyl alcohol (2-propanol) through seven brands of surgical gloves.[36] The two standards differ in the flow rates of the collection medium and in the chemical permeation rate at which the breakthrough time (BT) is detected. No statistical difference could be observed between the BT values obtained with the two standard methods.[11] When dental gloves made of NRL (powdered or unpowdered), PVC (powdered), nitrile, and synthetic elastomer were exposed to 5 mL of a hand disinfectant, it was found that after only 2 min the PVC and one nitrile glove were permeated by ethanol. After 10 min, all other gloves and types were permeated by ethanol. Powder seemed to not influence the permeation of ethanol. Some NRL gloves showed a low rate of permeation, while PVC and nitrile gloves had a much higher rate of permeation. The synthetic elastomer was the only glove with a significantly lower permeation even after 2–8 h.[37]

Phalen et al.[38] investigated the permeation of ethanol through disposable NRL, nitrile, and PVC gloves exposed to simulated hand movement. Regardless of the influence of movement, the BTs were all less than 15 min on average. The nitrile glove performed the best with an average BT of about 12 min but was more affected by movement (BT about 8 min; a 31% decrease). The average BT for the NRL glove was about 3 min without movement and decreased to 2.5 min with movement (a 23%

decrease). The PVC glove was not affected by movement, but the average BT was less than 2 min. The one caveat here is that permeation testing was performed under conditions of continuous contact and thus may not be representative of glove exposures involving intermittent exposure or during conditions of use.

As previously discussed concerning COVID-19, several recent studies have been conducted on the effects of common disinfectants on glove integrity, both physical and mechanical. These studies can provide some insight into the compatibility of disinfectants with medical exam gloves. For disposable NRL medical gloves, mechanical integrity (i.e., elastic modulus or stiffness) was not significantly affected by repeated treatments with an ABHR, soap and water, or dilute bleach per CDC crisis capacity guidelines.[18] However, disposable nitrile medical gloves were not appropriate for soap and water or dilute bleach treatments, and fewer treatments (not to exceed five) with an ABHR were recommended. The changes observed were related to the degradation of the glove material within 1 h of treatment. In a companion study, up to ten repeated treatments with dilute bleach had the least impact on the physical integrity of NRL and nitrile gloves, as evaluated using a water leak test.[19] Thus, it appears that up to five repeated treatments with ABHR are appropriate for disposable nitrile exam gloves, whereas up to ten repeated treatments with a dilute bleach solution are appropriate for disposable NRL exam gloves.

At this time, it must be assumed that disposable medical gloves should be used only for incidental contact with chemicals and promptly removed and replaced following contact. This is a similar recommendation for disposable gloves used in other industries and/or occupations.

26.5   SELECTION OF GLOVES

To meet the varying needs in different healthcare settings, the availability of a wide selection of high-quality gloves made of different materials is of the utmost importance.

The permeability to air and water increases after use, approximately ten times for NRL and 10–20 times for PVC.[39] Double gloves are often used in surgical procedures, and this reduces the risk of puncturing the inner glove by half. An inner glove of different colors can facilitate the discovery of a punctured outer glove. It is not known what impact the material of the inner glove has on the protection against bloodborne infections, but in surgical procedures, which involve irritant or allergenic chemicals such as acrylates in bone cement the glove materials have to meet the appropriate standards.

The efficacy of medical gloves against bloodborne infections is sometimes debated. A literature survey shows that only a few studies have been done and that they are small. They often lack important data on the water and air permeability of the gloves tested, and the methods have not been standardized. The methods used vary, from air or water permeability[39] to methods using various particles with different sizes.[25,40,41] In most examination gloves from well-reputed manufacturers less than 1%–2% show permeability. This is when the gloves are new and unused, but long-term usage decreases the protective effect. About 10% of NRL gloves and up to 60% of PVC gloves can then let through virus particles.[41] The conclusion is that gloves should be worn for a short time during well-defined work tasks with known or strongly suspected risk of contamination. Experimental studies show that longer-term exposure to chemicals such as ethanol and sodium hypochlorite can reduce the barrier properties of medical gloves of NRL as well as PVC.[40,42] The effect of organic solvents commonly used in health care on medical gloves needs to be studied under conditions that are close to the ordinary work situation. Medical gloves have for a long time been an important part of the precautions against bloodborne infections. According to the CDC,[43] in the USA, 57 healthcare personnel have been documented as having seroconverted to HIV following occupational exposures. After 1999, no new cases have been reported, aside from a possible case in 2009. Thus, the risk of being infected with HIV via the skin should be almost negligible if protected by gloves of PVC or NRL.

Nonsterile examination gloves have today in many cases replaced sterile operation gloves during clean work, such as child delivery, urine catheterization, and the dressing of central venous catheters. These gloves are considered clean enough to be used for this kind of work.[44] However, powdered gloves may have high amounts of mold and *Bacillus* spores, and in open containers, high amounts of *S. aureus* and coagulase-negative staphylococci have been found. Nonsterile products that are used for clean work should be virtually clean and not hold more than 100 colony-forming units per product. The package has to be designed so as not to allow contamination of the gloves remaining in the box.[44]

26.6 CONCLUSIONS

1. Gloves are an important part of barrier precautions to protect patients and staff against transmission of infection, both in surgery and with patient care.
2. Gloves are tested according to available standards for durability and resistance to penetration of fluids, which can aid in the selection process.
3. Additional standards for bloodborne pathogens and microorganism (e.g., viral) penetration are available and can provide a higher level of protection.
4. Intact PVC gloves provide protection comparable to latex gloves. Nitrile gloves seem to have leakage rates that approximate those of latex gloves. Standardized testing can help ensure gloves meet minimum standards for leakage and durability.
5. A selection of gloves must be available, to ensure the selection of type and size of gloves are suitable for the healthcare worker and the patient-care activity.
6. Disposable exam gloves often do not provide adequate chemical protection and should be used for incidental contact. Contaminated gloves should be promptly removed, discarded, and replaced.
7. The compatibility of glove materials with common disinfectants could be an important consideration, especially during crisis capacity scenarios involving glove shortages and extended use of gloves.

REFERENCES

1. Boyce, J.M., and Pittet, D. 2002. Healthcare Infection Control Practices Advisory Committee; HICPAC/SHEA/APIC/IDSA Hand Hygiene Task Force, Guideline for Hand Hygiene in Health-Care Settings. Recommendations of the Healthcare Infection Control Practices Advisory Committee and the HIPAC/SHEA/APIC/IDSA Hand Hygiene Task Force. *Am J Infect Control* 30:Sl–46.
2. Weber, D.J., and Rutala, W.A. 2016. Occupational health update: Focus on preventing the acquisition of infections with pre-exposure prophylaxis and postexposure prophylaxis. *Infect Dis Clin North Am* 30(3):729–757. DOI: 10.1016/j.idc.2016.04.008.
3. Denault, D., and Gardner, H. 2021. OSHA bloodborne pathogen standards. [Updated 2021 April 16]. In *StatPearls* [Internet]. Treasure Island, FL: StatPearls Publishing. Available from: https://www.ncbi.nlm.nih.gov/books/NBK570561/.
4. Centers for Disease Control and Prevention (CDC). 2002. Guideline for hand hygiene in health-care settings: Recommendations of the Healthcare Infection Control Practices Advisory Committee and the HICPAC/SHEA/APIC/IDSA Hand Hygiene Task Force. *MMWR* 51:RR16.
5. World Health Organization. 2009. *WHO Guidelines on Hand Hygiene in Health Care (WHO/IER/PSP/2009/01)*. Geneva: World Health Organization (WHO).
6. Spirling, L.I., and Daniels, I.R. 2002. William Stewart Halsted — Surgeon extraordinaire: A story of "drugs, gloves and romance." *J R Soc Health* 122:122–124.
7. Weber, L.W. 2003. Evaluation of the rate, location, and morphology of perforations in surgical gloves worn in urological operations. *Appl Occup Environ Hyg* 18:65–73.
8. Dexter, F., Parra, M.C., Brown, J.R., and Loftus, R.W. 2020. Perioperative COVID-19 defense: An evidence-based approach for optimization of infection control and operating room management. *Anesth Analg* 131(1):37–42. DOI: 10.1213/ANE.0000000000004829.
9. Tenorio, A.E., Badri, S.M., Sahgal, N.B., Hota, B., Matushek, M., Hayden, M.K., Trenholme, G.M., and Weinstein, R.A. 2001. Effectiveness of gloves in the prevention of hand carriage of vancomycin-resistant *Enterococcus* species by health care workers after patient care. *Clin Infect Dis* 32:826–829.
10. Doebbeling, B.N., Pfaller, M.A., Houston, A.K., and Wenzel, R.P. 1988. Removal of nosocomial pathogens from the contaminated glove. *Ann Intern Med* 109:394–398.
11. Centers for Disease Control and Prevention (CDC). 2020. Strategies for optimizing the supply of disposable medical gloves. Available at: https://www.cdc.gov/coronavirus/2019-ncov/hcp/ppe-strategy/gloves.html.
12. Gao, P., Horvatin, M., Niezgoda, G., Weible, R., and Shaffer, R. 2016. Effect of multiple alcohol-based hand rub applications on the tensile properties of thirteen brands of medical exam nitrile and latex gloves. *J Occup Environ Hyg* 13(12):905–914. DOI: 10.1080/15459624.2016.1191640.
13. Kampf, G., and Lemmen, S. 2017. Disinfection of gloved hands for multiple activities with indicated glove use on the same patient. *J Hosp Infect* 97(1):3–10. DOI: 10.1016/j.jhin.2017.06.021.
14. Esmizadeh, E., Chang, B.P., Jubinville, D., Seto, C., Ojogbo, E., Tzoganakis, C., and Mekonnen, T.H. 2021. Stability of nitrile and vinyl latex gloves under repeated disinfection cycles. *Materials Today Sustain* 11–12:100067. DOI: 10.1016/j.mtsust.2021.100067.
15. Garrido-Molina, J.M., Márquez-Hernández, V.V., Alcayde-García, A., Ferreras-Morales, C.A., García-Viola, A., Aguilera-Manrique, G., and Gutiérrez-Puertas, L. 2021. Disinfection of gloved hands during the COVID-19 pandemic. *J Hosp Infect* 107:5–11. DOI: 10.1016/j.jhin.2020.09.015.

16. Mansfield, S., Patterson, J., Cuadros Olave, J., Phalen, R.N., and Hamidi, Y.K. 2021. Repeated bleach sanitization effects on medical exam glove mechanical properties. *Am J Adv Res* 5(1):13–17. DOI: 10.5281/zenodo.5817219.

17. Patterson, J., Mansfield, S., Cuadros Olave, J., Phalen, R.N., and Hamidi, Y.K. 2021. Mechanical performance of latex and nitrile medical exam gloves under repeated soap and water treatment. *Am J Adv Res* 5(1):01–05. DOI: 10.5281/zenodo.5112602.

18. Phalen, R., Patterson, J., Cuadros Olave, J., Mansfield, S., Shless, J., Crider, Y., Pitchik, H.O., Qazi, A.S., Styczynski, A., LeMesurier, R., Haik, D., Kwong, L.H., LeBoa, C., Bhattacharya, A., and Hamidi, Y.K. 2021. Evaluation of the effects of repeated disinfection on medical exam gloves: Part 2. Changes in mechanical properties. *J Occup Environ Hyg* 13:1–14. DOI: 10.1080/15459624.2021.2015073.

19. Shless, J., Crider, Y., Pitchik, H., Qazi, A., Styczynski, A., LeMesurier, R., Haik, D., Kwong, L.H., LeBoa, C., Bhattacharya, A., Hamidi, Y.K., and Phalen, R.N. 2021. Evaluation of the effects of repeated disinfection on medical exam gloves: Part 1. Changes in physical integrity. *J Occup Environ Hyg* 13:1–11. DOI: 10.1080/15459624.2021.2015072.

20. Picheansanthian, W., and Chotibang, J. 2015. Glove utilization in the prevention of cross transmission: A systematic review. *JBI Database System Rev Implement Rep* 13(4):188–230. DOI: 10.11124/jbisrir-2015-1817.

21. Alshehari, A.A., Park, S., and Rashid, H. 2018. Strategies to improve hand hygiene compliance among healthcare workers in adult intensive care units: A mini systematic review. *J Hosp Infect* 100(2):152–158. DOI: 10.1016/j.jhin.2018.03.013.

22. Mitchell, R., Roth, V., Gravel, D., Astrakianakis, G., Bryce, E., Forgie, S., Johnston, L., Taylor, G., and Vearncombe, M. 2013. Are health care workers protected? An observational study of selection and removal of personal protective equipment in Canadian acute care hospitals. *Am J Infect Control* 41(3):240–244. DOI: 10.1016/j.ajic.2012.04.332.

23. Brown, L., Munro, J., and Rogers, S. 2019. Use of personal protective equipment in nursing practice. *Nursing Standard* 34:59–66. DOI: 10.7748/ns.2019.e11260.

24. Mast, S.T., Woolwine, J.D., and Gerberding, J.L. 1993. Efficacy of gloves in reducing blood volumes transferred during simulated needle-stick injury. *J Infect Dis* 168:1589–1592.

25. Dalgleish, A.G., and Malkovsky, M. 1988. Surgical gloves as a mechanical barrier against human immunodeficiency viruses. *Br J Surg* 75:171–172.

26. Code of Federal Regulations. 2017. *21 CFR 800.20: Patient Examination Gloves and Surgical Gloves; Sample Plans and Test Method for Leakage Defects; Adulteration.* Washington, DC: U.S. Government Printing Office.

27. ASTM International. 2019. *ASTM D 5151–19: Standard Test Method for Detection of Holes in Medical Gloves.* Philadelphia, PA: ASTM International.

28. CEN (European Standard). 2020. *EN 455-1:2020: Medical Gloves for Single Use - Part 1: Requirements and Testing for Freedom from Holes.* Brussels: Comité Européen De Normalisation (CEN).

29. ASTM International. 2013. *ASTM F1671/F1671M-13: Standard Test Method for Resistance of Materials Used in Protective Clothing to Penetration by Blood-Borne Pathogens Using Phi-X174 Bacteriophage Penetration as a Test System.* Philadelphia, PA: ASTM International. DOI: 10.1520/F1671_F1671M-13.

30. ASTM International. 2013. *ASTM F1342/F1342M-05(2013)e1: Standard Test Method for Protective Clothing Material Resistance to Puncture.* Philadelphia, PA: ASTM International. DOI: 10.1520/F1342_F1342M-05R13E01.

31. ASTM International. 2019. *ASTM F2878-19: Standard Test Method for Protective Clothing Material Resistance to Hypodermic Needle Puncture.* Philadelphia, PA: ASTM International. DOI: 10.1520/F2878-19.

32. ANSI. 2016. *ANSI/ISEA 105-2016: American National Standard for Hand Protection Classification.* Washington, DC: American National Standards Institute (ANSI).
33. NFPA. 2018. *NFPA 1999: Standard on Protective Clothing and Ensembles for Emergency Medical Operations.* Quincy, MA: National Fire Protection Association (NFPA).
34. Duxbury, M., Brown, C., and Lambert, A. 2003. Surgical gloves. How do you change yours? *Br J Perioper Nurs* 13:17–20.
35. Nelson, G.O., Priante, S.J., Strong, M., Anderson, D., and Fallon-Carine, J. 2000. Permeation of substituted silanes and siloxanes through selected gloves and protective clothing. *Am Ind Hyg Assoc J* 61:709–714.
36. Mäkelä, E.A., Vainiotalo, S., and Peltonen, K. 2003. Permeation of 70% isopropyl alcohol through surgical gloves: Comparison of the Standard Methods ASTM F 739 and EN 374. *Ann Occup Hyg* 47:305–312.
37. Baumann, M.A., Rath, B., Fischer, J.H., and Iffland, R. 2000. The permeability of dental procedure and examination gloves by an alcohol based disinfectant. *Dent Mater* 16:139–144.
38. Phalen, R.N., Le, T., and Wong, W.K. 2014. Changes in chemical permeation of disposable latex, nitrile, and vinyl gloves exposed to simulated movement. *J Occup Environ Hyg* 11(11):716–721. DOI: 10.1080/15459624.2014.908259.
39. Douglas, A., Simon, T.R., and Goddard, M. 1997. Barrier durability of latex and vinyl medical gloves in clinical settings. *Am Ind Hyg Assoc J* 58:672–676.
40. Klein, R.C., Party, E., and Gershey, E.L. 1990. Virus penetration of examination gloves. *Biotechniques* 9:196–199.
41. Korniewicz, D.M., Laughon, B.E., Butz, A., and Larson, E. 1989. Integrity of vinyl and latex procedures gloves. *Nurs Res* 38:144–146.
42. Richards, J.M., Sydiskis, R.J., Davidson, W.M., Josell, S.D., and Lavine, D.S. 1993. Permeability of latex gloves after contact with dental materials. *Am J Orthod Dentofacial Orthop* 104:224–229.
43. Centers for Disease Control and Prevention (CDC). 2010. Surveillance of occupationally acquired HIV/AIDS in healthcare personnel, as of December 2010. Available at: https://www.cdc.gov/hai/organisms/hiv/surveillance-occupationally-acquired-hiv-aids.html.
44. Rossoff, L.J., Lam, S., Hilton, E., Borenstein, M., and Isenberg, H.D. 1993. Is the use of boxed gloves in an intensive care unit safe? *Am J Med* 94:602–607.

Section V

Special Topics

27 Hydro-Alcoholic Gels and Glove Use

J.-M. Lachapelle

CONTENTS

27.1 INTRODUCTION

The worldwide pandemic of COVID-19 infection has deeply modified the life of millions of people. The routes of transmission of the virus can be direct, i.e. vectored by airborne drops (diameter < 5 μm; airborne > 1 μm) or by airborne droplets (diameter > 5 μm; airborne < 1 m). They can also be indirect, i.e. by direct contact with

DOI: 10.1201/9781003126874-32

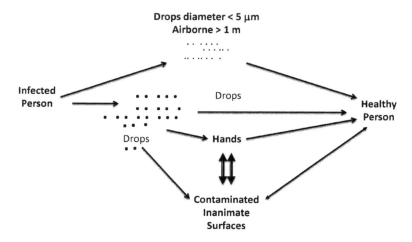

FIGURE 27.1   COVID-19: direct and indirect routes of transmission.

contaminated hands or by indirect contact with contaminated inanimate surfaces.[1] This is illustrated in Figure 27.1.

The airborne contaminated drops or droplets, as well as those deposited on hands or inanimate surfaces, are the forms of transmission to the airways (nasal and oral mucosa or eyes). The consequences are often dramatic, namely in the lungs; like other viruses, COVID-19 has a tropism for epithelial cells of the airways and alveoli, causing necrosis of the epithelium and leading to a respiratory distress syndrome (ARDS).[1] When the first symptoms appear, it is imperative to hospitalize the patient and treat him (or her) in an intensive care unit to provide oxygen as soon as possible.

Another clinical sign is the presence of chilblain-like lesions on the fingers and toes (similar to those observed in lupus erythematosus).[2]

They are consecutive to two sequential processes: (a) the sticking of COVID-19 to the surface of the endothelial cells of the vessels and (b) after the destruction of the cells, the development of thrombosis that provokes the aforementioned lesions.[3] Therefore, the systematic use of an anticoagulant (such as rivaroxaban) is highly recommended.

On the other hand, no drug has been found effective against COVID-19. Hydroxychloroquine has been disqualified as a potential candidate. The advent of mutants of the virus, which seem to be more contagious (i.e. British or South-African variants), creates an additional fear among the population and the prospect is none too promising. Nevertheless, the development of vaccines stimulates immunization, and let us hope that all will be the best! For the time being, prevention of any contact with the virus is the weapon to reduce the spread of the pandemic.

Four protective measures have been proposed and are now mandatory in many countries: (a) respect for a physical distance (>1.5 m) between individuals, (b) wearing a facial mask, (c) ventilation, and (d) application of hydro-alcoholic gels on the hands.

27.2   PREVENTIVE MEASURES

27.2.1   Respect for Physical Distance between Individuals

The respect for a physical (also called social) distance between people is imperative (>1.5 m). This clearly defined measure is aimed at avoiding contact with airborne drops or droplets contaminated by COVID-19 (see Figure 27.1). It includes the closure of non-essential shops such as public houses, restaurants, bars, cafeterias, and banqueting halls. Some sports activities are also canceled. All these measures can differ from country to country and also depend on a wave of momentary contagiousness in a defined area. The non-respect of rules determined by the authorities such as forbidden mass demonstrations and/or political gatherings can be severely punished.

27.2.2   Ventilation

The efficacy of ventilation was underestimated during the first epidemic of the COVID-19 infection. It is now considered important; it consists of opening doors and/or windows of premises for short periods (a few minutes). This allows the transport of contaminated drops or droplets from inside to outside and reduces the risks of spreading infection.

27.2.3   Wearing a Facial Protective Medical Mask

Wearing a disposable facial protective mask is considered fundamental in the strategy of avoiding COVID-19 infection.[1] It permits the filtering of many contaminated airborne drops or droplets disseminated from the oral mucosa and/or the nostrils. Some recommendations of use are listed in Table 27.1.

27.2.4   Hydro-Alcoholic Gels for the Protection of the Hands against COVID-19 Infection

The COVID-19 pandemic has emphasized the role of adequate hygiene and hand sanitizers in controlling the spread of infection in public places and healthcare

---

TABLE 27.1

Facial Protective Masks: Recommendations of Use

- The most recommended masks are those labeled FFP2 and FFP5 (European) or NIOSH-approved N95 (USA). They fit firmly for isolation of the nose and mouth. Acceptable masks will filter >90% of airborne contaminated drops and droplets.
- The so-called "surgical" masks are also convenient, they are disposable, and so they are used once or twice. Filtration efficiency is typically less than FFP2, FFP5, or N95 respirators.
- "Home-made" masks are not recommended and even forbidden nowadays in some countries, due to their insufficient filtration effect.
- After use, the masks have to be thrown away in dustbins to avoid pollution of the atmosphere.

---

institutions. Hands can be infected either by direct contact with airborne contaminated drops or by indirect contact with an inanimate surface (see Figure 27.1). The use of an efficient antiseptic was considered mandatory, and the choice turned to hydro-alcoholic gels, which are now the gold standard all over the world.[4] There has been a great surge in demand for these hand sanitization products leading to shortages in their supply. A consequent increase of substandard products in the market has raised safety concerns, but the problem is now partially solved. Hand sanitization will remain at the forefront of infection prevention measures. Moreover, it is reasonable to speculate that the current awareness of the general public of the importance of hand disinfection will remain assimilated and will become an integral part of people's hygiene practices, even post-COVID-19 era.

In conclusion, hydro-alcoholic gels, also called hand sanitizers, are "alcohol-based hand rubs (ABHRs)" and are the most effective and convenient infection prevention measures until the mass vaccination of the population is implemented and considered efficacious in the vast majority of patients. Directing the correct dose/amount is needed to achieve adequate sanitization. The choice of container, closure, and dispenser is also vital in dispensing the correct amounts of sanitizer for each use. All infectiologists insist on the methodology of rubbing the skin; in fact, the sanitizer has to be applied on all parts of the backs and palms of the hands.

27.2.5 INGREDIENTS THAT ENTER IN THE COMPOSITION OF HYDRO-ALCOHOLIC GELS

27.2.5.1 Ethanol

It is universally agreed that ethanol is the best antiseptic to be used in hydro-alcoholic gels.[4] The concentration of ethanol (65%–95%) is a crucial condition to ensure efficacy. The gels have reduced efficacy against COVID-19 when ethanol is used at lower concentrations.

Peroxide of hydrogen is sometimes added to the formulation.

27.2.5.2 Emollients (Humectants)

Ethanol in hand rubs can cause skin dryness, particularly over frequent exposures. Emollients have been shown to decrease the drying effect of ethanol on the skin.

Glycerin is the most commonly used humectant in hand sanitizers. The incorporation of glycerin in hand rubs promotes hand hydration. Reducing glycerin content to concentrations of 0.50%–0.73% has been proposed as the best compromise in maintaining antimicrobial activity while still offering the needed skin protection.[4,5]

Propylene glycol is the second most used humectant, and it is generally used for this purpose in hand sanitizers at concentrations of 2%–5%.[4]

Aloe vera gel is also used as a humectant, being able to retard water evaporation from formulations, yet to a lower extent than glycerol and propylene glycol.[4] Aloe vera can be used in combination with glycerin and propylene glycol to improve their water evaporation retardation effect. Its specificity is most probably related to an increasing interest of consumers toward natural products. Thus, the incorporation of aloe vera (or *Aloe barbadensis* leaf extract) may justify its use in hand rubs.

27.2.5.3 Viscosity Enhancers

For the consumer market, gel formulations are more portable and convenient to use than solutions. There is a low risk of spillage compared to liquid-based products. Moreover, gel-based formulations also reduce the evaporation rate of ethanol and help it to spread and penetrate through contaminating organisms, including COVID-19.[4] The list of viscosity enhancers is huge, but some of them are particularly advised: carbomer, hydroxyethylcellulose, hydroxypropylmethylcellulose, and sodium carboxymethylcellulose.[4]

27.2.5.4 Miscellaneous

Some ingredients, added to the basic list, have no practical interest. They are included for cosmetic reasons, but some display allergenic properties and are not to be recommended. The most frequently used are perfumes, dyes, linalool, citronellol, geraniol, citral, and limonene, but many others could be included.[4]

27.2.6 SKIN LESIONS OF THE HANDS RELATED TO HYDRO-ALCOHOLIC GELS

27.2.6.1 Skin Dryness Linked with the Application of Ethanol

Ethanol (mainly at a concentration of 70%–90%), when it evaporates after application on the skin, entails dryness. This is well documented, despite the fact that emollients and viscosity enhancers incorporated in the hydro-alcoholic gels tend to delay this evaporation. Xerosis affects symmetrically the backs of the hands, but not the palms. Dryness is the first step of the evolution of events, leading to irritant contact dermatitis.

27.2.6.2 Irritant Contact Dermatitis

Irritant contact dermatitis (ICD) is the most common side effect provoked by hydro-alcoholic gels.[6] The lesions are invariably localized on the skin surmounting the metacarpophalangeal joints (Figure 27.2) and undoubtedly result from frictions and the chemical irritancy of ethanol. In other words, a mixture of frictional and chemical irritation. The lesions are well demarcated, oblong, and deep red. Sub-acute or chronic ICD is characterized by hyperkeratosis, fissuring, glazed, or scalded appearance of the skin.

27.2.6.3 Atopic Subjects

Atopic subjects are more prone to develop ICD to hydro-alcoholic gels.[6] The symptoms are quite similar to those observed in non-atopics.

27.2.6.4 For All Patients, Atopic or Not, the Nuisance Is Quite Obvious

Pruritus is the main subjective symptom, but lesions can also become painful when chaps and cracks do occur. Work may be disturbed; complaints are very frequent, and there is no real way to alleviate the complaints. The use of emollients, corticosteroid-based creams, and/or ointments is indeed not very efficient.

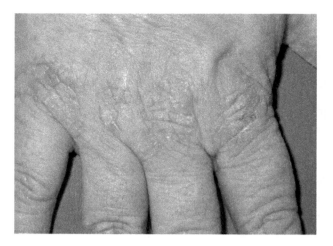

FIGURE 27.2   Irritant contact dermatitis provoked by applications of hydro-alcoholic gels. Lesions are limited to the skin surmounting metacarpophalangeal joints.

In summary, ICD lesions are undoubtedly related to the use of hydro-alcoholic gels, and their disagreement and severity are increased by several potential factors:

- Too drastic rubbing when gels are applied on the skin
- Long periods of application of the gel
- Number of daily applications (sometimes more than 15)

27.2.7   Use of Gloves in Occupational Medicine

The use of gloves is universally considered essential and even mandatory in various occupations. The interest in this use is self-evident and broadly explained in many chapters of the book. Certain specific aspects have to be pointed out.

First of all, gloves prevent cuts when workers are in contact with sharp objects. When this protection measure is forgotten, industrial injuries cannot be avoided.

There is a large variety of gloves, each being adapted to a well-defined workplace. When in doubt, the factory doctor or the safety officer is advised to refer to catalogs, usually full of all types of information.

Skin side effects of gloves are well known; for example, they include allergic contact dermatitis, immunological contact urticarial, or protein contact dermatitis provoked by natural rubber gloves (proteins of latex).[6]

27.2.8   The Concomitant Use of Hydro-Alcoholic Gels and Gloves against COVID-19

The first line of protection against COVID-19 is achieved by the use of hydro-alcoholic gels applied on the hands and is at the forefront of infection prevention measures. The use of viscosity enhancers in the formulation reduces the evaporation of ethanol and helps ethanol to spread and penetrate through contaminated organisms. As the COVID-19 is concerned, its activity is markedly decreased ($\pm$99%) by an effective blockade of its proliferation. Thus, this first line of protection is aimed to annihilate the viral infection but not to create a "barrier" to chemicals. In European countries, 10% povidone–iodine is dissolved in a 70% ethanol–water solution (trade name: Betadine®), largely used in hospitals.[7] It is a viricide but transfers to the skin a dark yellow color, which limits its use.

The second line of protection consists in wearing gloves impermeable to hydro-alcoholic gels. This occlusion enhances the sudation, mainly in a warm environment. Sweat dissolves the remaining ingredients of the gel, allowing their penetration into the skin.

27.2.9 SKIN LESIONS OF THE HANDS DUE TO GLOVES USED SIMULTANEOUSLY WITH HYDRO-ALCOHOLIC GELS

Lesions due to the use of gloves in those circumstances are the result of physical factors, i.e. pressure and friction, more or less important according to the type of gloves.[6]

In practice, classical lesions related to hydro-alcoholic gels are usually extended to the entirety of the backs of both hands.

Palms are sometimes also affected, and the lesions are characteristic: clinical signs and symptoms include painful, dry, erythematous, and scaly lesions with fissuring (Figure 27.3).[6]

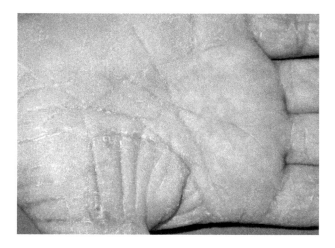

FIGURE 27.3 Palmar irritant contact dermatitis provoked by the concomitant use of gloves and hydro-alcoholic gels.

REFERENCES

1. Nigro, F., Tavares, M., Sato de Souza de Bustamante Monteiro, M., Toma, H.K., Faria de Freitas, Z.M., de Abreu Garófalo, D., Geraldes Bordalo MontáAlverne, M.A., Barros Dos Passos, M.M., Pereira Dos Santos, E., and Ricci-Júnior, E. 2020. Changes in workflow to a university pharmacy to facilitate compounding and distribution of antiseptics for use against COVID-19. *Res Social Adm Pharm* 17:1997–2001. DOI: 10.1016/j.sapharm.2020.09.016.

2. Landa, N., Mendieta-Eckert, M., Fonda-Pascual, P., and Aguirre, T. 2020. Chilblain-like lesions on feet and hands during the COVID-19 pandemic. *Int J Dermatol* 59(6):739–743. DOI: 10.1111/ijd.14937.

3. Jin, Y., Ji, W., Yang, H., Chen, S., Zhang, W., and Duan, G. 2020. Endothelial activation and dysfunction in COVID-19: From basic mechanisms to potential therapeutic approaches. *Signal Transduct Target Ther* 5(1):293. DOI: 10.1038/s41392-020-00454-7.

4. Berardi, A., Perinelli, D.R., Merchant, H.A., Bisharat, L., Basheti, I.A., Bonacucina, G., Cespi, M., and Palmieri, G.F. 2020. Hand sanitisers amid COVID-19: A critical review of alcohol-based products on the market and formulation and approaches to respond to increasing demand. *Int J Pharm* 30:584-119431.

5. Alpaslan, D., Ersen Dudu, T., and Aktas, N. 2021. Synthesis and characterization of novel organo-hydrogel based agar, glycerol and peppermint oil as a natural drug carrier/release material. *Mater Sci Eng C Mater Biol Appl.* 118:111534. DOI: 10.1016/j.msec.2020.111534.

6. Alikhan, A., Lachapelle, J.-M., and Maibach, H.I. 2014. *Textbook of Hand Eczema*. Berlin, Heidelberg: Springer-Verlag.

7. WHO. 2006. *WHO Guidelines on Hand Hygiene in Healthcare: Global Patient Safety Challenge 2005–2006: "Clean Care is Safer Care"*. Geneva, Switzerland: World Health Organization (WHO) Press.

28 Clinical Relevance of Masks in the Operating Room*

H.N. Mechels and H.I. Maibach

CONTENTS

28.1 INTRODUCTION

Face mask use in the operating room (OR) dates back to Germany in the nineteenth century.[1] Current recommendations are for all persons to be masked for sterile procedures.[2] While many studies have explored the microbiology of wearing a mask in the OR,[3,4] few have explored their clinical relevance. Here we systematically review randomized control trials on mask efficacy in the operating room as a means of preventing surgical site clinical infection.

28.2 MATERIALS AND METHODS

The Preferred Reporting Items for Systematic Review and Meta-Analysis guidelines were followed for this systematic review.[5]

28.2.1 SEARCH STRATEGY

A literature search utilized PubMed, Google Scholar, Web of Science, and National Institute for Occupational Safety and Health Publications and Products on March 1,

---

* Reprinted with permission from authors. Burdick, H.N. and Maibach, H. 2021. Clinical relevance of masks in the operating room? A systematic review. *Clinical Infect Practice* (Open Access) 12:100087.

DOI: 10.1201/9781003126874-33

2021, using the search terms "mask use" and "surgical site" and "infection," "face mask use" and "surgeons," and "mask" and "splash" and "surgery."

28.2.2 ELIGIBILITY

Articles were included if they fit the criteria of: (1) randomized control trial, (2) clinical patient outcomes, (3) mask efficacy, (4) surgery setting, (5) in vivo, and (6) article was in English.

28.2.3 DATA SCREENING

Title and abstract screening was completed using Covidence. References from the included articles were checked and included if they met the inclusion criteria.

28.2.4 DATA EXTRACTION

Data were extracted on the study and patient characteristics, type of surgery, the proportion of emergent procedures, primary outcomes, and results.

28.3 RESULTS

There were 717 articles uploaded, and 201 duplicates were removed. There were 516 titles and abstracts screened with 488 being found irrelevant and 68 being screened for full text. After the full-text review, two articles filled the inclusion criteria and an additional two articles were included based on findings in the references. Table 28.1 summarizes the results. The findings with NR stand for not related.

Overall, the results indicate no difference in surgical site infections between the operations where masks were worn versus the operations where no mask was worn. However, this is of limited evidence as there have been few studies that were randomized control trials focused on clinical outcomes. There were 3924 patients in all of the studies combined, a small amount when considering that surgical masks have been around since the nineteenth century.

Webster et al.[8] combined their studies and Tunevall et al.'s[7] and found a statistically significant result that favored not wearing a mask.

28.4 DISCUSSION

For something that is recommended in everyday practice, there is little evidence to support the continued use of surgical face masks in the operating room from an infection standpoint. Orr[6] found that there was actually a decrease in surgical site infection. One proposed hypothesis is that masks may increase surgical site infections by the rubbing of the mask against skin-releasing organisms such as staphylococci,[7] a known cause of surgical site infections.[10] With such limited evidence and the great cost that accrues from purchasing face masks for all surgical staff, we hope

TABLE 28.1

Data Extraction Results

Author	Date	Surgical Fields	Patients (No.)	Age	Sex	Emergent	Primary Outcome	Results
Neil Orr[6]	1981	General Surgery	NR	NR	NR	NR	Surgical site infection	No increase in wound infections with a significant ($p < 0.05$) decrease in surgical site infection with no mask.
Th. Göran Tunevall[7]	1991	General Surgery	3088	58 years mask, 57 years in unmasked	NR	6% masked and 5.4% not masked	Surgical site infection	No statistically significant differences in wound infection rates ($p > 0.5$). In the masked group, the infection rate was 4.7% (3.7–5.8%, 95% CI) and in the unmasked group, 3.5% (2.6%–4.5%, 95% CI).
Joan Webster et al.[8]	2009	Gynecology, Obstetric, General Surgery, and Urology	827	45.4 years in no mask, 44.7 years in mask	Male: 18.1% in no mask, 21.4% in mask	23.4% in no mask, 23.8% in mask	Surgical site infection	11.5% infection rate in mask group and 9.0% infection rate in no mask group, but the difference was not statistically significant (OR 0.77 95 CI 0.49–1.21)..
Geoffery V. Chamberlain and Elizabeth Houang[9]	1984	Gynecology	9	NR	100% Female	NR	Surgical site infection	3/5 patients in the no mask group had an infection and 0/4 in the mask group had an infection. The study was discontinued due to the three infections occurring early in the study.

for larger, well-designed randomized control trials to evaluate the true clinical efficacy of surgical masks in the operating room.

REFERENCES

1. Matuschek, C., Moll, F., Fangerau, H., Fischer, J.C., Zänker, K., van Griensven, M., Schneider, M., Kindgen-Milles, D., Knoefel, W.T., Lichtenberg, A., Tamaskovics, B., Djiepmo-Njanang, F.J., Budach, W., Corradini, S., Häussinger, D., Feldt, T., Jensen, B., Pelka, R., Orth, K., Peiper, M., Grebe, O., Maas, K., Bölke, E., and Haussmann, J. 2020. The history and value of face masks. *Eur J Med Res* 25:23. DOI: 10.1186/s40001-020-00423-4.
2. Siegel, J.D., Rhinehart, E., Jackson, M., and Chiarello, L. 2007. Health Care Infection Control Practices Advisory Committee. 2007 guideline for isolation precautions: Preventing transmission of infectious agents in health care settings. *Am J Infect Control* 35(10 Suppl 2):S65–S164. DOI: 10.1016/j.ajic.2007.10.007.
3. McLure, H.A., Talboys, C.A., Yentis, S.M., and Azadian, B.S. 1998. Surgical face masks and downward dispersal of bacteria. *Anaesthesia* 53(7):624–626.
4. Howard, B.E. 2020. High-risk aerosol-generating procedures in COVID-19: Respiratory protective equipment considerations. *Otolaryngol Head Neck Surg* 163(1):98–103. DOI: 10.1177/0194599820927335.
5. Moher, D., Liberati, A., Tetzlaff, J., Altman, D.G., and PRISMA Group. 2009. Preferred reporting items for systematic reviews and meta-analyses: The PRISMA statement. *PLOS Med* 6(7):e1000097. DOI: 10.1371/journal.pmed.1000097.
6. Orr, N.W. 1981. Is a mask necessary in the operating theatre?. *Ann R Coll Surg Engl* 63(6):390–392.
7. Tunevall, T.G. 1991. Postoperative wound infections and surgical face masks: A controlled study. *World J Surg* 15(3):383–387; discussion 387–388. DOI: 10.1007/BF01658736.
8. Webster, J., Croger, S., Lister, C., Doidge, M., Terry, M.J., and Jones, I. 2010. Use of face masks by non-scrubbed operating room staff: A randomized controlled trial. *ANZ J Surg* 80(3):169–173. DOI: 10.1111/j.1445-2197.2009.05200.x.
9. Chamberlain, G.V., and Houang, E. 1984. Trial of the use of masks in the gynaecological operating theatre. *Ann R Coll Surg Engl* 66(6):432–433.
10. Anderson, D.J., and Kaye, K.S. 2009. Staphylococcal surgical site infections. *Infect Dis Clin North Am* 23(1):53–72. DOI: 10.1016/j.idc.2008.10.004.

29 Are Masks Effective as Source Control in Index Influenza Patients? A Review*

H.N. Mechels and H.I. Maibach

CONTENTS

29.1 INTRODUCTION

The use of facemasks for infection prevention dates back to the nineteenth century in Germany in operating rooms.[1] With time and further research, the use of masks became widely accepted. The use of facemasks has been studied in various settings, including the respiratory infection agent influenza. Annual influenza epidemics are common, but several influenza pandemics have occurred in history starting in 1580,[2] and most recently in 2009 with the H1N1 strain.[3] Each year, influenza carries a significant burden for morbidity and mortality, with the Centers for Disease Control and Prevention (CDC) estimating that between 140,000 and 810,000 hospitalizations and 12,000 and 61,000 deaths have occurred annually since 2010.[4]

Influenza is spread by indirect or direct contact, droplet, or aerosol transmission,[5] and facemasks have been identified as a potential non-pharmacological intervention. A plethora of studies assess the efficacy of masks in the prevention of influenza in

* Reprinted with permission from authors. Burdick, H.N. and Maibach, H. 2021. Are masks effective as source control in index influenza patients? A systematic review. *Clinical Infect Practice* (Open Access) 12:100097.

DOI: 10.1201/9781003126874-34

terms of the type of mask used and randomization of hospital and community populations.[6–10] However, studies on mask use by index patients as a means for source control are limited. The current recommendation by the CDC includes influenza-infected patients wearing masks when seen in a medical setting.[11] Here we systematically reviewed randomized control trials on mask efficacy in index influenza patients to prevent transmission.

29.2   MATERIALS AND METHODS

The Preferred Reporting Items for Systematic Review and Meta-Analysis guidelines were followed for this review.[12]

29.2.1   Search Strategy

A literature search utilized PubMed, Google Scholar, and Web of Science on March 28, 2021, using the search terms "influenza" AND "infected patient" AND "control trial" AND "mask," "infected patient" AND "source control" OR "reduce transmission" AND "mask" AND "controlled trial" AND "influenza," and "index patient" AND "influenza" AND "mask" AND "control trial." Clinicaltrials.gov was also searching using the terms "influenza" AND "mask."

29.2.2   Eligibility

Articles were included if they fit the criteria of: (1) randomized control trial, (2) influenza, (3) mask efficacy, (4) influenza patients with masks for source control, (5) in vivo, and (6) article was in English.

29.2.3   Data Screening

Title and abstract screening was completed using Covidence. References from the included articles were checked and included if they met the inclusion criteria.

29.2.4   Data Extraction

Data were extracted on the study and patient characteristics, type of masks studied, setting in which mask efficacy was studied, primary outcomes, and results.

29.3   RESULTS

There were 179 articles uploaded, and 23 duplicates were removed. There were 156 titles and abstracts screened, with 124 being found irrelevant and 32 being screened for full text. After the full-text review, six articles filled the inclusion criteria and no additional articles were found to fit the inclusion criteria after reviewing the references. Table 29.1 summarizes the results. The findings with NR stand for not reported.

TABLE 29.1

Data Extraction Results

Author	Date	Index/ Contact Patients (No.)	Age (Years)	Sex (Male)	Type of Mask	Interventions Studied	Setting	Influenza or Influenza- Like Illness	Confirmation of Diagnosis	Results
Cowling et al.[13]	2009	407/764	Index Med.: 9–12 Contacts Med.: 38–40	319	Surgical facemask	Hand hygiene (HH) and HH plus facemask	Community	Influenza	RT-PCR for primary analysis and clinical definition for secondary analysis	No stat. sig. difference between randomized groups
MacIntyre et al.[14]	2009	274	NR	NR	Surgical facemask and P2 facemask	Two different types of masks	Community	Influenza- like illness	Clinical definition or one symptom and a laboratory positive test result	No stat. sig. diff. between interv. arms. But, study reported low adherence rates
Canini et al.[15]	2010	105/306	Interv.: 25 Control: 28	Interv.: 99 Control: 107	Surgical facemask	Mask	Community	Influenza- like illness	Clinical definition	No stat. sig. diff. between interv. arms
Simmerman et al.[16]	2011	465/1147	Med.: 34	Index: 192 Contacts: 362	Surgical facemask	Hand washing (HW) and HW plus facemask	Community	Influenza	RT-PCR and serological testing	No stat. sig. diff. between interv. arms

(Continued)

TABLE 29.1 (CONTINUED)
Data Extraction Results

Author	Date	Index/ Contact Patients (No.)	Age (Years)	Sex (Male)	Type of Mask	Interventions Studied	Setting	Influenza or Influenza- Like Illness	Confirmation of Diagnosis	Results
Suess et al.[17]	2012	84/218	Index Med.: 7–8 Contacts Med.: 34–38	Index: 39 Contacts: 106	Surgical facemask	Mask and mask plus hygiene	Community	Influenza	RT-PCR for primary outcome and clinical infection as a secondary outcome	No stat. sig. diff. between interv. arms. But, stat. sig. reduction in secondary attack rates when both the mask and mask plus hygiene groups combined
MacIntyre et al.[18]	2016	245/597	Interv. index mean: 40.2 Control index mean: 39.7 Interv. contact mean: 38.3 Control contact mean: 36.4	Index: 101 Contacts: 317	Surgical mask	Mask	Community	Influenza-like illness	Clinical infection or laboratory-confirmed infection	No stat. sig. diff. as source control between interv. arms

Overall, the results point to no difference in influenza transmission between medical mask and control groups. Suess et al.[17] did mention having a statistically significant reduction in secondary attack rates when mask intervention and mask plus hand hygiene intervention were combined. However, this highlights the difficulty in assessing the true efficacy of masks when multiple interventions were implemented in an intervention group.

29.4   DISCUSSION

The evidence supporting the recommendation for masked influenza patients is weak at best, as shown by this review's findings. Several reasons were proposed in the articles for the lack of substantial benefit. Some reasons include the need for earlier intervention,[17] low rates of adherence,[13] and small populations studied.

Additionally, these studies were relatively small and few have been conducted when considering the lengthy mask use history. All of these studies occurred in the community setting, which creates a challenge in extrapolating the results to the clinical setting. This review brings to attention the lack of information on the efficacy of masks for source control in influenza patients. We hope for larger, randomized control trials in the hospital setting that evaluate the efficacy of masks as a means of source control in influenza-infected patients.

REFERENCES

1. Matuschek, C., Moll, F., Fangerau, H., Fischer, J.C., Zänker, K., van Griensven, M., Schneider, M., Kindgen-Milles, D., Knoefel, W.T., Lichtenberg, A., Tamaskovics, B., Djiepmo-Njanang, F.J., Budach, W., Corradini, S., Häussinger, D., Feldt, T., Jensen, B., Pelka, R., Orth, K., Peiper, M., Grebe, O., Maas, K., Bölke, E., and Haussmann, J. 2020. The history and value of face masks. *Eur J Med Res* 25(1):23. DOI: 10.1186/s40001-020-00423-4.
2. Potter, C.W. 2001. A history of influenza. *J Appl Microbiol* 91(4):572–579. DOI: 10.1046/j.1365-2672.2001.01492.x.
3. CDC. 2019. 2009 H1N1 PANDEMIC (H1N1pdm09 virus). (2019, June 11). Centers for Disease Control and Prevention. Retrieved April 27, 2021, from https://www.cdc.gov/flu/pandemic-resources/2009-h1n1-pandemic.html.
4. CDC. 2020. Disease burden of influenza. (2020, October 05). Centers for Disease Control and Prevention. Retrieved April 27, 2021, from https://www.cdc.gov/flu/about/burden/index.html.
5. Brienen, N.C., Timen, A., Wallinga, J., van Steenbergen, J.E., and Teunis, P.F. 2010. The effect of mask use on the spread of influenza during a pandemic. *Risk Anal* 30(8):1210–1218. DOI: 10.1111/j.1539-6924.2010.01428.x.
6. Long, Y., Hu, T., Liu, L., Chen, R., Guo, Q., Yang, L., Cheng, Y., Huang, J., and Du, L. 2020. Effectiveness of N95 respirators versus surgical masks against influenza: A systematic review and meta-analysis. *J Evid Based Med* 13(2):93–101. DOI: 10.1111/jebm.12381.
7. Loeb, M., Dafoe, N., Mahony, J., John, M., Sarabia, A., Glavin, V., Webby, R., Smieja, M., Earn, D.J., Chong, S., Webb, A., and Walter, S.D. 2009. Surgical mask vs N95 respirator for preventing influenza among health care workers: A randomized trial. *JAMA* 302(17):1865–1871. DOI: 10.1001/jama.2009.1466.

8. Radonovich, L.J.J., Bessesen, M.T., Cummings, D.A., Eagan, A., Gaydos, C., Gibert, C., Gorse, G.J., Nyquist, A.C., Reich, N.G., Rodrigues-Barradas, M., Savor-Price, C., Shaffer, R.E., Simberkoff, M.S., and Perl, T.M. 2016. The Respiratory Protection Effectiveness Clinical Trial (ResPECT): A cluster-randomized comparison of respirator and medical mask effectiveness against respiratory infections in healthcare personnel. *BMC Infect Dis* 16:243. DOI: 10.1186/s12879-016-1494-2.

9. Radonovich, L.J.J., Simberkoff, M.S., Bessesen, M.T., Brown, A.C., Cummings, D.A.T., Gaydos, C.A., Los, J.G., Krosche, A.E., Gibert, C.L., Gorse, G.J., Nyquist, A.C., Reich, N.G., Rodriguez-Barradas, M.C., Price, C.S., Perl, T.M., and ResPECT investigators. 2019. N95 respirators vs medical masks for preventing influenza among health care personnel: A randomized clinical trial. *JAMA* 322(9):824–833. DOI: 10.1001/jama.2019.11645.

10. Aiello, A.E., Perez, V., Coulborn, R.M., Davis, B.M., Uddin, M., and Monto, A.S. 2012. Facemasks, hand hygiene, and influenza among young adults: A randomized intervention trial. *PLoS One* 7(1):e29744. DOI: 10.1371/journal.pone.0029744.

11. CDC. 2018. Prevention strategies for seasonal influenza in healthcare settings. (2018, October 30). Centers for Disease Control and Prevention. Retrieved April 27, 2021, from https://www.cdc.gov/flu/professionals/infectioncontrol/healthcaresettings.htm.

12. Moher, D., Liberati, A., Tetzlaff, J., Altman, D.G., and PRISMA Group. 2009. Preferred reporting items for systematic reviews and meta-analyses: The PRISMA statement. *PLOS Med* 6(7):e1000097. DOI: 10.1371/journal.pmed.1000097.

13. Cowling, B.J., Chan, K.-H., Fang, V.J., Cheng, C.K., Fung, R.O., Wai, W., Sin, J., Seto, W.H., Yung, R., Chu, D.W., Chiu, B.C., Lee, P.W., Chiu, M.C., Lee, H.C., Uyeki, T.M., Houck, P.M., Peiris, J.S., and Leung, G.M. 2009. Facemasks and hand hygiene to prevent influenza transmission in households: A cluster randomized trial. *Ann Intern Med* 151(7):437–446. DOI: 10.7326/0003-4819-151-7-200910060-00142.

14. MacIntyre, C.R., Cauchemez, S., Dwyer, D.E., Seale, H., Cheung, P., Browne, G., Fasher, M., Wood, J., Gao, Z., Booy, R., and Ferguson, N. 2009. Face mask use and control of respiratory virus transmission in households. *Emerg Infect Dis* 15(2):233–241. DOI: 10.3201/eid1502.081167.

15. Canini, L., Andréoletti, L., Ferrari, P., D'Angelo, R., Blanchon, T., Lemaitre, M., Filleul, L., Ferry, J.P., Desmaizieres, M., Smadja, S., Valleron, A.J., and Carrat, F. 2010. Surgical mask to prevent influenza transmission in households: A cluster randomized trial. *PLoS One* 5(11):e13998. DOI: 10.1371/journal.pone.0013998.

16. Simmerman, J.M., Suntarattiwong, P., Levy, J., Jarman, R.G., Kaewchana, S., Gibbons, R.V., Cowling, B.J., Sanasuttipun, W., Maloney, S.A., Uyeki, T.M., Kamimoto, L., and Chotipitayasunondh, T. 2011. Findings from a household randomized controlled trial of hand washing and face masks to reduce influenza transmission in Bangkok, Thailand. *Influenza Other Respir Viruses* 5(4):256–267. DOI: 10.1111/j.1750-2659.2011.00205.x.

17. Suess, T., Remschmidt, C., Schink, S.B., Schweiger, B., Nitsche, A., Schroeder, K., Doellinger, J., Milde, J., Haas, W., Koehler, I., Krause, G., and Buchholz, U. 2012. The role of facemasks and hand hygiene in the prevention of influenza transmission in households: Results from a cluster randomised trial; Berlin, Germany, 2009–2011. *BMC Infect Dis* 12:26. DOI: 10.1186/1471-2334-12-26.

18. MacIntyre, C.R., Zhang, Y., Chughtai, A.A., Seale, H., Zhang, D., Chu, Y., Zhang, H., Rahman, B., and Wang, Q. 2016. Cluster randomised controlled trial to examine medical mask use as source control for people with respiratory illness. *BMJ Open* 6(12):e012330. DOI: 10.1136/bmjopen-2016-012330.

30 Extended Use and Disinfection of N95 Respirators and Exam Gloves During a Pandemic*

R.N. Phalen, J-M. Lachapelle, and Y.K. Hamidi

CONTENTS

30.1 INTRODUCTION

On March 3, 2020, at the beginning of the COVID-19 pandemic, the World Health Organization (WHO) called for a significant increase in the manufacturing of personal protection equipment to meet rising demand and protect healthcare workers and their patients.[1] The WHO estimated that up to 89 million medical masks and 76 million exam gloves were needed each month. In the USA, the Centers for Disease Control and Prevention (CDC) issued crisis capacity strategies to help address the

---

* Printed with permission of the American Industrial Hygiene Association. Adapted from Phalen, R.N. and Hamidi, Y.K. 2021. Extended Use and Disinfection of PPE: A Summary of Current Research on N95 Respirators and Exam Gloves. *Synergist* Dec. 2021:30–34.

DOI: 10.1201/9781003126874-35

shortages of N95 respirators and disposable medical exam gloves.[2,3] These strategies included extended use and reuse of personal protective equipment (PPE).

Over the following months, healthcare providers and hospitals around the world were overwhelmed with patients, which strained the global supply chain for PPE. Both N95 respirators and medical exam gloves are critical PPE components for healthcare workers, helping protect against the spread of respiratory diseases to and from patients. N95 respirators are designed to filter small airborne respiratory droplets, including those associated with coughs, sneezes, breathing, and speech, and therefore provide a higher level of protection to healthcare workers than surgical masks and cloth face masks. If used appropriately, disposable medical exam gloves can provide additional protection against the transmission of most airborne viruses, including SARS-CoV-2.

Since the supply of PPE had returned to normal levels towards the end of 2021, the CDC no longer recommended crisis capacity strategies such as extended use and reuse of PPE. But knowledge about these strategies will help healthcare providers protect their workers and their patients in the event of future shortages.

30.2   EXTENDED USE OF N95 RESPIRATORS

The CDC has continued to update its "Strategies for Optimizing the Supply of N95 Respirators," which specifies guidelines on the limited reuse of N95 respirators during known shortages.[2] It includes the following recommendations for users:

- Consult with the manufacturer regarding the maximum number of reuse and donning activities that can be performed with its N95 respirator. Redonning an N95 respirator could reduce its fit and effectiveness.
- As a default, the CDC recommends that N95 respirators not be reused or redonned more than five times. A proper pre-use inspection and user seal check should occur prior to each reuse.
- Protect against contamination by wearing a face shield or face mask over the N95 respirator.
- As a limited reuse strategy, rotate products to reduce the risk of self-contamination between uses. The CDC recommends rotating N95 respirators with at least 72 hours of storage in a breathable paper bag before reuse. This recommendation is based on evidence that the SARS-CoV-2 virus would no longer be viable after this time has elapsed. However, as the CDC acknowledges, evidence in the peer-reviewed literature suggests a storage time of seven days may be more appropriate.[4]
- When a shortage exists and rotation is not feasible, seek proper decontamination methods. The CDC first recommends consulting the manufacturer or third-party expert organizations or laboratories for information on how to decontaminate the specific N95 respirator without affecting its performance. In the absence of these guidelines, the decontamination strategies recommended by the National Institute for Occupational Safety and Health

(NIOSH) include ultraviolet germicidal irradiation, vaporous hydrogen peroxide, and moist heat. This chapter provides additional details on the decontamination of N95 respirators.

30.3　SUPPORTING RESEARCH ON N95 RESPIRATORS

Since the COVID-19 pandemic started, researchers and experts have worked to address critical gaps in knowledge on extending the use of N95 respirators under crisis conditions. One such group that industrial hygienists and healthcare providers should be aware of is N95DECON, a collective of over 100 scientists, engineers, clinicians, and professionals from around the world focused on providing stakeholders valuable information on the decontamination and reuse of N95 respirators. The organization's website (n95decon.org) provides a repository for peer-reviewed research and technical reports on the subject as well as important considerations regarding a method's effectiveness, effects on respirator filtration efficiency and fit, available guidance and protocols, associated hazards, and costs. Below is a summary of recent work posted to n95decon.org. Key papers in the peer-reviewed literature are listed in Table 30.1.

TABLE 30.1
Essential Publications on N95 Decontamination

Room Temperature
- Smullin, S.J., Tarlow, B.D., and the N95DECON Consortium. 2021. Room temperature wait and reuse for bioburden reduction of SARS-CoV-2 on N95 filtering facepiece respirators. *Appl Biosafety* 26(2):103–111. DOI: 10.1089/apb.20.0055.

Heat and Humidity
- Anderegg, L., Doyle, J., Gardel, M.L., Gupta, A., Hallas, C., Lensky, Y., et al. 2021. Heat and humidity for bioburden reduction of N95 filtering facepiece respirators. *Appl Biosafety* 26(2):80–89. DOI: 10.1089/apb.20.0053.

Hydrogen Peroxide
- Rempel, D., Henneman, J., Agalloco, J., Crittenden, J., and the N95DECON Consortium. 2021. Hydrogen peroxide methods for decontaminating N95 filtering facepiece respirators. *Appl Biosafety* 26(2):71–79. DOI: 10.1089/apb.20.0042.

UV-C
- Grist, S.M., Geldert, A., Gopal, A., Su, A., Balch, H.B., Herr, A.E., and the N95DECON Consortium. 2021. Current understanding of ultraviolet-C decontamination of N95 filtering facepiece respirators. *Appl Biosafety* 26(2):90–102. DOI: 10.1089/apb.20.0051.
- Geldert, A., Balch, H.B., Gopal, A., Su, A., Grist, S.M., and Herr, A.E. 2021. Best practices for germicidal ultraviolet-C dose measurement for N95 respirator decontamination. *J Res Nat Inst Standards Technol* 126:1–14. DOI: 10.6028/jres.126.020.

Comparison of Methods
- N95DECON. 2021. Publications. Available at: https://www.n95decon.org/publications.

30.3.1 N95 Methods Implemented in Hospitals

The primary methods used in hospital settings for disinfecting and reuse of N95 respirators include ultraviolet C (UV-C) irradiation within a room or cabinet,[5,6] vaporized hydrogen peroxide or hydrogen peroxide gas plasma,[7] and heated convection chamber.[8] All these methods are well supported in the peer-reviewed literature and by regulatory guidance.

UV-C irradiation at a peak wavelength of 254 nm and a dose of at least 1.0 Joules per square centimeter (J/cm^2) shows significant germicidal effectiveness against SARS-CoV-2 with certain N95 respirators.[5,6] The dose of UV-C must be delivered uniformly to all surfaces of the respirator, which can be challenging. Significantly higher doses of UV-C may damage the respirator and thus are not recommended. Furthermore, the elastic straps may require additional chemical disinfection. The primary advantages of this method are that it does not affect filter performance or respirator fit and leaves no chemical residue. Therefore, the number of reuses is likely to be limited by fit diminution caused by donning and doffing.

Hydrogen peroxide vapor and gas plasma methods have been shown to effectively inactivate SARS-CoV-2.[7] These methods are specific to tested brands of N95 respirators, and their implementation involves an additional chemical hazard that requires the use of trained personnel and adequate facilities. A chemical residue can remain on the respirators, so adequate off-gas time is required to protect users. But compared to other methods, hydrogen peroxide vapor and some gas plasma applications provide a higher level of disinfection, and repeated treatments are less likely to affect filtration efficiency and fit.

The use of heat, combined with humidity, has the potential for an inexpensive decontamination treatment, especially for hospitals and other settings where cost and ease of implementation are limiting factors. Evidence suggests that incubation for more than 30 minutes at 70–85 C and greater than 50% relative humidity is likely to sufficiently inactivate SARS-CoV-2.[4] In contrast to heat alone, the addition of humid conditions has shown promise with multiple enveloped and non-enveloped viruses, but data are limited for SARS-CoV-2. It is likely this method will not sterilize an N95 respirator and may affect filter efficiency and fit over time. Only validated methods specific to the respirator brand and infectious agent should be used.

30.3.2 N95 Methods under Investigation

Of the several methods currently under investigation, those showing promise include a 2- to 3-minute microwave-generated steam treatment and a room-temperature treatment with a waiting time of up to seven days for SARS-CoV-2 inactivation.[9] The CDC provides guidance on room-temperature treatment, but supporting evidence in the peer-reviewed literature appears limited at this time.[2]

30.3.3 N95 Methods Not Recommended

Several methods are not recommended, primarily due to their failure to effectively inactivate SARS-CoV-2, issues with compromised filter efficiency or fit, or the presence of a chemical residue or hazard.[9] Some of these methods include submersion in alcohol, bleach, or soapy water. Ethylene oxide and formaldehyde vapor treatments are not recommended primarily for the residual hazard to users. Exposure to sunlight has also been shown to neither effectively decontaminate N95 respirators nor inactivate SARS-CoV-2.

30.4   EXTENDED USE OF DISPOSABLE EXAM GLOVES

The CDC has also continued to update its "Strategies for Optimizing the Supply of Disposable Medical Gloves," which specifies guidelines on methods for sanitizing gloved hands to extend the use of gloves during known shortages.[3] The guidelines include the following recommendations for users:

- Disinfection and extended use of disposable medical exam gloves is not a recommended standard practice and should only be considered during extreme shortages.
- Reuse and repeated donning and doffing of disposable gloves is not recommended, as this could affect the integrity of the gloves. Disinfection should only be performed on gloved hands for extended use. Once removed, the gloves should be discarded.
- Before disinfection, gloves need to be inspected and discarded if signs of damage or degradation are present. Signs of damage include tearing or holes. Signs of degradation include tackiness, changes in elasticity such as increased stiffness or softness, discoloration, and cracking.
- Visibly soiled gloves should be discarded.
- Published research shows that up to six repeated disinfection cycles with an alcohol-based hand sanitizer (ABHS) do not significantly affect the mechanical integrity of latex and nitrile gloves.[10,11] The CDC's "Hand Hygiene in Healthcare Settings" recommends standard guidelines on the use of an ABHS.[10] The agency cites a 2016 paper that reported less changes in tensile strength for both latex and nitrile gloves resulting from the use of an ethanol-based ABHS compared to an isopropanol-based ABHS.[11]
- When an ABHS is not available, soap and water can be used to clean and remove contamination from the gloves for up to ten repeated treatments.[10] Long-cuffed gloves are recommended to prevent soap and water from entering the glove. No supporting literature was cited by the CDC on the integrity of latex or nitrile gloves exposed to repeated treatments with soap and water, but recent studies address this subject and are discussed later in this chapter.[12,13]
- Based on limited data, an alternative of up to ten repeated disinfection cycles with dilute bleach (for example, a 0.1% sodium hypochlorite solution) can be considered. Once again, long-cuffed gloves are recommended to protect the hands inside the gloves. The treatment involves dipping the gloved hands in a dilute bleach solution for five seconds, allowing 1 minute of contact time in the air, then rinsing with water and blotting dry with a

paper towel. This treatment is based on a CDC report of a manufacturer's permeation data for a nitrile glove exposed to a more concentrated 10%–13% bleach solution.[10] However, it must be noted that permeation is a different process than degradation. A recently published study on the integrity of disposable exam gloves exposed to repeated bleach treatments is discussed later in this chapter.[14]

30.5 SUPPORTING RESEARCH ON EXAM GLOVES

Several recent studies have investigated the physical and mechanical integrity of latex and nitrile gloves repeatedly treated with ABHS, dilute bleach, and soap and water. The two critical factors evaluated in these investigations include:

1. The physical integrity and penetration of gloves via holes or tearing, which can be measured using a standardized water leak test. For example, the Acceptable Quality Level (AQL)—a measure of the percentage of defects or of gloves that fail the water leak test—for non-sterile medical exam gloves varies from about 1.0 to 2.5.[15] Significant changes in the physical integrity during use would be a cause for concern.
2. The mechanical integrity of gloves via degradation and changes in the polymer structure, which can be measured as a change in tensile strength, elastic modulus (stiffness), or elongation at break (ductility). These tests can indicate if a glove is likely to fail under conditions of use.

Key papers on the effects of disinfection on medical exam gloves are listed in Table 30.2.

30.5.1 PHYSICAL INTEGRITY

Shless et al.[12] evaluated latex and nitrile exam gloves sourced from the USA and India. The researchers found that up to ten applications of a dilute bleach solution had the least impact on physical integrity, as compared to repeated applications of an ABHS or soap and water. However, significant variation was observed, and the results were inconclusive. Thus, the authors recommended that specific glove and disinfectant combinations be tested when facing shortages and extended use is necessary.

30.5.2 MECHANICAL INTEGRITY

In addition to the studies cited by the CDC in support of their recommendations for ABHS,[3] three recently published studies evaluated repeated treatments with ABHS, dilute bleach, and/or soap and water.[13,14,16]

Phalen et al.[13] evaluated the effects of repeated disinfection treatments with an ethanol-based ABHS, diluted bleach, and soap and water on the elastic modulus of latex and nitrile exam gloves. Treatments were performed per the CDC recommendations.

TABLE 30.2

Key Publications on Medical Exam Glove Decontamination

Physical Integrity

- Pitten, F.A., Müller, P., Heeg, P., Kramer, A. 1999. Untersuchungen zur wiederholten Desinfizierbarkeit von Einweghandschuhen während des Tragens [The efficacy of repeated disinfection of disposable gloves during usage]. *Zentralbl Hyg Umweltmed* 201(6):555–562.
- Pitten, F-A., Herdemann, G., Kramer, A. 2000. The integrity of latex gloves in clinical dental practice. *Infection* 28(6):388–392. DOI: 10.1007/s150100070011.
- Shless, J., Crider, Y., Pitchik, H., Qazi, A., Styczynski, A., LeMesurier, R., et al. 2021. Evaluation of the effects of repeated disinfection on medical exam gloves: Part 1. Changes in physical integrity. *J Occup Environ Hyg* Dec 13:1–11. DOI: 10.1080/15459624.2021.2015072.

Mechanical Integrity

- Gao, P., Horvatin, M., Niezgoda, G., Weible, R., and Shaffer, R. 2016. Effect of multiple alcohol-based hand rub applications on the tensile properties of thirteen brands of medical exam nitrile and latex gloves. *J Occup Environ Hyg* 13(12):905–914. DOI:10.1080/15459624.2016.1191640.
- Esmizadeh, E., Chang, B.P., Jubinville, D., Seto, C., Ojogbo, E., Tzoganakis, C., Mekonnen, T.H. 2021. Stability of nitrile and vinyl latex gloves under repeated disinfection cycles. *Mater Today Sustain* 11–12:100067. DOI: 10.1016/j.mtsust.2021.100067.
- Garrido-Molina, J.M., Márquez-Hernández, V.V., Alcayde-García, A., Ferreras-Morales, C.A., García-Viola, A., Aguilera-Manrique, G., Gutiérrez-Puertas, L. 2021. Disinfection of gloved hands during the COVID-19 pandemic. *J Hosp Infect* 107:5–11. DOI: 10.1016/j.jhin.2020.09.015.
- Phalen, R.N., Patterson, J., Cuadros Olave, J., Mansfield, S.A., Shless, J.S., Crider, Y.S., et al. 2021. Evaluation of the effects of repeated disinfection on medical exam gloves: Part 2. Changes in mechanical properties. *J Occup Environ Hyg* Jan 13:1–11. DOI: 10.1080/15459624.2021.2015073.
- Mansfield, S., Patterson, J., Cuadros Olave, J., Phalen, R.N., Hamidi, Y.K. 2021. Repeated bleach sanitization effects on medical exam glove mechanical properties. *Amer J Adv Research* 5(1):13–17. DOI: 10.5281/zenodo.5817219.
- Patterson, J., Mansfield, S., Cuadros Olave, J., Phalen, R.N., Hamidi, Y.K. 2021. Mechanical performance of latex and nitrile medical exam gloves under repeated soap and water treatment. *Amer J Adv Research* 5(1):01–05. DOI: 10.5281/zenodo.5112602.

The latex gloves performed well with six repeated treatments for an ethanol-based ABHS and ten repeated treatments of dilute bleach or soap and water. However, the nitrile exam gloves showed significant changes in elastic modulus, and the results among brands were more inconclusive. Nitrile glove performance was generally poor for the dilute bleach and soap and water treatments. Ultimately, their results supported the use of five repeated treatments of an ethanol-based ABHS with nitrile exam gloves, which was a lower threshold than recommended by the CDC.

Mansfield et al.[14] found that latex gloves performed well with no significant change in elastic modulus after ten repeated treatments with dilute bleach. In contrast, two of the three nitrile glove brands exhibited significant decreases in elastic modulus of about 50% or greater. The general recommendation was to not use dilute bleach treatments with nitrile gloves.

Patterson et al.[16] found that latex gloves performed well with no significant change in elastic modulus beyond 26% after up to 20 treatments with soap and water. However, nitrile glove brands exhibited significant changes in elastic modulus above 40% after as few as five repeated treatments. In general, soap and water did not appear to be an appropriate disinfection method for nitrile gloves.

Overall, it appears that latex and nitrile exam gloves can be treated up to five times with an ABHS, whereas only latex exam gloves appear suitable for dilute bleach and soap and water treatments as outlined in the CDC guidelines. The results of these studies indicate that more research on the effects of water-based disinfectants on the mechanical integrity of nitrile exam gloves is needed. Water absorption alone may be a contributing factor to the degradation of nitrile gloves.[13]

30.6   ADDITIONAL ISSUES DURING THE PANDEMIC

The shortages of N95 respirators, medical exam gloves, surgical masks, and sanitizers gave rise to the distribution of counterfeit products on the market. The NIOSH National Personal Protective Technology Laboratory (NPPTL) issued a guide and tips on how to identify NIOSH-approved respirators (www.cdc.gov/niosh/npptl).[17] They also provided details on counterfeit N95 and KN95 products on the market at the time. Some of the signs that a respirator may be counterfeit included:

1. Lack of markings on the filtering facepiece respirator, such as an approval (TC) number on the filtering facepiece respirator or headband, or a NIOSH identifier.
2. Incorrect spelling of NIOSH.
3. Decorative fabric or other decorative add-ons (e.g., sequins).
4. Filtering facepiece respirator has ear loops instead of headbands.
5. Claims of approval for use with children (NIOSH does not approve any type of respiratory protection for children).
6. Claims that the product was tested by NPPTL.
7. The producer is not listed as a NIOSH approval holder or private label assignee.

Additionally, the World Customs Organization reported an alarming number of fraudulent activities and seizures of counterfeit medical supplies, including surgical face masks and sanitizers, during the peak of the COVID-19 pandemic.[18]

Ultimately, healthcare providers and the general public need to exercise caution when purchasing medical supplies from unknown sources, especially online and during times when there is a supply-chain crisis.

30.7   CONCLUSIONS

The extended use and reuse of disposable N95 respirators and medical exam gloves are not recommended practices. Nevertheless, during the COVID-19 pandemic, many authorities endeavored to address shortages of PPE critical for infection control, which included the establishment of guidelines for extended use and reuse of disposable PPE. Several viable methods have been established for N95 respirators. However, we reference an important cautionary fact sheet, in several languages, concerning the decontamination of N95 respirators.[19] While more research is needed on disposable exam gloves, CDC guidelines appear favorable for extended use and reuse of latex exam gloves. Caution should be applied with nitrile exam gloves, especially when turning to methods other than alcohol-based hand sanitizers. Ethanol-based sanitizers appear to affect glove integrity less than isopropanol-based sanitizers.

Additionally, the shortages of medical supplies during the pandemic gave rise to the distribution of counterfeit products on the market, which required healthcare organizations to exercise caution when purchasing medical supplies from unknown sources, especially online.

REFERENCES

1. WHO. 2020. *Shortage of personal protective equipment endangering health workers worldwide* [News Release 3 March 2020]. Geneva: World Health Organization (WHO).
2. CDC. 2021. *Strategies for optimizing the supply of N95 respirators* [Online]. Washington, DC: U.S. Centers for Disease Control and Prevention (CDC). Available at: https://www.cdc.gov/coronavirus/2019-ncov/hcp/respirators-strategy/index.html.
3. CDC. 2020. *Strategies for optimizing the supply of disposable medical gloves* [Online]. Washington, DC: U.S. Centers for Disease Control and Prevention (CDC). Available at: https://www.cdc.gov/coronavirus/2019-ncov/ppe-strategy/gloves.html.
4. Smullin, S.J., Tarlow, B.D., and the N95DECON Consortium. 2021. Room temperature wait and reuse for bioburden reduction of SARS-CoV-2 on N95 filtering facepiece respirators. *Appl Biosafety* 26(2):103–111. DOI: 10.1089/apb.20.0055.
5. Grist, S.M., Geldert, A., Gopal, A., Su, A., Balch, H.B., Herr, A.E., and the N95DECON Consortium. 2021. Current understanding of ultraviolet-C decontamination of N95 filtering facepiece respirators. *Appl Biosafety* 26(2):90–102. DOI: 10.1089/apb.20.0051.
6. Geldert, A., Balch, H.B., Gopal, A., Su, A., Grist, S.M., and Herr, A.E. 2021. Best practices for germicidal ultraviolet-C dose measurement for N95 respirator decontamination. *J Res Nat Inst Standards Technol* 126:1–14. DOI: 10.6028/jres.126.020.
7. Rempel, D., Henneman, J., Agalloco, J., Crittenden, J., and the N95DECON Consortium. 2021. Hydrogen peroxide methods for decontaminating N95 filtering facepiece respirators. *Appl Biosafety* 26(2):71–79. DOI: 10.1089/apb.20.0042.
8. Anderegg, L., Doyle, J., Gardel, M.L., Gupta, A., Hallas, C., Lensky, Y., Love, N., Lucas, B., Mazenc, E., Meisenhelder, C., Pillarisetti, A., Ranard, D., Squires, A., Vechakul, J., Vilas, N., Williams, S., Wilson, D., Chen, T., Abbas, M., and Yang, H. 2021. Heat and humidity for bioburden reduction of N95 filtering facepiece respirators. *Appl Biosafety* 26(2):80–89. DOI: 10.1089/apb.20.0053.
9. N95DECON. 2021. *Publications*. Available at: https://www.n95decon.org/publications.
10. CDC. 2021. *Hand hygiene in healthcare settings* [Online]. Washington, DC: U.S. Centers for Disease Control and Prevention (CDC). Available at: https://www.cdc.gov/handhygiene/index.html.
11. Gao, P., Horvatin, M., Niezgoda, G., Weible, R., and Shaffer, R. 2016. Effect of multiple alcohol-based hand rub applications on the tensile properties of thirteen brands of medical exam nitrile and latex gloves. *J Occup Environ Hyg* 13(12):905–914. DOI: 10.1080/15459624.2016.1191640.

12. Shless, J., Crider, Y., Pitchik, H., Qazi, A., Styczynski, A., LeMesurier, R., Haik, D., Kwong, L.H., LeBoa, C., Bhattacharya, A., Hamidi, Y.K., and Phalen, R.N. 2021. Evaluation of the effects of repeated disinfection on medical exam gloves: Part 1. Changes in physical integrity. *J Occup Environ Hyg* 13:1–11. DOI: 10.1080/15459624.2021.2015072.
13. Phalen, R.N., Patterson, J., Cuadros Olave, J., Mansfield, S.A., Shless, J.S., Crider, Y.S., Pitchik, H.O., Qazi, A.S., Styczynski, A., LeMesurier, R., Haik, D., Kwong, L.H., LeBoa, C., Bhattacharya, A., and Hamidi, Y.K. 2021. Evaluation of the effects of repeated disinfection on medical exam gloves: Part 2. Changes in mechanical properties. *J Occup Environ Hyg* 13:1–11. DOI: 10.1080/15459624.2021.2015073.
14. Patterson, J., Mansfield, S., Cuadros Olave, J., Phalen, R.N., and Hamidi, Y.K. 2021. Mechanical performance of latex and nitrile medical exam gloves under repeated soap and water treatment. *Am J Adv Res* 5(1):01–05. DOI: 10.5281/zenodo.5112602.
15. Code of Federal Regulations. 2017. *21 CFR 800.20: Patient examination gloves and surgical gloves; sample plans and test method for leakage defects; adulteration.* Washington, DC: U.S. Government Printing Office.
16. Mansfield, S., Patterson, J., Cuadros Olave, J., Phalen, R.N., and Hamidi, Y.K. 2021. Repeated bleach sanitization effects on medical exam glove mechanical properties. *Am J Adv Res* 5(1):13–17. DOI: 10.5281/zenodo.5817219.
17. CDC. 2021. *Counterfeit respirators/misrepresentation of NIOSH-approval.* Washington, DC: U.S. Centers for Disease Control and Prevention (CDC), National Institute for Occupational Safety and Health (NIOSH). Available at: https://www.cdc.gov/niosh/npptl/usernotices/counterfeitResp.html.
18. World Customs Organization. 2020. *COVID-19 urgent notice: Counterfeit medical supplies and introduction of export controls on personal protective equipment.* 23 March 2020. Available at: http://www.wcoomd.org/en/media/newsroom/2020/march/covid_19-urgent-notice-counterfeit-medical-supplies.aspx.
19. N95DECON. 2020. *COVID-19 N95 decon and reuse: Caution when reusing* [Online]. Available at: https://www.n95decon.org/files/cautionary-fact-sheet.

Index

Printed in the USA
CPSIA information can be obtained
at www.ICGtesting.com
LVHW011642120124
768841LV00005B/426

9 780367 649005